D0908981

Gynecology
for the
Primary Care Physician
Second Edition

Editors

Thomas G. Stovall, MD
Clinical Professor
Department of Obstetrics and Gynecology
Vanderbilt University School of Medicine
Women's Health Specialists, PLLC
Germantown, Tennessee
Clinical Professor
Department of Obstetrics and Gynecology
University of Tennessee College of Medicine
Memphis, Tennessee

Frank W. Ling, MD
Clinical Professor
Department of Obstetrics and Gynecology
Vanderbilt University School of Medicine
Women's Health Specialists, PLLC
Germantown, Tennessee

Nikki B. Zite, MD, MPH
Assistant Professor
Residency Program Associate Director
Department of Obstetrics and Gynecology
Division of Education
University of Tennessee School of Medicine
Knoxville, Tennessee

Alice W. Chuang, MD
Assistant Professor
Department of Obstetrics and Gynecology
Division of Women's Primary Healthcare
University of North Carolina
Chapel Hill, North Carolina

Todd D. Tillmanns, MD
Assistant Professor
Department of Obstetrics and Gynecology
University of Tennessee
Health Sciences Center
Gynecologic Oncologist
Department of Gynecology/Oncology
The West Clinic
Memphis, Tennessee

With 57 Contributors
Developed by
Current Medicine Group LLC
Philadelphia

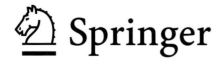

Current Medicine Group LLC
a division of
Springer Science+Business Media LLC

CURRENT MEDICINE GROUP LLC
A DIVISION OF SPRINGER SCIENCE+BUSINESS MEDIA LLC

400 Market Street, Suite 700 • Philadelphia, PA 19106

Senior Developmental Editor:	Anthony Mirra
Editorial Assistant:	Juleen Deaner
Cover Design:	Daniel J. Britt
Design and Layout:	Daniel J. Britt and Theresa Englehart
Illustrators:	Daniel J. Britt, Kim Broadbent, Theresa Englehart, Wieslawa Langenfeld, Maureen Looney, and Andrea Penko
Creative Director:	Wendy Vetter
Assistant Production Manager:	Megan Charlton
Indexer:	Holly Lukens

ISBN-10 1-57340-295-8
ISBN-13 978-1-57340-295-8
ISSN 1939-778X

Although every effort has been made to ensure that drug doses and other information are presented accurately in this publication, the ultimate responsibility rests with the prescribing physician. Neither the publishers nor the authors can be held responsible for errors or for any consequences arising from the use of information contained herein. Products mentioned in this publication should be used in accordance with the prescribing information prepared by the manufacturers. No claims or endorsements are made for any drug or compound at present under clinical investigation.

For more information, please call 1 (800) 427-1796 or (215) 574-2266 or email us at inquiry@phl.cursci.com

www.currentmedicinegroup.com

10 9 8 7 6 5 4 3 2 1

Printed in the United States by IPC Print Services

This book was printed on acid-free paper

Preface

Gynecology for the Primary Care Physician was conceived and written to address what we believe is a growing concern for primary care physicians. Managed care continues to alter patient choice and requires the primary care physician to diagnose and treat a broader array of gynecologic problems than ever before. Therefore, there is a need for a book that provides the information needed in a format that is easy to use. We believe that *Gynecology for the Primary Care Physician* does just this.

The topics included in this text were selected because they represent those clinical situations that are faced by primary care physicians every day. The authors were selected not only for their expertise and academic credibility, but also because they are front-line practitioners who see and care for patients. Furthermore, each chapter was arranged in such a fashion that the material is organized in a standardized format and answers those questions and clinical situations most commonly encountered.

The above Preface was included in the first edition of *Gynecology for the Primary Care Physician*. The Editors of the current edition still see the same challenges for primary care providers with an ever-enlarging body of knowledge.

The updated version of the text includes important advances in gynecology that every provider needs to be aware of to fully care for their female patients. With a continued emphasis on prevention, this text outlines novel contraceptive options, changes in Papanicoloau screening recommendations, and the human papillomavirus vaccine, while continuing to provide the information needed to treat and diagnose a wide array of gynecologic problems. Since the first edition, the volume and content of data surrounding menopause treatment have exploded, and these changes are reflected in this edition. Many authors updated their chapters from the first edition, while for other topics we solicited the expertise of new authors. We maintained the standardized format and emphasize situations that are frequently encountered.

We are once again indebted to all the authors for their time and expertise in creating this functional reference. It is our hope that you will find this book invaluable and utilize it frequently in caring for your patients.

Thomas G. Stovall, MD
Frank W. Ling, MD
Nikki B. Zite, MD, MPH
Alice W. Chuang, MD
Todd D. Tillmanns, MD

Contributors

Deborah Bartz, MD, MPH
Clinical Fellow
Department of Obstetrics and
 Gynecology
Division of Family Planning
Brigham and Women's Hospital
Harvard Medical School
Boston, Massachusetts

Paula H. Bednarek, MD
Assistant Professor
Department of Obstetrics and
Gynecology
Oregon Health and Sciences
 University
Portland, Oregon

Abbey B. Berenson, MD
Professor
Department of Obstetrics and
 Gynecology
Chief
Division of Pediatric and
 Adolescent Gynecology
Director
Center for Interdisciplinary Research
 in Women's Health
University of Texas Medical Branch
 at Galveston
Galveston, Texas

Kelly A. Best, MD
Assistant Professor
Department of Obstetrics and
 Gynecology
University of Florida
College of Medicine, Jacksonville
Jacksonville, Florida

Sarah J. Betstadt, MD
Instructor
Department of Obstetrics and
 Gynecology
Boston University
School of Medicine
Boston, Massachusetts

Lynn Borgatta, MD, MPH
Department of Obstetrics and
 Gynecology
Boston Medical Center
Associate Professor
Boston University
 School of Medicine
Boston, Massachusetts

C. Bryce Bowling, MD
Fellow
Department of Graduate Medical
 Education
University of Alabama at
 Birmingham
Birmingham, Alabama

Dalia Brahmi, MD, MPH
Assistant Professor
Department of Family and
 Social Medicine
Albert Einstein College of Medicine
Bronx, New York

Candace Brown, MSN, PharmD
Professor
Departments of Pharmacy,
 Obstetrics and Gynecology,
 and Psychiatry
University of Tennessee
 Health Science Center
Memphis, Tennessee

Michael E. Carney, MD
Associate Professor,
 Gynecologic Oncology
Department of Obstetrics,
 Gynecology and Women's Health
John A. Burns School of Medicine
Kapi'olani Medical Center
University of Hawaii at Manoa
Honolulu, Hawaii

C. James Chuong, MD, MPH
Medical Director
Cooper Institute for Advanced
 Reproductive Medicine
Houston, Texas

AnnaMarie Connolly, MD
Associate Professor
Department of Obstetrics and
 Gynecology
University of North Carolina
Chapel Hill, North Carolina

Allison A. Cowett, MD, MPH
Clinical Assistant Professor
Department of Obstetrics and
 Gynecology
Director
Center for Reproductive Health
University of Illinois at Chicago
Chicago, Illinois

Patrick Duff, MD
Professor and Residency Program
 Director
Associate Dean for Student Affairs
Department of Obstetrics and
 Gynecology
University of Florida
 College of Medicine
Gainesville, Florida

Adjoa B. Duker, MD
Assistant Professor
Department of Family and
 Social Medicine
Albert Einstein College of Medicine
Bronx, New York

Rodney K. Edwards, MD
Assistant Professor
Department of Obstetrics and
 Gynecology
Division of Maternal-Fetal Medicine
University of Florida
 College of Medicine
Gainesville, Florida

David B. Engle, MD
Clinical Instructor
Obstetrics and Gynecology
University of Wisconsin School of
 Medicine and Public Health
Madison, Wisconsin

Christopher M. Estes, MD
Fellow
Department of Obstetrics and
 Gynecology
Columbia University
New York, New York

**Francisco A. R. Garcia,
MD, MPH**
Associate Professor and Director
University of Arizona
National Center of Excellence in
 Women's Health
College of Medicine
Tucson, Arizona

Kamini Geer, MD, MPH
Clinical Instructor
Department of Family and
 Social Medicine
Albert Einstein College of Medicine
Medical Director
Beth Israel Residency in
 Urban Family Health
New York, New York

Lynda Gioia-Flynt, MD
Clinical Instructor
Department of Obstetrics and
  Gynecology
University of Tennessee
  Health Science Center
Memphis, Tennessee

Marji Gold, MD
Professor
Department of Family and
  Social Medicine
Albert Einstein College of Medicine
Bronx, New York

James A. Hall, MD
Women's Health Center of
Logansport
Logansport, Indiana

Jennifer L. Hardman, PharmD
University of Illinois at Chicago
College of Pharmacy
Department of Pharmacy Practice
Chicago, Illinois

William H. Hindle, MD
Director
Breast Diagnostic Center
Women's and Children's Hospital
LAC & USC Medical Center
Emeritus Professor
Department of Obstetrics and
  Gynecology
University of Southern California
Los Angeles, California

Emily Jackson, MD
Assistant Professor
Department of Family and
  Social Medicine
Albert Einstein College of Medicine
Bronx, New York

Jeffrey T. Jensen, MD, MPH
Director
Women's Health Research Unit
Leon Speroff Professor of Obstetrics
  and Gynecology
Departments of Obstetrics and
  Gynecology and Public Health
  and Preventive Medicine
Oregon Health and
  Science University
Portland, Oregon

Beth Y. Karlan, MD
Director
Women's Cancer Research
  Institute and Division of
  Gynecologic Oncology
Cedars-Sinai Medical Center
Professor of Obstetrics and
  Gynecology
Geffen School of Medicine at UCLA
Los Angeles, California

Andrew M. Kaunitz, MD
Professor and Assistant Chairman
Medical Director-Menopause
  and Gynecology
Department of Obstetrics and
  Gynecology
Southside Women's Health
University of Florida
  College of Medicine-Jacksonville
Jacksonville, Florida

Melissa Kottke, MD
Associate Family Planning Clinical
  Care and Research Fellow
Department of Gynecology and
  Obstetrics
Emory University School of
  Medicine
Atlanta, Georgia

John A. Lamont, MD
Professor Emeritus
Department of Obstetrics and
  Gynecology
McMaster University
Hamilton, Ontario, Canada

Lisa M. Landrum, MD, PhD
Fellow, Gynecologic Oncology
Department of Obstetrics and
Gynecology
University of Oklahoma
Health Science Center
Oklahoma City, Oklahoma

Frank W. Ling, MD
Clinical Professor
Department of Obstetrics and
  Gynecology
Vanderbilt University
  School of Medicine
Women's Health Specialists, PLLC
Germantown, Tennessee

Gary H. Lipscomb, MD
Professor and Vice-Chair for
  Clinical Affairs
Department of Obstetrics and
  Gynecology
University of Tennessee
  Health Science Center
Memphis, Tennessee

Ginat W. Mirowski, DMD, MD
Associate Professor of Dermatology
Feinberg School of Medicine
Northwestern University
Chicago, Illinois
Adjunct Associate Professor
Department of Oral Pathology,
  Medicine, Radiology
Indiana University
  School of Dentistry
Indianapolis, Indiana

Amy L. Mitchell, MD
Assistant Professor of Clinical
  Obstetrics and Gynecology
Department of Obstetrics and
  Gynecology
University of Arizona
  Health Sciences Center
Tucson, Arizona

Kelly L. Molpus, MD
Director
Division of Gynecologic Oncology
Department of Oncology
Halifax Medical Center
Daytona Beach, Florida

M. Cristina Muñoz, MD
Assistant Professor
Department of Obstetrics and
  Gynecology
University of North Carolina
Chapel Hill, North Carolina

David Muram, MD
Professor of Obstetrics and
  Gynecology
State University of New York,
  Downstate
Health Sciences Center at Brooklyn
Brooklyn, New York

Ringland S. Murray, Jr., MD
Assistant Professor
Department of Obstetrics and
  Gynecology
University of Tennessee
Physician
Fertility Associates of Memphis
Memphis, Tennessee

Deborah L. Myers, MD
Associate Professor and Director
Division of Urogynecology and
  Reconstructive Pelvic Surgery
Department of Obstetrics and
  Gynecology
Warren Alpert Medical School of
  Brown University
Women and Infants' Hospital
Providence, Rhode Island

Thao Nguyen, MD
Fellow and Clinical Instructor
Department of Obstetrics and
  Gynecology
Division of Urogynecology and
  Reconstructive Pelvic Surgery
University of North Carolina at
  Chapel Hill
Chapel Hill, North Carolina

Deborah L. Nucatola, MD
Medical Director
Planned Parenthood of
Santa Barbara, Ventura, and
  San Luis Obispo Counties
Santa Barbara, California

Joquetta D. Paige, MD, MPH
Assistant Professor
Department of Family and
  Social Medicine
Albert Einstein College of Medicine
Bronx, New York

James C. Pavelka, MD
Fellow
Department of Obstetrics and
  Gynecology
David Geffen School of Medicine at
  University of California
Fellow
Department of Obstetrics and
  Gynecology
Division of Gynecologic Oncology
Cedars-Sinai Medical Center
Los Angeles, California

C. Paul Perry, MD
Director
C. Paul Perry Pelvic Pain Center
Birmingham, Alabama

Brook A. Saunders, MD
Fellow
Division of Gynecologic Oncology
University of Kentucky
Medical Center
Lexington, Kentucky

Erin J. Saunders, MD
Instructor
Department of Obstetrics and
  Gynecology
University of Kentucky
Lexington, Kentucky

M. Mercedes Sayago, MD
Department of Obstetrics and
  Gynecology
University of Tennessee
Memphis, Tennessee

Roger P. Smith, MD
Professor, Vice Chair and
Program Director
Department of Obstetrics and
  Gynecology
University of Missouri-Kansas City
Kansas City, Missouri

Xavier L. Smith, MD
Department of Obstetrics and
  Gynecology
University of Tennessee
Memphis, Tennessee

Thomas G. Stovall, MD
Clinical Professor
Department of Obstetrics and
  Gynecology
Vanderbilt University
School of Medicine
Women's Health Specialists, PLLC
Clinical Professor
Department of Obstetrics and
  Gynecology
University of Tennessee
  College of Medicine
Germantown, Tennessee

Aya Sultan, MD, PhD
Department of Obstetrics and
  Gynecology and Women's Health
University of Hawaii
Honolulu, Hawaii

Robert L. Summitt, Jr., MD
Clinical Professor
Department of Obstetrics and
  Gynecology
Vanderbilt University
School of Medicine
Women's Health Specialists, PLLC
Germantown, Tennessee

Todd D. Tillmanns, MD
Assistant Professor
Department of Obstetrics and
Gynecology
University of Tennessee
Health Sciences Center
Gynecologic Oncologist
Department of
Gynecology/Oncology
The West Clinic
Memphis, Tennessee

Renée M. Ward, MD
Fellow
Division of Urogynecology and
  Reconstructive Pelvic Surgery
Department of Obstetrics and
  Gynecology
Warren Alpert Medical School of
  Brown University
Women and Infants' Hospital
Providence, Rhode Island

Matthew A. Will, MD
Resident Physician
Department of Obstetrics and
  Gynecology
Indiana University
  School of Medicine
Indianapolis, Indiana

Contents

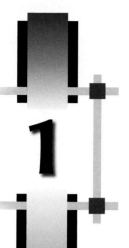

1 Breast Pain (Mastalgia)

David B. Engle and William H. Hindle

- Most women of reproductive age experience cyclic breast pain at some time.
- Fear of breast cancer motivates many women to seek urgent medical attention when they experience pain in their chest.
- Breast pain without a palpable mass is rarely a sign of cancer.
- The definitive diagnosis of a palpable breast mass takes precedence over evaluation of breast pain.
- After thorough evaluation, including mammography, most women with breast pain can be appropriately managed by reassurance that they have no evidence of breast cancer.

Most women at some time experience breast pain (mastalgia), a common symptom that is usually physiologic but can be pathologic. Although mastalgia is commonly seen during a woman's later reproductive (menstruating) years, it can occur at any age. Cyclic mastalgia is the most common variant of breast pain. Noncyclic mastalgia can be related specifically to abscess, costal chondritis (Tietze syndrome), cyst, fibroadenoma, mastitis, trauma, or other breast pathology (Figure 1-1). True mastalgia occurs within the breast tissue and must be differentiated from pain elsewhere in the anterior chest. Primary care physicians can appropriately evaluate women with breast pain, reassure those with benign findings, and expeditiously refer the few with lesions that may be breast cancer. Because pain anywhere in the anterior chest heightens a woman's concern and anxiety, it is compassionate and humane to expedite the evaluation of any woman's complaint of breast pain.

Incidence and Epidemiology

As many as 70% of women experience bothersome mastalgia at some point in their lives [1]. Approximately two thirds of these patients experience cyclic mastalgia [2]. In a study of questionnaire responses, more than 20% of women described their mastalgia as "severe," but only half of those so reporting had consulted a physician for their symptoms [3]. A long-term follow-up of women presenting to the Cardiff Breast Clinic (Wales, UK) revealed that in more than 40%, the mastalgia persisted until menopause [4]. A recent descriptive questionnaire study of 1171 women documented premenstrual mastalgia in 69%, of whom 36% (25% of the total population surveyed) had sought medical attention for their breast pain [5]. Any woman presenting with a primary complaint of breast pain requires a complete evaluation and explanation. Once a specific cause of breast pain is determined, appropriate treatment or referral should be carried out in a timely manner. In the past, unless an associated breast mass was present, mastalgia was often thought to be medically insignificant, and the complaint received little clinical attention. Now, however, with the current emphasis on a healthy lifestyle and increased breast awareness, mastalgia is considered a valid reason for a woman to consult her physician. Lifestyle impairments cited by women with mastalgia include sexual activity (48%), physical activity (37%), social functioning (12%), and interference with work or school (8%) [5]. Additionally, the stress placed on a woman with severe breast mastalgia has been found in one study to be as severe as the stress on women waiting to undergo breast cancer surgery [6].

Pathophysiology

Mastalgia is rarely the sole sign of breast cancer. If cancer is present, there is usually an associated palpable mass. When breast cancer advances to involvement of the bone, chest wall, muscle, or skin, pain may be an additional symptom. Nipple retraction of recent onset is occasionally painful and can be a sign of a nonpalpable tumor, which usually is identified on mammography.

CYCLICAL

Most cyclic mastalgia has no associated characteristic, histologic findings or demonstrable pathophysiology. The pain is usually the result of cyclical rise and fall of sex hormones during the menstrual cycle. The pain can also be caused be exogenous hormones such as those found in birth control pills. Ductal elements of the breast are stimulated by estrogen, while progesterone has a stimulatory effect on the stroma. The typical symptoms of cyclical mastalgia occur after ovulation, as progesterone and estradiol are rising during the luteal phase. The pain usually will stop with the onset of menstruation, as both sex hormones nadir.

Clinical cyclic mastalgia has been defined by Ader and Browne [5] to be pain of four of 10 on a visual analog scale lasting at least 7 days per month. However, cyclical breast pain may not necessitate such a strict criteria. Cyclical mastalgia is often bilateral and may be diffuse or localized more to the upper outer quadrants.

Fibrocystic breast disease is another common cause of cyclical breast pain. It is caused by increased amounts of fibrous tissue or cysts within the stroma of the breast tissue. The fibrous tissue can be either epithelial or fibrous in nature. The cysts can be either large or small and are formed by ductal occlusion. The pain associated is often from ductal dilation, inflammation, and edema.

Occasional cases of sclerosing adenosis are associated with cyclic, generally diffuse, mastalgia [7]. This process now carries a small increased risk of malignancy, whereas in the past it was believed to be a benign condition [8••].

Causes of Anterior Chest Pain That May Be Perceived By A Woman As Breast Pain

Achalasia

Cervical radiculitis

Cervical spondylosis (C6-C7)

Cervical rib

Cholelithiasis

Coronary artery disease

Costal chondritis (Tietze syndrome)

Herpes zoster virus (shingles)

Hiatal hernia

Infected epidermal inclusion cyst (skin)

Myalgia

Neuralgia

Phantom pain

Pleurisy

Psychologic pain

Trauma

Tuberculosis

Figure 1-1. Causes of anterior chest pain that may be perceived by a woman as breast pain.

NONCYCLICAL

Noncyclical mastalgia accounts for only approximately one third of mastalgia complaints. By report their symptoms can be constant or come and go. However, the pain is not associated with the menstrual cycle. The engorgement of the breasts that occurs in pregnancy and lactation can result in mastalgia that, in some cases, is severe enough to require symptomatic treatment. These symptoms more commonly occur in the early postpartum period, and the cause is generally from an obstruction in the lactation ducts. The stasis from this obstruction can then become seeded by skin bacteria, such as *Streptococcus* or *Staphylococcus*. In mastitis the whole breast is warm, swollen, and red. This is compared with a breast abscess, in which a specific area of the breast develops a fluctuance, with the surrounding area showing signs of infection.

Some women with mammary duct ectasia (periductal mastitis) have associated localized noncyclic pain in addition to the typical spontaneous dark-green nipple discharge from multiple duct openings on the nipple. The involved dilated ducts may be tender and palpable below the areola.

A cyst in the breast can present with localized cyclic or noncyclic mastalgia and a tender palpable mass. A fibroadenoma can present in a similar manner, though less commonly. Cysts and fibroadenomas can become painful and tender in estrogen-deficient women who are placed on estrogen-replacement therapy. However, the mastalgia associated with estrogen replacement is usually diffuse, bilateral, and not associated with specific localized histopathology.

When oral contraceptives contained higher dosages of estrogen than are presently manufactured, bilateral diffuse mastalgia was common when beginning oral contraceptive therapy. This bothersome side effect is much less common (and less severe when it does occur) with the low-dose oral contraceptives currently in use.

Trauma can cause localized breast pain. The cause of an ecchymosis is usually evident by recent history. Fat necrosis secondary to previous trauma can be painful, however, and may mimic cancer by examination and mammography. Fewer than 10% of women with invasive breast cancer present with pain, and those that do usually have a readily palpable breast mass [9]. In rare cases, a nonpalpable breast tumor has been coincidentally discovered by diagnostic mammography as part of a breast evaluation of a woman presenting with breast pain.

Referred Pain

Pain in the anterior chest need not be from only breast origin. Pain can be referred from cardiac, pulmonary, chostochondritis (Tietze syndrome), chest wall muscle (*eg*, strain from strenuous upper body exercise), or gastric to name a few (Figure 1-1). However, a careful history and physical can usually isolate the responsible system.

DIAGNOSTIC STUDIES, HISTORY, AND CLINICAL PRESENTATION

When a patient presents with a perceived breast mass and mastalgia, the urgent diagnosis of the mass takes precedence and becomes the primary focus of the breast evaluation. When a woman's primary presenting complaint is breast pain, the key questions to ask are whether the pain is cyclic or noncyclic and whether it is diffuse or localized. Noncyclic breast pain can be constant or intermittent. The patient can usually pinpoint localized breast pain with the tip of her index finger. Further questions include the following: 1) What makes the pain better or worse?; 2) On a scale of 1 to 10, how severe is the pain?; 3) How long has it been present?; 4) How does the pain compare with that of headaches, backaches, or menstrual cramps? The patient may describe the pain as sharp, aching, drawing, itching, throbbing, or stabbing and as tenderness, heaviness, or pressure. Radiating pain, particularly if beyond the breast, suggests that the pain is not true mastalgia but rather has a nonbreast related cause. The history should include inquiry about any recent change in bras, swimwear, undergarments, athletic wear, or constricting garments and about any trauma to the breast. The patient should be asked whether she is taking psychotropic or estrogenic medications (including complementary or alternative therapies, such as ginseng or black cohosh), which can correlate with the onset of mastalgia. A mastalgia calendar on which the patient can record the day and severity of her breast pain is helpful for women who do not respond to reassurance and symptomatic care, that is, those requiring pharmacologic therapies. A visual linear analog scale can be used to quantitate the severity of the pain [10]. Some authorities advise using a prospective daily visual analog scale for reproducible results [11]. The patient should record the occurrence of breast pain on the mastalgia calendar for at least 2 months before pharmacologic therapy, during the therapy, and for several months after the therapy is completed or otherwise discontinued. However, such a detailed calendar is usually not necessary for most cases of mastalgia.

PHYSICAL EXAMINATION
A complete bilateral clinical breast examination including the axillary and supraclavicular areas should be performed [12]. Gentle, firm compression by the flat open palms held above and below the breast perpendicular to the chest wall usually elicits true mastalgia.

LABORATORY STUDIES
Generally, specific laboratory tests are not indicated in the evaluation of mastalgia. Estrogen, progesterone, prolactin, follicle-stimulating hormone, luteinizing hormone, and thyroid-stimulating hormone tests are rarely of clinical value, and therefore, are not cost-effective in the evaluation of mastalgia [10].

IMAGING
Unless recent films are available for review, mammography should be ordered for all women over the age of 35 years who present with mastalgia to screen for nonpalpable lesions that may be present. However, mammography rarely contributes directly to the mastalgia evaluation, except for localized lesions, such as cysts or fibroadenomas. Although breast ultrasound can be useful in the imaging evaluation of young women with dense breasts, to the degree that the density prevents adequate mammographic evaluation, ultrasound is otherwise not essential to the evaluation of mastalgia. The exception is when a nonpalpable mass is perceived on mammography, in which case ultrasound can differentiate a cyst from a solid mass. A 1998 case-control study looking at imagining for breast pain, found that there were equal number of malignancies found in the painful breast (0.4) and in the asymptomatic breast (0.4). There was also no difference in this group compared with healthy control subjects undergoing routine screening. The authors of this study felt the value of breast imaging for mastalgia lay in patient reassurance [13].

Treatment

After complete evaluation and explanation, reassurance that there is no evidence of breast cancer is effective treatment for more than 85% of women who present with mastalgia [3,10]. Another study found that reassurance helped more than half the women with severe mastalgia [14]. When treatment beyond reassurance is required, a step-wise progression of therapy should be undertaken [15]. Physical measures (eg, a professionally fitted bra), salt restriction (particularly premenstrual), intermittent analgesia (eg, nonsteroidal over-the-counter medications), should be tried before prescription medication. Furthermore, the treatment should be tailored to the exact type of pain [16].

For women whose pain is severe enough to impair their lifestyle, pharmacologic therapy has been shown to be effective in 77% with cyclic mastalgia and 44% of those with noncyclic mastalgia [17]. More than 20% of the women presenting with mastalgia who were followed by the Cardiff Breast Clinic had spontaneous resolution of their breast symptoms without treatment [4,10]. Placebo therapy is effective in clearing more than 25% of mastalgia cases [10]. To be truly effective pharmacology, a mastalgia treatment should resolve more than half of cases. Although nonsteroidal analgesics are generally recommended for pain management, any analgesic can be used. Asking the patient what she has found to be most effective for pain relief often leads to the optimal analgesia for that particular patient.

A randomized control trial of topical diclofenac versus placebo for cyclical and noncyclical breast pain was reported in 2004. In this study, 108 women were randomized to either arm of the study. After 6 months, those patients in the diclofenac arm had gone from a pretreatment pain score of 7.13 to a score of 1.27 after 6 month ($P = 0.00001$). In the placebo arm the average pain score only changed from 7.23 to 5.93 [18]. Another study found more than an 80% satisfactory response had been reported with the topical application of NSAIDs [19].

Tamoxifen, an antiestrogen, has been shown, in randomized trials, to reduce breast pain in up to 90% of women with mastalgia over a period of some 3 to 6 months [20–23]. Additionally, it was shown in a separate randomized trial that 10 mg was as effective as 20 mg [21]. Although there is always a fear with the use of tamoxifen for either endometrial hyperplasia or thrombotic event, this risk does not seem to appear in premenopausal patients younger than age 49 [24••]. Tamoxifen has been shown to be just as effective in the treatment of breast pain as danazol [25].

Unfortunately, almost half of patients on tamoxifen experience side effects. Some of the most common include vaginal discharge, gastrointestinal upset, and hot flashes. These effects can possibly be lessened by using tamoxifen only for the 10 to 14 days after ovulation [26].

Bromocriptine is marketed as a 5 mg capsule or a scored 2.5 mg tablet that can be broken in half. An initial 1.25 mg per day is increased by 1.25 mg per day every 2 weeks until a total dose of 5 mg per day (if tolerated) is achieved [27]. Approximately half of woman with cyclic mastalgia respond to bromocriptine therapy. Nausea is a prominent side effect in more than 25% of cases. The oral tablets can be inserted in the vagina with effective absorption and less nausea. However, because of its side effects, bromocriptine is rarely used today.

Gonadotropin-releasing hormone analogs have been reported in European studies as an effective therapy for cyclic mastalgia [28,29]. Amenorrhea is a common side effect with prolonged therapy. Within 6 months of stopping pharmacologic therapy for cyclic mastalgia, as many as 70% of women have recurrent symptoms [10,29]. Use longer than 6 months should be avoided, if possible, due to bone loss.

Currently the only US Food and Drug Administration–approved medication for breast pain is danazol. Danazol is marketed in 50-, 100-, and 200-mg capsules. As many as 90% of women with cyclic mastalgia respond to danazol therapy, although only approximately 40% of noncyclic mastalgia patients respond [10,30]. Danazol is first given in a dose of 100 mg orally twice daily, with sequential increases up to 400 mg per day until symptoms are controlled. This may take several months. Once the mastalgia is controlled for several months, the dose of danazol can usually be sequentially decreased to 100 mg per day or even 50 mg per day as long as symptom control is maintained. For more than 30% of women taking danazol, masculinizing side effects are so bothersome that they discontinue therapy. If voice changes occur, danazol should immediately be discontinued because the changes can be permanent.

The Cardiff Breast Clinic documented a 60% response to oil of evening primrose (linoleic acid) in women with cyclic mastalgia and a more than 40% response in women with noncyclic mastalgia [10]. These women were treated with 500 mg of linoleic acid given orally three times daily for 4 months (500-mg capsules can be found in most health food stores). In some cases, 1000 mg given three times daily is necessary for symptom relief. The reported side effects are minimal [31]. However, in two recent randomized controlled trials, linoleic acid showed no difference from placebo [32,33••].

Although some of the published study results conflict, generally progesterone (oral, intramuscular, or locally applied cream) has not proven to be effective therapy for mastalgia [34]. Despite anecdotal reports of efficacy, therapy with vitamins A, B complex, B_6, C, or E and dietary elimination of caffeine (methylxanthine) has not been proven effective in multicenter scientific clinical trials for the treatment of mastalgia [10,35–42]. On occasion, however, a woman with mastalgia has had what appears to be resolution of her symptoms using one of these therapies. Except in the rare case of mastalgia associated with clinical thyroid disorders, thyroid therapy is not effective treatment. Diuretics are of no proven value in the treatment of mastalgia [10]. For patients with premenstrual swelling and tension (which is often associated with cyclic mastalgia), salt restriction is innocuous and can be as effective as a diuretic.

Referral

If the primary care physician is unable to establish a definite diagnosis, or if step-wise therapy is unsuccessful in controlling the patient's symptoms, then the woman with breast pain should be referred to a medical breast specialist. Such specialists are usually found in comprehensive breast centers, often associated with medical schools. It is imperative that any woman with an undiagnosed palpable breast mass be urgently referred to a breast specialist.

References

Papers of particular interest have been highlighted as follows:
• Of interest
•• Of outstanding interest

1. Gateley CA, Mansel RE: Management of cyclical breast pain. Br J Hosp Med 1990, 43:300–332.

2. Wetzig NR: Mastalgia: a 3-year Australian study. Aust N Z J Surg 1994, 64:329–331.

3. Maddox PR, Mansel RE: Management of breast pain and nodularity. World J Surg 1989, 13:699–705.

4. Wisbey JR, Kumar S, Mansel RE, et al.: Natural history of breast pain. Lancet 1983, ii:672–674.

5. Ader DN, Browne MW: Prevalence and impact of cyclic mastalgia in a United States clinic-based sample. Am J Obstet Gynecol 1997, 177:126–132.

6. Ramirez AJ, Jarret SR, Hamed H: Psychosocial distress associated with severe mastalgia. In Recent Developments in the Study of Benign Breast Disease. Edited by Mansel RE. London: Parthenon; 1994.

7. Preece PE: Sclerosing adenosis. World J Surg 1989, 13:721–725.

8.•• Santen RJ, Mansel R: Benign breast disease. N Engl J Med 2005, 353:275.
Excellent in-depth article concerning benign breast lesions and their treatment.

9. Smallwood JA, Kye DA, Taylor I: Mastalgia: is this commonly associated with operable breast cancer? Ann R Coll Surg Engl 1986, 68:262–263.

10. Hughes LE, Mansel RE, Webster DJT: Breast pain and nodularity. In Benign Disorders and Diseases of the Breast. Edited by Hughes LE, Mansel RE, Webster DJT. London: Bailliere Tindall; 1989:75–92.

11. Tavaf-Motamen H, Ader DN, Browne MW, et al.: Clinical evaluation of mastalgia. Arch Surg 1998, 133:211–213.

12. Hindle WH: The diagnostic evaluation. In Breast Disease. Edited by Marchant DJ. Philadelphia: WB Saunders; 1997:69–82.

13. Duijm LE, Guit GL, Hendriks JH, et al.: Value of breast imaging in women with painful breast: observational follow up study. BMJ 1998; 317:1492.

14. Barros ACSD, Mottola J, Ruiz CA, et al.: Reassurance in the treatment of mastalgia. Breast J 1999, 5:162–165.

15. Goodwin PJ, Neelan M, Boyd NF: Cyclical mastopathy: a critical review of therapy. Br J Surg 1988, 75:837–844.

16. Steinbrunn BS, Zera RT, Rodriguez JL: Mastalgia: tailoring treatment to type of breast pain. Postgrad Med 1997, 102:183–184.

17. Gateley CA, Mansel RE: Management of painful and nodular breast. Br Med Bull 1991, 47:284–294.

18. Colak T, Ipek T, Kanik A, et al.: Efficacy of topical nonsteroidal anti-inflammatory drugs in mastalgia treatment. J Am Coll Surg 2003, 196:525–530.

19. Irving AD, Morrison SL: Effectiveness of topical non-steroidal anti-inflammatory drugs in the management of breast pain. J R Coll Surg Edinb 1998, 43:158–159.

20. Fentiman IS, Caleffi M, Brame K, et al.: Double blind controlled trial of tamoxifen therapy for mastalgia. Lancet 1986, i:287–288.

21. Fentiman IS, Caleffi M, Hamed H, et al.: Dosage and duration of tamoxifen treatment for mastalgia: a controlled trial. Br J Surg 1988, 75:845–846.

22. Grio R, Cellura A, Geranio R, et al.: Clinical efficacy of tamoxifen in the treatment of premenstrual mastodynia. Minerva Ginecol 1998, 50:101–103.

23. Gong C, Song E, Jia W, et al.: A double-blind randomized controlled trial of toremifen therapy for mastalgia. Arch Surg 2006,141:43–47.

24.•• Fisher B, Costantino JP, Wickerham DL, et al.: Tamoxifen for the prevention of breast cancer: current status of the National Surgical Adjuvant Breast and Bowel Project P-1 study. J Natl Cancer Inst 2005, 97:1652.

Tamoxifen study that looks at a large number of patients with breast pain and their response to the selective estrogen receptor modulator.

25. Kontostolis E, Stefanidis K, Navrozoglou I, et al.: Comparison of tamoxifen with danazol for treatment of cyclical mastalgia. Gynecol Endocrinol 1997, 11:393–397.

26. GEMB Group: Tamoxifen therapy for cyclical mastalgia: dose randomised trial. Breast 1997, 5:212–213.

27. Mansel RE, Dogliotti L: European multi-center trial of bromocriptine in cyclical mastalgia. Lancet 1990, 335:190–193.

28. Hamed H, Caleffi M, Chaudary MA, et al.: LHRH analogue for treatment of recurrent and refractory mastalgia. Ann R Coll Surg Engl 1990, 72:221–224.

29. Mansel RF, Goyal A, Preece P, et al.: European randomized, multicenter study of goserelin (Zoladex) in the management of mastalgia. Am J Obstet Gynecol 2004, 191:1942–1949.

30. Mansel RE, Wisbey JR, Hughes LE: Controlled trial of the antigonadotropin danazol in painful nodular benign breast disease. Lancet 1982, 1:928–930.

31. Holland PA, Gateley CA: Drug therapy of mastalgia: what are the options? Drugs 1994, 48:709–716.

32. Blommers J, de Lange-De Klerk ES, Kuik DJ, et al.: Evening primrose oil and fish oil for severe chronic mastalgia: a randomized, double-blind, controlled trial. Am J Obstet Gynecol 2002, 187:1389–1394.

33.•• Goyal A, Mansel RE, on behalf of the Efamast Study Group: A randomized multicenter study of gamolenic acid (Efamast) with and without antioxidant vitamins and minerals in the management of mastalgia. Breast J 2005, 11:41–47.

Large multicenter randomized trial that looked at several nutritional supplements and their effect on breast pain.

34. Maddox PR, Harrison BJ, Horobin JM, et al.: A randomized controlled trial of medroxyprogesterone acetate in mastalgia. Ann R Coll Surg Engl 1990, 72:71–76.

35. Minton JP, Foecking MK, Webster DJT, et al.: Response of fibrocystic disease to caffeine withdrawal and correlation of cyclic nucleotides with breast disease. Am J Obstet Gynecol 1979, 135:157–158.

36. Minton JP, Abou-Isa H, Reiches N, et al.: Clinical and biochemical studies in methylxanthine-related fibrocystic breast disease. Surgery 1981, 90:299–304.

37. Ernester VL, Mason L, Goodson WH III, et al.: Effects of caffeine free diet on benign breast disease: a randomized trial. Surgery 1982, 91:263–267.

38. Marshall J, Graham S, Swanson M: Caffeine consumption and benign breast disease: a case-control comparison. Am J Public Health 1982, 72:610–612.

39. Lubin F, Ron E, Wax Y, et al.: A case-control study of caffeine and methylxanthines in benign breast disease. JAMA 1985, 253:2388–2392.

40. Schairer C, Brinton LA, Hoover RN: Methylxanthines and benign breast disease. Am J Epidemiol 1986, 124:603–611.

41. Rohan TE, Cook MG, McMichael AJ: Methylxanthines and benign proliferative epithelial disorders of the breast in women. Int J Epidemiol 1989, 18:626–633.

42. Allen SS, Froberg DC: The effect of decreased caffeine consumption on benign proliferative breast disease: a randomized clinical trial. Surgery 1986, 101:720–730.

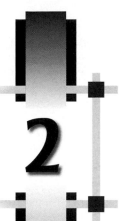

Galactorrhea and Nipple Discharge

David B. Engle and James A. Hall

- Galactorrhea results from elevated prolactin levels and the lactogenic effect on the breasts, not from intrinsic breast disease.
- Pathologic nipple discharge results from a disease process within a specific area of the breast.
- Carcinoma is the least likely cause of pathologic nipple secretion.
- The differentiation between galactorrhea and pathologic nipple secretion can be based on the history and physical examination.
- Prolactinomas are treated medically and rarely require surgery.

Introduction

Fluid discharged from the nipple can be a common occurrence among women. The fluid discharge can be classified as either galactorrhea (milk expression) or as pathologic nipple discharge (PND). Up to 80% of women in the premenopausal years can express some fluid from the nipple. Whereas nipple discharge can be disconcerting for patients, it is a very unlikely symptom of breast cancer.

Incidence and Epidemiology

Ten percent of nonpuerperal women experience spontaneous nipple discharge. Nipple discharge can be differentiated into galactorrhea and PND on the basis of the history and physical examination. Galactorrhea is caused by an elevation in prolactin levels and is nearly always induced, bilateral, and from multiple duct openings on the nipple. The secretion is watery or milky and does not contain blood or pus.

PND is spontaneous, unilateral, and from a single duct opening on the nipple. The secretion is bloody, serous, serosanguinous, purulent, or watery. The most common cause of PND is a benign papilloma (35% to 48% of cases). Duct ectasia (17% to 36% of cases) is the next most common cause and results from a benign chronic inflammatory condition of the duct wall. Carcinoma is the least often observed cause of PND (5% to 21% of cases) [1].

Gullay et al. [2] reported on a series of 448 women with nipple discharge from 1959 to 1991. Biopsy was performed in 115 women with spontaneous discharge and in 25 with discharge seen only with expression. Forty-five percent of the biopsy specimens were benign papillomas. Carcinoma was found in 14% of the spontaneous group and in 3% of the provoked group. Carcinoma was found in 61.5% of the patients with both discharge and a mass and in only 6% of those with nipple discharge alone. Another study that looked at more than 1100 women with nipple discharge found that only about 5% of them had an underlying malignancy [3].

Finally, age at the time of the nipple discharge is important. One study found that as the age of the women with the nipple discharge increased, so does the risk of malignancy [4]. In this study, the risk of cancer was 3% in those under age 40, 10% for those age 40 to 60, and 32% for those greater than 60 years old.

Pathophysiology

GALACTORRHEA

The patient history and physical examination can differentiate between PND and galactorrhea. PND is a unilateral, single-duct nipple discharge from a localized abnormality within the breast. Galactorrhea is a nonpuerperal, milky, or watery secretion that is usually bilateral and from multiple duct openings. Galactorrhea results from elevated serum prolactin levels that are lactogenic to the breast. An algorithm of nipple discharge causes is seen in Figure 2-1.

Knowledge of breast anatomy is essential to differentiate between PND and galactorrhea (Figure 2-2). The breasts are modified sebaceous glands within the superficial fascia of the anterior chest wall. Approximately 20% of the breast tissue is glandular and the remaining 80% is fatty. The breast is composed of 15 to 20 lobes arranged in a radial fashion extending from the nipple. Each lobe is divided into 20 to 40 lobules, and each lobule is subdivided into 10 to 100 alveoli. Each lobe has one unique terminal excretory duct or collecting duct. The collecting ducts are 2 mm in diameter and converge into subareolar lactiferous sinuses that are 5 mm to 8 mm in diameter. Five to 10 ducts ultimately drain to the outside through the nipple.

Knowing that each lobe has a single terminal duct is important when trying to identify the origin of single duct nipple discharge. Determining the location of the duct opening on the nipple from which the secretion is seen can lead to identification of the involved lobe. For example, a nipple duct opening at the 5 o'clock position drains a lobe from near the 5 o'clock

position within the breast. Most PND abnormalities originate in a duct that is under or very near the nipple-areola complex. PND usually results from an abnormality within a single lobe of the breast. Although carcinoma is the least likely cause of PND, a thorough diagnostic evaluation is essential.

Galactorrhea is a nonpuerperal, milky secretion from multiple duct openings in both breasts. The color is clear, milky, green, gray, or brown. The secretion does not contain blood or pus. Galactorrhea results from the lactogenic effect of increased serum prolactin levels. Prolactin is synthesized and released from the anterior pituitary gland, and is controlled by central nervous system neurotransmitters from the hypothalamus. The control of prolactin is from inhibition. Dopamine, a prolactin-inhibiting factor (PIF), is the major inhibitor of prolactin release. A specific hypothalamic prolactin-releasing factor (PRF) has not

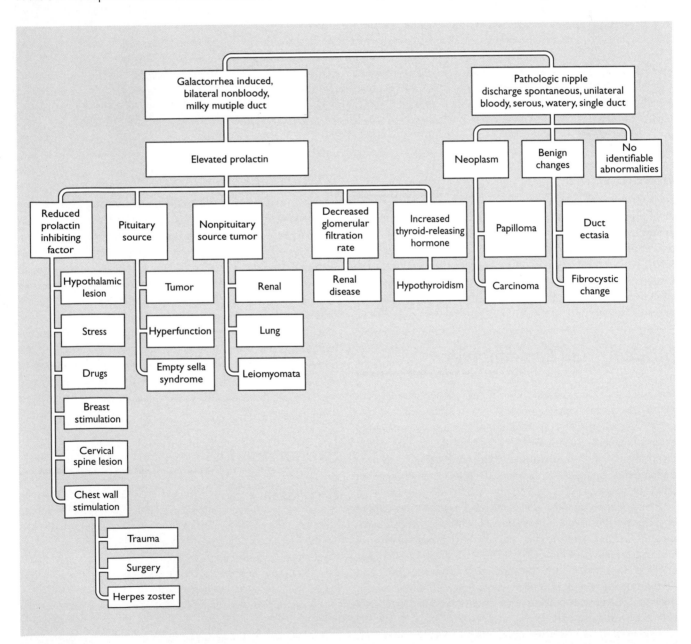

Figure 2-1. Etiology of nipple discharge.

been isolated. Serotonin and thyrotropin-releasing factor stimulate prolactin release. Because thyrotropin-releasing factor stimulates minimally, it is thought that serotonin is the primary PRF.

Prolactin levels fluctuate throughout the day, with the highest levels occurring during the night because of serotonin production. A smaller increase occurs in the early afternoon. Prolactin levels are also increased if drawn from a patient who recently awoke, exercised, or had breast stimulation. The optimal time to obtain prolactin samples is during the morning.

The ultimate cause of galactorrhea is an increased level of prolactin-stimulating secretion from both breasts. Conversely, about 66% of women with hyperprolactinemia do not have galactorrhea [3,5•]. Hyperprolactinemia has many causes. Estrogen suppresses the hypothalamus, resulting in lowered production of PIF, and thus, increased levels of prolactin. The effect on estrogen to the hypothalamus also explains the increase of prolactin at puberty and during the third trimester of pregnancy (approximately 200 ng/mL). Because estrogen also inhibits the action of prolactin on the breast, lactation usually does not occur early in pregnancy or with estrogen hormonal products such as birth control pills. Reduction in PIF also may result from hypothalamic neoplasm, cervical spine lesions, emotional stress, breast stimulation, or chest wall stimulation by trauma, surgery, or herpes zoster virus infection.

Many drugs (Figure 2-3) inhibit hypothalamic production of PIF or act directly on the pituitary. Phenothiazines, reserpine derivatives, opiates, diazepam, butyrophenones, methyldopa, and tricyclic antidepressants may also stimulate galactorrhea. Phenothiazine-stimulated prolactin levels can approach but do not exceed 100 ng/mL. Hypothyroidism may result in hyperprolactinemia and galactorrhea because low thyroxine levels result in an increase in thyroid-releasing hormone, which mimics and acts as prolactin-releasing hormone. Hyperprolactinemia can result

from nonpituitary sources, such as lung and renal tumors, as well as from uterine leiomyoma. Renal disease with a decreased glomerular filtration rate may elevate prolactin levels. The pituitary gland may produce excess prolactin as a result of tumor, hyperplasia, or empty sella syndrome. The most common pituitary tumors are benign prolactinomas, of which approximately 80% secrete prolactin.

Half of women with hyperprolactinemia have a prolactinoma, and the incidence is higher in those whose prolactin level exceeds 100 ng/mL. Twenty percent of women with galactorrhea and 35% of women with amenorrhea and galactorrhea have evidence of pituitary tumor. Approximately 20% of women with hyperprolactinemia and menstrual irregularities, but without galactorrhea, have pituitary tumors. It has been postulated that prolactinomas alter dopamine regulation of prolactin secretion, resulting in elevated levels. Prolactinomas are defined as microadenomas if the diameter is less than 1 cm and macroadenomas if the diameter is 1 cm or larger.

The empty sella syndrome is a benign clinical situation in which there is intrasellar extension of the subarachnoid space, and this causes increased pressure in the sella resulting in compression of the pituitary gland and an enlarged sella turcica. Radiographically, this will appear as an "empty sella" because of the pituitary being compressed, usually along the inferior wall. In this syndrome, pituitary function is normal except for elevated prolactin levels. Figure 2-4 lists sellar and suprasellar tumors and conditions that may result in hyperprolactinemia.

Pathologic Nipple Discharge

Breast papilloma is usually a benign growth of papilloma cells into the ductal lumen and is the most common cause

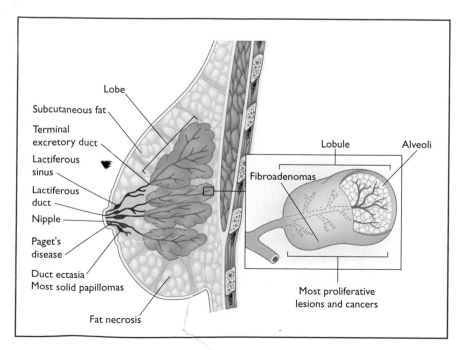

Figure 2-2. Breast anatomy and associated pathology.

of PND. This discharge is often times a sticky straw colored fluid. This fluid is essentially plasma, since arterial blood flow to the papilloma is unimpeded while the capillaries and venous drainage are often compressed by the papilloma itself. This will lead to increased venous resistance, and therefore, "leaking" plasma into the ducts which result in a nipple discharge. Papillomas are not considered precancerous unless they contain atypical hyperplasia [6]. Patients with atypical hyperplasia have a fourfold increased risk of developing cancer.

Duct ectasia is the second most common cause of PND. It is a benign condition in which the large ducts under the areola become dilated and results in periductal fibrosis. These larger ducts can then fill with fluid and become infected causing nipple discharge, pain, fever, and tenderness. One study showed that as many as 12% of all women undergoing breast surgery had histologic evidence of duct ectasia [7]. However, only 4% of these women had clinical symptoms.

DIFFERENTIAL DIAGNOSIS

Figure 2-5 lists some causes of hormone-induced galactorrhea from hyperprolactinemia and some causes of PND.

Drugs Affecting Prolactin Secretion

Stimulators
  Anesthetics
  Psychotropics
    Phenothiazines
    Tricyclic antidepressants
    Opiates
    SSRI antidepressants
  Hormones
    Estrogen
    Thyrotropin-releasing hormones
  Antihypertensives
    Methyldopa
    Reserpine
    Verapamil
  Antiemetics
    Sulpiride
    Metoclopramide
  H2 receptor antagonist
    Cimetidine
Inhibitors
  L-dopa
  Dopamine

Figure 2-3. Drugs affecting prolactin secretion. SSRI—selective serotonin reuptake inhibitors.

DIAGNOSTIC STUDIES

A thorough history and physical examination can help differentiate between galactorrhea and PND. Galactorrhea secondary to increased prolactin is nearly always provoked (induced through stimulation), bilateral, nonbloody, and expressed from multiple openings on the nipple. PND from a breast abnormality can be spontaneous or induced, unilateral, and comes from a single duct opening on the nipple. PND from benign disease is often green, gray, or brown. Malignant nipple discharge is more likely to be bloody, serosanguinous, or watery and is often associated with a palpable breast mass.

Sellar or Supersellar Tumors and Conditions That May Result in Hyperprolactinemia

Abscess
Aneurysm
Arachnoid cyst
Cephalocele
Chloroma (granulocytic sarcoma)
Colloid cyst
Craniopharyngioma
Dermoid
Ectopic neurohypophysis
"Empty" sella
Epidermoid tumor
Germinoma
Hamartoma (tubercinereum or hypothalamus)
Histiocytosis
Hyperplasia
Lipoma
Lymphoma
Meningioma
Meningitis (bacterial, fungal, or granulomatous)
Metastasis
Mucocele
Nasopharyngeal carcinoma
Opticochiasmatic-hypothalamic glioma
Osteocartilaginous tumor
Paracystic cyst
Pars intermedia cysts
Pituitary adenoma
Rathke's cleft cyst
Sarcoidosis

Figure 2-4. Sellar or supersellar tumors and conditions that may result in hyperprolactinemia. (*Adapted from* Hershlag and Peterson [9].)

Laboratory evaluation for galactorrhea includes serum prolactin and thyroid-stimulating hormone (TSH) levels. Treatment of hypothyroidism returns the prolactin levels to normal. Elevated TSH but normal triiodothyronine and thyroxine levels may indicate a rare TSH-secreting pituitary adenoma. Patients with elevated prolactin levels should have imaging studies of the sella to evaluate for neoplasm or empty sella syndrome. MRI is the imaging modality of choice because it provides the best resolution (1 mm) and avoids irradiation. Coned-down CT studies have high false-negative and false-positive rates, and the radiation exposure may exceed 20 cGy. CT scanning offers resolution closer to MRI, but the radiation approximates 3 cGy per study. The primary risk associated with cumulative radiation exposure is cataracts. Although most prolactinomas result in prolactin levels of more than 100 ng/mL, small increases over normal may result from microadenomas, macroadenomas, other sellar or suprasellar tumors, or other central nervous system abnormalities.

Pathologic nipple discharge should be evaluated with mammography and physical examination. Guaiac testing of the secretion may help identify occult bleeding. Microscopic evaluation in the office may help with the diagnosis by identifying fat globules or white blood cells. Otherwise, cytology of the nipple discharge has little value. Groves *et al.* reported on 338 patients who had nipple discharge cytology during a 10-year period [8]. Less than half of the carcinomas were identified, and there was one false-positive result. The most important mammographic finding is microcalcification along a duct, suggesting carcinoma or a suspicious mass. Galactography is a radiographic procedure involving cannulization of a single duct with injection of water-soluble dye. Papillomas and carcinomas may be identified, but the procedure lacks specificity. Clot and debris may mimic tumor, and dilated ducts may make identification of neoplasm impossible. The involved duct is nearly always under the nipple-areola complex, making identification of the abnormal area possible by careful physical examination. Therefore, galactography is reserved for unusual cases or peripheral lesions. Sequential palpation around the areola usually produces nipple discharge from the location of the involved duct. Thus, with physical examination alone, the site of an abnormality or neoplasm can usually be localized. A palpable mass deserves immediate evaluation. An algorithm for evaluation of galactorrhea and PND is shown in Figure 2-6.

Treatment

Treatment of galactorrhea depends on the patient's findings and tolerance of the secretions. Alteration in medications or decreased breast stimulation may return prolactin levels to normal. Women with functional hyperprolactinemia, empty sella syndrome, or microadenoma who do not wish to conceive or are not concerned by the breast secretion do not require treatment and should be followed clinically with prolactin levels. Headaches, visual changes, or prolactin levels higher than 100 ng/mL increase the likelihood of microadenoma or other significant sellar and suprasellar tumors. Microadenomas rarely enlarge, and many regress over time. Pregnancy, oral contraceptives, and hormonal replacement do not stimulate growth and are not contraindicated. The risk of osteoporosis is increased with hyperprolactinemia-induced estrogen deficiency, and estrogen or oral contraceptives may be indicated if the patient has amenorrhea or irregular menses. Nonlactotroph pituitary tumors or other central nervous system disorders require referral. Microadenomas are treated with dopamine agonists and rarely require surgery. Prolactin-secreting microadenomas rarely cause complications

Differential Diagnosis	
Hormone-induced Galactorrhea from Hyperprolactinemia	**Pathologic Nipple Discharge**
Common causes	Common causes
Emotional stress	Benign papilloma
Breast stimulation	Duct ectasia
Drugs	Fibrocystic changes
Pituitary tumor	Least likely causes
Pituitary hyperplasia	Carcinoma
Empty sella syndrome	Nonidentifiable cause
Hypothyroidism	
Least likely causes	
Hypothalamic lesions	
Cervical spine lesions	
Chest wall stimulation	
Nonpituitary source of prolactin (lung, kidney, fibroid)	
Decreased glomerular filtration rate	

Figure 2-5. Differential diagnosis.

in pregnancy. Serial prolactin levels during pregnancy are of no value because of the expected rise. Monitoring during pregnancy includes visual field and funduscopic examinations. Abnormal findings or persistent headaches should be investigated with MRI to rule out tumor growth. Medical management with dopamine agonists is the cornerstone of therapy.

Bromocriptine was approved for use in the United States in 1985 and decreases prolactin levels. Its half-life is 3.5 hours, resulting in depressed prolactin levels for 14 hours, and twice-daily dosing is required. The doses start at 1.25 mg per day and generally increase to 2.5 mg per day. The lowest effective dose is best. Side effects include nausea, headaches, hypotension, fatigue, dizziness, nasal congestion, and drowsiness. Vaginal administration of bromocriptine may reduce side effects. Carbergoline is a longer-acting dopamine agonist, and dosing starts at 0.25 mg given twice weekly. MRI should be repeated after 1 year of medical therapy with further scans done only to evaluate new symptoms or elevations in prolactin levels. Because some adenomas regress or cease to function, an attempt at discontinuation of medications is possible after 2 to 3 years. Although bromocriptine is not known to affect pregnancy outcome adversely, therapy is usually discontinued in pregnant patients.

Macroadenomas are also treated with dopamine agonists. Surgery is reserved for those who fail to respond to therapy or have persistent visual field loss. Recurrence of hyperprolactinemia and tumor growth is not uncommon after surgical resection. An MRI scan obtained 6 months after therapy is initiated to evaluate for regression, stabilization, or growth. Serial MRI scans and prolactin levels are obtained every 6 months. Approximately half of macroadenomas treated with bromocriptine reduce in size by 50%, and another one fourth reduced by 30%. Long-term therapy is usually required, however, because more than 60% of patients experience tumor regrowth after discontinuation of bromocriptine. It is recommended that medical therapy be discontinued after conception and reinstituted if headaches or changes in visual field develop. Breastfeeding is not contraindicated with either microadenomas or macroadenomas.

Treatment of pathologic nipple discharge is surgical excision when either benign or breast neoplasm is suspected. Outpatient excision with an excellent cosmetic result is possible using a circumareolar incision because the involved duct is usually under or near the nipple-areola complex. An incision away from the areola may be necessary if the preoperative evaluation suggests a more peripheral lesion. For patients who desire to maintain their ability to breastfeed, either a wide excision of the terminal ducts or selective duct excision is appropriate.

Referral

Referral is indicated if there is uncertainty about the diagnosis or need for neurosurgical (sellar and suprasellar tumor) or breast surgeon (breast neoplasm) consultation.

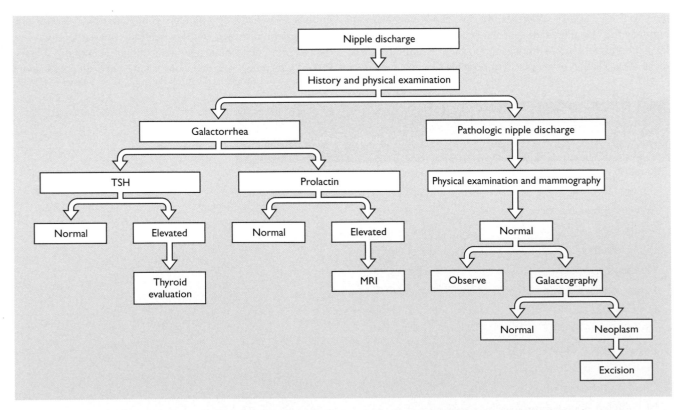

Figure 2-6. Diagnostic evaluation of galactorrhea and pathologic nipple discharge. TSH—thyroid-stimulating hormone.

Prevention

The primary preventative suggestion for galactorrhea is to avoid excessive breast and nipple stimulation. Using a properly supportive bra during athletic training and adjustment in breast stimulation during sex may eliminate or prevent galactorrhea. Vigorous attempts to elicit nipple discharge during breast self-examination or physical examination is painful and unnecessary and may stimulate galactorrhea.

References

Papers of particular interest are highlighted as follows:
- • Of interest
- •• Of outstanding interest

1. Winchester D: Nipple discharge. In *Diseases of the Breast*. Edited by Harris J, Lippman M, Morrow M, Hellman S. Philadelphia: Lippincott-Raven; 1996:106–119.

2. Gullay H, Bora S, Kilioturgay S, *et al*.: Management of nipple discharge. *J Am Coll Surg* 1994, 178:471–474.

3. Murad TM, Contesso G, Mouriesse H: Nipple discharge from the breast. *Ann Surg* 1982, 195:259.

4. Seltzer MH, Perloff LJ, Kelley RI, *et al*.: The significance of age in patients with nipple discharge. *Surg Gynecol Obstet* 1970, 131:519.

5.• Mishell D: Hyperprolactinemia, galactorrhea, and pituitary adenoma. In *Comprehensive Gynecology*. Edited by Mishell D, Stenchever M, Droegemueller W, Herbst A. St. Louis: CV Mosby; 1997:1069–1086.
Excellent textbook review chapter on etiology, diagnosis, clinical effect, and management of hyperprolactinemia and pituitary disorders.

6. Page DL, Salhany KE, Jensen RA, Dupont WD: Subsequent breast carcinoma risk after biopsy with atypia in a breast papilloma. *Cancer* 1996, 15:258–266.

7. Browning J, Bigrigg A, Taylor I: Symptomatic and incidental mammary duct ectasia. *J R Soc Med* 1986, 79(12):715–716.

8. Groves AM, Carr M, Wadhera V, *et al*.: An audit of cytology on the evaluation of nipple discharge: a retrospective study of 10 years' experience. *Breast J* 1996, 5:96–99.

9. Hershlag A, Peterson CM: Endocrine disorders. In *Novak's Gynecology*. Edited by Berek J, Adashi E, Hillard P. Baltimore: Williams & Wilkins; 1996:833–864.

3 | Breast Masses

David B. Engle

- Breast masses are a common cause of concern for patients and are usually diagnosed as fibrocystic changes, fibroadenoma, cysts, or malignancy.
- In 2006, it is estimated that there will be over 214,000 new cases of breast cancer and over 41,000 deaths.
- Routine breast screening by history and physical as well as appropriately-timed mammography are essential for early detection of breast cancers.

Introduction

A breast mass is any palpable, distinct mass within the breast tissue. However, because normal breast tissue often contains irregularities, especially in the premenopausal breast, breast masses may be hard to differentiate. Whereas breast masses may be just normal breast tissue or possible benign changes within the breast such as fibrocystic changes or breast cysts, it is essential to rule out malignancy.

Epidemiology

In women over the age of 40 whose primary complaint was a breast mass, 11% were diagnosed with breast cancer [1]. The overall majority of breast masses are fibrocystic changes or simple cysts. It is estimated there will be 214,640 new breast cancer diagnoses and 41,430 breast cancer deaths for the United States in 2006 [2]. A woman's lifetime risk of developing breast cancer is 12.5%. White women have a slightly higher risk of breast cancer at 13% than black women, whose risk is 10% [2]. As age increases, so does the risk of breast cancer; the median age of diagnosis is 61. In fact, 75% of women diagnosed with breast cancer are older than 50 years of age.

Risk factors other than age have been identified (Figure 3-1), yet 75% of women diagnosed with breast cancer have no identifiable risk factors [3]. The most common risk factor is family history, but only 7% of cases are thought to be genetically linked. The most common specific gene mutations associated with familial breast cancer are located on the BRCA-1 and BRCA-2 tumor suppressor genes. BRCA-1 is located on chromosome 17, whereas BRCA-2 is located on chromosome 13, and both genes are autosomal dominant. BRCA-1 carries a lifetime risk of 87% for breast cancer and 44% for ovarian cancer [4,5]. It is believed that BRCA-1 and 2 are responsible for 90% of all hereditary breast cancers [6]. Other inheritable causes of breast cancer include Li-Fraumeni syndrome and hereditary nonpolyposis colon cancer.

Extensive counseling, preferably by a genetic specialist, should be provided to the patient and her family before undergoing genetic testing. It is important for the patient to understand that a negative test does not eliminate the risk of developing breast cancer. Additionally, a positive test may have unfortunate social and insurability ramifications. Several groups have recommendations regarding the use of BRCA testing. The recommendations from the United States Preventive Services Task Force for offering BRCA testing are listed in Figure 3-2 [7].

Risk Profile for Development of Breast Cancer

Increasing age

Family history of breast cancer (twofold to threefold increased risk if mother or sister has breast cancer)

Reproductive history

Early menarche (before 11 years of age)

Nulliparity

Older than 30 years of age at first full-term pregnancy

Late menopause (after 50 years of age)

Figure 3-1. Risk profile of development of breast cancer.

In 2002, the Women's Health Initiative reported an increased risk of breast cancer among postmenopausal women who had taken conjugated equine estrogen 0.625 mg and medroxyprogesterone acetate 2.5 mg for more than 5 years [8]. This increase in invasive breast cancer caused the study to be halted. The study reported eight more breast cancers in 10,000 women per year compared to the control population, leading to a hazard ratio of 1.26. The increase in breast cancer was not seen until the patients had been on this hormone replacement regimen for 5 years. These results have lead many gynecologists to recommend the lowest effective dose of hormone replacement therapy necessary for women with bothersome menopausal symptoms. It is also recommended that the treatment duration be as short as possible. Interestingly, in the estrogen-only Women's Health Initiative trial for hysterectomized women, no increased risk of breast cancer was found [9].

Pathophysiology

Fibrocystic breast disease is the most common cause of breast complaints. Half of all women between the ages of 25 and 50 have signs of fibrocystic disease [10]. The disease is caused by increased amounts of fibrous tissue or cysts within the stroma of the breast tissue. The fibrous tissue can be epithelial or fibrous in nature. The multiple cysts can be large or small and are formed by ductal occlusion. The pain associated is usually a result of ductal dilation, inflammation, and edema. The pain and size of the cysts often fluctuate during the menstrual cycle, and the majority of fibrocystic disease subsides with menopause.

Fibroadenomas are the most common type of benign breast mass, and they usually occur in women who are in their teens or early 20s. The masses are rubbery, solid, mobile, and solitary 80% of the time. Their size can vary, but the average is approximately 2.5 cm. Fibroadenomas are not usually painful, and they do not change with the menstrual cycle.

US Preventive Services Task Force *BRCA* Screening Recommendations

Two first-degree relatives with breast cancer, one of whom received the diagnosis at the age of 50 or younger

Combination of three or more first- or second-degree relatives with breast cancer regardless of age at diagnosis

Combination of breast and ovarian cancer among first- and second-degree relatives

First-degree relative with bilateral breast cancer

Combination of two or more first- or second-degree relatives with ovarian cancer regardless of age at diagnosis

First- or second-degree relative with breast and ovarian cancer at any age

History of breast cancer in a male relative

Figure 3-2. US Preventive Services Task Force *BRCA* screening recommendations.

Approximately 30% will completely regress. Fibroadenomas without complex histology features or proliferative disease in the adjacent parenchyma are not associated with an increased risk of breast cancer [11].

Breast cysts are also a common finding in the premenopausal breast. They can be solitary or multiple, in either or both breasts. As the term implies, they are simple fluid-filled cysts that respond to hormone changes during the menstrual cycle. There can be cyclic pain associated with the cysts. Patients can be reassured that simple fluid-filled cysts do not increase the risk of breast cancer and can usually be treated, if necessary, in the office.

Breast cancer accounts for more than 30% of all new cancer diagnoses in women. It is second only to lung cancer as the leading cause of cancer death in women. A woman's lifetime risk of developing breast cancer is one in eight. Any suspicious breast mass should be considered malignant until proven otherwise.

Histologically, breast cancers usually arise from the lobules or the ducts. Like many other cancers, breast cancer can be invasive or in situ. The most common type is infiltrating ductal carcinoma. Location can also be important because 60% of all breast cancers are found in the upper outer quadrant.

Work-up

HISTORY AND PHYSICAL EXAMINATION
The first step in the evaluation of a patient with a breast mass is to take a thorough history from the patient. The history needs to assess not only the symptoms of the mass but also the patient's breast cancer risk. The medical record should include the patient's menstrual and reproductive history, including the age at first full-term delivery and lactation history. The family history of breast cancer should include maternal and paternal relatives and the ages at diagnosis of affected individuals. Personal history of breast disease should include pathologic diagnoses of prior biopsy specimens; history of hormone use, including oral contraceptive pills, hormone replacement therapy, and testosterone, exposure to diethylstilbestrol, and exposure to radiation.

The physical examination must include a clinical breast examination. A clinical breast examination includes visual and tactile examination of both breasts and axillae (Figure 3-3). The visual inspection should look for obvious asymmetry, bulging of the skin, nipple retraction, peau d'orange (orange peal appearance), and nipple ulceration. The examination should continue with palpation of the breast, nipple, and Tail of Spence. Nodal tissue should also be palpated in the supraclavicular region as well as the axillae. Worrisome findings on palpation include nodules that are hard, fixed, irregular in shape, solitary, and greater than 2 cm. Pain on palpation is not typical of breast cancer but does not exclude it. As a final part of the examination, nipple discharge should be looked for, with the finding of bloody discharge being the most concerning (*see* Chapter 2 for additional details).

IMAGING

Mammography is used not only as a screening tool, but also for diagnostic work up of a breast mass. Mammography is usually used for women age 35 and older because younger women's breasts are usually too dense to evaluate properly. Whereas the images from a mammogram are good, especially with the newer digital image machines, they still cannot completely differentiate between a benign and malignant mass. Furthermore, mammography has been reported to miss up to 20% of palpable breast masses [12]. Figure 3-4 lists the current American Cancer Society guidelines for the early detection of breast cancer.

Screening mammograms have 82% sensitivity and 91% specificity, whereas diagnostic mammograms for patients with a breast mass have a sensitivity and specificity of 87% and 84%, respectively [12]. Breast imaging reporting and data system is used to report mammogram results, which are based on the chance of the findings being cancer [13]. The scale is from 0 to 5, where zero represents an incomplete study and 5 represents "highly suggestive" for malignancy. Figure 3-5 shows the breast imaging reporting and data system scale.

During the workup for a palpable mass, an ultrasound of the mass can help differentiate the mass further after mammography. If the patient is under 35 years of age, it is recommended to go directly to ultrasound, bypassing mammography because of dense breast tissue. Ultrasound images of the breast mass can help differentiate solid versus cystic breast masses. The risk of cancer in a simple cyst is extremely low [14]. Ultrasound not only helps to determine the makeup of the mass, but also to determine the type of work-up that should follow.

SAMPLING

Fine needle aspiration (FNA) is a simple procedure that can be done in the office with or without local anesthesia. The cyst should be stabilized with one hand. Then, using a small-gauge needle (22 or 24) on a syringe, the cyst is aspirated. If clear or "straw" colored fluid is obtained, the patient can be reassured that the lesion is not cancerous, and the sample does not need to go for cytologic review [15,16]. The patient should be followed up in 4 to 6 weeks to see if the mass has completely resolved or reformed.

However, if the fluid is bloody, it should be sent for cytologic review. Of patients with bloody cyst fluid, approximately 7% will be found to have cancer [16]. Furthermore, if the mass turns out to be solid, and no fluid can be aspirated, the cells that are aspirated can be fixed on a slide and sent for cytologic review.

Diagnostic triad refers to the use of clinical breast exam, mammography, and FNA for the initial workup of a breast mass. The diagnostic triad has been reported to have a negative predictive value of near 100% [17]. It has also been shown that the FNA can be done before the mammogram without interfering with the results [18]. If the results of all three are negative, then the patient can be seen safely in 3 to 6 months for follow-up. If all three are positive, the patient needs to be referred to a breast specialist for histologic diagnosis and treatment. If there is conflict between the three different tests, the patient should undergo biopsy for definitive results.

American Cancer Society Guidelines for Early Detection of Breast Cancer

Annual mammography for women beginning at 40 years of age

No age at which screening should be terminated

Clinical breast examination close to time of mammogram

Figure 3-4. American Cancer Society guidelines for early detection of breast cancer.

American College of Radiology Breast Imaging Reporting and Data System of Mammogram Reporting

Category 0 designates an incomplete assessment, and additional imaging is necessary

Category 1 is a negative finding

Category 2 designates a benign finding

Category 3 is a probable benign finding, and short follow-up interval is suggested

Category 4 is a suspicious abnormality for which biopsy should be considered

Category 5 is a highly suspicious finding, and appropriate action should be taken

Figure 3-5. American College of Radiology Breast Imaging Reporting and Data System of mammogram reporting.

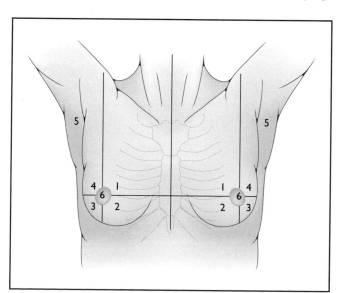

Figure 3-3. A drawing of the breast divided into various segments. The physical findings can be noted on this chart, which will be an easy reference point at the time of the next examination.

Treatment

Fibrocystic disease requires no treatment except for symptomatic pain. Over-the-counter analgesics and nonsteroidal anti-inflammatory drugs (oral or topical) are usually sufficient. Oral contraceptive pills may be of benefit if over-the-counter treatment is insufficient. For more severe cases, tamoxifen, danazol, or even gonadotropin-releasing hormone agonists may be required (see Chapter 1 for more details on treatment of breast pain).

Fibroadenomas, once the diagnosis is made, can be followed knowing that 30% will resolve and more than 10% will decrease in size over time. Definitive therapy may be necessary for larger masses as well as in those cases needing conclusive diagnosis. In this case, an open breast biopsy or lumpectomy can be undertaken.

Breast cysts can be observed or drained with a fine needle aspiration. If the fluid is nonbloody, it can be discarded, and the patient reassured that cysts are a common finding. Patients should be warned that cysts can recur up to 30% of the time, and they may require repeat drainage. For cysts that do recur, it may become necessary for surgical biopsy to remove the cyst wall.

The treatment and prognosis of invasive breast cancer depends on the initial stage of disease. Figure 3-6 shows the Tumor, Node, Metastasis staging classification for breast cancer. The most important independent variable in predicting prognosis is the status of the axillary lymph nodes [19].

A Tumor, Node, Metastasis Staging System for Breast Cancer

Primary tumor (T)

TX	Primary tumor cannot be assessed
T0	No evidence of primary tumor
Tis	Carcinoma in situ; intraductal carcinoma, lobular carcinoma in situ, or Paget's disease of the nipple with no tumor
T1	Tumor 2 cm or less in greatest dimension
T1mic	Microinvasion 0.1 cm or less in greatest dimension
T1a	Tumor more than 0.1 cm, but not more than 0.5 cm in greatest dimension
T1b	Tumor more than 0.5 cm, but not more than 1 cm in greatest dimension
T1c	Tumor more than 1 cm, but not more than 2 cm in greatest dimension
T2	Tumor more than 2 cm, but not more than 5 cm in greatest dimension
T3	Tumor more than 5 cm in greatest dimension
T4	Tumor of any size with direct extension to 1) chest wall or 2) skin, only as described below
T4a	Extension to chest wall
T4b	Edema (including peau d'orange) or ulceration of the skin of the breast or satellite skin nodules confined to the same breast
T4c	Both T4a and T4b
T4d	Inflammatory carcinoma

Regional lymph nodes (N)

NX	Regional lymph nodes cannot be assessed (eg, previously removed)
N0	No regional lymph node metastasis
N1	Metastasis to movable ipsilateral axillary lymph node(s)
	Metastasis to ipsilateral axillary lymph node(s) fixed to one another or other structures
N3	Metastasis to ipsilateral internal mammary lymph node(s)

Distant metastasis (M)

MX	Distant metastasis cannot be assessed
M0	No distant metastasis
M1	Distant metastasis (includes metastasis to ipsilateral supraclavicular lymph node[s])

B Tumor, Node, Metastasis Staging System for Breast Cancer

Stage Grouping

0	Tis	N0	M0
I	T1a	N0	M0
IIA	T0	N1	M0
	T1a	N1b	M0
	T2	N0	M0
IIB	T2	N1	M0
	T3	N0	M0
IIIA	T0	N2	M0
	T1*	N2	M0
	T2	N2	M0
	T3	N1	M0
	T3	N2	M0
IIIB	T4	Any N	M0
	Any T	N3	M0
IV	Any T	Any N	M1

*T1 includes T1mic.

Figure 3-6. A and **B**, Tumor, Node, Metastasis staging system for breast cancer.

Treatment begins with ipsilateral surgical excision and axillary lymph node biopsy and continues with radiation therapy, adjuvant chemotherapy, or both.

Studies have shown comparable survival data between mastectomy (radical or modified radical) and conservative surgical management (lumpectomy, axillary node dissection, and radiotherapy) [20]. The primary advantage of breast conservation therapy is cosmetic and psychologic. Requirements for breast conservation therapy include a tumor that can be reduced to a microscopic size with lumpectomy, a patient who is able to undergo radiation treatment, and a strong likelihood that follow-up mammograms and physical examinations will detect recurrence. Therefore, the contraindications to breast conservation therapy include diffuse suspicious calcifications or multicentric disease, previous radiation treatment, or the first or second trimester of pregnancy [20].

In women with early-stage disease, morbidity of the staging procedure relates primarily to the axillary node dissection. Forty percent of patients develop acute arm lymphedema, 20% develop paresthesias, and 5% develop chronic lymphedema [21]. Surgical advances have developed minimally invasive techniques to assess the status of the axillary lymph nodes. These techniques are based on the theory that the lymphatic drainage of a primary tumor is to a specific set of regional lymph nodes and then to the remainder of the nodal basin. The specific node or set of nodes is termed the *sentinel node*. If the surgeon can identify the sentinel node, and the pathologist can determine that it is free of disease, the remainder of the nodal basin is likely to be free of metastatic disease [21,22].

The sentinel node technique involves injecting vital dye and radioisotope around the breast lesion. After 2 to 6 hours, a gamma probe is used to detect the sentinel lymph node, and biopsy of that node is performed. In a recent multicenter trial, the sentinel node was detected in 93% of patients and was 97% accurate in predicting the status of the axillary nodes. The success of this technique varies with the experience of the surgeon and is years away from becoming the standard of care [23]. It holds great promise, however, for patients with small tumors and early disease in decreasing the morbidity of breast cancer staging procedures.

Prevention

In the general premenopausal population, there is little that can be recommended for breast cancer prevention. However, for women at increased risk of breast cancer due to age, *BRCA* receptor positive status, nulliparity, first-degree relatives with breast cancer, or other factors, there have been two developments. In 1998, the National Surgical Adjuvant Breast and Bowel Project released the results of its randomized prospective trial of using tamoxifen versus placebo for prevention of breast cancer in at-risk patients [24]. This trial of over 13,000 women showed over 5 years a 50% reduction in invasive and noninvasive breast cancers with estrogen receptor positive status. There was no difference in the rates of estrogen receptor negative tumors. Unfortunately, due to tamoxifen's

stimulatory properties in the uterus, these women had a 2.5 times increased risk of endometrial cancer. Also there was an increase in cataracts, deep vein thrombosis, and cerebrovascular accident in the tamoxifen group, but this was limited to patients over the age of 50. Tamoxifen is currently approved by the US Food and Drug Administration for breast cancer prevention in at-risk women.

After the conclusion of the above trial, the National Surgical Adjuvant Breast and Bowel Project started a second trial comparing tamoxifen to raloxifene (Evista; Eli Lilly and Co., Indianapolis, IN) for the prevention of breast cancer in at-risk women [25••]. The STAR trial, as it was referred to, included almost 20,000 women with an increased 5-year risk of breast cancer. Raloxifene was found to be just as effective at preventing breast cancers with a lower risk of thrombotic events, cataracts, and endometrial cancer. In December 2006, Eli Lilly submitted a new drug application for raloxifene for risk reduction of breast cancer in the postmenopausal patient.

Aromatase inhibitors are currently used in the treatment of estrogen receptor positive breast cancers. Currently there are several trials underway to examine their use in breast cancer prevention. At this time, their use is still considered experimental.

Prophylactic salpingo-oophorectomy in *BRCA*-positive patients has been shown to reduce the risk of breast cancer by 50% to 80% [26]. Additionally, it reduces the risk of *BRCA*-related ovarian cancer by 96% [27,28]. Whereas the use of current low-dose oral contraceptive pills do not change the risk of developing breast cancer in *BRCA*-positive patients, it does reduce the risk of ovarian cancer by 50% after 5 years of use [29••].

References

Papers of particular interest are highlighted as follows:
- *Of interest*
- •• *Of outstanding interest*

1. Barton MB, Elmore JG, Fletcher SW: Breast symptoms among women enrolled in a health maintenance organization: frequency, evaluation, and outcome. *Ann Intern Med* 1999, 130:651–657.

2. National Cancer Institute: SEER Database. Available at www.cancer.gov.

3. Landis S, Murray T, Bolden S, *et al.*: Cancer statistics, 1998. *CA Cancer J Clin* 1998, 48:6–29.

4. Ford D, Easton D, Bishop D, *et al.*: Risks of cancer in BRCA 1 mutation carriers. *Lancet* 1994, 343:692–695.

5. Easton D, Bishop D, Ford D, Crockford G: Genetic linkage analysis in familial breast and ovarian cancer: results from 214 families. *Am J Hum Genet* 1993, 52:678–701.

6. Mann GB, Borgen PI: Breast cancer genes and the surgeon. *J Surg Oncol* 1998, 67:267–274.

7. US Preventive Services Task Force: Genetic risk assessment and BRCA mutation testing for breast and ovarian caner susceptibility: recommendation statement. *Ann Int Med* 2005, 143:355–361.

8. Rossouw JE, Anderson GL, Prentice RL, *et al.*: Risks and benefits of estrogen plus progestin in healthy postmenopausal women. *JAMA* 2002, 288:321–333.

9. The Women's Health Initiative Steering Committee: Effects of conjugated equine estrogen in postmenopausal women with hysterectomy: the Women's Health Initiative randomized controlled trial. *JAMA* 2004, 291:1701–1712.

10. Giuliano AE: Fibrocystic disease of the breast. In *Current Surgical Therapy II*. Edited by Cameron JL. Toronto: DC Decker, 1986:315–317.

11. Dupont WD, Page Dl, Parl FF, *et al.*: Long-term risk of breast cancer in women with fibroadenomas. *N Engl J Med* 1994, 331:10–15.

12. Barlow WE, Lehman CD, Zheng Y, *et al.*: Performance of diagnostic mammography for women with signs or symptoms of breast cancer. *J Natl Cancer Inst* 2002, 94:1151–1159.

13. *Breast Imaging Reporting and Data System (BI–RADS) Atlas*, edn 4. Reston: American College of Radiology, 2003.

14. Sickles EA, Filly RA, Callen PW: Benign breast lesions: ultrasound detection and diagnosis. *Radiology* 1984, 151:467–470.

15. Hindle WH, Arias RD, Florentine B, Whang J: Lack of utility in clinical practice of cytologic examination of nonbloody cyst fluid from palpable breast cysts. *Am J Obstet Gynecol* 2000, 182:1300.

16. Ciatto S, Cariaggi P, Bulgaresi P: The value of routine cytologic examination of breast cyst fluids. *Acta Cytol* 1987, 31:301–304.

17. Chaiwun B, Thorner P: Fine needle aspiration for evaluation of breast masses. *Curr Opin Obstet Gynecol* 2007, 19:48–55.

18. Hindle WH, Chen EC: Accuracy of mammographic appearances after breast fine-needle aspiration. *Am J Obstet Gynecol* 1997, 176:1286–1290; discussion 1290–1292.

19. Carcinoma of the breast. *ACOG* 1991, 158:1–7.

20. Hansen N, Morrow M: Breast disease. *Med Clin North Am* 1998, 2.

21. Reintgen D, Joseph E, Lyman G, *et al.*: The role of selective lymphadenectomy in breast cancer. *Cancer Control* 1997, 3:211–219.

22. Krag DN, Ashikaga T, Harlow S, *et al.*: Development of sentinel node targeting technique in breast cancer patients. *Breast J* 1998, 2:67–74.

23. Krag DN, Weaver D, Ashikaga T, *et al.*: The sentinel node in breast cancer. *N Engl J Med* 1998, 14:941–946.

24. Fisher B, Costantino JP, Wickerham DL, *et al.*: Tamoxifen for prevention of breast cancer: report of the National Surgical Adjuvant Breast and Bowel Project P-1 Study. *JNCI* 1998; 90:1371–1388.

25.•• Vogel VG, Constantino JP, Wicherham DL, *et al.*: Effects of tamoxifen vs. raloxifene on the risk of developing invasive breast cancer and other disease outcomes. *JAMA* 2006, 295:2727–2741.

Large double-blind, randomized trial comparing tamoxifen to raloxifene for prevention of breast cancer.

26. Kauf ND, Satagopan JM, Rovson ME, *et al.*: Risk reducing salpingo-oophorectomy in women with a *BRCA*-1 or *BRCA*-2 mutation. *N Engl J Med* 2002, 346:1609–1615.

27. Rebbeck TR, Lynch HT, Neuhausen SL, *et al.*: Prophylactic oophorectomy in carriers of *BRCA*-1 or *BRCA*-2 mutations. *N Engl J Med* 2002, 346:1616–1622.

28. Haber D: Prophylactic oophorectomy to reduce the risk of ovarian and breast cancer in carriers of *BRCA* mutations. *N Engl J Med* 2002, 346:1660–1662.

29.•• Use of hormonal contraception in women with coexisting medical conditions. ACOG Practice Bulletin No. 73. *Obstet Gynecol* 2006, 107:1453–1472.

Authoritative review of the use of hormonal contraception in women with other medical conditions.

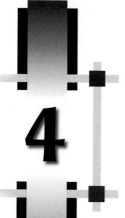

4 Ectopic Pregnancy

Thomas G. Stovall

- Ectopic pregnancy treatment has moved from an inpatient surgical standard to an outpatient medical treatment in many cases.
- The death ratio from ectopic pregnancies has decreased because of better and faster diagnoses.
- Plateaued human chorionic gonadotropin titers are the most predictive measures of an ectopic pregnancy.
- Management includes surgical treatment or medical therapy with methotrexate.

Incidence

The incidence of ectopic pregnancy in the United States has increased threefold during the past 20 years. More than 80,000 women are diagnosed with an ectopic pregnancy each year. During this same time, the death-to-case ratio declined from 3.6 to 0.9. Death from ectopic pregnancy in the United States today is a rare event. Nationwide, 1% of all pregnancies are ectopic gestations, with an incidence in some communities as high as one in 45. Several factors responsible for the rise in incidence are previous laparoscopically proven pelvic inflammatory disease, previous tubal pregnancy, current use of an intrauterine device, and previous tubal surgery. Other factors include progestin-only contraception, history of ectopic pregnancy, history of infertility, and smoking [1–3]. In light of the increasing incidence, the continued decrease in the death-to-case ratio is certainly a result of more sensitive and specific radioimmunoassays for the beta-subunit human chorionic gonadotropin (hCG), serum progesterone screening, high resolution transvaginal sonography, and the widespread availability of laparoscopy.

Diagnostic Methods

Serum and urine hCG assays are virtually always positive in the patient with an ectopic pregnancy, although it is possible to have an ectopic pregnancy with a negative hCG titer [6–8]. A single hCG titer is of limited usefulness so several titers are necessary. Human chorionic gonadotropin is detectable in maternal serum 8 days after the leuteinizing hormone (LH) surge. It rises exponentially to peak approximately at 8 to 10 weeks' gestation (dated from last menstrual period); and thereafter falls to a nadir between 16 and 24 weeks of gestation. At a serum concentration of greater than 10,000 mIU/mL, the doubling time of the hCG among different individuals is more varied. However, its doubling time above 2500 mIU/mL is of little practical importance because at levels above this critical cut-off, transvaginal ultrasound is the diagnostic tool of choice. In ectopic pregnancy, hCG generally increases more slowly than during normal pregnancy. If the hCG titer rises 50% over 48 hours, the pregnancy is considered nonviable. Plateaued levels are the most predictive of ectopic pregnancy [9–11].

Figure 4-1 shows a nonsurgical protocol utilizing hCG, transvaginal ultrasound, progesterone, and dilation and curettage [4,5•] Progesterone was dropped later from the algorithm because it was not found to be 100% accurate in determining abnormal pregnancies. Human chorionic gonadotropin is used in the nonlaparoscopic algorithm for several reasons (Figure 4-1):

1. To document an abnormal gestation (persistent abnormal rise of less than 50% in 48 hours).

2. To time the vaginal ultrasound. At an hCG level of 2000 mIU/mL or greater, transvaginal ultrasound can visualize an intrauterine sac in all normal, viable intrauterine pregnancies.

3. To follow the hCG levels after completion of a dilation and curettage. A fall in hCG level following this procedure is indicative of a completed abortion while a plateaued or rising

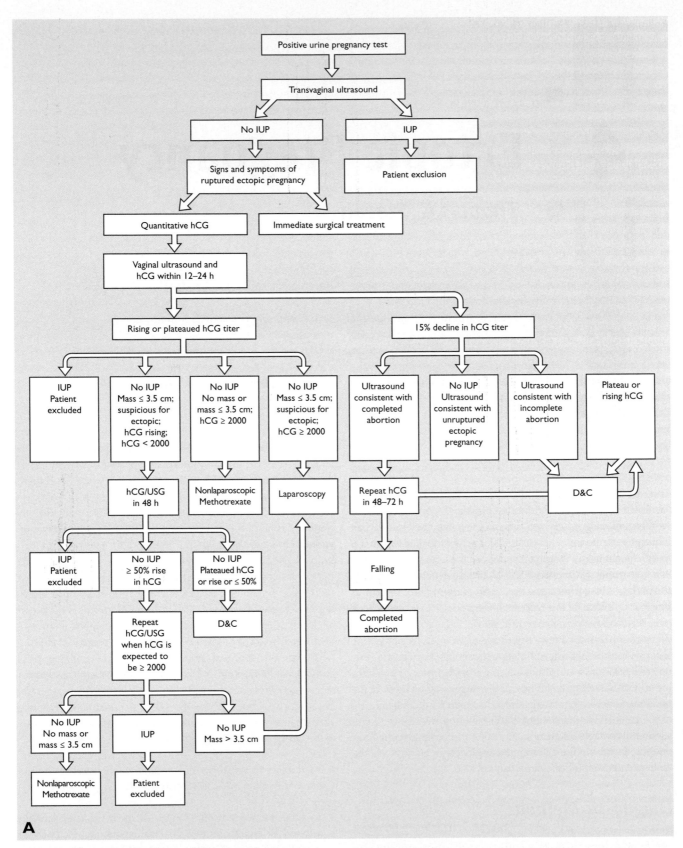

Figure 4-1. A and **B**, Diagnostic algorithm for ectopic pregnancy. D&C—dilation and curettage; hCG—human chorionic gonadotropin; IUP—intrauterine pregnancy; USG—ultrasonography.

Continued on the next page

level after dilation and curettage indicates persistent tropho-blastic tissue, and is diagnostic of an extrauterine pregnancy.

4. To screen for viable pregnancy. An hCG titer greater than 50,000 is rarely associated with an ectopic pregnancy.

Progesterone concentrations in patients with an ectopic pregnancy are usually lower than in patients with a viable intra-uterine pregnancy. In retrospective studies, Yeko et al. [12] and Matthews et al. [13] demonstrated that all ectopic pregnancies were associated with a serum progesterone less than 15 ng/mL, whereas all normal intrauterine pregnancies had progesterone levels greater than 15 ng/mL. An initial prospective study using serum progesterone revealed considerable overlap in proges-terone values for normal and abnormal pregnancies [14–16].

Additional studies of serum progesterone concentrations in 10,000 first-trimester pregnancies confirm several important concepts. Progesterone can be used as a screening test for nor-mal and abnormal pregnancy. Only 1% to 2% of abnormal pregnancies (abortions or ectopic pregnancies) are associated with a progesterone greater than 25 ng/mL. But serum proges-terone is not as helpful in identifying a nonviable pregnancy. Although it is uncommon (one in 10,000) to identify a viable pregnancy in association with a serum progesterone less than 5.0 ng/mL, two such cases have been reported. Both patients had a viable intrauterine pregnancy in association with a serum progesterone of 3.9 ng/mL.

Vaginal ultrasound permits identification of a gestational sac at a much lower hCG titer than transabdominal scanning. The minimal hCG titer at which a sac should always be seen is not yet clear, but a transvaginal sonogram should always visualize a viable intrauterine pregnancy at an hCG titer of greater than 2000 mIU/mL. Vaginal ultrasound can also image oviducts and ovaries so that masses and their dimension can be defined with increasing reliability. The addition of color Doppler evaluation aids in earlier detection of an intrauterine gestation and allows better visualization of an ectopic gestation [17].

The role of transvaginal ultrasound using the nonsurgical alternative is:

1. To identify an intrauterine gestational sac that essentially excludes a diagnosis of ectopic pregnancy.

2. To identify ectopic pregnancy greater than 3.5 to 4.0 cm in greatest dimension. This finding represents a contraindication to medical therapy.

3. Identify adnexal cardiac activity in the ectopic gestation, which is a relative contraindication to medical therapy.

4. Color Doppler scanning helps to differentiate between a completed abortion, incomplete abortion and an early intra-uterine pregnancy before visualization of a gestational sac in many patients. However, from a clinical standpoint, hCG

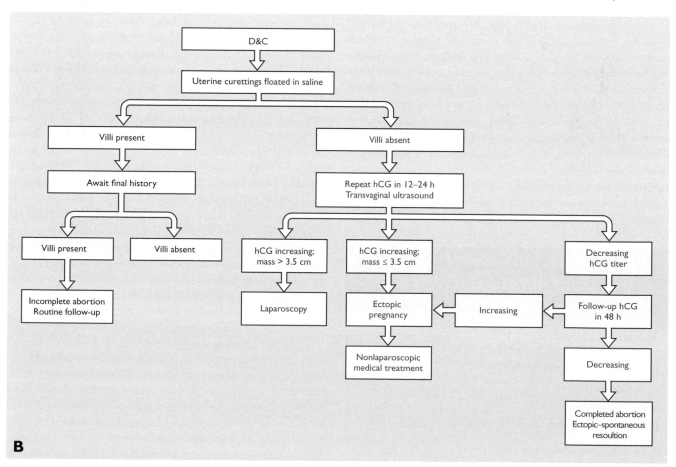

B

Figure 4-1. *(Continued)*

confirmation is necessary to make certain that the diagnosis is absolutely correct.

Culdocentesis (evacuation of fluid from the peritoneal cavity) is useful for the diagnosis of hemoperitoneum. However, there is a false-positive rate of up to 15% with a positive culdocentesis [18]. In reality, there is no actual use for culdocentesis when considering nonsurgical diagnosis and therapy because 45% to 60% of unruptured ectopic pregnancies eligible for methotrexate will have a positive culdocentesis.

Dilation and suction curettage is a useful part of the nonsurgical algorithm in patients with a confirmed abnormal gestation with an associated hCG titer 2000 mIU/mL. The identification of chorionic villi essentially eliminates the diagnosis of ectopic pregnancy (one in 15,000). Furthermore, its use eliminates giving methotrexate to a patient with an abnormal intrauterine pregnancy.

Laparoscopy remains the gold standard for the diagnosis of ectopic pregnancy. However, we have now moved to a point at which laparoscopy is a surgical modality and rarely necessary as a diagnostic tool for ectopic gestation. As one eliminates laparoscopy, the risks, costs, and morbidity of medical therapy are decreased.

Treatment

SURGICAL MANAGEMENT

Surgical management of an ectopic pregnancy has in the past been the mainstay of treatment and is the standard to which other treatments are compared. While all ectopic pregnancies can be managed surgically, under certain circumstances surgical management is the only alternative. Obviously, if a patient presents to the emergency department in hypovolemic shock, the need for surgical intervention is not questioned. However, in the stable individual, indications for the use of surgery are outlined in Figure 4-2. Other than the unstable patient in shock, most women with ectopic pregnancies are candidates for laparoscopic intervention. It is estimated that 4% to 5% of women with ectopic pregnancies present in shock. Excluding another 5% to 10% who would require conversion from laparoscopy to laparotomy, over 80% of women could be treated with laparoscopy [19•,20,21]. In the hands of an experienced laparoscopist, the rate of conversion to laparotomy should remain low.

There are several published reports comparing laparoscopy with laparotomy for the treatment of ectopic pregnancy in women who are hemodynamically stable. Outcome factors such as days of hospitalization, blood loss, operating time, cost, pain medication use, adhesion formation, and subsequent pregnancies have been studied.

Vermesh et al. [19•] randomized 60 women with unruptured ectopic pregnancies less than 5 cm to laparoscopic or laparotomy linear salpingostomy. Mean blood loss was statistically less for laparoscopy (79 mL) when compared with laparotomy (195 mL). However, two patients in the laparoscopy group required laparotomy to achieve hemostasis after the salpingostomy was performed. No differences were noted in postoperative fever or wound infection. One patient in each group required a second operation for rising hCG levels after surgery. Hospital stay was shorter (1.4 vs 3.3 days) for laparoscopy. This translated to a $1500 savings. Postoperative hysterosalpingogram showed patency in the involved tube in 16 of 20 (80%) laparoscopy patients and 17 of 19 (89%) laparotomy patients. Subsequent pregnancy rates also were not different.

Brumsted et al. [20] compared laparoscopy and laparotomy for the treatment of ectopic pregnancy, randomizing 25 women to each group. The postoperative length of stay was significant shorter in the laparotomy group (1.34 vs 3.42 days), as was return to normal activity (8.7 vs 25.7 days). Postoperative pain as measured by the number of doses of intramuscular/intravenous analgesia was also significantly less in the laparoscopy group (0.84 vs 4.64).

Murphy et al. [21] prospectively assigned women with suspected ectopic pregnancies to laparoscopy ($n = 26$) or laparotomy ($n = 37$), in a university based residency training program. Operative and postoperative parameters were similar to previously reported studies. Patients treated by laparoscopy had reduced estimated blood loss (62 vs 115 mL), reduced need for analgesia (26 vs 58 mg). The length of stay was also shorter (26 vs 634 hours), as were the patient hospital charges ($5528 vs $6793). Finally patients who underwent laparoscopy have a shorter time to the return of normal activity (17 vs 62 days). In summary, the laparoscopic approach is associated with equal to shorter operating times, shorter hospital stays and convalescence, lower analgesic needs, and potentially lower costs. However, other factors must be considered.

Sultana et al. [22] reviewed 126 cases of ectopic pregnancy at the Cleveland Clinic Foundation and compared rates of pregnancy and term deliveries among women who had laparoscopic salpingostomy, laparotomy with salpingostomy, and laparotomy with salpingectomy. Crude pregnancy rates were no different among the three study groups. A history of infertility was a significant predictor of subsequent pregnancy rates. As noted earlier, Vermesh et al. [19•] found no difference in subsequent outcomes in women having salpingostomy by laparoscopy or laparotomy.

Indications for Surgical Treatment of Ectopic Pregnancy in the Stable Patient

1. Refuses medical management
2. Ectopic > 3.5–4.0 cm in greatest dimension by ultrasound
3. Evidence of rupture by ultrasound
4. Unsure diagnosis
5. Prior tubal ligation
6. Contraindication to medical therapy

Figure 4-2. Indications for surgical treatment of ectopic pregnancy in the stable patient.

There is evidence to suggest that the conservative laparoscopic approach of salpingostomy has a higher incidence of persistent trophoblast than laparotomy. Seifer *et al.* [23] found 15.5% (16 of 103) women undergoing laparoscopic salpingostomy had persistent hCG levels compared with only 1.8% (one of 54) of women having salpingostomy via laparotomy. Murphy *et al.* [21] found three patients with laparoscopic salpingostomy to have persistent hCG titer compared with none undergoing laparotomy. However, the study group of Vermesh *et al.* [19•] showed no differences in persistent hCG levels after laparoscopy or laparotomy; although the incidence of persistent trophoblast is lower after laparoscopic salpingostomy. Regardless of the method of treatment, hCG levels must be followed until negative so that persistence can be diagnosed and treated.

Lundorff *et al.* [24] performed second look laparoscopy on 73 women who had been treated by laparoscopy or laparotomy for ectopic pregnancy. Adhesions were statistically more common on the involved and contralateral sides in women undergoing laparotomy.

NONSURGICAL MANAGEMENT

In an effort to eliminate the risk of surgery, a number of medical regimens and agents have been studied. At the present time, methotrexate, a folic analogue that inhibits dihydrofolate reductase and thereby blocks DNA synthesis, appears to be the agent of choice for medical management. Potential side effects include leukopenia, thrombocytopenia, bone marrow suppression, stomatitis, and gastrointestinal upset; however, few such effects have been reported with the doses necessary for ectopic pregnancy treatment.

Methotrexate has been used extensively for the treatment of trophoblastic disease, and for the treatment of placental tissue left in situ after exploration for an abdominal pregnancy [25–27]. In 1982, Tanaka *et al.* [28] treated an unruptured interstitial ectopic gestation with a 15-day course of intramuscular methotrexate. Following this, a few case reports described limited experience of methotrexate in unusual presentations of ectopic pregnancies [29–33]. Miyazaki [34] in 1983 and Ory *et al.* [35] in 1986 published the first clinical studies utilizing methotrexate as primary treatment for ectopic pregnancy.

To capitalize on the generally favorable published outcomes, we began a prospective outpatient treatment protocol [36]. Our initial report detailed 36 patients who were treated with methotrexate and citrovorum factor, 34 (94.4%) of which were successful with completed resolution of their ectopic pregnancy. Two patients experienced rupture after chemotherapy and one patient experienced rupture 23 days after treatment. There were no major chemotherapy-related side effects, and only three of 36 (8.3%) experienced a minor side effect. From this study, we concluded that: 1) individualized dosing of outpatient methotrexate and citrovorum could be safely managed on an outpatient basis, even in an indigent population; 2) ectopic pregnancy rupture could still occur up to 23 days after chemotherapy initiation; and 3) fetal cardiac activity is a relative contraindication to medical therapy.

One hundred patients were treated with the multidose outpatient protocol with a 96% success rate [37]. Cardiac activity in the ectopic is not an absolute contraindication to medical therapy. The multidose protocol is shown in Figure 4-3 [37]. When using this protocol, citrovorum should be given on the day after the methotrexate dose, even if no further methotrexate will be indicated. Patients are instructed to refrain from sexual intercourse until there is complete resolution of the ectopic pregnancy (hCG < 15 mIU/mL), to avoid vitamins containing folic acid, and not to use alcohol while receiving methotrexate. In addition, as a precaution, patients are asked to use oral contraceptives or double-barrier contraception for 1 to 2 months after treatment, or until a hysterosalpingogram can be obtained (usually after the first or second menstrual period after treatment completion). Patients with iron deficiency anemia are given iron sulfate, 325 mg two or three times per day. Rh immune globulin is given if the patient is Rh-negative. Absolute contraindications to methotrexate therapy include active liver or renal disease, and tubal rupture. Using this protocol, our incidence of methotrexate-related side effects is approximately 3% to 4%, all of which are mild, and the incidence of failure (nonresponders or tubal rupture) is approximately 3% to 4%.

Weekly intramuscular methotrexate without citrovorum factor (Figure 4-4) has been reported for the treatment of nonmetastatic gestational trophoblastic disease. Single-dose methotrexate for ectopic pregnancy was first reported by Stovall *et al.* [38,39]. The initial report detailed 31 patients treated with a single injection of methotrexate (50 mg/m²) without citrovorum factor rescue, utilizing the same criteria as the multidose protocol. Twenty-nine of 30 (96.7%) patients were successfully treated. No patients experienced side effects. The number of patients was expanded to include 120 patients treated using

Outpatient Multidose Protocol for Methotrexate Treatment*

Day	Time	Variable
1	Variable	CBC, SGOT, MTX, β-hCG, blood type +Rh, BUN, creatinine
2	8:00 AM	CF, β-hCG
3	8:00 AM	MTX, β-hCG
4	8:00 AM	CF, β-hCG
5	8:00 AM	MTX, β-hCG
6	8:00 AM	CG, β-hCG
7	8:00 AM	MTX, β-hCG
8	8:00 AM	CF, β-hCG

*MTX is alternated with CF until there is a decrease in the hCG titer. If MTX has been given, it is always followed by CG.

Figure 4-3. Outpatient multidose protocol for methotrexate (MTX) treatment. β-hCG—quantitative beta-human chorionic gonadotropin, mIU/mL; BUN—blood urea nitrogen; CBC—complete blood count with differential and platelet count; CF—intramuscular citrovorum 0.1 mg/kg; SGOT—serum glutamine oxalacetic transaminase, U/L.

this protocol. Patients had a mean hCG titer before treatment initiation of 3950 plus 1193 mlU/mL. Transvaginal ultrasound visualized cardiac activity in 14 (11.9%) patients, with ectopic pregnancies more visualized in 113 (94.2%). Of these 120 patients, 113 (94.2%) were successfully treated, with four (3.3%) of these patients requiring a second dose on day 7. The mean time to achieve pregnancy was 3.1 plus 1.1 months [39]. Similar results have now been reported with 315 patients [40•].

Ransom et al. [41] reported that serum progesterone 10 ng/mL was useful in predicting the resolution of ectopic pregnancy when treated with methotrexate, whereas a serum progesterone greater than10 ng/mL was associated with methotrexate treatment failure. Henry and Gentry [42] reported 61 patients with a gestational sac size less than 3.5 cm. Of the 61 patients, 16 required a second dose, and 52 (85%) were successfully treated. Human chorionic gonadotropin was measured on days 1, 4, 7, and 10 and patients were given a second dose for any two rising hCG titers or for a plateauing hCG after day 7. Four of nine patients who were operated on had an unruptured ectopic pregnancy. Dilation and curettage was not done pretreatment with an hCG titer less than 2000. The pretreatment hCG level is also an important predictor of successful treatment outcome. Various cut-off levels have been supported. The largest database shows that when the hCG level is above 10,000 mlU/mL there is a decrease in treatment success. However, even at this level most patients can be successfully treated.

Reproductive function after methotrexate-citrovorum treatment was recently studied in a group of 57 patients who were successfully treated. Reproductive function was assessed by studying time to resolution, return of menses, tubal patency on hysterosalpingogram, time to pregnancy, and pregnancy outcome. In this study, methotrexate-citrovorum treatment of unruptured ectopic pregnancy assists in the restoration of tubal anatomy and does not impair return of menses. Most important, pregnancy rates following this form of therapy appear to be better than those achieved by traditional surgical methods, and comparable to laparoscopic salpingostomy.

Pregnancy outcome after systemic therapy was reported by Stovall et al. [37,43] in two separate reports. The first was a group of 14 patients attempting pregnancy after multidose intramuscular methotrexate. Of 44 patients available for follow-up, 14 desired and were attempting pregnancy. Of the 14 patients, 11 (78.6%) became pregnant with 10 of 11 (90.9%) having an intrauterine pregnancy, with one (9.1%) being extrauterine. The mean time in this group from first attempting pregnancy to achieving pregnancy was 2.3 months. More recently, Stovall et al. [43] reported a group of 49 patients attempting pregnancy after completion of single-dose intramuscular methotrexate. Of these 49 women, 39 (79.6%) became pregnant with 34 (87.2%) intrauterine and five (12.8%) ectopic pregnancies. The mean time from attempting pregnancy to achieving pregnancy was 3.2 plus 1.1 months. Currently, the intrauterine pregnancy rate remains at 86%, with an ectopic pregnancy recurrence rate of 14%.

Injection of methotrexate into the tubal gestation by an ultrasonographic guided needle or at laparoscopy has been described with successful outcome. There have been numerous reports showing varying degrees of success [43–54]. Potential advantages to this technique include a one-time injection, with the avoidance of potential systemic complications of methotrexate. The use of laparoscopy has the obvious disadvantage of requiring laparoscopy, and the results to date have not been as good as with intramuscular administration of methotrexate. Because the success rate for this method is not equivalent to intramuscular methotrexate, this form of treatment cannot be recommended until further studies are undertaken. Other agents used have included potassium chloride, prostaglandins, and hyperosmolar glucose [55–68].

Graczykowski and Mishell [68] reported a group of 116 women who were randomized to receive a single dose of methotrexate (n = 54) or to function as control group (n = 62). Persistence was defined as a rise in the serum hCG level or a decline of less than 20% between two consecutive measurements taken three days apart. One woman in the prophylactic group (1.9%) and nine in the control group (14.5%) had persistence. Although this difference is significant, if one treats all laparoscopic salpingostomies with methotrexate, one would be treating 85% of patients who would otherwise not require the treatment for the benefit of the 15%. Whether this is the correct approach remains controversial.

Methotrexate Versus Laparoscopic Salpingostomy

Hajenius et al. [69••] recently reported a randomized trial in which 51 patients were treated with methotrexate and 49 underwent laparoscopic salpingostomy. Of the 51 patients, 46 (90.2%) were successfully treated. Of the 49 patients allocated to laparoscopic salpingostomy, 35 (72%) were treated by laparoscopy alone, and 10 (20%) needed methotrexate.

Single-dose Methotrexate Protocol*

Day	Therapy
0	hCG, D&C, CBC, SGOT, BUN, creatinine, blood type +Rh
1	MTX, hCG
4	hCG
7	hCG

*If there is no decline in the hCG titer between days 4 and 7, give a second dose of MTX 50 mg/m² on day 7. If ≥ 15% decline in hCG titer between days 4 and 7, follow weekly until hCG < 10 mlU/mL. If < 15% decline, repeat 50 mg/m² dose on day 7. In those patients not requiring D&C (hCG > 2000 mlU/mL) before treatment initiation, day 0 and day 1 were combined. Endometrial curettage done only on patients with an hCG titer < 2000 mlU/mL at the time of treatment initiation.

Figure 4-4. Single-dose methotrexate protocol. BUN—blood urea nitrogen; CBC—complete blood count; D&C—dilation and curettage; hCG—human chorionic gonadotropin; SGOT—serum glutamine oxalacetic transaminase, U/L.

In all, the tube was preserved in 90% of the patients treated with methotrexate and 92% of the patients treated surgically. In follow-up, tubal patency was documented in 55% and 59% of the patients treated with methotrexate or surgery, respectively. The authors concluded that the two treatment methods were similar with respect to treatment outcome and both represent viable alternatives to therapy. This study confirms yet again that methotrexate represents an alternative to surgery in those patients who meet the selection criteria. Methotrexate should be seen as a complementary form of treatment rather than a replacement for surgical management.

Summary

Salpingostomy or salpingectomy performed by laparoscopy or laparotomy is the mainstay of treatment for ectopic pregnancy when medical therapy is not indicated. However, in those patients meeting the criteria for methotrexate treatment, medical management offers specific advantages and should be considered as the treatment of choice when the appropriate criteria are met. In patients undergoing laparoscopic salpingostomy, the use of methotrexate prophylaxis should be considered.

References

Papers of particular interest have been highlighted as follows:
• Of interest
•• Of outstanding interest

1. Ectopic Pregnancy: United States, 1990-1992. Centers for Disease Control, Current Trends. *MMWR Morbid Mortal Weekly* 1995, 44:46–48.

2. Westrom L, Bengtsson LPH, Mardh PA: Incidence, trends, and risks of ectopic pregnancy in a population of women. *BMJ* 1981, 282:15.

3. DeStefano F, Peterson HB, Layde PM, Rubin GL: Risk of ectopic pregnancy following tubal sterilization. *Obstet Gynecol* 1982, 60:326.

4. Stovall TG, Ling FW, Carson SA, Buster JE: Nonsurgical diagnosis and treatment of tubal pregnancy. *Fertil Steril* 1990, 54:537–538.

5.• Stovall TG, Ling FW: Ectopic pregnancy: diagnostic and therapeutic algorithms minimizing surgical intervention. *J Reprod Med* 1993, 38:807–812.
The study outlines the protocol for the nonsurgical diagnosis of ectopic gestation using a combination of diagnostic modalities.

6. Maccato ML, Estrada R, Faro S: Ectopic pregnancy with undetectable serum and urine beta hCG levels and detection of beta hCG in the ectopic trophoblast by immunocytochemical evaluation. *Obstet Gynecol* 1993, 81:878.

7. Lonky NM, Sauer MV: Ectopic pregnancy with shock and undetectable beta human chorionic gonadotropin: a case report. *J Reprod Med* 1987, 32:559.

8. Uribe MA, Dunn RC, Buttram VC: Tubal pregnancy with normal hysterosalpingogram and negative serum pregnancy test. *Obstet Gynecol* 1990, 75:483.

9. Fritz MA: Doubling time of human chorionic gonadotropin (hCG) in early normal pregnancy: relationship to hCG concentration and gestational age. *Fertil Steril* 1987, 47:584–589 .

10. Kadar N, Freedman M, Zacher M: Further observation on the doubling time of human chorionic gonadotropin in early asymptomatic pregnancy. *Fertil Steril* 1980, 54:783–787.

11. Kadar N, Caldwell BV, Romero R: A method of screening for ectopic pregnancy and its indications. *Obstet Gynecol* 1981, 58:162–166.

12. Yeko TR, Gorrill JM, Hughes LH, et al.: Timely diagnosis of ectopic pregnancy using a single blood progesterone measurement. *Fertil Steril* 1987, 48:1049.

13. Matthews CP, Coulson PB, Wild RA: Serum progesterone levels as an aid in the diagnosis of ectopic pregnancy. *Obstet Gynecol* 1986, 68:390.

14. Stovall TG, Ling FW, Cope BJ, Buster JE: Preventing ruptured ectopic pregnancy with a single serum progesterone. *Am J Obstet Gynecol* 1989, 160:1425–1431.

15. Stovall TG, Kellermann AL, Ling FW, Buster JE: Emergency department diagnosis of ectopic pregnancy. *Ann Emerg Med* 1990, 19:1098–1103.

16. Stovall TG, Ling FW, Carson SA, Buster JE: Serum progesterone and uterine curettage in the differential diagnosis of ectopic pregnancy. *Fertil Steril* 1992, 57:456–458.

17. Emerson DS, Cartier MS, Alter LA, et al.: Diagnostic efficacy of endovaginal color Doppler through imaging in an ectopic pregnancy screening program. *Radiology* 1992, 183:413.

18. Vermesh M, Graczyhowski JW, Sauer MV: Re-evaluation of the role of culdocentesis in the management of ectopic pregnancy. *Am J Obstet Gynecol* 1990, 162:411.

19.• Vermesh M, Silva PD, Rosen GF, et al.: Management of unruptured ectopic gestation by linear salpingostomy: a prospective, randomized clinical trial of laparoscopy versus laparotomy. *Obstet Gynecol* 1989, 73:400–404.
This is one of several studies to compare in a randomized format patients undergoing surgery for the treatment of tubal ectopic pregnancy.

20. Brumsted J, Kessler C, Gibson C, et al.: A comparison of laparoscopy and laparotomy for the treatment of ectopic pregnancy. *Obstet Gynecol* 1988, 71:889–892.

21. Murphy AA, Nager CW, Wujek JJ, et al.: Operative laparoscopy versus laparotomy for the management of ectopic pregnancy: a prospective trial. *Fertil Steril* 1992, 57:1180–1185.

22. Sultana CJ, Easley K, Collins RL: Outcome of laparoscopic versus traditional surgery for ectopic pregnancies. *Fertil Steril* 1992, 57:285–289.

23. Seifer DB, Gutmann JN, Grant MD, et al.: Comparison of persistent ectopic pregnancy after laparoscopic salpingostomy versus salpingostomy at laparotomy for ectopic pregnancy. *Obstet Gynecol* 1993, 81:378–382.

24. Lundorff P, Hahlin M, Kalifelt B, et al.: Adhesion formation after laparoscopic surgery in tubal pregnancy: a randomized trial versus laparotomy. *Fertil Steril* 1991, 55:911–915.

25. Hreshchyshyn MM, Naples JD Jr, Randle CL: Amethopterin in abdominal pregnancy. *Am J Obstet Gynecol* 1965, 93:286.

26. Latrop JC, Bowles GE: Methotrexate in abdominal pregnancy: report of a case. *Obstet Gynecol* 1968, 32:81.

27. St. Clair JT, Whealer DA: Methotrexate in abdominal pregnancy. *JAMA* 1969, 21:529.

28. Tanaka T, Hayaski H, Kutsuzawa T, *et al.*: Treatment of interstitial ectopic pregnancy with methotrexate: report of a successful case. *Fertil Steril* 1982, 37:851.

29. Farabow WS, Fulton JW, Fletcher V Jr, *et al.*: Cervical pregnancy treated with methotrexate. *N C Med J* 1983, 44:910.

30. Chotiner JC: Nonsurgical management of ectopic pregnancy associated with severe hyperstimulation syndrome. *Obstet Gynecol* 1985, 66:740.

31. Brandes MC, Youngs DD, Goldstein DP, Parmby TH: Treatment of cornual pregnancy with methotrexate: case report. *Am J Obstet Gynecol* 1986, 1551:655.

32. Higgins KA, Schwartz MB: Treatment of persistent trophoblastic tissue after salpingostomy with methotrexate. *Fertil Steril* 1986, 45:427.

33. Cowan BD, McGehee RP, Gates GH: Treatment of persistent ectopic pregnancy with methotrexate and leucovorin rescue: a case report. *Obstet Gynecol* 1986, 67:50S.

34. Miyazaki Y: Nonsurgical therapy of ectopic pregnancy. *Hokkaido Igaku Zasshi* 1983, 58:132.

35. Ory SJ, Villanueva AL, Sand PK, Tamura RK: Conservative treatment of ectopic pregnancy with methotrexate. *Am J Obstet Gynecol* 1986, 154:1299.

36. Stovall TG, Ling FW, Buster JE: Outpatient chemotherapy of unruptured ectopic pregnancy. *Fertil Steril* 1989, 51:435.

37. Stovall TG, Ling FW, Gray LA, *et al.*: Methotrexate treatment of unruptured ectopic pregnancy: a report of 100 cases. *Obstet Gynecol* 1991, 77:749.

38. Stovall TG, Ling FW, Gray LA: Single dose methotrexate for ectopic pregnancy. *Obstet Gynecol* 1991, 77:754.

39. Stovall TG, Ling FW: Single dose methotrexate: an expanded clinical trial. *Am J Obstet Gynecol* 1993, 168:1759–1762.

40.• Lipscomb GH, Bran D, McCord ML, *et al.*: Analysis of three hundred fifteen ectopic pregnancies treated with single-dose methotrexate. *Am J Obstet Gynecol* 1998, 178:1354-1358.

The study represents the most recent experience with a large group of patients undergoing medical therapy with single-dose methotrexate for the treatment of ectopic gestation.

41. Ransom MX, Garcia AJ, Bohrer M, *et al.*: Serum progesterone as a predictor of methotrexate success in the treatment of ectopic pregnancy. *Obstet Gynecol* 1994, 83:1033–1037.

42. Henry MA, Gentry WL: Single injection of methotrexate for treatment of ectopic pregnancies. *Am J Obstet Gynecol* 1994, 171:1584–1587.

43. Stovall TG, Ling FW, Buster JE: Reproductive performance after methotrexate treatment of ectopic pregnancy. *Am J Obstet Gynecol* 1990, 162:1620.

44. Menard A, Cruquat J, Mandelbrot L, *et al.*: Treatment of unruptured tubal pregnancy by local injection of methotrexate under transvaginal sonographic control. *Fertil Steril* 1990, 54:47–50.

45. Feichtinger W, Kemetre P: Conservative treatment of ectopic pregnancy by transvaginal aspiration under sonographic control and methotrexate injection. *Lancet* 1987, i:381.

46. Leeton J, Davison G: Nonsurgical management of unruptured tubal pregnancy with intra-amniotic methotrexate; preliminary report of two cases. *Fertil Steril* 1988, 50:167.

47. Robertson De, Moye MA, Hansen JH, *et al.*: Reduction of ectopic pregnancy by injection under ultrasound control. *Lancet* 1987, 1:974–975.

48. Tulandi T, Bret PM, Atri M, Senterman M: Treatment of ectopic pregnancy by transvaginal intratubal methotrexate administration. *Obstet Gynecol* 1991, 77:627–630.

49. Clark LC, Raymond S. Stanger J, Jackel G: Treatment of ectopic pregnancy with intraamniotic methotrexate: a case report. *Aust N Z J Obstet Gynaecol* 1989, 29:84–85.

50. Timor-Tritsch IE, Montequdo A, Matera C, Veit CR: Sonographic evolution of cornual pregnancies treated without surgery. *Obstet Gyencol* 1992, 79:1044–1049.

51. Mottla GL, Rulin MC, Guzick DS: Lack of resolution of ectopic pregnancy by intratubal injection of methotrexate. *Fertil Steril* 1992, 57:685–687.

52. Porreco RP: Percutaneous, ultrasound-directed ablation of ectopic pregnancy with methotrexate: a report of three cases. *J Reprod Med* 1992, 37:363–366.

53. Zilber U, Pansky M, Bukovsky I, Golan A: Laparoscopic salpingostomy versus laparoscopic local methotrexate injection in the management of unruptured ectopic gestation. *Am J Obstet Gynecol* 1996, 175:600–602.

54. Tulandi T, Atri M, Bret P, Falcone T, *et al.*: Transvaginal intratubal methotrexate treatment of ectopic pregnancy. *Fertil Steril* 1992, 58:98–100.

55. Ribic Paucel JM, Novak-Antolic Z, Urhovec I: Treatment of ectopic pregnancy with prostaglandin E2. *Clin Exp Obstet Gynecol* 1989, 16:106–109.

56. Lindblom B, Lakklfelt B, Hahlin M, Hamberger L: Local prostaglandin F2 injection for termination of ectopic pregnancy. *Lancet* 1987, 1:776.

57. Egarter C, Husslein P: Treatment of tubal pregnancy by prostaglandins. *Lancet* 1988, 1:1104–1105.

58. Egarter C, Fitz R, Spona J, *et al.*: Treatment of tubal pregnancy with prostaglandins: a multicenter study. *Geburstshilfe Fauenheilkd* 1989, 49:808–812.

59. Vetorp M, Vejerslev LO, Ruge S: Local prostaglandin treatment of ectopic pregnancy. *Hum Reprod* 1989, 4:464–467.

60. Lang P, Weiss PAM, Mayer HO: Local application of hyperosmolar glucose solution in tubal pregnancy. *Lancet* 1989, 2:922–923.

61. Feichtinger W, Kemeter P: Treatment of unruptured ectopic pregnancy by needling of sac and injection of methotrexate or PGE$_2$ under transvaginal sonography control. *Arch Gynecol Obstet* 1989, 246:85–89.

62. Shalev E, Megory E, Romano S, Weiner E, *et al.*: Interstitial pregnancy: successful treatment with methotrexate. *Isr J Med Sci* 1989, 25:239–240.

63. Bengtsson G, Bryman I, Thorburn J, Lindblom B: Low dose oral methotrexate as second line therapy for persistent trophoblast after conservative treatment of ectopic pregnancy. *Obstet Gynecol* 1992, 79:589–591.

64. Yeko TR, Mayer JC, Parsons AK, Maroulis GB: A prospective series of unruptured ectopic pregnancies treated by tubal injection with hyperosmolar glucose. *Obstet Gynecol* 1995, 85:265–268.

65. Paulson G, Kuint S, Labecker B, *et al.*: Laparoscopic prostaglandin injection in ectopic pregnancy: success rate according to endocrine activity. *Fertil Steril* 1995, 63:473–477.

66. Laatikainen T, Tuomiuaara L, Käär K: Comparison of a local injection of hyperosmolar glucose solution with salpingostomy for the conservative treatment of tubal pregnancy. *Fertil Steril* 1993, 60:80–84.

67. Pansky M, Bukovsky J, Olin A, *et al.*: Reproductive outcome after laparoscopic local methotrexate injection for tubal pregnancy. *Fertil Steril* 1993, 60:85–87.

68. Graczykowski JW, Mishell DR: Methotrexate prophylaxis for persistent ectopic pregnancy after conservative treatment by salpingostomy. *Obstet Gynecol* 1997, 99:118–122.

69.•• Hajenius PJ, Engelsbel S, Mol BWJ, *et al.*: Randomised trial of systemic methotrexate versus laparoscopic salpingostomy in tubal pregnancy. *Lancet* 1997, 350:774.
This is the first randomized trial to compare laparoscopic surgery versus medical therapy. One hundred patients were randomly assigned to laparoscopic salpingostomy or methotrexate. The treatment outcomes in the two groups were similar.

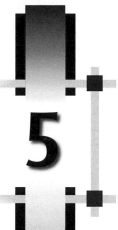

Abortion and Miscarriage

5

Kamini Geer and Marji Gold

- Early abortion care can be provided by primary care clinicians in the primary care setting. Medical abortion with mifepristone/misoprostol is an excellent treatment for primary care physicians to offer their patients.
- In early abortion, a woman's preference is the most important factor in determining the type of abortion.
- Cervical dilation is critical for safe and facile uterine evacuation procedures in the first and second trimesters and can be obtained by mechanical or osmotic methods.
- Ultrasound is an important diagnostic tool in assessing location and viability of pregnancy, as well as a useful adjunct during difficult uterine evacuation procedures. Indications for the use of ultrasound are determined by clinical assessment of the pregnant woman.

Abortion is part of the full spectrum of reproductive health care for women. Forty-nine percent of all pregnancies in the United States are unintended. Of these, 26.5% end in an abortion [1]. Physicians should never assume that a pregnant woman wanted to become pregnant or that she wants to remain pregnant. The patient should be approached nonjudgmentally and presented with all her options, including continuing the pregnancy and keeping the baby, continuing the pregnancy and placing the baby for adoption, and abortion.

Access to medical and procedural methods of abortion increases women's options. Many of the techniques that are used in medical and procedural abortion can be applied to the management of spontaneous pregnancy loss.

This chapter reviews the assessment of embryonic or fetal viability, the techniques used for uterine evacuation in first and second trimester pregnancies, the management of nonviable pregnancies, and the management of complications resulting from uterine evacuation procedures.

First Trimester Abortion

PREGNANCY DIAGNOSIS AND ASSESSMENT

Women usually present to their clinician's office when they are concerned about a missed or abnormal menstrual period. Many women begin to experience symptoms of pregnancy at or shortly after the time of the missed menses. These may include, but are not limited to, nausea, breast tenderness, food intolerance, mild alopecia, vaginal spotting, or abdominal discomfort or pain. When a woman of reproductive age presents with symptoms of pregnancy or missed menses, a qualitative urine human chorionic gonadotropin (hCG) assay should be obtained. Pregnancy, regardless of location or viability, will cause an increase in hCG levels. If the hCG is positive, the patient is assumed to be pregnant, although the location or future viability of the gestation cannot yet be determined [2].

Ultrasound is recommended in the first trimester for specific indications [3]. The clinician should assess the patient and her clinical findings to determine if an ultrasound is necessary. The following are reasons to consider obtaining an ultrasound: uncertain last menstrual period, use of hormonal birth control at the time of conception, abdominal pain, vaginal bleeding, history of prior ectopic pregnancy, size/dates discrepancy on bimanual examination, and pelvic examination in which an adnexal mass is found. If a sonogram is performed, the fetal location, the presence of a fetal heart rate, number of fetuses, placental locations or abnormalities (eg, hematoma), and significant maternal structural findings, such as ovarian cysts or uterine fibroids should be documented.

The majority of abortions in the United States occur in the first trimester, with 87% occurring before the 13th week [4•]. There are two methods for first trimester abortions available to patients in the United States: medical and aspiration. Abortion can be provided as soon as the woman has a positive pregnancy test. Medical abortions can be performed up to 9 weeks' gestational age. Aspiration abortions are generally performed up to 12 to 13 weeks. These are very different options, and patients should be presented with the details of each so that they can make an informed choice.

Physicians performing any abortion should obtain a comprehensive history from all patients to identify any potential risks or problems. Pre-abortion counseling, including a thorough review of the risks of the abortion, is then provided. A targeted physical examination is performed before the procedure, and information concerning the patient's hematocrit and Rh status is obtained; other tests may be warranted according to the individual patient's past medical or surgical history. All women undergoing an abortion have to sign a document, such as a patient agreement, for medical abortion, or an informed consent document for procedural abortions, indicating that they elect to have the abortion.

Medical Abortion

In 2000, the US Food and Drug Administration (FDA) approved mifepristone (formerly RU-486) for commercial use, marketed under the brand name Mifeprex (Danco Laboratories, New York, NY). Mifepristone inhibits the activity of endogenous or exogenous progesterone by competitive interaction with progesterone at progesterone-receptor sites. Since 2000, medical abortions have been offered in the United States to patients in their primary care physician's office and at dedicated abortion clinics [5•]. Contraindications to the use of mifepristone are listed in Figure 5-1 [6].

The FDA approved medical abortions with mifepristone for pregnancies less than 50 days' gestation. The FDA regimen is 600 mg of oral mifepristone followed 2 days later by 400 μg of oral misoprostol. Data from multiple studies have demonstrated that different regimens are up to 99.5% effective [5•,7–12]. Most medical abortions in the United States are provided using alternate protocols. These alternate protocols use a lower dose (200 mg) of oral mifepristone, followed in 6 to 48 hours by a vaginal or buccal dose of 800 μg of misoprostol, self-administered by the woman at home. The buccal route has been shown effective for pregnancies less than 57 days' gestation [13•], and the vaginal route is effective for pregnancies of 63 days or less.

The use of ultrasound is optional in medical abortion. The FDA and the National Abortion Federation guidelines state that the physician must determine gestational age and rule out ectopic pregnancy. An ultrasound-as-needed protocol, accompanied by sequential serial hCG monitoring, has been shown to be as efficacious and as safe as protocols that involve the utilization of routine ultrasound before and after the medical abortion. Figure 5-2 lists the indications for sonography in the ultrasound-as-needed protocol [14•].

Many women choose medical abortion because it offers them more control and privacy, it feels more natural, safer, and less invasive than an aspiration procedure, and it allows them to avoid the instrumentation and anesthesia associated with suction abortions [15••,16••]. The most important aspect of medical abortion care is the counseling given to patients about the timing and use of the misoprostol. The process for medical abortion with mifepristone/misoprostol includes an initial office visit, self-administration of the misoprostol at home, and a follow-up visit to confirm the success of the treatment. After the woman swallows the mifepristone in her physician's office, she can continue her regular activities. Most women have no effects from this medication, although some patients will have minimal vaginal bleeding. Six to 48 hours later, depending on the exact regimen the patient is using, she will self-administer 800 μg of misoprostol at home [12,13•]. Two to 6 hours after using misoprostol, most women will begin to experience uterine cramping and bleeding; she can use high-dose ibuprofen or a mild narcotic to alleviate the cramping and should receive prescriptions for these medications at the initial visit [17]. Most women will experience the heaviest uterine bleeding within the first 24 hours after using

Contraindications to the Use of Mifepristone

Confirmed or suspected ectopic pregnancy

Intrauterine device in place

Chronic adrenal failure

Concurrent long-term corticosteroid therapy

History of allergy to mifepristone, misoprostol, or other prostaglandins

Hemorrhagic disorders

Concurrent anticoagulant therapy

Inherited porphyria

Figure 5-1. Contraindications to the use of mifepristone.

Indications for Sonography for Medical Abortion

Pre-abortion

  Uterine size discrepant with gestational age

  Uncertain date of last menstrual period

  Amenorrhea postpartum, postabortion, or after discontinuing depomedroxyprogesterone acetate

  Adnexal mass or pain

  Provider uncertainty with uterine size by pelvic examination

  History of previous ectopic pregnancy

Post-abortion

  History not consistent with successful medical abortion (no cramping, no bleeding)

  Woman still feels pregnant

  Serum human chorionic gonadotropin not declining

  Provider uncertainty with history

Figure 5-2. Indications for sonography for medical abortion.

misoprostol and the average duration of heavy bleeding is 3 to 5 hours. Patients should be informed that the bleeding during this initial few hours will be heavier than their usual period, and they may pass large clots. Patients should be reassured that they will not see fetal parts. The majority of women will continue to have some vaginal bleeding for an average of 16 days, although this is usually intermittent spotting to mild bleeding. To confirm the success of the medical abortion, two quantitative beta hCG levels are drawn, one at the time of the administration of the mifepristone, and another at 1 to 2 weeks after the use of the misoprostol. A decrease in this level of at least 50% demonstrates a successful completion of a medication abortion [18]. Fiala *et al.* [19•] have demonstrated that an hCG level after medical abortion that is no more than 20% of the original level has a positive predictive value of 0.995 for a successful abortion.

Some centers use a pre- and postmedical abortion ultrasound to document the completion of the medical abortion. At the time of the initial visit, Rh immune globulin should be administered if the patient is Rh negative. If the medical abortion is not successful, the patient should have a suction procedure. The ability to offer medical abortion in primary care clinics offers patients a safe and effective option to increase their access to reproductive health services [20•]. Many patients appreciate that this option is available at their primary care physician's office [21].

There are other medical abortion protocols besides the mifepristone/misoprostol regimens discussed above. One protocol involves the use of methotrexate and misoprostol, which is 84% effective at terminating pregnancies that are 49 days' gestational age or less [22,23]. Other regimens involve the use of misoprostol only. Several studies have demonstrated 90.8% to 93% effectiveness of repeated doses of intravaginal misoprostol in terminating pregnancies of less than 63 days' gestational age [24•,25,26]. The determination of which medical abortion protocol to use depends on the practitioner, the woman, and their resources.

COMPLICATIONS FROM MEDICAL ABORTION

The major risks from medical abortion are vaginal bleeding that lasts more than 4 weeks and continuing viable pregnancy. In the United States, only 0.5 out of 1000 women who received mifepristone/misoprostol for medication abortion needed a transfusion for severe blood loss [27]. The rate of continuing viable pregnancy is 0.5% to 1% [9,10–12,28•]. Suction curettage can be done in the primary care setting to treat prolonged bleeding and to complete the abortion [29••].

Four cases of fatal sepsis have been documented in women who have used mifepristone for medical abortion in the United States. Since 1 million women have used mifepristone/misoprostol for medical abortion, this represents a case fatality rate of 1.1 per 100,000, no higher than that associated with surgical abortion; the infectious agent was determined to be *Clostridium sordelli*. This is a rare human pathogen that has been associated with deaths after other obstetric events, such as childbirth [30,31]. There are many theories as to why these deaths occurred, but none have been proven. In order to reduce the possibility of *C. sordelli* sepsis, many providers of medical abortion have decided to recommend the buccal instead of the vaginal route for misoprostol [32].

Aspiration for Uterine Evacuation

SUCTION CURETTAGE

As of 2002, suction curettage was the most commonly used method of uterine evacuation in the United States, with up to 91% of abortions done through this method [33]. The procedure is usually performed between the gestational ages of 6 to 13 weeks. This procedure is usually provided in an ambulatory setting, except in high-risk cases, such as patients with a bleeding disorder.

Women should be counseled before the procedure on options for pain control that are available during suction curettage. These options include oral ibuprofen, paracervical block, conscious sedation, and general anesthesia. Higher levels of anesthesia require monitoring equipment and trained personnel. Each clinician should be aware of the types of abortion and anesthesia techniques offered in their own practice and/or in surrounding clinics, so that they can present all options to their patients, ensuring that their patients can make an informed choice.

For suction curettage, the endocervical canal is manually dilated using instrument sets that have progressively increasing diameters. The most commonly used are Pratt or Denniston dilators. After dilation of the endocervical canal has been achieved, a suction curette (without suction having been started) is inserted into the uterine cavity. Choice of suction curette size is dependent on gestational age. The diameter of the suction curette usually equals the gestational age (in weeks) of the pregnancy. For example, a number 8 suction curette (8-mm diameter) would be used to evacuate an 8-week pregnancy. Suction is then applied using a device that creates a vacuum; once applied, the curette is rotated on its axis with little motion along the longitudinal axis of insertion during tissue aspiration. This axis rotation of the curette reduces the likelihood of instrument perforation of the uterine fundus. When no further tissue can be aspirated, the curette is withdrawn. The vacuum can be created using either an electrical or hand-held device. The manual vacuum aspiration syringe is a small plastic instrument that allows the creation of suction without electricity. The manual vacuum aspiration syringe is usually used up to 10 weeks' gestational age [34•]. One of the benefits of manual vacuum aspiration is that it can be used safely and effectively in primary care offices and in low resource settings [35]. An electric vacuum aspiration machine also can be used. The device that is used to create the suction is dependent on the clinical setting and the practitioner.

The aspirated uterine contents are placed in a dish containing a small amount of sterile water or saline to examine them for pregnancy tissue. Absence of such may indicate incomplete abortion, ectopic pregnancy, or inaccurate dating of the pregnancy. Appropriate diagnostic measures, such as ultrasound and serial hCG levels, should be performed if there is inadequate tissue.

After the procedure, the patient is monitored for at least 30 minutes for hemorrhage or changes in vital signs. Women who are Rh negative and not sensitized receive Rh immune globulin after the abortion. Prophylactic antibiotics have been demonstrated to be effective in preventing infection, and doxycycline and its analogues are usually given to patients after the procedure [36].

Complications resulting from suction curettage can be categorized as being either immediate or delayed and are listed in Figure 5-3. Most complications should be preventable. Careful dilation can decrease the risk of cervical laceration. Examination of the tissue obtained by suction curettage can signal an unsuccessful uterine evacuation procedure resulting from an ectopic pregnancy or retained intrauterine contents. Failure to obtain chorionic villi necessitates an ultrasound examination. If an intrauterine pregnancy is visualized, ultrasonography should be used to guide the repeat procedure. Women with suspected ectopic pregnancies should be carefully monitored with serial hCG levels and ultrasound, with a low threshold for hospitalization. Although surgical interventions (eg, salpingectomy, salpingostomy) traditionally have been used to treat ectopic pregnancy, nonsurgical regimens using methotrexate are being used with success, moving the management of ectopic pregnancy to the outpatient setting [37].

Overall, suction curettage is a safer method for pregnancy termination than sharp curettage. Abortions performed using local anesthesia are safer than those done with general anesthesia. Abortions performed in ambulatory clinics and offices are safer than those performed in hospitals [38••]. In 2000, 93% of abortions were performed in free standing clinics. These clinics are at risk from antichoice protestors and violence [35]. The overall death rate from abortions has been less than 0.8 per 100,000 abortions since the 1980s [33]. To further put this in perspective, the risk of death from pregnancy is 11 times higher than the risk of death from an abortion [35]. However, women who have second trimester abortions have a risk of death that exponentially

increases 38% with each additional week of gestation beyond 8 weeks. This illustrates the importance of improving access to first trimester abortion [39•].

Second Trimester Abortion

Second trimester abortion can be performed in most states up to 24 weeks, but the gestational limit varies state by state.

EXTRACTION PROCEDURES

In the United States, dilatation and evacuation is the most common technique used for second trimester pregnancy termination and can be performed in an outpatient setting [40]. Second trimester extraction requires dilation of the cervix prior to performing the procedure. Although careful manual dilation can achieve sufficient cervical dilation to permit uterine evacuation in many cases, this technique carries a significantly increased risk of cervical laceration, hemorrhage, and unsuccessful uterine evacuation. The preferred technique employs synthetic cervical dilators that gradually expand within the endocervical canal [29••]. Synthetic dilators (eg, polyacrylonitrile [Dilapan; FEMA International, Kendall Park, NJ]; magnesium sulfate sponge [Lamicel; Cabot Medical Corp., Langhorne, PA]) or the laminaria seaweed dilator can be used. These osmotic tools dilate the endocervical canal by absorbing cervical moisture. This uptake in water and the resulting expansion of the dilator produce a softening of the cervix and dilation of the endocervical canal to two to three times the original diameter. The number of synthetic dilators used depends on the gestational age, with more dilators being used for larger gestational ages.

Products of conception are evacuated using instruments specifically designed to extract intrauterine contents at this stage of gestation. At 13 to 16 weeks, the products of conception can be removed with a 12 to 16 mm vacuum cannula, although some physicians prefer to use the ovum forceps and the vacuum cannula as an adjunct. At 17 weeks and above, forceps such as the Sopher (Figure 5-4), Bierer, and Hern ovum forceps are primarily used, with vacuum as an adjunct [29••].

Complications of Suction Curettage

Immediate complications

 Hemorrhage

 Uterine perforation

 Cervical laceration

 Uterine atony

 Postoperative pain and hematometra

 Broad ligament hematoma

Delayed complications

 Fever and infection

 Hemorrhage

 Retained products of conception

 Hematometra and postabortal syndrome

 Broad ligament hematoma

Figure 5-3. Complications of suction curettage.

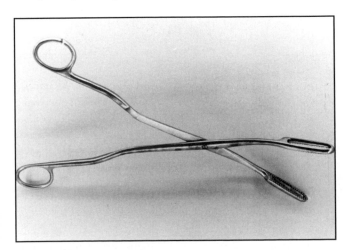

Figure 5-4. Ovum forceps.

Concurrent ultrasonography also is helpful in facilitating uterine evacuation. Although ultrasound guidance is not essential for safe and successful uterine evacuation, it often facilitates the evacuation procedure, particularly in problematic cases, such as patients with severe uterine anteversion or anteflexion or uterine fibroids.

Labor induction is another method of second trimester abortion. Medications that induce labor include hypertonic saline, systemic prostaglandins, misoprostol, mifepristone and prostaglandins, high dose oxytocin, and feticidal agents such as intra-amniotic or fetal intracardiac injections of digoxin [29••].

Selective reduction involves the intracardiac injection of potassium chloride to decrease the number of fetuses in a multiple gestation pregnancy. This increases the survival of the remaining fetuses and can also be done in the case of a single anomalous fetus in a multiple gestation. This technique has become more common as more fertility agents are utilized [41].

The choice of technique for second trimester uterine evacuation should rely on the indication for uterine evacuation, availability of skilled personnel, and advantages of extraction (eg, outpatient procedure, less expensive to perform) compared with other second trimester uterine evacuation techniques.

The psychological benefits of a rapid outpatient method have also been documented. Second trimester extraction requires less time to complete than labor induction methods [42], although this difference may be less in cases of fetal demise. Kaltreider et al. [43] reported that 30 patients undergoing second trimester extraction experienced less postoperative pain, anger, and depression than 20 women undergoing labor induction methods. Other authors have documented similar findings in patients [44,45•].

COMPLICATIONS OF SECOND TRIMESTER ABORTION

Complications of second trimester abortion procedures are listed in Figure 5-5. The major complication is hemorrhage resulting from uterine perforation. Although osmotic dilation of the cervix, concurrent ultrasound, inspection of the products of conception, and postoperative administration of antibiotics and methylergonovine reduce the incidence of complications, some invariably occur. Physicians must be prepared to administer resuscitation maneuvers necessary for stabilizing such patients and to manage any complications. Physicians also should be prepared to perform laparotomy in the case of bowel injury. In addition, the risk for disseminated intravascular coagulation, although rare, is higher in second trimester procedures than in first trimester abortions [29••].

Physicians who elect to use labor induction methods (eg, intra-amniotic or intravaginal prostaglandin) after detection of fetal demise or for other pregnancy termination indications must be able to provide sharp and suction curettage or manual uterine evacuation using ovum forceps. Retained placenta or other products of conception occur relatively commonly after labor induction methods and prostaglandin abortions. Inability to complete the uterine evacuation in a timely fashion could result in serious complications resulting from hemorrhage or infection [29••].

When performed by an experienced clinician, second trimester dilatation and evacuation carries significantly lower morbidity and mortality rates than those methods requiring labor induction. For example, at 16 to 20 weeks, the mortality for dilatation and evacuation is 6.5 per 100,000, compared with induction, which is 7.9 per 100,000 [46]. Because of these safety concerns, uterine induction accounted for less than 0.8% of abortions performed in the United States as of 2002 [33].

As indicated above, the mortality associated with abortion increases with increasing gestational age. For example, at or before 8 weeks, there are 0.1 deaths per 100,000 legal induced abortions. At 16 to 20 weeks, this increases to 3.4 deaths per 100,000 legal abortions, and at 21 weeks or more, there are 8.9 deaths per 100,000 legal abortions [39]. The pregnancy-related mortality rate is 11.8 per 100,000 live births, indicating that all second trimester abortions have a lower risk of mortality than childbirth [47].

Spontaneous Pregnancy Loss

FIRST TRIMESTER

The most common symptom of miscarriage in the first trimester is vaginal bleeding. Women who present with this complaint should be evaluated by ultrasound for a viable intrauterine pregnancy. Fetal cardiac activity generally can be detected by endovaginal ultrasound in most 6- to 7-week gestations. If no fetal heart activity is detected, consideration of waiting 7 to 10 days may be warranted, especially if the predicted gestational age is less than the actual fetal or embryonic size and especially if it is a desired pregnancy. If fetal viability is not confirmed, a discussion with the patient concerning her options should be undertaken. Clinicians should be aware that spontaneous miscarriage

Complications of Second Trimester Evacuation Procedures

All techniques
  Retained products of conception
  Infection
  Hemorrhage
  Uterine atony
  Cervical laceration
  Disseminated intravascular coagulation
Dilation and evacuation
  Uterine or cervical perforation
  Labor induction
  Incomplete abortion
  Bowel injury

Figure 5-5. Complications of second trimester evacuation procedures.

is a loss for the woman and her partner, and thus should demonstrate appropriate behavior, empathy, and respect with patients and their families at all times. Women who are clinically stable do not require immediate evacuation of the uterus and can be given the choice of three options. Expectant management allows her to wait for the pregnancy to be expelled on its own. Medical management utilizes misoprostol in doses similar to the treatment for induced abortion. Pain medications, such as ibuprofen and hydrocodone, are given to women who choose expectant or medical management. A third option is aspiration, which can be done easily in the primary care office, using the hand-held syringe [48•,49•].

FETAL DEMISE: SECOND AND THIRD TRIMESTERS

Detection of fetal demise in the second or third trimester is usually heralded by perceived changes in fetal movement. In such cases ultrasonography is the standard to assess fetal viability and should include a full survey of the fetus, placenta, and maternal pelvic organs [50].

In cases of fetal loss, determination of the specific uterine evacuation procedure should be based on the gestational size of the fetus as well as the technical experience of the clinician. Induction techniques are reserved for almost all fetal demise at or after 24 weeks. Dilation and evacuation has the lowest mortality rate of all second trimester uterine evacuation procedures for fetal demise and comparable morbidity to other second trimester techniques [51]. Second trimester extraction procedures can be performed in an ambulatory setting, unlike labor induction methods; accordingly, extraction procedures are less expensive to perform than labor induction techniques [52].

Conclusion

There are several abortion methods available to patients depending on the gestational age. The critical part of the process is providing empathetic and complete counseling so that the women can make truly informed decisions about pregnancy management. Early abortion care and miscarriage management can be provided by trained primary care clinicians in the primary care setting.

References

Papers of particular interest have been highlighted as follows:
• Of interest
•• Of outstanding interest

1. Henshaw SK: Unintended pregnancy in the United States. *Fam Plan Prespect* 1998, 30:24–29.

2. Mishell DR Jr: Spontaneous and recurrent abortion: etiology, diagnosis and treatment. In *Comprehensive Gynecology*. Edited by Mishell DR Jr, Stenchever MA, Droegemueller W, *et al.* St Louis: CV Mosby; 1997.

3. COG Practice Bulletin: Ultrasonagraphy in Pregnancy. *Obstet Gynecol* 2004, 104:1449–1458.

4.• Strauss LT, Herndon J, Chang J: Abortion Surveillance United States 2002. *MMWR Morbid Mortal Wkly Rep.* CDC Surveillance Summaries 2005, 54:1–37.
MMWR outlining pregnancy and abortion demographics and trends in 2002.

5.• Fiala C, Gemzell-Danielsson K: Review of medical abortion using mifepristone in combination with a prostaglandin analogue. *Contraception* 2006, 74:66–86.
A review of the medication, abortion demographics, and techniques.

6. Davey A: Mifepristone and prostaglandin for termination of pregnancy: contraindications for use, reasons and rationale. *Contraception* 2006, 74:16–20.

7. Marions L: Mifepristone dose in the regimen with misoprostol for medical abortion. *Contraception* 2006, 74:21–25.

8. Spitz IM, Bardin CW, Benton L, *et al.*: Early pregnancy termination with mifepristone and misoprostol in the United States. *N Engl J Med* 1998, 338:1241–1247.

9. Ashok PW, Penney GC, Flett GM, *et al.*: An effective regimen for early medical abortion: a report of 2000 consecutive cases. *Hum Reprod* 1998, 13:2962–2965.

10. Schaff EA, Eisinger SH, Stadalius LS, *et al.*: Low-dose mifepristone 200 mg and vaginal misoprostol for abortion. *Contraception* 1999, 59:1–6.

11. Schaff EA, Fielding SL, Westhoff C, *et al.*: Vaginal misoprostol administered 1, 2, or 3 days after mifepristone for early medical abortion: a randomized trial. *JAMA* 2000, 284:1948–1953.

12. Creinin MD, Fox MC, Teal S, *et al.*: A randomized comparison of misoprostol 6 to 8 hours versus 24 hours after mifepristone for abortion. *Obstet Gynecol* 2004, 103:850–859.

13.• Middleton T, Schaff E, Fielding SL, *et al.*: Randomized trial of mifepristone and buccal or vaginal misoprostol for abortion through 56 days last menstrual period. *Contraception* 2005, 72:328–332.
This article demonstrated that medication abortion could be done as early as 56 days through last menstrual period.

14.• Clark W, Panton T, Hann L, *et al.*: Medication abortion employing routine sequential measurements of hCG and sonography only when indicated. *Contraception* 2007, 75:131–135.
This article demonstrated that the feasibility and safety of the ultrasound as a needed protocol.

15.•• Winikoff B: Acceptability of medical abortion in early pregnancy. *Fam Plan Prespect* 1995, 185:142–148.
This article demonstrated that women found medication abortion to be an acceptable option.

16.•• Fielding SL, Edmunds E, Shcaff EA: Having an abortion using mifepristone and home misoprostol: a qualitative analysis of women's experiences. *Perspect Sex Reprod Health* 2002, 34:34–40.
A qualitative study that provided data on why women would choose a medication abortion.

17. Penney G: Treatment of pain during medical abortion. *Contraception* 2006, 74:45–47.

18. Schaff E, Walker K, Fielding S, *et al.*: Monitoring serum chorionic gonadotropin levels after mifepristone abortion. *Contraception* 2001, 64:271–273.

19.• Fiala C, Safar P, Bygdeman M, *et al.*: Verifying the effectiveness of medical abortion: ultrasound versus hCG testing. *Europe J Obstet Gynecol Reprod Biol* 2003, 109:190–195.
This article demonstrated the hCG level percentage decrease that assures the clinician of 99.5% certainty that the medication abortion is complete.

20.• Prine L, Lesnewski R, Gold M: Medical abortion in family practice: a case series. *J Am Board Fam Pract* 2003, 16:290–295.
This article demonstrated that family medicine physicians who provide abortions increases access and options for women.

21. Rubin SE, Godfrey EM, Gold M: Abstract: Integration of early abortion into primary care: an acceptability survey of female patients. *Contraception* 2006, 74:189–190.

22. Borgotta L, Burnhill MS, Tyson J, *et al.*: Early medical abortion with methotrexate and misoprostol. *Obstet Gynecol* 2001, 97:11–16.

23. Crenin MD, Potter C, Holovanisin M, *et al.*: Mifepristone and misoprostol and methotrexate/misoporstol in clinical practice for abortion. *Am J Obstet Gynecol* 2003, 188:664–669.

24.• Borgotta L, Mullaly B, Vragovic, *et al.*: Misoprostol as the primary agent for medical abortion in a low income urban setting. *Contraception* 2004, 70:121–126.
This article demonstrated that misoprostol could be used alone for medication abortion.

25. Carbonell JL, Rodriguez J, Aragon S, *et al.*: Vaginal misoprostol 1000 micrograms for early abortion. *Contraception* 2001, 63:131–136.

26. Singh K, Fong YF, Dong F: A viable alternative to surgical vacuum aspiration: repeated doses of intravaginal misoprostol over 9 hour for medical termination of pregnancies up to 8 weeks. *Br J Obstet Gynecol* 2003, 110:175–180.

27. Henderson JT, Hwang AC, Harper CC: Safety of mifepristone abortion in clinical use. *Contraception* 2005, 72:175–178.

28.• Spitz IM, Bardin CW, Benton L, *et al.*: Early pregnancy termination with mifepristone and misoprostol in the United States. *N Engl J Med* 1998, 338:1241–1247.
This article demonstrated the effectiveness of medication abortion.

29.•• Stubblefield PG, Carr-Ellis S, Borgotta L: Methods for induced abortion. *J Obstet Gynecol* 2004, 104: 174–185.
This article is a good review of the abortion methods that are available in the United States.

30. US FDA Public Health Advisory: Sepsis and Medical Abortion. Available at: http://www.fda.gov/cder/drug/advisory/mifeprex.htm.

31. Fischer M, Bhatnagar J, Guarner J: Fatal toxic shock syndrome associated with *Clostridium sordellii* after medical abortion. *N Engl J Med* 2005, 353:2352–2360.

32. Winikoff B: *Clostridium sordelli* infection in medical abortion. *Clin Infect Dis* 2006, 43.

33. Strauss LT, Herndon J, Chang, J: Abortion surveillance United States 2002. *MMWR Morbid Mort Wkly Rep* 2005, 54:1–37.

34.• Lichtenberg ES, Paul M, Jones H: First trimester surgical abortion practices: a survey of National Abortion Federation members. *Contraception* 2001, 64:345–352.
This article is a survey of the mehtods used by abortion providers who are members of the National Abortion Federation.

35. Harper CC, Henderson JT, Darney PD: Abortion the in the United States. *Ann Rev Public Health* 2005, 26: 501–512.

36. Sawaya GF, Grady D, Kerlikowske K, *et al.*: Antibiotics at the time of induced abortion: the case for universal prophylaxis based on a meta-analysis. *Obstet Gynecol* 1996, 87:884–890.

37. Carr RJ, Evans P: Ectopic pregnancy. *Prim Care* 2000, 27:169–183.

38.•• Cates W, Grimes D, Schulz KF: Abortion surveillance at the CDC: creating public health light out of political heat. *Am J Public Health* 2000, 19:12–17.
This article demonstrated the public health importance of abortion surveillance and the political ramifications of this surveillance.

39.• Bartlett LA, Berg CJ, Shulman HB, *et al.*: Risk factors for legal induced abortion related mortality in the United States. *Obstet Gynecol* 2004,103:729–737.
This article demonstrated that the risk for mortality from an abortion increases as the gestational age increases.

40. Elam-Evans LD, Strauss LT, Herndon J, *et al.*: Abortion surveillance 2000. *MMWR Morbid Mortal Wkly Rep* 2003, 52:1–32.

41. Evans MI, Goldberg JD, Horenstein J, *et al.*: Selective termination for structural, chromosomal and mendelian anomalies. *Am J Obstet Gynecol* 1999, 181:893–897.

42. Grimes DA, Hulka JF, McCutchen ME: Midtrimester abortion by dilatation and evacuation versus intra-amniotic instillation of prostaglandin F2a: a randomized clinical trial. *Am J Obstet Gynecol* 1980, 137:785.

43. Kaltreider NB, Goldsmith S, Margolis AJ: The impact of midtrimester abortion techniques on patients and staff. *Am J Obstet Gynecol* 1979, 135:235.

44. Freeman EW: Abortion: subjective attitudes and feelings. *Fam Plan Perspect* 1978, 10:150–155.

45.• Rooks JB, Cates W: Emotional impact of D and E versus instillation. *Fam Plan Perspect* 1977, 9:276–277.
This article demonstrated the experiences of women with different techniques of second trimester abortion.

46. Lawson HW, Fyre A, Atrash HK, *et al.*: Abortion mortality: United States 1972-1987. *Am J Obstet Gynecol* 1994, 171:1365–1372.

47. Chang J, Elam-Evans LD, Berg CJ, *et al.*: Pregnancy-related mortality surveillance: United States, 1991–1999. *MMWR Morbid Mortal Wkly Rep* 2003, 52:1–8.

48.• Blanchard K, Clark S, Winikoff B, *et al.*: Misoprostol for women's health: a review. *Obstet Gynecol* 2002, 99:316–332.
This article demonstrated the many applications of misoprostol in reproductive health care.

49.• Griebel, CP Halvorsen J, Golemon TB, *et al.*: Management of spontaneous abortion. *Am Fam Physician* 2005, 72:1243–1253.
This article is a good review of the primary care management of spontaneous pregnancy loss.

50. ACOG Practice Bulletin: antepartum fetal surveillance. *Int J Gynecol Obstet* 2000, 68:175–185.

51. Stubblefield PG: Midtrimester abortion by curettage procedures: an overview. In *Abortion and Sterilization: Medical and Social Aspects*. Edited by Hodgson JE. San Diego: Academic Press; 1981:277.

52. Crist T, Williams P, Lee SH, *et al.*: Midtrimester pregnancy termination: a study of the cost effectiveness of dilatation and evacuation in a free-standing facility. *North Carolina Med J* 1983, 44:549.

6 | Gonorrhea

M. Cristina Muñoz

- Gonorrhea is a common sexually transmitted infection with extreme disparities in incidence among different groups. Rates are high in women who are young, black, and those who live in disadvantaged urban or rural communities. The chance of acquiring gonorrhea depends on personal behaviors and the incidence of gonorrhea in the community.
- A woman with gonorrhea often carries other sexually transmitted diseases. Gonorrhea increases the chance of acquiring and spreading HIV, and HIV increases gonorrhea transmission.
- The clinical picture of gonorrhea varies from obvious infection with discharge of copious pus to asymptomatic infection that can only be diagnosed by screening. Ascending genital infection causes endometritis, salpingitis, tubo-ovarian abscess, and peritonitis.
- Disseminated gonococcal infection is caused by different types of *Neisseria gonorrhoeae* than complex pelvic infection.
- *Neisseria gonorrhoeae* rapidly evolves antibiotic resistance; a high proportion of isolates are currently resistant to entire classes of drugs.
- Gonococcal ophthalmia neonatorum can cause blindness in newborns; antibiotic prophylaxis is given routinely at birth. After the newborn period, gonorrhea in children implies sexual abuse.
- Public health efforts are crucial in gonorrhea for surveillance of incidence among communities, diagnosis of antibiotic resistance and spread, treatment recommendations, and social or policy interventions to reduce the disease.

Introduction

The clinical syndrome of gonorrhea ("flow of semen") has been known since biblical times. In 2005, there were 339,593 cases of gonorrhea reported in the United States [1] of an estimated 600,000 new infections [2]. Worldwide, there are approximately 60 million infections yearly [3], making it the most common bacterial sexually transmitted infection. Gonorrhea in men, with the obvious symptom of penile discharge, is usually rapidly apparent, prompting treatment. Gonorrhea in women is now more common than in men. Early symptoms may be absent or unnoticed, leading to a long course of infection and serious morbidity from ascending infection. Women are often harmed more by sexually transmitted diseases, including gonorrhea, than men are, because of asymptomatic infection, lack of power in their relationships (eg, they cannot make their partner use a condom or remain monogamous), and inadequate access to treatment.

The diseases caused by *Neisseria gonorrhoeae* are fascinating not only for their microbiology and pathogenesis, but also because of the complex relationships between individual behavior, community characteristics, and public health interventions that affect their spread.

Epidemiology

Although gonorrhea is common, its incidence and prevalence vary widely throughout the world and among different populations in each country. The rate in the United States (Figures 6-1 and 6-2) is the highest among industrialized countries and is 50 times greater than that of Sweden [4]. Rates range from a low of 8.5 cases per 100,000 in Idaho to 247 per 100,000 in Mississippi. Age is a potent risk factor. Adolescent women 15 to 19 years old have 625 cases per 100,000, higher than any other age or gender [1].

Reported rates of gonorrhea among African-Americans are 30 times higher than rates among whites and 11 times that of nonblack Hispanics. This is partly because of differences in reporting, as minority group members are more likely to use public clinics that consistently report cases of sexually transmitted infections. Other factors contributing to the disparity may include access to health care, health-seeking behaviors, prevalence of sexually transmitted infections within a person's social group, level of drug and alcohol use, and availability of education about prevention [4]. Personal risk factors for gonorrhea include a previous gonorrhea infection, other sexually transmitted infections, new or multiple sex partners, inconsistent condom use, commercial sex work, and drug use [5••].

Gonorrhea and chlamydia are similar in their modes of transmission, affected populations, symptoms (or lack thereof), and long-term sequelae. Coinfection is common. In one study of juvenile detention facilities, 54% of girls infected with gonorrhea also had chlamydia [6].

Gonorrhea and HIV infection also occur concurrently [7]. In epidemiologic studies, gonorrhea was associated with increased transmission of HIV, perhaps because HIV shedding is increased in persons with cervicitis or urethritis. Women with gonorrhea are also several times more likely to acquire HIV than uninfected women exposed to HIV.

Pathophysiology

Gonorrhea is transmitted through sexual intercourse, and the columnar epithelium of the cervix is the most common site of initial infection in women. In adolescents, ectopy of the squamocolumnar junction may increase susceptibility to infection. Pharyngeal gonorrhea occurs after oral sex, whereas rectal gonorrhea may result from anal sex or from autoinoculation from the vagina. Transmission is extremely efficient; a woman has a 50% or greater chance

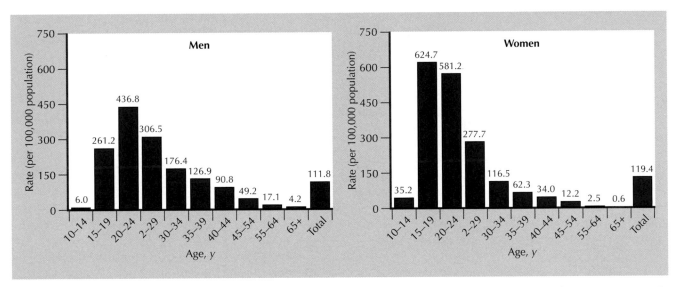

Figure 6-1. Age- and gender-specific rates for gonorrhea in the United States. (*Adapted from* Centers for Disease Control and Prevention [1].)

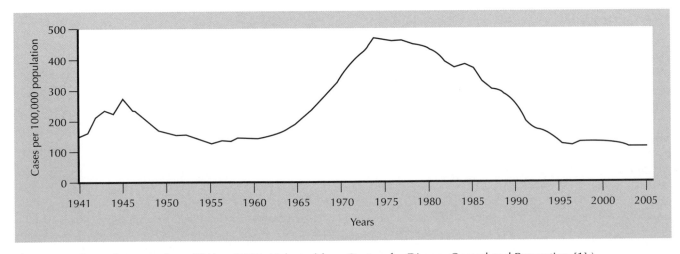

Figure 6-2. Gonorrhea rates from 1941 to 2005. (*Adapted from* Centers for Disease Control and Prevention [1].)

of becoming infected from just one act of intercourse with an infected man [8]. *N. gonorrhoeae* attaches to cervical columnar epithelial cells and induces membrane ruffling, resulting in macropinocytosis without inflammation, causing asymptomatic infection. This contrasts greatly with its invasion into male urethral epithelium or the upper female genital tract, where infection triggers autolysis, cytokine release and inflammation, with damage of nearby epithelial cells and release of bacteria into the subepithelial tissue. Different strains of *N. gonorrhoeae* vary in their ability to adhere to epithelial cells, to invade host tissues, and to cause an inflammatory response, largely due to the membrane proteins expressed on the cell surface.

Neisseria gonorrhoeae may spread via septic emboli to distant locations in the body, causing skin lesions and polyarticular tenosynovitis or arthritis, especially of the hands and feet. Rare sequelae include endocarditis, meningitis, and myocarditis. Intrauterine fetal infection has been reported. Disseminated gonococcal infection occurs in only 0.5% to 3% of infected persons. Causative strains are able to evade host defenses because they are resistant to complement [9].

Clinical Manifestations

Most women with gonorrhea are asymptomatic. They may be diagnosed (and treated) upon routine screening during annual exams or prenatal care, through contact tracing of an infected partner, or at entry into the military, training programs, or incarceration. Women with gonococcal cervicitis may have white or yellow vaginal discharge with onset from 2 to 10 days after exposure. Oropharyngeal infection causes pharyngitis whereas rectal infection causes proctitis. Gonococcal infection ascends from the cervix to the upper genital tract about 20% of the time, often coinciding with the first menses after infection is acquired. Endometritis causes pelvic pain, dyspareunia, dysmenorrhea, and abnormal menstrual bleeding, whereas salpingitis can cause infertility, ectopic pregnancy, or tubo-ovarian abscesses. Infection in the peritoneal cavity may cause pelvic adhesions or perihepatitis (Fitz-Hugh-Curtis syndrome), though the latter is five times more likely to result from chlamydia than gonorrhea.

Pelvic inflammatory disease (PID), infection of the upper genital tract encompassing endometritis, salpingitis and/or peritonitis is a polymicrobial infection that often follows gonococcal cervicitis. In addition to *Neisseria gonorrhoeae*, other pathogens isolated in PID include *Chlamydia trachomatis*, aerobic gram-negative rods such as *Escherichia coli*, anaerobes such as *Bacteroides* species, and occasionally mycoplasmas, ureaplasmas, and gram-positive organisms. *N. gonorrhoeae* is recovered from the cervix in 30% to 80% of women with PID, depending on the population studied [10]. PID has significant consequences, including an increased risk of ectopic pregnancy that is six to 10 times greater than background. The rate of tubal infertility is 8% after one episode of PID, 20% after two episodes, and 40% after 3 episodes. Subclinical pelvic

inflammatory disease, that is, the presence of neutrophils and plasma cells in an endometrial biopsy specimen from a woman with cervicitis, may cause prolonged infection and subsequent tubal damage.

Diagnostic Methods

The symptoms of gonorrhea may be mild or absent, so it is important to screen populations at risk using sensitive tests. Routine screening may detect only 65% to 85% of infected women. Incidence varies by age, sex, race, residence, and other characteristics, so it is important to know which groups in a region are at greatest risk. Sexual habits may increase risk, *eg*, early age at first intercourse, inconsistent or absent condom use, trading sex for money or drugs, or having a partner who is older or has been incarcerated. Discomfort with discussing sexual behavior may keep providers from asking about such risks, but failure to take a sexual history may lead to missed diagnosis.

In women with vaginal discharge or cervicitis, clinical suspicion plus confirmation with culture or a sensitive non-culture test will diagnose gonorrhea. PID is diagnosed clinically and treated empirically, but tests for *N. gonorrhoeae* and *C. trachomatis* should be sent. Ultrasound is helpful in diagnosing causes of abdominal pain such as appendicitis, ectopic pregnancy, and tubo-ovarian abscesses. Laparoscopy may be useful in cases where the diagnosis is unclear. In disseminated infection, culture of the inflamed tissue and exudates (including joint fluid) and the rapid response to antibiotic treatment help make the diagnosis.

Differential Diagnosis

When the cervix is inflamed or bleeds upon manipulation and has a yellow-white creamy exudate, a clinical diagnosis of cervicitis is made. Usually no causative organism is found. *Trichomonas vaginalis*, bacterial vaginosis, and *Candida albicans* may be identified by characteristic discharge, vaginal pH, and findings on saline wet mount and potassium chloride preparations of vaginal discharge. *C. trachomatis* may cause mucopurulent discharge, a mixture of mucus and pus arranged in twisted stripes, and often causes a friable cervix. Herpes viruses may be associated with classic painful vulvar ulcers and can be cultured on appropriate media.

Cystitis and urethritis caused by gonorrhea have similar symptoms to other urinary tract infections, though the discharge of gonorrhea may be more copious or purulent.

Women with lower abdominal pain and cervical motion tenderness and cervical discharge are diagnosed clinically with PID. The differential diagnosis includes appendicitis, gastroenteritis, inflammatory bowel disease, gastroenteritis, pyelonephritis, nephrolithiasis, dysmenorrhea, ectopic pregnancy, threatened abortion, and cystic or solid ovarian mass with or without torsion.

Oropharyngeal gonorrhea has variable appearance ranging from mild erythema to severe ulceration, resembling many viral and bacterial infections.

Laboratory Testing

Traditionally, gonorrhea could be presumptively diagnosed by identifying typical gram-negative diplococci within abundant polymorphonuclear leukocytes in a patient with a discharge and a history of sexual contact. *N. gonorrhoeae* grows in culture in a CO_2 enriched atmosphere in media containing blood and antibiotics to inhibit the growth of competing organisms. *N. gonorrhoeae* can be distinguished from *Neisseria meningitidis* and nonpathogenic *Neisseria* species by the appearance (pigmentation and opacity) of colonies in culture and by its ability to ferment glucose, but not mannose, lactose, sucrose, or maltose. Culture is more sensitive in women with symptomatic gonorrhea than in asymptomatic women, and Gram stain is insensitive even in symptomatic women.

In recent years, modern nonculture tests have become the first-line tests for screening programs and for diagnosis of genital symptoms. These tests may cost less than culture and do not require viable organisms for culture, making them more reliable in areas where culture is difficult or unavailable. Early nonculture tests for *N. gonorrhoeae* include enzyme immunoassays (EIAs), which detect specific gonococcal antigens in cervical swabs or urine, and nucleic acid hybridization probes, which highlight specific DNA or RNA sequences. Nucleic acid amplification tests (NAATs) amplify *N. gonorrhoeae*-specific DNA or RNA sequences in endocervical swabs, self-collected vaginal specimens, urine or urethral swabs in men, and in the remaining fluid from liquid-based Papanicolaou testing. Self-collected vaginal swabs or urine can even be collected at home and sent out for testing. Nucleic acid amplification tests are more sensitive than cultures, and current NAAT of the cervix are 99% specific [11].

Nucleic acid amplification tests are not approved for use in children or in extragenital sites because of cross-reactivity with *N. meningitidis* and nonpathogenic bacteria found in those sites. Additionally, testing for antibiotic susceptibility requires culturing the organism, so cultures remain important both for treatment of individuals who fail initial therapy and for surveillance of antibiotic resistance patterns throughout the world.

Given the high rate of coinfection and similar risk factors, patients at risk for gonorrhea should be tested for other sexually transmitted infections, particularly chlamydia and HIV.

Treatment

Treatment guidelines are frequently updated to reflect knowledge of gonorrhea epidemiology, especially development of resistance in different regions and groups. The Centers for Disease Control and Prevention regularly publishes guidelines that outline the best available treatments. Special populations are addressed, including adolescents (the largest group affected by gonorrhea), pregnant women, and children, among others. These guidelines can be used with populations outside the United States, as long as resistance patterns are known. Some of the recommended treatments, *eg*, spectinomycin or cefixime, are currently unavailable in the United States.

For uncomplicated gonorrhea of the cervix, urethra, rectum, or pharynx, a third generation cephalosporin such as ceftriaxone is preferred, though quinolones may be used in areas where the organism remains susceptible. Treatment with azithromycin or doxycycline is given concurrently to treat chlamydial infection. Single-dose treatments administered in the office are preferred, because they increase the likelihood of cure.

Pelvic inflammatory disease is diagnosed clinically, and empiric treatment should include coverage for gonorrhea, chlamydia, and anaerobes. Prompt treatment for salpingitis usually prevents tubal infertility if started before the development of a mass.

Disseminated gonococcal infection is treated with intravenous antibiotics, including third-generation cephalosporins and quinolones. The treatment is given until symptoms such as fever are resolved for 24 to 48 hours, and then oral medications are given for another week. Meningitis caused by *N. gonorrhoeae* should be treated with intravenous ceftriaxone 1 to 2 g every 12 hours for 10 to 14 days.

Sexual partners of patients with gonorrhea should also be treated to protect them, to prevent rapid reinfection of the index patient, and to protect their other partners. Expedited treatment, providing medication for partners without meeting or examining them, is more effective than asking patients to refer their partners and is legally permitted in many states [12,13].

Neisseria gonorrhoeae is a versatile, rapidly evolving pathogen that efficiently infects humans while rapidly evolving resistance to antibiotics. Gonorrhea was one of the first infections to be treated with sulfonamides in the 1930s and with penicillin the 1940s, but these antibiotics are no longer used because of the development of resistant strains. Resistance arises through mutations or acquisition of plasmids. Lactamase (penicillinase)–producing strains of *N. gonorrhoeae* (PPNG) first appeared in the 1970s. Tetracycline resistance is common, whereas resistance to modern antibiotics such as the quinolones and azithromycin is increasing as these drugs are used for therapy. Use of antibiotics for other infections, for example, prophylaxis of peripartum Group B streptococcus infection or ineffective prescribing for viral upper respiratory infection, may cure gonorrheal infections in a patient who is unaware of her infection. Alternatively, use of antibiotics can add to the development of resistance by partially treating asymptomatic gonorrhea.

Prevention

There are currently no vaccines to prevent gonorrhea. Condoms, when used correctly and consistently, significantly decrease the incidence of gonorrhea [5••,14] and other sexually transmitted infections, as well as sequelae such as chronic pelvic pain and infertility [15].

Public health interventions to screen and treat individuals at risk, especially those who are likely to infect others, have been very effective in lowering the rate of gonorrhea. For example, in the United States between 1975 and 1997, there was a 74% drop in the reported incidence of gonorrhea, largely as a result of programs to screen at-risk populations and treat infected individuals. Such programs lower the burden of disease in individuals who would have been diagnosed late or not at all in the absence of screening.

Referrals

Most gonorrheal infections can be treated successfully by primary care physicians and other trained providers. Laparoscopy may be needed for patients diagnosed with PID if they do not respond to antibiotics or if a surgical emergency (such as appendicitis) cannot be ruled out. Examination by an ophthalmologist is useful in cases of suspected gonococcal ophthalmia. Disseminated gonococcal infection may be difficult to diagnose, and a rheumatologist can help greatly with differential diagnosis.

References

Papers of particular interest have been highlighted as follows:
- Of interest
- •• Of outstanding interest

1. Centers for Disease Control and Prevention: Trends in Reportable Sexually Transmitted Diseases in the United States, 2005, National Surveillance Data for Chlamydia, Gonorrhea, and Syphilis. Atlanta. US Department of Health and Human Services, 2006.

2. Centers for Disease Control and Prevention: Sexually Transmitted Disease Surveillance, 2005. Atlanta: US Department of Health and Human Services, 2006.

3. Tapsall JW: What management is there for gonorrhea in the postquinolone era? *Sexually Transmitted Diseases* 2006, 33:8–10.

4. Centers for Disease Control and Prevention: Tracking the Hidden Epidemics, Trends in STDs in the United States 2000. Atlanta. US Department of Health and Human Services, 2000, 9–10.

5.•• Workowski KA, Berman SM: Sexually transmitted diseases treatment guidelines, 2006. *MMWR Recomm Rep* 2006, 55:1.
The treatment guidelines are evidence-based recommendations that are updated regularly and are always available through a variety of print and electronic media. When possible, multiple options for treatment are listed. Special populations such as pregnant women, newborns, and men who have sex with men are addressed.

6. Kahn RH, Mosure DJ, Blank S, *et al.*: Jail STD prevalence monitoring project: *Chlamydia trachomatis* and *Neisseria gonorrhoeae* prevalence and coinfection in adolescents entering selected US juvenile detention centers, 1997-2002. *Sexually Transmitted Diseases* 2005, 32:255–259.

7. Cohen MS: HIV and sexually transmitted diseases: lethal synergy. *Top HIV Med* 2004, 12:104–107.

8. Lin JS, Donegan SP, Heeren TC, *et al.*: Transmission of *Chlamydia trachomatis* and *Neisseria gonorrhoeae* among men with urethritis and their female sex partners. *J Infect Dis* 1998, 178:1707.

9. Brunham RC, Plummer F, Slaney L, *et al.*: Correlation of auxotype and protein 1 type with expression of disease due to *Neisseria gonorrhoeae*. *J Infect Dis* 1985, 152:339.

10. McNeeley S: Gonococcal infections in women. *Obstet Gynecol Clin North Am* 1989, 16:467.

11. Schachter J, Morse SA: Nucleic acid amplification tests in the diagnosis of bacterial STDs. *Infect Med* 2005, 22:323–326; discussion 329–331.

12. Golden MR, Whittington WL, Handsfield HH, *et al.*: Expedited treatment of sex partners in cases of persistent gonorrhea and chlamydial infection. *N Engl J Med* 2005, 352:676.

13. Centers for Disease Control and Prevention: Expedited partner therapy in the management of sexually transmitted diseases. Atlanta: US Department of Health and Human Services, 2006.

14. Paz-Bailey G, Koumans EH, Sternberg M, *et al.*: The effect of correct and consistent use on chlamydial and gonococcal infection among urban adolescents. *Arch Pediatr Adolesc Med* 2005, 159:536–542.

15. Ness RB, Randall H, Richter HE, Peipert JF, *et al.*: Pelvic Inflammatory Disease Evaluation and Clinical Health Study Investigators: Condom use and the risk of recurrent pelvic inflammatory disease, chronic pelvic pain, or infertility following an episode of pelvic inflammatory disease. *Am J Public Health* 2004, 94:1327–1329.

Recommended Reading

•• Handsfield H: *Color Atlas and Synopsis of Sexually Transmitted Disease*, edn 2. New York: McGraw-Hill Professional; 2000.
In addition to good-quality photographs of different manifestations of sexually transmitted diseases, this book includes succinct information on their epidemiology, diagnosis, and treatment.

•• Holmes K: *Sexually Transmitted Diseases*, edn 4. New York, McGraw-Hill Professional; 2007.
This encyclopedic reference covers all sexually transmitted diseases, and includes detailed information about the causative organisms, pathogenesis, epidemiology, and treatment of sexually transmitted diseases. New developments in research and social issues related to sexually transmitted diseases are addressed.

US Preventive Services Task Force: *Screening for Gonorrhea*. Rockville, MD: Agency for Healthcare Research and Quality; 2006. Available at http://ww.ahrq.gov/clinic/uspstf/uspsgono.htm.

7 | Chlamydia

Melissa Kottke

- Most women with chlamydial infection do not have symptoms.
- *Chlamydia trachomatis* infection can cause pelvic inflammatory disease with subsequent infertility and ectopic pregnancy.
- Identification and treatment of infected women reduces the rate of long-term complications.
- Sexually active women younger than 25 years should be routinely screened for *C. trachomatis*.
- Nonpregnant women with uncomplicated chlamydial infection treated with recommended regimens do not need to return for a test of cure.
- Testing for *C. trachomatis* should be performed even when patients are treated presumptively.

Incidence and Epidemiology

Chlamydia trachomatis is the most common bacterial infectious disease reported to state health departments and the Centers for Diseased Control and Prevention (CDC) [1••], with an estimated 2.8 to 4 million infections occurring annually [2••,3]. As of 2000, all 50 states and the District of Columbia had regulations requiring the reporting of chlamydia. From 1987 through 2005, the annual reported rate of chlamydial infections increased from 47.8 to 332.5 cases per 100,000 [1••]. This likely reflects increased screening and reporting, improved sensitivity of diagnostic tests, and possibly increased burden of disease.

The prevalence of chlamydial infection varies greatly by age, race, the population screened, and the geographic area of the participating subjects. The most important of these is age [1••,4]. The prevalence of female patients with positive cervical cultures is highest in teenaged girls and declines as women age (Figure 7-1). The prevalence of serum antibody to *C. trachomatis* increases with age until about 30 years, when it plateaus near 50% [5]. In the United States, 41.6% of diagnoses of *C. trachomatis* were in African-Americans. In 2005, the rate for African-American women was 1729 *C. trachomatis* cases per 100,000 women compared to 1177.7 for American Indian/Alaska Native females, 733.2 for Hispanic females, 237.2 for white females, and 222.3 for Asian/Pacific Islander women [1••,4]. More than 20% of women presenting for treatment at sexually transmitted disease (STD) clinics tested positive for *C. trachomatis* [5]. In contrast, the overall prevalence of chlamydial infection was 9.2% in new female Army recruits [6,7]. In 2005, the median state-specific rate of *C. trachomatis* was 6.3% (range 3.0%–20.3%) in family planning clinics and 8.0% (range 2.8%–16.9%) in prenatal clinics [1••,4]. The southern region of the United States has the highest reported prevalence. The states with the highest prevalence of chlamydial infection are listed in Figure 7-2. Risk factors for chlamydial infection are listed in Figure 7-3.

Most cases of chlamydial infection are asymptomatic. Unfortunately, this correlates with high numbers of infectious people sustaining transmission in a community as well as a lack of seeking treatment to prevent sequelae. In a large epidemiologic study, concordant infection was found in 10.7% of couples. Male-to-female and female-to-male transmission frequencies were equal at 68% [8]. In contrast, a recent study found a much higher couple concordance of 75% [9]. Pelvic inflammatory disease (PID) is one of the most serious complications of chlamydial infection and is associated with 2.5 million outpatient medical visits yearly [10,11]. Including PID sequelae of infertility, chronic pelvic pain, and ectopic pregnancy, the estimated annual cost of treating chlamydial infection exceeds $2.4 billion [12]. Chlamydial infections in pregnant women can lead to preterm labor, premature rupture of membranes, low birth weight, neonatal conjunctivitis and pneumonia, as well as increasing the likelihood of postpartum endometritis [13].

Pathophysiology

C. trachomatis is an obligatory intracellular gram negative bacterium. Infection is initiated by specific attachment of the elementary body to sites on susceptible host cells. The initial site of infection is usually the cervix, although the urethra and rectum may also be infected. The chlamydial particles are then taken up by the host cell in a process similar to phagocytosis. The remainder of the lifecycle takes place within a cytoplasmic vacuole called the reticulate body. Within the reticulate bodies, replication and reorganization into small elementary bodies occurs. After 2 to 3 days, the cell ruptures, releasing new

infectious particles [5]. These intracellular inclusions permit identification of infected cells by light or fluorescence microscopy and are often visualized in culture (Figure 7-4).

Diagnosis

PRESENTATION

The spectrum of clinical disease caused by *C. trachomatis* is broad (Figure 7-5). As many as 70% to 80% of infected women do not have symptoms. When symptoms do occur, patients typically present with vaginal discharge and dysuria.

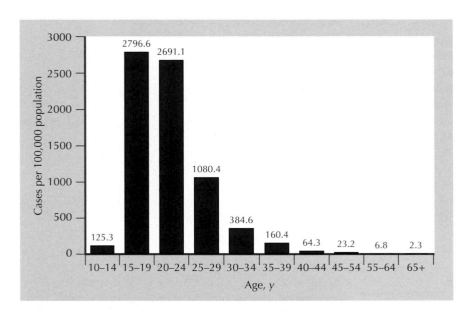

Figure 7-1. Prevalence of *Chlamydia trachomatis* cervical infection by age in women attending a sexually transmitted disease clinic. (*Adapted from* Stamm and Holmes [5].)

States with the Highest Prevalence of Chlamydial Infection in Women, 2005

Ranking	State	Rate per 100,000 Population
1	Mississippi	732.6
2	Alaska	664.4
3	New Mexico	444.3
4	South Carolina	435.8
5	Hawaii	434.7
6	Delaware	408.5
7	Illinois	397.7
8	Tennessee	391.2
9	Missouri	388.7
10	Michigan	383
	United States Total	332.5

Figure 7-2. States with the highest prevalence of chlamydial infection in women, 2005. (*Adapted from* Centers for Disease Control and Prevention [1••].)

Risk Factors for Chlamydial Infection in Women

Age ≤ 25 years

Minority race

More than one sex partner in previous 90 days

New sex partner in previous 90 days

Having a partner who did not always use condoms in previous 90 days

Having ever had a sexually transmitted disease

Use of oral contraceptives

Symptomatic male partner

Cervical ectopy > 25%

Figure 7-3. Risk factors for chlamydial infection in women. (*Data from* Gaydos *et al.* [6], Quinn *et al.* [7], and Marrazzo *et al.* [34].)

Patients with cervicitis may present with lower abdominal pain, endocervical bleeding, mucopurulent endocervical discharge, and cervical edema. Gram stain of the discharge often finds 10 or more polymorphonuclear leukocytes per high-power field. Symptoms of acute dysuria and urinary frequency are associated with chlamydial urethritis. Differential diagnosis of cervicitis, mucopurulent discharge, and urethritis are listed in Figure 7-6. Infection of Bartholin's ducts can cause pain, swelling, and exudative discharge from the ducts.

Infections can ascend to involve the upper genital tract. Salpingitis and endometritis can result from chlamydial infection. Eighty-six percent of women with cervical infection have evidence of infection in the uterus and fallopian tubes [13]. Because of the importance of PID, it is discussed in detail in Chapter 10. The sequelae of fallopian tube infection, even those that are subclinical as is often seen with *C. trachomatis*, include chronic pain, infertility, and ectopic pregnancy (discussed in Chapter 4). Approximately 17% of women treated for PID experience chronic pelvic pain, and an equal percentage are infertile. Of those women who do conceive, as many as 10% have an ectopic pregnancy [18]. In 5% to 15% of women with PID, *C. trachomatis* may also cause perihepatic inflammation, called Fitz-Hugh-Curtis syndrome. This should be suspected in young sexually active women with right upper quadrant pain and signs of lower genital infection [5].

Pregnant women with chlamydial infection of the lower genitourinary tract have similar symptoms to their nonpregnant counterparts. Like nonpregnant women, the majority will be asymptomatic. Unique findings in this population include increased rates of preterm delivery [14,15] and more frequent postpartum endometritis [2••]. Vertical transmission is uncertain but is likely near 50% [16]. *C. trachomatis* is the most common identifiable cause of neonatal conjunctivitis and results from perinatal transmission from an infected gravida. Symptoms begin on days 5 to 12 of life. It can also cause subacute, afebrile pneumonia in newborns, generally from 1 to 3 months of age [17••].

LYMPHOGRANULOMA VENEREUM

The invasive serotypes of *C. trachomatis*, L1, L2, or L3, cause lymphogranuloma venereum (LGV), a rare disease in the United States. Generally, LGV does not present as genital ulcer disease in women. The self-limited genital ulcer has usually resolved when most adults seek medical care. The most common signs are tender unilateral inguinal or femoral adenopathy. Other presentations include proctocolitis or fistulas and strictures from inflammatory involvement of perirectal and perianal lymphatic tissues. The diagnosis of LGV is usually made serologically and by exclusion of other causes of inguinal adenopathy or genital lesions. Treatment of LGV cures infection and prevents ongoing tissue damage but may not prevent scarring. Buboes may require aspiration through intact skin to prevent the formation of inguinal or femoral ulcerations. The preferred treatment is doxycycline, 100 mg orally twice a day for 21 days [17••].

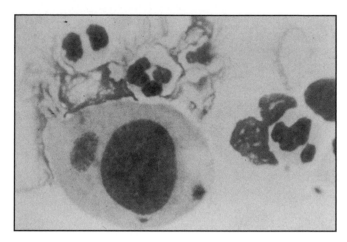

Figure 7-4. Photomicrograph of intracellular chlamydial inclusions.

Clinical Spectrum of Chlamydial Infection in Women

Asymptomatic

Mucopurulent cervicitis

Urethritis

Bartholinitis

Endometritis: chronic and postpartum

Acute salpingitis and pelvic inflammatory disease

Perihepatitis (Fitz-Hugh-Curtis syndrome)

Lymphogranuloma venereum

Conjunctivitis

Pharyngitis

Figure 7-5. Clinical spectrum of chlamydial infection in women.

Differential Diagnosis of Chlamydial Infections

Urethritis

Bacterial cystitis

Trichomonas species infection

Cervicitis

Neisseria gonorrhoeae infection

Trichomonas species infection

Herpes simplex virus

Mucopurulent discharge

Inflammation induced by an intrauterine device

Fistulas from pelvic tuberculosis

Bacterial vaginosis

Figure 7-6. Differential diagnosis of chlamydial infections. (*Adapted from* Gaydos *et al.* [6], Centers for Disease Control and Prevention [18], Watson *et al.* [20], and Steece [21].)

Diagnostic Studies

For many years, culture was considered the gold standard for diagnosis of chlamydial infection. The past 20 years have seen an evolution of techniques involving detection of organisms by antigens and by nucleic acids (Figure 7-7). Even if a presumptive diagnosis of *C. trachomatis* is made by clinical evaluation and treatment with partner referral is made, chlamydial detection tests should be performed. The test results help to ensure appropriate medical care, particularly if symptoms persist despite therapy. Additionally, counseling of the patient and accurate reporting are facilitated, and firm ground for partner notification is established [2••].

CULTURE

Compared to the other methods of detection, a major advantage of culture is a specificity that approaches 100%. The disadvantages of cell culture include the inherent time delay required to make the diagnosis. Additionally, because of the necessity of viable organisms, specimen collection, transport, and processing, requirements are stringent. In experienced laboratories, the sensitivity of culture is 70% to 85% [18••,21]. The culture process involves inoculation of the specimen into cell culture. Viable organisms reproduce, and intracytoplasmic inclusions (*see* Figure 7-4) are subsequently visualized by staining the infected cells with fluorescently labeled antibodies to chlamydial lipopolysaccharide (LPS) or major outer membrane protein-1 (MOMP-1). The LPS antibodies are not specific for *C. trachomatis*; therefore, MOMP-1 antibody is the preferred method used for the detection of *C. trachomatis* isolated in cell culture. Antibiotic sensitivity testing of specimens with *C. trachomatis* is generally not performed because of a high susceptibility to recommended agents for treatment. Of special note, culture is the preferred method of diagnosis of chlamydial infection in cases of potential sexual abuse or assault because of its 100% specificity [18••] (*see* Chapter 46).

Test Method	Sensitivity, %	Specificity, %
Culture	70–85	100
Nucleic acid amplification tests*	90–96	98–100
Direct fluorescent antibody	68–85	96–99.5
Enzyme immunoassay	52–84	95–99
Nucleic acid hybridization	60–83	96–100

*Sensitivities for nucleic acid amplification tests on urine samples are somewhat lower.

Figure 7-7. Common chlamydial diagnostic tests.

NUCLEIC ACID AMPLIFICATION TESTS

Nucleic acid amplification tests (NAATs) have largely replaced culture as the diagnostic method of choice secondary to their high sensitivity and specificity. These tests are able to produce positive results from a single copy of DNA or RNA and do not require viable organisms. There are several different amplification techniques used by different commercial tests. They include polymerase chain reaction, transcription mediated amplification, and strand displacement amplification. Ligase chain reaction was the basis for some of the earlier NAATs; these have been removed from the market. All methods of amplification result in very high sensitivities (90%–96%) and specificities (> 98%). Many of the NAATs have received US Food and Drug Administration approval for chlamydial detection in urine samples [18••,19–21].

Other Diagnostic Methods

Before nucleic acid amplification test development, several other diagnostic tests were developed to circumvent the challenges of culture. Most are currently not recommended for screening because of lower sensitivities. Please see Figure 7-7 for a comparison of diagnostic methods. For accurate patient counseling, it is prudent to be familiar with the method of *C. trachomatis* detection your lab uses.

Direct fluorescent antibody tests involve direct examination of specimens stained with chlamydia-specific antibodies. Several different tests are available with antibodies directed against MOMP-1 or LPS. As with culture, antibodies to MOMP-1 are more specific to *C. trachomatis* [18••, 21].

Enzyme immune assay uses enzyme-labeled antibodies to LPS, but the sensitivity of this assay is limited because of potential cross-reactivity of LPS antibodies with gram negative bacteria. This technique has been adapted for use in rapid tests, which can be performed at the bedside and results read qualitatively in approximately 30 minutes. Performance of a test while the patient waits on the result, or point of care testing, can be useful in settings where immediate treatment decisions are necessary. These tests should only be used when a patient is going to wait on the results, otherwise the decreased sensitivity and specificity, as well as increased cost, are inappropriate [18••,21].

Nucleic acid hybridization tests use a chemiluminescent DNA probe that hybridizes to a specific sequence of chlamydial RNA. These tests have improved sensitivity compared with most enzyme immunosorbent assay tests. The test kit includes collection swab and transport media. This test does not require cold transport and storage. In addition, when used in conjunction with a probe to detect *Neisseria gonorrhoeae*, a single swab can be used for both assays [18••, 21].

Serologic testing for acute chlamydial infection is limited because of the persistence of immunoglobulin G antibodies. The use of immunoglobulin M to diagnose infection in adults is also limited because of an anamnestic response, which yields false negative results. Chlamydial antibodies have been associated with tubal factor infertility [22].

SPECIMEN COLLECTION

Proper specimen collection and handling is critical in all the methods that are used to identify *C. trachomatis*. Because chlamydiae are obligate intracellular organisms, optimal results are obtained when the specimen contains cellular material. The type of swab used for specimen collection is important; those with wooden shafts should be avoided because they may contain inhibitors to the bacterium. The best swabs for the isolation of chlamydiae (and other sexually transmitted pathogens) have cotton, rayon, or Dacron tips with plastic or aluminum shafts. For nonculture tests, the appropriate swab is often included in the test kit. For cervical sampling, secretions and discharge should be removed; the swab is then inserted into the endocervical canal 1 to 2 cm above the squamocolumnar junction. The swab is rotated for 15 to 30 seconds and removed without touching any vaginal surfaces. To sample the urethra, the swab should be inserted about 1 to 2 cm, rotated once for 5 seconds, and removed. There are also specific recommendations regarding transport of specimens with which clinicians should become familiar [18••,21].

If a woman is symptomatic, a pelvic exam and endocervical sampling as above is prudent. However, in asymptomatic patients, less invasive means of screening for *C. trachomatis* are desirable. Because of the very high sensitivity and potential amplification of a single bacterium, *C. trachomatis* can be detected using nucleic acid amplification tests with great accuracy from a first catch urine stream [18••,19]. This has been found to be acceptable to patients and has utility in large scale screening of asymptomatic persons. Self-collected vaginal swabs also show high acceptability to patients [23,24]. Most commercial tests do not currently have US Food and Drug Administration approval for self-collected vaginal swabs. Detecting *C. trachomatis* from ophthalmic, pharyngeal, or rectal specimens generally requires culture [18••].

Treatment

Treatment of chlamydial infection in women reduces complications for the patient, prevents transmission to sexual partners, and reduces transmission of *C. trachomatis* to neonates of pregnant women. An investigation of patients in a health maintenance organization demonstrated that screening and treatment of women with cervical infection may significantly reduce the likelihood of PID [25].

Recent recommendations for the treatment of genital chlamydial infection have been published [17••] and are outlined in Figure 7-8. Steps should be taken to maximize compliance with treatment regimens, including dispensing medications on-site and direct observation of the first dose. In settings of positive gonorrhea testing, presumptive diagnosis and treatment of *C. trachomatis* is appropriate unless simultaneous nucleic acid hybridization test is negative for *C. trachomatis* [17••].

The results of clinical trials indicate that azithromycin and doxycycline are equally efficacious in populations with good compliance, with bacteriologic cures exceeding 95% [17••,26]. Doxycycline has been used extensively and is significantly less expensive than azithromycin. However, in populations with erratic health care–seeking behavior, poor compliance, or minimal follow-up, azithromycin may be more cost-effective because it provides single-dose, directly observed therapy. A similar percentage of patients have gastrointestinal and other side effects from doxycycline and azithromycin [26]. Available formulations of azithromycin include 250-mg capsules and 1-g powder mix. Erythromycin is less efficacious than azithromycin or doxycycline, and gastrointestinal side effects are common. Ofloxacin and levofloxacin are effective but expensive and do not offer an improvement in dosage scheduling [17••].

Recommended therapies for infection in pregnant patients are outlined in Figure 7-9. Because of the toxicity of tetracyclines to the developing fetus, doxycycline is not used in pregnancy. Azithromycin and amoxicillin are recommended instead.

Several studies have evaluated the safety and efficacy of azithromycin in pregnancy [27–30]. Two randomized trials comparing amoxicillin with azithromycin show similar efficacy and tolerance rates [29,30].

Patients should be counseled to abstain from sexual intercourse for 7 days after the single-dose therapy or until completion of a 7-day regimen. In addition to counseling about abstinence and methods of future STD prevention, patients should be instructed to have their sexual partners tested and treated. This includes persons having sexual contact with the

Treatment of Chlamydial Infections in Nonpregnant Women

Recommended Regimens	Alternative Regimens
Azithromycin 1 g PO as a single dose	Erythromycin base 500 mg PO four times daily for 7 days
Doxycycline 100 mg PO twice daily for 7 days	Erythromycin ethylsuccinate 800 mg PO four times daily for 7 days
	Ofloxacin 300 mg PO twice daily for 7 days
	Levofloxacin 500 mg PO daily for 7 days

Figure 7-8. Treatment of chlamydial infections in nonpregnant women. PO—by mouth. (*Adapted from* Centers for Disease Control and Prevention [17••].)

infected patient during the 60 days preceding the onset of symptoms in the patient or the diagnosis of chlamydial infection. Health-care providers should treat the most recent sex partner even if the last contact was more than 60 days before onset or diagnosis [17••]. The most effective manner of partner notification and treatment is unclear. Expedited partner therapy with patient-delivered partner therapy may be of benefit for *C. trachomatis*; however, it presents several implementation issues [31]. Further research in this area is needed.

A test of cure is not necessary after a nonpregnant patient has completed treatment with recommended or alternate therapy, unless symptoms persist, antibiotic compliance is questioned, or reinfection is suspected because these therapies are highly efficacious [17••]. However, there is a recommendation for repeat testing after 3 months because reinfection is not only common, but also more likely to be associated with PID and other complications [32]. Reinfection often occurs secondary to not having one's partner tested and treated or by infection from a new partner. The Centers for Disease Control and Prevention does recommend test of cure on pregnant patients 3 to 4 weeks after therapy secondary to possible vertical transmission and neonatal infection. Nonculture tests should not be used as a test of cure sooner than 3 weeks after completion of therapy because false-positive results can result from continued excretion of dead organisms [17••,18••].

Chlamydial ophthalmia neonatorum and infant pneumonia may be treated with erythromycin base, 50 mg/kg/d orally divided into four doses daily for 10 to 14 days. Efficacy in both settings is approximately 80%, so a second course of therapy may be required. The mothers of infants who have chlamydial infection and their sex partners should be evaluated and treated. Although infants born to women with known untreated chlamydial infection are at risk, the efficacy of prophylactic therapy is unknown. Therefore, the neonates should be given only routine newborn ophthalmic prophylaxis (*see* Chapter 6) and observed as outpatients for infection [17••]. The management of chlamydial infection in children, which may be a result of sexual abuse, is outlined in Chapter 46.

Referral

The primary care provider in the outpatient setting can treat women with asymptomatic disease and those with cervical infection in the absence of upper tract symptoms. When clinical signs of pelvic inflammatory disease are present, the provider may choose to consult a specialist depending on the familiarity of the provider with treatment of pelvic infection (*see* Chapter 10). Referral should be considered for patients whose symptoms persist after adequate treatment. Dermatologic or infectious disease consultation should be obtained if the diagnosis of lymphogranuloma venereum is considered. As noted previously, the Centers for Disease Control and Prevention recommends referral and treatment of the sexual partners of infected patients. All patients should be offered counseling and testing for HIV and other sexually transmitted infections.

Prevention

The principal goals of strategies to prevent chlamydial infection are to prevent both overt and silent chlamydia salpingitis and its sequelae and to prevent perinatal and postpartum infection. Primary and secondary prevention strategies are necessary [12].

Primary prevention strategies are efforts to prevent chlamydia infection. Behavioral changes that reduce the risk of acquiring or transmitting infection should be promoted. These behaviors include abstinence, delaying the age of first intercourse, reduction in the number of sexual partners, careful partner selection, and the use of condoms, which act as a barrier to STD acquisition.

Secondary prevention strategies are efforts to prevent complications among patients already infected with *C. trachomatis* [2••]. Strategies are needed to identify and treat chlamydial infection before the infection of sex partners or neonates. Additionally, early detection and treatment of STDs, including chlamydial infections, may help to reduce

Treatment of Chlamydial Infections in Pregnant Women	
Recommended Regimens	**Alternative Regimens**
Azithromycin 1 g PO as a single dose	Erythromycin base 500 mg PO four times per day for 7 days
Amoxicillin 500 mg PO three times per day for 7 days	Erythromycin base 250 mg PO four times per day for 14 days*
	Erythromycin ethylsuccinate 800 mg PO four times per day for 7 days
	Erythromycin ethylsuccinate 400 mg PO four times per day for 14 days*

These regimens are used when only erythromycin can be used and a patient cannot tolerate higher-dose erythromycin schedules.

Figure 7-9. Treatment of chlamydial infections in pregnant women. PO—by mouth. (*Adapted from* Centers for Disease Control and Prevention [17••].)

the risk of HIV sexual transmission. Any STD, ulcerative or nonulcerative, that causes genital inflammation may increase local HIV load in infected adults. In noninfected persons, genital infection can disrupt epithelial and mucosal barriers to infection and may increase a person's susceptibility to HIV infection [33].

Secondary prevention efforts require active screening and referral of sex partners. Because most women infected with *C. trachomatis* do not have symptoms, population-based screening is vital. The optimal screening strategy for an individual practitioner depends largely upon the prevalence of infection in the population to be screened.

Several studies have investigated the performance and cost-effectiveness of selective versus universal screening. In one study, universal screening was more cost effective than selective screening when the prevalence of chlamydial infection was greater than 3.1% in family planning clinics and greater than 7% in STD clinics [34]. Other evaluations of the cost efficacy of screening indicate that the natural history of asymptomatic infection is unclear, clouding the picture of cost efficacy [35–36].

General screening guidelines based on current estimates of prevalence, natural history, and cost efficacy from the Centers for Disease Control and Prevention and US Preventive Services Task Force are summarized in Figure 7-10. As age is the primary risk factor for chlamydial infection, those under age 26 should be screened annually. Women 26 and over can be screened based on risk factors [18,37]. Beyond these guidelines, clinicians should be aware of local prevalence of disease and determine appropriate screening strategies within their own communities. Greater availability of rapid, effective screening and the education of patients and their sexual partners are important strides in reducing the incidence of chlamydial infection. Continued efforts are necessary to reduce the heavy personal and economic toll of this insidious disease.

Screening Recommendations

All sexually active women age ≤ 25 years

Sexually active women age > 25 years who are at high risk of acquiring an STI

Substance abuse

History of sexually transmitted disease

Having new or multiple sexual partners

Inconsistent condom use

From community with high rate of sexually transmitted disease

Women entering a correctional or detention facility

Women with HIV infection

Figure 7-10. Screening recommendations. STI—sexually transmitted infection. (*Adapted from* Centers for Disease Control and Prevention [18] and US Preventive Services Task Force [37].)

References

Papers of particular interest have been highlighted as follows:
•   *Of interest*
••   *Of outstanding interest*

1.•• Centers for Disease Control and Prevention Division of STD Prevention: Sexually Transmitted Disease Surveillance, 2005. US Department of Health and Human Services, Public Health Service. Atlanta: Centers for Disease Control and Prevention; December, 2006.
This is an annual report of STD burden in the United States. The epidemiology STDs is well represented.

2.•• Centers for Disease Control and Prevention: Recommendations for the prevention and management of Chlamydia trachomatis infections, 1993. *MMWR Morb Mortal Wkly Rep* 1993, 42:1–27.
This reference is an excellent resource for strategies to reduce the morbidity of chlamydial infections and to prevent transmission to uninfected persons.

3. Groseclose SL, Zaidi AA, DeLisle SJ, et al.: Estimated incidence and prevalence of genital *Chlamydia trachomatis* infections in the United States, 1996. *Sex Transm Dis* 1999, 26:339–344.

4. Centers for Disease Control and Prevention: Sexually Transmitted Disease Surveillance 2005 Supplement, Chlamydia Prevalence Monitoring Project Annual Report 2005. Atlanta: US Department of Health and Human Services, Centers for Disease Control and Prevention; 2006.

5. Stamm WE, Holmes KK: *Chlamydia trachomatis* infections of the adult. In *Sexually Transmitted Diseases*, edn 3. Edited by Holmes KK, Mårdh PA, Sparling PF, et al. New York: McGraw-Hill; 1999:407–422.

6. Gaydos CA, Howell MR, Dare B, et al.: *Chlamydia trachomatis* infections in female military recruits. *N Engl J Med* 1998, 339:739–744.

7. Morrison CS, Wong P, Kwok C, et al.: Hormonal contraceptive use, cervical ectopy, and the acquisition of cervical infections. *Sex Transm Dis* 2004, 31:561–567.

8. Quinn TC, Gaydos C, Shepherd M, et al.: Epidemiologic and microbiologic correlates of *Chlamydia trachomatis* infection in sexual partnerships. *JAMA* 1996, 276:1737–1742.

9. Markos AR: The concordance of *Chlamydia trachomatis* genital infection between sexual partners in the era of nucleic acid testing. *Sexual Health* 2005, 2:23–24.

10. Washington A, Johnson R, Sanders L: *Chlamydia trachomatis* infections in the United States: what are they costing us? *JAMA* 1987, 257:2070–2072.

11. Rolfs RT, Galaid EI, Zaidi AA: Pelvic inflammatory disease: trends in hospitalization and office visits, 1979 through 1988. *Am J Obstet Gynecol* 1992, 166:983–990.

12. Eng TR, Butler WT, for the Institute of Medicine, Committee on Prevention and Control of Sexually Transmitted Diseases: *The Hidden Epidemic: Confronting Sexually Transmitted Diseases*. Washington, DC: National Academy Press; 1997.

13. Mårdh PA, Ripa T, Svensson L, et al.: *Chlamydia trachomatis* infection in patients with acute salpingitis. *N Engl J Med* 1977, 296:1377–1379.

14. Mardh PA: Influence of infection with *Chlamydia trachomatis* on pregnancy outcome, infant health and life-long sequelae in infected offspring. *Best Pract Res Clin Obstet Gynecol* 2002, 16:847–864.

15. Martin DH, Koutsky L, Eschenbach DA, *et al*.: Prematurity and perinatal mortality in pregnancies complicated by maternal *Chlamydia trachomatis* infections. *JAMA* 1982, 247:1585–1588.

16. Norman J: Epidemiology of female genital *Chlamydia trachomatis* infections. *Best Pract Res Clin Obstet Gynecol* 2002, 16:775–787.

17.•• Centers for Disease Control and Prevention: 2006 Guidelines for treatment of sexually transmitted disease. *MMWR Morb Mortal Wkly Rep* 2006, 55:38–43.

This paper is an excellent resource for current recommendations regarding diagnosis, treatment, and follow-up.

18.•• Centers for Disease Control and Prevention: Screening tests to detect *Chlamydia trachomatis* and *Neisseria gonorrhoeae* infections—2002. *MMWR* 2002, 51:1–48.

This is a great paper that discusses the different testing options for chlamydia. It also gives details and background behind the Centers for Disease Control and Prevention screening recommendations.

19. Gaydos CA: Nucleic acid amplification test for gonorrhea and chlamydia: practice and applications. *Infect Dis Clin N Am* 2005, 19:367–386.

20. Watson EJ, Templeton A, Russell I, *et al*.: The accuracy and efficacy of screening tests for Chlamydia trachomatis: a systematic review. *J Med Microbol* 2002, 51:1021–1031.

21. Steece R: *Chlamydia Testing Technologies. Infertility Prevention Project*. Bethesda: Centers for Disease Control and Prevention; 2004.

22. Persson K: The role of serology, antibiotic susceptibility testing and serovar determination in genital chlamydial infections. *Best Pract Res Clin Obstet Gynecol* 2002, 16:801–814.

23. Hoebe CJ, Rademaker CW, Brouwers EE, *et al*.: Acceptability of self-taken vaginal swabs and first-catch urine samples for the diagnosis of urogenital *Chlamydia trachomatis* and *Neisseria gonorrhoeae* with an amplified DNA assay in young women attending a public health sexually transmitted disease clinic. *Sex Transm Dis* 2006, 33:491–495.

24. Schachter J, McCormack WM, Chernesky MA, *et al*.: Vaginal swabs are appropriate specimens for diagnosis of genital tract infection with *Chlamydia trachomatis*. *J Clin Microbiol* 2003, 41:3784–3789.

25. Scholes D, Stergachis A, Heidrich FF, *et al*.: Prevention of pelvic inflammatory disease by screening for cervical chlamydial infection. *N Engl J Med* 1996, 334:1362–1366.

26. Martin DH, Mroczkoswki TF, Dalu ZA, *et al*.: A controlled trial of a single dose of azithromycin for the treatment of chlamydial urethritis and cervicitis. *N Engl J Med* 1992, 327:921–925.

27. Adair CD, Gunter M, Stovall TG, *et al*.: Chlamydia in pregnancy: a randomized trial of azithromycin and erythromycin. *Obstet Gynecol* 1998, 91:165–168.

28. Bush MR, Rosa C: Azithromycin and erythromycin in the treatment of cervical chlamydial infection during pregnancy. *Obstet Gynecol* 1994, 84:61–63.

29. Kacmar J, Cheh E, Montagno A, Peipert JF: A randomized trial of azithromycin versus amoxicillin for the treatment of Chlamydia trachomatis in pregnancy. *Infect Dis Obstet Gynecol* 2001, 9:197–202.

30. Jacobson GF, Autry AM, Kirby RS: A randomized controlled trial comparing amoxicillin and azithromycin for the treatment of *Chlamydia trachomatis* in pregnancy. *Am J Obstet Gynecol* 2001, 184:1352–1354.

31. Centers for Disease Control and Prevention. Expedited partner therapy in the management of sexually transmitted diseases. Atlanta: US Department of Health and Human Services; 2006.

32. Hillis SD, Owens M, Marchbanks PA, *et al.:* Recurrent chlamydial infections increase the risks of hospitalization for ectopic pregnancy and pelvic inflammatory disease. *Am J Obstet Gynecol* 1997, 196:103–107.

33. Centers for Disease Control and Prevention: HIV prevention through early detection and treatment of other sexually transmitted diseases-United States. *MMWR Morb Mortal Wkly Rep* 1998, 47(RR-12):13–15.

34. Marrazzo JM, Celum CL, Hillis SD, *et al.:* Performance and cost-effectiveness of selective screening criteria for Chlamydia trachomatis infection in women: implications for a national chlamydia control strategy. *Sex Transm Dis* 1997, 24:131–141.

35. Hu D, Hook EW, Goldie SJ: The impact of natural history parameters on the cost-effectiveness of Chlamydia trachomatis screening strategies. *Sex Transm Dis* 2006, 33:428–436.

36. Roberts TE, Robinson S, Barton P, *et al.:* Screening for Chlamydia trachomatis: a systematic review of the economic evaluations and modeling. *Sex Transm Infect* 2006, 82:193–200.

37. US Preventive Services Task Force: Screening for chlamydial infection: recommendations and rationale. *Am J Prev Med* 2001, 20(Suppl):90–94.

8 Human Papillomavirus and Genital Warts

Francisco A. R. Garcia and Amy L. Mitchell

- Human papillomavirus is a ubiquitous viral pathogen that infects that vast majority of sexually active individuals at some point in their lives.
- Most immunologically intact individuals will clear the infection spontaneously without intervention.
- Genital warts are the consequence of infection with low oncogenic risk human papillomavirus types 6 and 11.
- Among the variety of efficacious treatments for genital warts, selection should be guided by availability, patient preference, and provider experience.
- Primary prevention with the prophylactic quadrivalent human papillomavirus vaccination is recommended for all 11- to 12-year-old girls and should be considered up to 18 years of age.

Condyloma acuminata is the term used to describe benign epithelial or fibroepithelial tumors of the skin and contiguous mucous membranes caused by human papillomavirus (HPV). Condyloma acuminata, or genital warts, tend to occur as multiple lesions that may coalesce to form large masses in the vulvar, vaginal perineal, or anal areas.

Condyloma acuminata were first described in 25 AD by Celsius, but an understanding of the etiology of this condition is relatively recent. In 1907, skin warts were experimentally produced by inoculation of extracts of penile warts into nongenital epithelium. However, as recently as the 1960s, dirt and genital secretions were still being implicated in the development of genital warts. In 1949, electron microscopy demonstrated the presence of viral particles in wart tissue, suggesting its etiology, and sexual transmission of genital warts was confirmed in 1954. More recently, the identification of multiple HPV types using recombinant DNA analysis has led to the conclusion that certain types have predilections for specific epithelial surfaces [1]. It is a small group of low oncogenic risk HPV types that are responsible for external genital warts.

Epidemiology

Human papillomavirus is probably the most common sexually transmitted infection worldwide. Each year in the United States more than 6 million people are infected with genital HPV.

Recent estimates suggest that at any one time approximately 15% of the US population—or nearly 20 million individuals—is infected, as evidenced by the recovery HPV DNA from genital specimens [2,3]. Nearly half of these infections occur among individuals between 15 and 25 years of age, in which the point prevalence can range from 27% to 46% [4–7]. Conservative estimates suggest that at least half of all sexually active men and women are exposed to HPV at some point in their life, and approximately 80% of sexually active women will become infected by the age of 50 [8].

Genital HPV is transmitted by genital to genital contact, most commonly through vaginal or anal intercourse, and usually sometime shortly after the onset of insertional sexual activity. Among college-aged women, nearly 40% will be infected within 24 months of the initiation of sexual activity, and by 48 months, more than 50% will be infected [9]. At 5 to 7 years after beginning intercourse, 70% of women will have been exposed to the virus [10]. Transmission by non-insertional genital contact, although rare, has been reported in women who denied intercourse [9,11]. Rarely oral-genital and hand to genital transmission is possible [9]. Vertical transmission at delivery although not well characterized is probably uncommon, but may occur especially among women with large exophytic lesions in the setting of protracted labor and prolonged ruptured membranes. In such cases, infants may develop juvenile laryngeal or respiratory papillomatosis [12]. Laryngeal papillomatosis occurs in about 1 in 200,000 children under age

18 years, the vast majority before 4 years of age. This condition is characterized by HPV 6- and HPV 11-related, recurrent benign tumors of the upper airway that are occasionally obstructive and require surgical resection [13].

Genital warts are very common with more than 0.5 million new cases diagnosed annually, and as many as 1.4 million individuals in this United States have genital warts at any one time [14]. Peak attack rates occur in females from 15 to 24 years of age and in males between 20 to 29 years of age [14], and approximately 10% of men and women develop genital warts at some point in their lives. The overwhelming majority (> 90%) of genital warts is related to HPV 6 or HPV 11 infection, but 20% to 50% may be associated with a high-risk type coinfection [15]. Vulvar cancer may rarely occur as a result of malignant transformation of genital warts. Among younger women these tumors and their precursors are HPV (types 16, 18, and, rarely, 6 and 11) [16,17] related in most (60%–90%) of cases, whereas in older women, HPV infection is less commonly (10%) associated with malignancy [18].

Pathophysiology

Papillomaviridae are a family of DNA viruses that infect almost every mammalian species. HPV is an 8000 base-pair circular DNA molecule wrapped in a protein capsid [18]. More than 100 HPV types infect humans, and 40 of these HPV types infect the lower genital tract epithelium [18]. Viral types are grouped according to oncogenic potential as high or low risk. Infection with one of 15 carcinogenic or high-risk types (16, 18, 31, 33, 35, 39,45, 51, 52, 56, 58, 59, 68, 73, 82, 23, 53, and 66) is required for the development of nearly all cervical cancer [19], whereas low oncogenic risk types are 6, 11, 40, 42, 43, 44, 54, 61, 70, 72, 81. The vast majority of HPV infections are transient, spontaneously resolving within approximately 18 months. These transient infections result frequently in minor cytologic (atypical squamous cells or low-grade squamous intraepithelial lesion) or histologic (cervical intraepithelial neoplasia [CIN] 1) abnormalities [5,20–23]. A small proportion of such infections do not clear spontaneously, and women with persistent carcinogenic HPV have the greatest risk of developing truly premalignant cervical lesions and ultimately cervical cancer (Figure 8-1) [24,25].

Human papillomavirus type 16 is the most commonly associated with preneoplastic cervical disease, high-grade cervical intraepithelial neoplasia (CIN 2/3), or cancer [25]. HPV 16 persistence is more commonly associated with CIN 3, and viral persistence is inversely related to spontaneous resolution of dis-

ease [5,25]. Not all persistent infections progress to high-grade lesions, and high-grade disease does not always lead to cancer. Most low-grade lesions are caused by high-risk viral types, but are themselves transient and resolve spontaneously without intervention in immune competent individuals (75% for adults and 90% for adolescents) [21]. Usually the development of cancer from HPV acquisition to invasion can require up to 20 years [26]. Carcinogenesis requires an accumulation of host gene mutations leading to integration of portions of the viral genome into the host. When that occurs, HPV E6 and E7 proteins disrupt the host cell regulatory machinery leading to aberrant cellular replication, and inconsistent repair or elimination of damaged DNA [27,28].

The female genital tract contains specialized epithelium that may be particularly susceptible to HPV infection. The cervix, vaginal walls, and vulvar vestibule are lined by a glycogenated, non-cornified, and stratified squamous epithelium. The labia minora, clitoris, and interlabial sulci are lined by thinly keratinized epithelium but no hair follicles or sweat glands. The labia majora, mons pubis, and perineal areas are fully keratinized and contain hair follicles and sebaceous and sweat glands. HPV infection occurs with the entry of the virion into the basal layer of the epithelium through micro-abrasions that occur as a result of sexual activity. Genital warts are established after 10 to 12 weeks. The highest amount of viral DNA and viral antigen production takes place in the most differentiated superficial cells. The sequence of events in tissues in which latency occurs is not known. After infection, the viral DNA becomes stabilized as an independent, replicating episome within the epithelial cell nucleus.

Genital warts are highly infectious with a transmission risk of 65% [15]. The period of incubation ranges between 3 to 32 weeks, and most susceptible individuals will develop warts between 2 to 3 months [29]. Once established, genital warts may remain stable, increase/proliferate or regress spontaneously. Based on placebo-controlled trials, complete spontaneous regression rates are low (5%) in the short term [15], and recurrence within 3 months may be as high as 25 to 67% [30]. It is not yet understood the proportion of infections that are cleared spontaneously and those that may remain latent, nor are the factors that are associated with these outcomes clear.

Diagnosis

The diagnosis of genital warts is usually made on the basis of history and careful physical examination of the lower genital tract. Patients typically complain of a palpable nonpainful genital lesions appearing 1 to 8 months after sexual exposure.

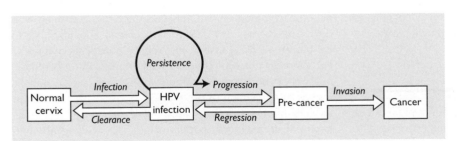

Figure 8-1. Natural history of human papillomavirus (HPV) and cervical cancer. (*Courtesy of* M. Schiffman.)

Warts are typically exophytic, moist, fleshy, pink or grey lesions of the epithelium of the vulva, labia, perianal region, and urethra (Figure 8-2A). Flat lesions can also occur in the vulva and may be hyperpigmented and raised (Figure 8-2B), or pink papular lesions found in the vagina, cervix, urethra, and anus. The location of warts is not typically tender, except for large lesions that may be susceptible to mechanical trauma and friction or may undergo bacterial superinfection. Biopsy is not required for diagnosis, but should be considered for atypical appearing lesions, when malignancy is suspected, for lesions in immune-compromised hosts, or those unresponsive and worsening with therapy. There is currently no role for HPV testing in the diagnosis or the management of genital warts [31].

Once an infection is established, the patient typically develops flat warts which may not change or even regress. The regression rate for external genital warts varies between 0% and 69% in placebo-treated patients. However, in up to 67% of patients, disease may recur, and in 45%, the infection may remain latent after treatment [32]. The genital warts may alternatively increase in size. Although most genital warts do not, in most cases, significantly enlarge during pregnancy, some patients do develop lesions that grow rapidly, becoming confluent over the vulva or even obstructing the birth canal. The theoretic cause of these enlargements may be related to the effect of increasing levels of progesterone. Eventually most external genital warts spontaneously resolve in the postpartum period. Malignant transformation of external genital warts although possible occurs relatively rarely and for unclear reasons.

The diagnosis of genital warts can usually be made on clinical grounds. There are important pathologic entities that may have similar presentations and differential diagnosis (Figure 8-3) should include the following considerations. A common error made in the diagnosis of genital warts is to confuse it with micropapillomatosis labialis; a normal anatomic variant characterized by small finger-like projections present on the medial aspect of the labial minora near the junction with the hymenal ring. By contrast condyloma lata caused by *Treponema pallidum* are broad-based, smooth, moist, multiple lesions that are heavily populated with spirochetes because they represent a manifestation of secondary

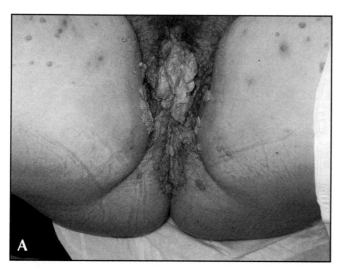
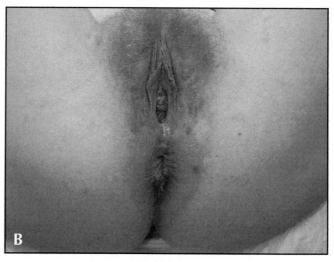

Figure 8-2. Warts are typically exophytic, moist, fleshy, pink or grey lesions of the epithelium of the vulva, labia, perianal region, and urethra (**A**). Flat lesions can also occur in the vulva and may be hyperpigmented and raised (**B**), or pink papular lesions found in the vagina, cervix, urethra, and anus. (*Courtesy of* K. Hatch.)

Differential Diagnosis of Genital Warts

Condition	Common	Description
Micropapillomatosis labialis	Yes	Papillary lesions on the epithelium of labia minor at junction with the hymen
Condyloma lata	No	Broad-based, raised lesions with smooth surface; moist; secondary to syphilis
Nevus, melanoma	Yes	Painful vesicular eruption with an erythematic base; may be ulcerated
Seborrheic keratoses	No	Raised on flat, dark-colored lesion
Giant condyloma	No	Hypertrophied lesion with rough surface; occurs in women older than 50 years
Molluscum contagiosum	Yes	Umbilicated yellowish papules with central waxy core
Bowenoid papulosis	No	Rough papules, 2–4 mm, flesh-colored to reddish-brown; resists treatment
Squamous cell carcinoma	No	Red, firm nodule forming shallow ulcer with indurated border

Figure 8-3. Differential diagnosis of genital warts.

syphilis. Any ulcerated lesion other than classic herpes simplex virus infection requires biopsy, whereas umbilicated lesions may be molluscum contagiosum.

Women with this clinical presentation should have a careful inspection of the entire vulva, perineum, and perianal area as well as the vagina and cervix. Additionally, screening should be performed for other sexually transmitted infections as well as for cervical cancer and its precursors.

Therapy

The recommendations for the treatment of genital warts provided by the Centers for Disease Control and Prevention are listed in Figure 8-4 [31]. The treatment of genital warts should be guided by the preference of the patient, the available resources, and the experience and knowledge of the health care provider. Factors that influence the selection of treatment modality include the size and number of warts, wart morphology, patient preference, cost of therapy, convenience, side effects, and provider experi-

ence. Therapeutic approaches may be divided into three broad categories: antiproliferative, immune therapies, and ablative or excisional modalities. Consistently, clinical studies demonstrated that available therapeutic techniques are 22% to 94% effective in clearing exophytic genital warts and that recurrence rates are high. In all cases the goals of therapy for external genital warts are removal of the lesion, amelioration of signs and symptoms and cosmesis.

Antiproliferative agents such as podophyllin and podophyllotoxin work by interfering with the host cellular mechanisms associated with keratinocyte differentiation and involved in HPV replication. These agents are widely used as cost effective first-line treatments for genital warts, with cure rates of 70% to 80% at 4 weeks for first-time use [14].

A variety of immune therapies have been used for the treatment of genital warts, although currently only the topical immune response modulator imiquimod is in common use. This agent acts by inducing a Th-1 cellular immune response. Imiquimod is associated with cure rates of more than 75% in women over 1 to 3 months [30]. This therapy is relatively

Centers for Disease Control and Prevention Recommendations for Treatment of Genital Warts: 2006

Patient-directed

Podofilox 0.5% solution/gel	Apply topically BID for 3 days, followed by 4 days off; repeat up to four cycles
Imiquimod 5% cream	Apply topically at bedtime three times per week for up to 16 weeks
Clinician-directed	
Podophyllin resin 10%–25%	Apply sparingly to lesions and allow to air dry; repeat weekly
Trichloroacetic acid/bichloracetic acid 10%–25%	Apply sparingly to lesions and air dry
Cryotherapy	Using liquid nitrogen or cryoprobe to lesion every 2 to 3 weeks
Surgical	Excision, curettage, or electrosurgical destruction

Figure 8-4. Centers for Disease Control and Prevention recommendations for treatment of genital warts. BID—twice daily. (*Data from* Centers for Disease Control and Prevention.)

American Cancer Society Recommendations for Human Papillomavirus Vaccine Use [36]

Routine HPV vaccination is recommended for girls ages 11 through 12

Girls as young as 9 years of age may receive HPV vaccination

HPV vaccination is also recommended for girls 13 through 18 years of age to catch up on missed vaccine or complete the vaccination series

There are currently insufficient data [1] to recommend for or against universal vaccination for women aged 19 through 26 in the general population; a decision about whether a woman aged 19 to 26 years should receive the vaccine should be based on an informed discussion between the woman and her health care provider regarding her risk of HPV exposure and potential benefit from vaccination; ideally, the vaccine should be administered before potential exposure to genital HPV through sexual intercourse, because the potential benefit is likely to diminish with increasing number of lifetime sexual partners

HPV vaccination is not currently recommended for women over the age of 26 and males

Screening for cervical intraepithelial neoplasia and cancer should continue in vaccinated and unvaccinated women according to current American Cancer Society early detection guidelines

Figure 8-5. American Cancer Society recommendations for human papillomavirus (HPV) vaccine use [1].

expensive compared with antiproliferative agents, but may be particularly useful for recalcitrant or recurrent disease.

Excisional or ablative therapies using electrical surgical approaches, laser ablation, or cryo destruction offer important benefits to women with large volume disease and disease that is refractory to alternative medical modalities. With good surgical technique, cosmetic results are excellent. Although comparatively better, recurrence rates continue to be significantly elevated.

Treatment is not recommended for subclinical HPV infection, in the absence of genital warts or high-grade squamous disease of the lower genital tract, because of the high rate of spontaneous clearance.

Referral to a specialist with experience in lower genital tract HPV related disease should be considered for patients with large volume disease, those with potentially premalignant conditions (vaginal and vulvar intraepithelial neoplasia), for immune compromised and pregnant patients, and for lesions refractory to standard therapies especially when invasive malignancy must be excluded.

Prevention

Recent US Food and Drug Administration approval of a prophylactic quadrivalent HPV vaccine (Gardasil; Merck and Co., Whitehouse Station, NJ) has created new and practical opportunities for the primary prevention of genital warts. This recombinant vaccine is formulated from L1 protein products that self-assemble into virus-like particles resembling the outer viral capsid shell. Vaccination elicits a sustained type-specific immunologic response. Randomized placebo-controlled trials have shown that prophylactic vaccines for HPV types 6, 11, 16, and 18 prevented persistent infection and related CIN2/3 [33–35]. More importantly for this discussion, however, the quadrivalent vaccine has been demonstrated to protect against HPV 6- and HPV 11-related external genital warts and vulvar and vaginal neoplasia. Guidelines for the use of this vaccine have been recently published by the American Cancer Society (Figure 8-5) [36]. Currently, there are no clinical outcome data for males although this is expected in the near future. However, at this time, vaccination is not recommended for this group.

In 3 years of follow-up, in subjects who completed the vaccination regimen and did not violate the protocol and who had no virologic evidence of infection with the respective HPV vaccine type at study entry through 1 month after the third vaccine dose (vaccine = 2261 vs placebo = 2279), vaccine efficacy was 100% for preventing HPV 6-, 11-, 16-, and 18-related external genital warts or vulvar/vaginal intraepithelial neoplasia of any grade [37].

An intent-to-treat analysis also was conducted to estimate the overall impact of Gardasil with respect to HPV 6-, 11-, 16-, and 18-related cervical and other genital disease in all women who were randomized into the trials and received at least one dose of vaccine. The overall vaccine impact on prevalent disease was estimated among women regardless of baseline HPV 6, 11, 16, or 18 PCR status (ie, current infection) and serostatus (ie, prior infection). The majority of CIN and lower

genital disease (ie, warts, vulvar intraepithelial neoplasia and vaginal intraepithelial neoplasia) detected in the group that received Gardasil occurred as a consequence of HPV infection that was present at enrollment. The efficacy for HPV 6-, 11-, 16-, and 18-related CIN or adenocarcinoma in situ was 55% [37]. More significant for this discussion, an efficacy of 73% was observed for HPV 6-, 11-, 16-, 18-related anogenital and vaginal lesions [37].

The exact duration of HPV vaccine-induced immunity and therefore long-term efficacy of vaccination is uncertain. It is equally unclear where and under what conditions booster vaccination may be necessary. Nevertheless, the quadrivalent vaccine creates new and practical opportunities for the primary prevention of HPV infection and its sequelae. For the first time women have realistic options for the prevention of HPV-related disease, beyond the recommendation of sexual abstinence or consistent condom use (which may decrease genital warts risk by 60%–70%) [38]. In this post-vaccine environment, the challenge is to provide the broadest rational vaccine coverage to the largest number of people and to do so in a way that is economical and achieves the greatest public health impact.

References

1. zur Hausen H, Meinhof W, Scheiber W, Bornkamm GW: Attempts to detect virus-specific DNA in human tumors. I. Nucleic acid hybridizations with complementary RNA of human wart virus. *Int J Cancer* 1974, 13:650–656.

2. Cates W, Jr.: Estimates of the incidence and prevalence of sexually transmitted diseases in the United States. American Social Health Association Panel. *Sex Transm Dis* 1999, 26(Suppl):S2–S7.

3. Koutsky L: Epidemiology of genital human papillomavirus infection. *Am J Med* 1997, 102:3–8.

4. Bauer HM, Ting Y, Greer CE, et al.: Genital human papillomavirus infection in female university students as determined by a PCR-based method. *JAMA* 1991, 265:472–477.

5. Ho GY, Bierman R, Beardsley L, et al.: Natural history of cervicovaginal papillomavirus infection in young women. *N Engl J Med* 1998, 338:423–428.

6. Kulasingam SL, Hughes JP, Kiviat NB, et al.: Evaluation of human papillomavirus testing in primary screening for cervical abnormalities: comparison of sensitivity, specificity, and frequency of referral. *JAMA* 2002, 288:1749–1757.

7. Richardson H, Kelsall G, Tellier P, et al.: The natural history of type-specific human papillomavirus infections in female university students. *Cancer Epidemiol Biomarkers Prev* 2003, 12:485–490.

8. Schootman M, Jeffe DB, Baker EA, Walker MS: Effect of area poverty rate on cancer screening across US communities. *J Epidemiol Community Health* 2006, 60:202–207.

9. Winer RL, Lee SK, Hughes JP, et al.: Genital human papillomavirus infection: incidence and risk factors in a cohort of female university students. *Am J Epidemiol* 2003, 157:218–226.

10. Moscicki AB, Hills N, Shiboski S, et al.: Risks for incident human papillomavirus infection and low-grade squamous intraepithelial lesion development in young females. *JAMA* 2001, 285:2995–3002.

11. Rylander E, Ruusuvaara L, Almstromer MW, et al.: The absence of vaginal human papillomavirus 16 DNA in women who have not experienced sexual intercourse. *Obstet Gynecol* 1994, 83:735–737.

12. Derkay CS, Darrow DH: Recurrent respiratory papillomatosis of the larynx: current diagnosis and treatment. *Otolaryngol Clin North Am* 2000, 33:1127–1142.

13. Lele SM, Pou AM, Ventura K, et al.: Molecular events in the progression of recurrent respiratory papillomatosis to carcinoma. *Arch Pathol Lab Med* 2002, 126:1184–1188.

14. Monteiro EF, Lacey CJ, Merrick D: The interrelation of demographic and geospatial risk factors between four common sexually transmitted diseases. *Sex Transm Infect* 2005, 81:41–46.

15. Lacey CJ, Lowndes CM, Shah KV: Burden and management of non-cancerous HPV-related conditions: HPV-6/11 disease. *Vaccine* 2006, 24(Suppl 3):S35–S41.

16. *Monographs on the Evaluation of Carcinogenic Risks to Humans*, vol 90. Lyon: International Agency for Research; 2007.

17. Tavassoli F, Devilee P: WHO classification of tumour, pathology and genetics of tumors of the breast and female genital organs. In *Monographs on the Evaluation of Carcinogenic Risks to Humans*. Lyon: International Agency for Research; 2003.

18. Munoz N, Castellsague X, de Gonzalez AB, Gissmann L: HPV in the etiology of human cancer. *Vaccine* 2006, 24(Suppl):S1–S10.

19. Munoz N, Bosch FX, de Sanjose S, et al.: Epidemiologic classification of human papillomavirus types associated with cervical cancer. *N Engl J Med* 2003, 348:518–527.

20. Cuschieri KS, Cubie HA, Whitley MW, et al.: Multiple high risk HPV infections are common in cervical neoplasia and young women in a cervical screening population. *J Clin Pathol* 2004, 57:68–72.

21. Moscicki AB, Shiboski S, Hills NK, et al.: Regression of low-grade squamous intra-epithelial lesions in young women. *Lancet* 2004, 364:1678–1683.

22. Winer RL, Kiviat NB, Hughes JP, et al.: Development and duration of human papillomavirus lesions, after initial infection. *J Infect Dis* 2005, 191:731–738.

23. Woodman CB, Collins S, Winter H, et al.: Natural history of cervical human papillomavirus infection in young women: a longitudinal cohort study. *Lancet* 2001, 357:1831–1836.

24. Nobbenhuis MA, Walboomers JM, Helmerhorst TJ, et al.: Relation of human papillomavirus status to cervical lesions and consequences for cervical-cancer screening: a prospective study. *Lancet* 1999, 354:20–25.

25. Wright TC, Jr., Schiffman M: Adding a test for human papillomavirus DNA to cervical-cancer screening. *N Engl J Med* 2003, 348:489–490.

26. Hildesheim A, Hadjimichael O, Schwartz PE, et al.: Risk factors for rapid-onset cervical cancer. *Am J Obstet Gynecol* 1999, 180:571–577.

27. Duensing S, Munger K: Mechanisms of genomic instability in human cancer: insights from studies with human papillomavirus oncoproteins. *Int J Cancer* 2004, 109:157–162.

28. Munger K, Howley PM: Human papillomavirus immortalization and transformation functions. *Virus Res* 2002, 89:213–228.

29. Reidy PM, Dedo HH, Rabah R, et al.: Integration of human papillomavirus type 11 in recurrent respiratory papilloma-associated cancer. *Laryngoscope* 2004, 114:1906–1909.

30. Lacey CJ: Therapy for genital human papillomavirus-related disease. *J Clin Virol* 2005, 32(Suppl 1):S82–S90.

31. Workowski KA, Berman SM: Sexually transmitted diseases treatment guidelines: 2006. *MMWR Recomm Rep* 2006, 55:1–94.

32. Ferenczy A, Mitao M, Nagai N, et al.: Latent papillomavirus and recurring genital warts. *N Engl J Med* 1985, 313:784–788.

33. Koutsky LA, Ault KA, Wheeler CM, et al.: A controlled trial of a human papillomavirus type 16 vaccine. *N Engl J Med* 2002, 347:1645–1651.

34. Mao C, Koutsky LA, Ault KA, et al.: Efficacy of human papillomavirus-16 vaccine to prevent cervical intraepithelial neoplasia: a randomized controlled trial. *Obstet Gynecol* 2006, 107:18–27.

35. Villa LL, Costa RL, Petta CA, et al.: Prophylactic quadrivalent human papillomavirus (types 6, 11, 16, and 18) L1 virus-like particle vaccine in young women: a randomised double-blind placebo-controlled multicentre phase II efficacy trial. *Lancet Oncol* 2005, 6:271–278.

36. Saslow D, Castle PE, Cox JT, et al.: American Cancer Society Guideline for human papillomavirus (HPV) vaccine use to prevent cervical cancer and its precursors. *CA Cancer J Clin* 2007, 57:7–28.

37. Garland SM, Hernandez-Avila M, Wheeler CM, et al.: Quadrivalent vaccine against human papillomavirus to prevent anogenital diseases. *N Engl J Med* 2007, 356:1928–1943.

38. Manhart LE, Koutsky LA: Do condoms prevent genital HPV infection, external genital warts, or cervical neoplasia? A meta-analysis. *Sex Transm Dis* 2002, 29:725–735.

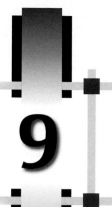

9 Herpes Simplex Virus Infections in Women

Rodney K. Edwards and Patrick Duff

- Herpes simplex virus infects regional sensory nerves and establishes a latent infection. Reactivation and recurrent infections may occur thereafter for the duration of the life of the host.
- Genital herpes is transmitted most often during periods of asymptomatic viral shedding.
- The diagnosis of genital herpes can be made by viral culture, polymerase chain reaction, Tzanck smear, or Papanicolaou smear. Laboratory confirmation of first-episode infections is recommended.
- Treatment of genital herpes in immunocompetent patients is recommended for first-episode but not necessarily recurrent infections. Patients who have frequent recurrences should be considered for chronic suppressive therapy.
- Patient education, especially regarding the importance of asymptomatic viral shedding, is paramount in preventing the spread of genital herpes.

Classification

Genital herpes simplex virus (HSV) infection is designated as primary, initial-nonprimary, or recurrent. A primary infection occurs when antibodies to HSV-1 and HSV-2 are absent at the time the patient acquires genital HSV. Initial nonprimary episodes occur when antibodies are present at the time of HSV acquisition but are directed at the other viral type (eg, a patient contracting a genital HSV-2 infection who has antibodies against HSV-1). Recurrent infections result from reactivation of genital HSV from a latent infection in regional sensory nerve ganglia. The viral type that is recovered from lesions is the same as the serum antibody present.

A patient's first clinical presentation may be a recurrent infection because of the possibility of asymptomatic initial infection. In general, primary infections tend to be more severe than recurrent infections, and initial nonprimary infections usually are of intermediate severity. Because serologic studies are not routinely performed, genital herpes is categorized clinically as a first-episode infection or a recurrent infection.

Virology

Herpes simplex virus-1 and HSV-2 are two of the eight identified human herpesviruses. The other members of this family are varicella-zoster virus, cytomegalovirus, Epstein-Barr virus, and three recently described viruses: herpesvirus types 6, 7, and 8 [1].

Herpes simplex virus is a double-stranded DNA virus. Its genome is surrounded by an icosahedral protein capsid that is covered by a lipid-containing envelope [2]. This envelope is derived from host cell nuclear membrane. Embedded in the envelope are viral glycoproteins that mediate such activities as host cell receptor attachment and cell penetration. There is an approximately 50% homology between the HSV-1 and HSV-2 genomes.

Crossreactivity to the glycoproteins in the envelope is common, but one of these—glycoprotein G—is an exception, because it exhibits little crossreactivity between the two viral subtypes. This differentiation serves as the basis for several type-specific assays [3]. Clinically, however, the human antibody response is directed against epitopes within areas of homology between the HSV-1 glycoprotein G (gG1) and the HSV-2 glycoprotein G (gG2). This crossreactivity explains to some degree why initial nonprimary infections are typically less severe than primary infections.

Cutaneous surfaces and mucous membranes are penetrated by HSV, where the virus replicates at the site of contact and then seeds and infects sensory nerves. A latent infection is established in the sensory nerve ganglion. Reactivation and recurrent infections occur thereafter for the duration of the life of the host. The ability to cause latent infection is a characteristic of all herpesviruses.

Epidemiology

Historically, HSV-1 has been associated with orolabial infection and HSV-2 with genital infection [4]. However, both viruses may cause genital or oropharyngeal lesions, which are indistinguishable clinically. Although in some populations, HSV-1 has been reported to account for 30% to 40% of new cases of genital herpes [5], the clinical recurrence of genital HSV-1 is much less common than that of HSV-2 [6].

Genital tract disease spread by sexual contact is primarily the result of HSV-2. The prevalence of serum antibodies against this virus is on the rise in the United States. During the period 1988 to 1994, 21.9% of the population age 12 years or older was found to be seropositive for HSV-2 [7]. This represents a 30% increase since the period 1976 to 1980 and corresponds to 45 million cases of infection. Higher rates are associated with female gender, black or Hispanic race, older age, lower socioeconomic status, and greater number of lifetime sexual partners.

Most people who are seropositive for HSV-2 have no history of genital herpes infection. However, most patients with serologic evidence of HSV-2 infection shed this virus [8,9] whether or not a clinically evident infection has previously occurred.

Genital herpes is transmitted most often during periods of asymptomatic viral shedding [10,11••]. Transmission is more likely to occur from men to women and in nonusers of barrier contraception. Asymptomatic viral shedding also has been shown to occur more often during the first 3 months after acquisition of HSV-2 than during later periods [12].

The presence of herpes genital lesions facilitates the transmission of HIV [13–15]. Ulcers caused by herpes infection serve as portals of entry for HIV particles. Also, large numbers of CD4-positive lymphocytes are present in the base of genital herpes ulcers. Additionally, in the presence of concurrent infection with HIV and HSV, reciprocal enhancement of viral replication occurs [16]. This finding has led some authorities to recommend routine suppression for HSV infection in patients who are seropositive for HIV. In addition, the presence of chronic, slow-healing herpetic ulcers in HIV-positive patients is included among the Centers for Disease Control and Prevention AIDS case definition [17].

Clinical Presentation

After an incubation period of 3 to 7 days, primary genital herpes presents as multiple vesicles of the skin in the genital region. In women, the lesions may involve the vulva, urethra, vagina, and cervix. These vesicles usually start out as papules, then progress to vesicles and finally to ulcers (Figure 9-1). The lesions are characteristically painful. After 4 to 6 weeks, the lesions typically resolve without scarring [18]. Lesions on keratinized skin become crusted before reepithelializing, whereas those on mucosal epithelium do not. Viral particles are actively shed from these lesions. Tender inguinal adenopathy may accompany local symptoms and persist into the third week of illness. Constitutional symptoms, such as fever, malaise, headache, and myalgias, often accompany primary infections and occur within the first few days of the illness [19].

Recurrent episodes of genital herpes are less likely to be accompanied by constitutional symptoms. The duration of illness is typically less than 2 weeks, and there are fewer lesions. In a study by Corey et al. [19], patients with primary HSV-2 infections had an average of 15.5 lesions covering 517 mm² and 11.8 days of pain. Their counterparts with recurrent disease had, on average, 9.5 lesions that covered only 158 mm² and 8.7 days of pain. Additionally, recurrent infections are often unilateral. However, the lesions in recurrent genital herpes infections may still be painful, especially in women. Approximately half of patients report a prodrome before a recurrent infection that lasts a few hours to 2 days and that consists of hyperesthesia at the site of vesicle development. Rates of recurrence vary widely among patients and with time in individual patients. As stated previously, recurrent genital infection is much more common with HSV-2.

Meningitis, encephalitis, and disseminated infection have been reported with primary episodes of genital herpes. These complications are rare in immunocompetent patients.

Diagnosis

Many patients present with genital herpes infection after the vesicles have evolved into ulcerative lesions. Therefore, clinical diagnosis based on the classic presentation of multiple, small, grouped vesicles that are painful has a low sensitivity and specificity. Because of this finding and the social and future implications of making the diagnosis of genital herpes infection, first-episode infections should be confirmed by laboratory methods.

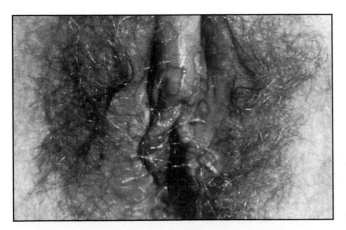

Figure 9-1. Typical clinical appearance of primary genital herpes simplex virus infection. (*Courtesy of* Glaxo-Wellcome.)

Although recent studies regarding the prevalence of HSV have used type-specific serologic assays, these assays are not widely available. Assays to detect antibody to HSV-1 or HSV-2 are commercially available, but they are not type specific [20]. Therefore, the gold standard for diagnosing acute HSV remains viral culture, the results of which can be reliably reported by 4 days after inoculation [21]. Culture of vesicular fluid gives the highest yield, and sensitivity decreases with the duration of active lesions.

The Tzanck smear is a rapid diagnostic test that can identify herpes infection. To perform this test, the base of a fresh ulcer or unroofed vesicle should be scraped and adherent cells spread on a glass slide. Staining with Wright's or Giemsa's stain reveals characteristic cytopathic changes, such as nuclear molding, multinucleated giant cells, cytoplasm with the appearance of "ground glass," or peripheral margination of nuclear chromatin (Figure 9-2) [22]. The Papanicolaou smear (Figure 9-3) may also show evidence of herpes infection. Neither of these tests can differentiate among HSV-1, HSV-2, and varicella-zoster virus infection, and neither has a sensitivity above 60%, making confirmation of positive findings by another diagnostic test, such as culture or polymerase chain reaction (PCR), advisable.

Polymerase chain reaction to detect HSV DNA probably is the most useful test available [22–24]. Results are available in a matter of hours rather than days, and PCR is at least equivalent to conventional culture techniques in identifying cases of HSV. The frequency of asymptomatic viral shedding of HSV particles, using PCR, has been shown to be eight times higher than that previously reported using culture alone.

Differential Diagnosis

Even though herpes simplex viruses are the most common cause of genital ulcers in developed countries, other possible etiologies should be considered. Syphilis, chancroid, lympho-

granuloma venereum, and granuloma inguinale are the other infections that typically cause genital ulcers. Other causes of genital ulceration not related to infection that should be considered are Behçet's disease, Crohn's disease, and trauma [3]. Attention to definitive diagnosis is especially important in patients infected with HIV. The clinical features used to discriminate between the etiologies of genital ulcers are often atypical in these patients.

Treatment

FIRST-EPISODE GENITAL HERPES
Acyclovir, a synthetic purine nucleoside analog, is available for topical, oral, or intravenous use. These preparations have not been compared directly in clinical trials, but evidence from three double-blind placebo-controlled trials indicates that systemic oral treatment is superior to topical therapy [25–27]. Topical therapy decreases the duration of viral shedding, time to complete healing of lesions, and local pain, but these effects are more pronounced with oral therapy. Additionally, only systemic therapy has been shown to decrease the duration of dysuria and the percentage of patients developing new crops of lesions after 48 hours of therapy.

Oral acyclovir is, therefore, the treatment of choice for most patients with first-episode genital herpes. The original recommended treatment regimen was 200 mg five times daily for 7 to 10 days. However, 400 mg three times daily for 7 to 10 days is equally effective and ensures greater compliance [28]. Higher doses, such as those used to treat herpes zoster (800 mg five times daily), are associated with gastrointestinal upset, but the standard doses to treat genital herpes are generally well tolerated. Most experts suggest treating until all lesions have healed rather than for an arbitrary length of time.

Intravenous acyclovir is normally reserved for patients who are hospitalized with severe first-episode genital herpes. Patients who are unable to tolerate oral medications because of vomiting, who develop complications such as disseminated

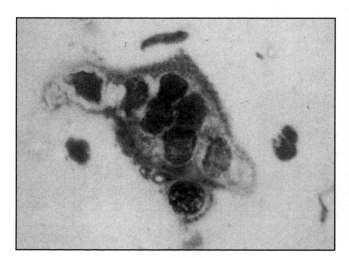

Figure 9-2. Tzanck smear showing the cytopathic changes associated with herpes simplex virus infection.

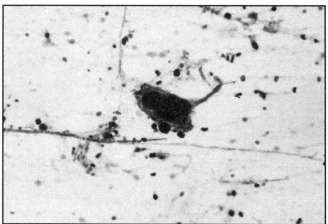

Figure 9-3. Papanicolaou smear showing cytopathic changes characteristic of herpes infection. (*Courtesy of* Nancy Hardt, MD.)

infection or encephalitis, or who are severely immunocompromised might also benefit from parenteral therapy.

Oral acyclovir is incompletely absorbed. Its L-valyl ester, valacyclovir, is more completely absorbed and is rapidly hydrolyzed to acyclovir in the intestinal wall and liver [29]. Valacyclovir is now available and licensed for treating first-episode genital herpes. A randomized, double-blind trial of 1000 mg of valacyclovir administered twice daily for 10 days showed it to be as effective and well tolerated as 200 mg of acyclovir administered five times daily for the same duration [30•].

Adverse effects reported with valacyclovir are similar to those seen with acyclovir. Although both are generally well tolerated, gastrointestinal disturbance, headache, and rash may occur. Concurrent use of cimetidine or probenecid may decrease the renal clearance of acyclovir and increase its plasma concentrations. Valacyclovir, in high doses, has been reported to cause a thrombotic thrombocytopenic purpura/hemolytic-uremic syndrome in some severely immunocompromised patients [29]. Comparison of the recommended treatment regimens is presented in Figure 9-4.

RECURRENT GENITAL HERPES

Treatment of recurrent genital herpes in an immunocompetent patient is optional. Although acyclovir has been shown to shorten the duration of viral shedding and duration of lesions, the duration of pain, itching, and the time to subsequent recurrence are not significantly affected [31]. A recent large trial of valacyclovir and acyclovir versus placebo for this indication showed a statistically significant difference for both of these drugs over placebo for pain duration [32]. However, the median values were 2 days for the active drugs and 3 days for placebo. The clinical significance of this difference is questionable. Valacyclovir at 1000 mg twice daily

[32] and 500 mg twice daily [33] for five days have been shown to be equivalent to 200 mg of acyclovir five times daily for 5 days in this setting.

Famciclovir, the oral prodrug of penciclovir, has been licensed recently for the treatment of recurrent genital herpes. The mechanism of action of penciclovir is similar to that of acyclovir. Compared with placebo, famciclovir has been shown to decrease significantly the duration of viral shedding, lesion persistence, and pain [34]. All dosage regimens studied (125 mg, 250 mg, and 500 mg all twice daily for 5 days) were effective. All of these regimens, if used, should be initiated by the patient at the first symptom of recurrence.

As stated previously, episodic treatment of recurrent genital herpes does not affect the time interval to next recurrence. Patients who have frequent recurrences (usually defined as six or more episodes per year) should be considered for chronic suppressive therapy. Acyclovir taken chronically has been shown to reduce significantly the number of recurrent genital herpes infections in patients who have frequent recurrences [35–37•]. For example, one study showed that acyclovir, 400 mg administered twice daily, was associated with an average of 1.8 recurrences over the course of a year, compared with 8.7 recurrences with placebo [37•]. Additionally, acyclovir suppressive therapy has been shown to be safe for up to 5 or 6 years without selection of resistant HSV strains [38,39•]. With continued use of acyclovir, recurrences become even less common than during the first year of suppression, and most patients become recurrence free.

Oral valacyclovir and famciclovir have proved to be similarly effective in suppression of recurrent genital herpes [40,41]. However, only valacyclovir shows a dosing schedule advantage over acyclovir. Figure 9-5 shows a comparison of suggested dosing regimens for suppression of recurrent genital herpes.

Recommended Oral Treatment Regimens for First-episode Genital Herpes with Cost Comparison

Drug	Dosage	Price (Per Month)
Acyclovir	200 mg five times daily for 7–10 days	$32.29–$49.50
Acyclovir	400 mg three times daily for 7–10 days	$37.60–$56.88
Valacyclovir	1000 mg twice daily for 7–10 days	$50.98–$72.83

Figure 9-4. Recommended oral treatment regimens for first-episode genital herpes with cost comparison.

Recommended Oral Treatment Regimens for Suppression of Recurrent Genital Herpes with Cost Comparison

Drug	Dosage	Price (Per Month)
Acyclovir	400 mg twice daily	$107.43–$113.77
Valacyclovir	500 mg once daily	$84.90
Famciclovir	250 mg twice daily	$191.00

Figure 9-5. Recommended oral treatment regimens for suppression of recurrent genital herpes with cost comparison.

Prevention

In addition to decreasing the number of clinical recurrences experienced by patients with genital herpes, suppressive therapy may prove beneficial in reducing its transmission. As alluded to previously, about 70% of HSV-2 infections are transmitted during periods of asymptomatic viral shedding [11•]. Suppressive therapy substantially reduces, but does not completely eliminate, subclinical shedding [42,43].

Patient education is essential in preventing transmission of genital herpes. Patients should be urged to use condoms even when they have no clinically apparent infection. Sexual contact should be avoided altogether during periods of recurrence. Additionally, patients should understand the possibility of genital transmissibility of orolabial herpes.

Vaccines hold promise for the future in terms of primary prophylaxis and immunotherapy of established infection. To date, however, no vaccines have been developed that are effective for either situation. Although vaccines have been shown to boost the immune response, no reduction in the frequency of recurrent infection has been demonstrated [44].

Special Considerations Related to Pregnancy

Although it is rare, neonatal herpes simplex virus infection carries a risk of mortality or major morbidity in excess of 40% [45]. Because vertical transmission is most likely to occur in an infant delivered vaginally through a birth canal with active infection, especially primary infection [46], Cesarean delivery is indicated when lesions are clinically apparent. However,

neonates have been documented to acquire herpes simplex virus infection in the presence of asymptomatic viral shedding in the parturient [47]. Suppressive therapy with acyclovir in gravidas with recurrent genital herpes has been investigated. Treatment with acyclovir, 400 mg three times daily, starting at 36 weeks' gestation significantly decreases the proportion of patients with clinically apparent lesions at the time of labor [48]. Therefore, the need for cesarean delivery for this indication is reduced. This strategy has been shown to be cost effective compared with cesarean delivery for all women presenting with genital herpes lesions in labor [49]. Figure 9-6 shows a management algorithm for pregnant patients with genital herpes.

Available evidence shows no increased risk for congenital defects in infants born to women receiving acyclovir during pregnancy [50]. Although there is no indication that the newer drugs valacyclovir and famciclovir pose more risk to the fetus, acyclovir remains the recommended drug for suppression of genital herpes in late gestation because it has been the most extensively studied.

Indications for Referral

Patients who experience complications of genital herpes infection, such as meningitis or encephalitis, may benefit from consultation with an infectious disease specialist. Referral to an obstetrician-gynecologist should be considered for pregnant patients with genital herpes, especially those having first-episode infections during the current pregnancy. Otherwise, genital herpes is a disease that can be managed effectively by primary care physicians.

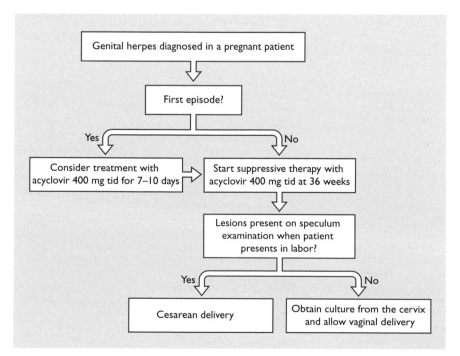

Figure 9-6. Algorithm for management of pregnant patients with genital herpes. tid—three times daily.

References

Papers of particular interest have been highlighted as follows:
- Of interest
- •• Of outstanding interest

1. Erlich KS: Management of herpes simplex and varicella-zoster virus infections. *West J Med* 1997, 166:211–215.

2. Corey L, Spear PG: Infections with herpes simplex viruses (first of two parts). *N Engl J Med* 1986, 314:686–691.

3. Schomogyi M, Wald A, Corey L: Herpes simplex virus-2 infection: an emerging disease? *Infect Dis Clin North Am* 1998, 12:47–61.

4. Nahmias AJ, Dowdle WR: Antigenic and biologic differences in herpesvirus hominis. *Prog Med Virol* 1968, 10:110–159.

5. Ross JDC, Smith IW, Elton RA: The epidemiology of herpes simplex types 1 and 2 infection of the genital tract in Edinburgh 1978–1991. *Genitourin Med* 1993, 69:381–383.

6. Lafferty WE, Coombs RW, Benedetti J, et al.: Recurrences after oral and genital herpes simplex virus infection: influence of site of infection and viral type. *N Engl J Med* 1987, 316:1444–1449.

7. Fleming DT, McQuillan GM, Johnson RE, et al.: Herpes simplex virus type 2 in the United States, 1976 to 1994. *N Engl J Med* 1997, 337:1105–1111.

8. Koutsky LA, Stevens CE, Holmes KK, et al.: Underdiagnosis of genital herpes by current clinical and viral isolation procedures. *N Engl J Med* 1992, 326:1533–1539.

9. Wald A, Zeh J, Selke S, et al.: Virologic characteristics of subclinical and symptomatic genital herpes infections. *N Engl J Med* 1995, 333:770–775.

10. Bryson Y, Dillon M, Bernstein DI, et al.: Risk of acquisition of genital herpes simplex virus type 2 in sex partners of persons with genital herpes: a prospective couple study. *J Infect Dis* 1993, 167:942–946.

11. •• Mertz GJ, Benedetti J, Ashley R, et al.: Risk factors for the sexual transmission of genital herpes. *Ann Intern Med* 1992, 116:197–202.

This prospective cohort study shows that the majority of transmission of genital herpes occurs during periods of asymptomatic viral shedding.

12. Koelle DM, Benedetti J, Langenberg A, et al.: Asymptomatic reactivation of herpes simplex virus in women after the first episode of genital herpes. *Ann Intern Med* 1992, 116:433–437.

13. Stamm WE, Handsfield HH, Rompalo AM, et al.: The association between genital ulcer disease and acquisition of HIV infection in homosexual men. *JAMA* 1988, 260:1429–1433.

14. Holmberg SB, Stewart JA, Geger AR, et al.: Prior HSV type 2 infection as a risk factor for HIV infection. *JAMA* 1988, 259:1048–1050.

15. Kreis J, Carael M, Meheus A: Role of sexually transmitted diseases in transmitting human immunodeficiency virus. *Genitourin Med* 1988, 64:1–2.

16. Heng MCY, Heng SY, Allen SG: Co-infection and synergy of human immunodeficiency virus-1 and herpes simplex virus-1. *Lancet* 1994, 343:255–258.

17. Centers for Disease Control: Revised classification system for HIV infection and expanded surveillance case definition for AIDS among adolescents and adults. *MMWR Morb Mortal Wkly Rep* 1992, 41(RR-17):15.

18. Landy HJ, Grossman JH: Herpes simplex virus. *Obstet Gynecol Clin North Am* 1989, 16:495–515.

19. Corey L, Adams HG, Brown ZA, et al.: Genital herpes simplex virus infections: clinical manifestations, course, and complications. *Ann Intern Med* 1983, 98:958–972.

20. Mertz GJ: Epidemiology of genital herpes infections. *Infect Dis Clin North Am* 1993, 7:825–839.

21. Yeager AS, Arrin AM, Hensleigh PA: The validity of reporting results of cultures for herpes simplex virus after four days. *J Reprod Med* 1982, 27:447–448.

22. Nahass GT, Goldstein BA, Zhu WY, et al.: Comparison of Tzanck smear, viral culture, and DNA diagnostic methods in detection of herpes simplex and varicella-zoster infection. *JAMA* 1992, 268:2541–2544.

23. Cone RW, Hobson AC, Brown Z, et al.: Frequent detection of genital herpes simplex virus DNA by polymerase chain reaction among pregnant women. *JAMA* 1994, 272:792–796.

24. Rogers BB, Josephson SL, Mak SK, et al.: Polymerase chain reaction amplification of herpes simplex virus DNA from clinical samples. *Obstet Gynecol* 1992, 79:464–469.

25. Corey L, Nahmias AJ, Guinan ME, et al.: A trial of topical acyclovir in genital herpes simplex virus infections. *N Engl J Med* 1982, 306:1313–1319.

26. Bryson YJ, Dillon M, Lovett M, et al.: Treatment of first episodes of genital herpes simplex virus infection with oral acyclovir: a randomized double-blind controlled trial in normal subjects. *N Engl J Med* 1983, 308:916–921.

27. Nilsen AE, Aasen T, Halsos AM, et al.: Efficacy of oral acyclovir in the treatment of initial and recurrent genital herpes. *Lancet* 1982, 2:571–573.

28. Drugs for non-HIV viral infections. *Med Lett* 1994, 36:27–32.

29. Valacyclovir. *Med Lett* 1996, 38:3–4.

30. • Fife KH, Barbarash RA, Rudolph T, et al.: Valacyclovir versus acyclovir in the treatment of first-episode genital herpes infection: results of an international, multicenter, double-blind, randomized clinical trial. *Sex Transm Dis* 1997, 24:481–486.

This multicenter, randomized, double-blind trial demonstrated valacyclovir to be as effective as acyclovir but with a more convenient dosing regimen.

31. Reichman RC, Badger GJ, Mertz GJ, et al.: Treatment of recurrent genital herpes simplex infections with oral acyclovir: a controlled trial. *JAMA* 1984, 251:2103–2107.

32. Tyring SK, Douglas JM, Corey L, et al.: A randomized, placebo-controlled comparison of oral valacyclovir and acyclovir in immunocompetent patients with recurrent genital herpes infections. *Arch Dermatol* 1998, 134:185–191.

33. Bodsworth NJ, Crooks RJ, Borelli S, et al.: Valacyclovir versus acyclovir in patient-initiated treatment of recurrent genital herpes: a randomised, double-blind clinical trial. *Genitourin Med* 1997, 73:110–116.

34. Sacks SL, Aoki FY, Diaz-Mitoma F, et al.: Patient-initiated, twice-daily oral famciclovir for early recurrent genital herpes: a randomized, double-blind multicenter trial. *JAMA* 1996, 276:44–49.

35. Straus SE, Takiff HE, Seidlin M, et al.: Suppression of frequently recurring genital herpes: a placebo-controlled double-blind trial of oral acyclovir. *N Engl J Med* 1984, 310:1545–1550.

36. Douglas JM, Critchlow C, Benedetti J, et al.: A double-blind study of oral acyclovir for suppression of recurrences of genital herpes simplex virus infection. *N Engl J Med* 1984, 310:1551–1556.

37.• Baker DA, Blythe JG, Kaufman R, *et al.*: One-year suppression of frequent recurrences of genital herpes with oral acyclovir. *Obstet Gynecol* 1989, 73:84–87.
This multicenter trial showed that acyclovir suppression of genital herpes recurrences was safe and effective for at least 1 year.

38. Goldberg LH, Kaufman R, Kurtz TO, *et al.*: Long-term suppression of recurrent genital herpes with acyclovir: a 5-year benchmark. *Arch Dermatol* 1993, 129:582–587.

39.• Fife KH, Crumpacker CS, Mertz GJ, *et al.*: Recurrence and resistance patterns of herpes simplex virus following cessation of > or = 6 years of chronic suppression with acyclovir. *J Infect Dis* 1994, 169:1338–1341.
In this study, the safety and efficacy of suppressive acyclovir were demonstrated for up to 6 years.

40. Mertz GJ, Loveless MO, Levin MJ, *et al.*: Oral famciclovir for suppression of recurrent genital herpes simplex virus infection in women: a multicenter, double-blind, placebo-controlled trial. *Arch Intern Med* 1997, 157:343–349.

41. Patel R, Bodsworth NJ, Woolley P, *et al.*: Valacyclovir for the suppression of recurrent genital HSV infection: a placebo controlled study of once daily therapy. *Genitourin Med* 1997, 73:105–109.

42. Wald A, Corey L, Cone R, *et al.*: Frequent genital herpes simplex virus 2 shedding in immunocompetent women: effect of acyclovir treatment. *J Clin Invest* 1997, 99:1092–1097.

43. Wald A, Zeh J, Barnum G, *et al.*: Suppression of subclinical shedding of herpes simplex virus type 2 with acyclovir. *Ann Intern Med* 1996, 124:8–15.

44. Straus SE, Wald A, Kost RG, *et al.*: Immunotherapy of recurrent genital herpes with recombinant herpes simplex virus type 2 glycoproteins D and B: results of a placebo-controlled vaccine trial. *J Infect Dis* 1997, 176:1129–1134.

45. Whitley R, Arvin A, Prober C, *et al.*: Predictors of morbidity and mortality in neonates with herpes simplex virus infections. *N Engl J Med* 1991, 324:450–454.

46. Brown ZA, Vontver LA, Benedetti J, *et al.*: Effects on infants of a first episode of genital herpes during pregnancy. *N Engl J Med* 1987, 317:1246–1251.

47. Brown ZA, Benedetti J, Ashley R, *et al.*: Neonatal herpes simplex virus infection in relation to asymptomatic maternal infection at the time of labor. *N Engl J Med* 1991, 324:1247–1252.

48. Scott LL, Sanchez PJ, Jackson GL, *et al.*: Acyclovir suppression to prevent cesarean delivery after first-episode genital herpes. *Obstet Gynecol* 1996, 87:69–73.

49. Randolph AG, Hartshorn RM, Washington AE, *et al.*: Acyclovir prophylaxis in late pregnancy to prevent neonatal herpes: a cost-effectiveness analysis. *Obstet Gynecol* 1996, 88:603–610.

50. Pregnancy outcomes following systemic prenatal acyclovir exposure: June 1, 1984–June 30, 1993. *MMWR Morb Mortal Wkly Rep* 1993, 42:806–809.

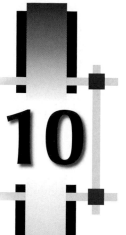

Pelvic Inflammatory Disease

10

Deborah Bartz

- Given the high disease prevalence and the long-term sequelae that can be reduced with prompt treatment, clinicians should have a high index of suspicion for pelvic inflammatory disease in patients with a wide spectrum of symptoms.
- Most cases of pelvic inflammatory disease are associated with more than one organism, which often includes *Chlamydia trachomatis*, *Neisseria gonorrhoeae*, and anaerobic and aerobic bacteria.
- Although there is a trend toward increased outpatient treatment of pelvic inflammatory disease, the clinician should choose a treatment option based on the patient, the clinical picture, and the medical environment in which they are practicing.
- Recent well-performed research on the association of pelvic inflammatory disease and the intrauterine device is reassuring, as there is good evidence that there is a slight increase in upper genital tract infection risk at the time of intrauterine device insertion only, and any risk of infection after the first 3 weeks of insertion is minimal.

Pelvic inflammatory disease (PID) is an acute infection in women located primarily within organs of the upper genital tract, including the uterus, fallopian tubes, and ovaries, with possible involvement of surrounding abdominal structures. The primary etiologic agents responsible for PID are sexually transmitted pathogens, including *Chlamydia trachomatis* and *Neisseria gonorrhoeae*, though nonsexually transmitted pathogens are often also involved. Given that sexually transmitted diseases (STDs) are the primary etiologic pathogens involved in PID, risk factors for the disease mimic risk factors associated with increased STD acquisition, primarily young age, multiple sexual partners, and poor use of barrier contraceptives. Although the exact incidence of PID is unknown, this disease has profound implications on the health of millions of women in the United States. Annually, PID accounts for 2.5 million outpatient visits, 350,000 emergency department visits, 200,000 hospitalizations, and 100,000 surgical procedures in the United States [1]. Long-term sequelae of PID, including infertility, chronic pelvic pain, and ectopic pregnancy also impose profound medical, economic, and emotional burden on women and their families.

The diagnosis of PID is not easy because the disease represents a spectrum of infection and resulting symptomatology—from subacute disease to surgical emergencies easily confused with other diagnoses. Given the high disease prevalence and the long-term sequelae that can be reduced with prompt diagnosis and treatment, clinicians should have a high index of suspicion for PID diagnosis and treatment. Therapy options are multiple, though all are directed at polymicrobial pathogens that include *N. gonorrhoeae* and *C. trachomatis* coverage. Medical professionals in many subspecialties can implement disease prevention through primary, secondary, and tertiary strategies in order to decrease the disease and economic burden of PID. This chapter will also address special concerns specific to PID including tubo-ovarian abscesses, intrauterine device (IUD) use and its effect on upper genital tract infections, and adolescents as a high-risk population with special prevention, diagnosis, and treatment needs.

Epidemiology and Risk Factors

Pelvic inflammatory disease is a disease that affects primarily young, sexually active, reproductive age women. The exact estimates of PID incidence and prevalence in the United States are unclear as 1) only two thirds of clinically diagnosed cases of PID demonstrate laparoscopic evidence of the disease [2]; 2) an unknown number of PID cases are erroneously diagnosed as some other disease; and 3) an unknown number of PID cases are a "silent" subclinical disease only to be diagnosed during an infertility or pelvic pain work-up. Estimates by the United States Center for Disease Control (CDC) indicate the PID incidence has been declining since the 1970s, with recent estimates of 780,000 new cases of PID diagnosed annually [3•].

As STDs, particularly *N. gonorrhoeae* and *C. trachomatis* are the most common etiologic agents for PID. Risk factors for developing PID are similar to those for STD acquisition. Demonstrated PID risk factors are listed in Figure 10-1. Being sexually active, particularly at a young age, is the greatest risk factor, as celibate women and women in long-standing monogamous relationships rarely develop PID. High-risk sexual behaviors such as intercourse with multiple sexual partners or absence of barrier contraceptives also increase PID risk. Current or prior STDs or PID further characterize high-risk populations.

Other risk factors have been proposed but remain unresolved regarding clear PID causality, including race, douching, or frequency of intercourse (Figure 10-1). The connection between bacterial vaginosis as a causative agent for STDs or PID has been debated and studied with conflicting results. No clear link has been demonstrated to date in the literature.

Pathogenesis and Microbiology

The normal, healthy vaginal flora contains a variety of potentially pathogenic bacteria including streptococci, staphylococci, enterobacteriaceae, and a variety of anaerobes. The endocervical canal acts as a barrier protecting the sterile upper genital tract from the organisms in the vagina. PID is thought to result from direct canalicular spread of organisms from the vagina and endocervix to the endometrium and fallopian tubes. *N. gonorrhoeae* and *C. trachomatis* commonly cause cervicitis. Between 10% and 40% of women not treated for their gonococcal or chlamydial cervicitis develop clinical manifestations of acute PID, and even higher rates of subclinical infection are diagnosed in these women by endometrial biopsies [4].

Four factors could contribute to the ascent of these bacteria to result in PID. First, uterine instrumentation, such as IUD insertion, facilitates upward spread of vaginal and cervical bacteria. Second, the hormonal changes that occur during menses, as well as the act of menstruation itself, lead to cervical alterations that may result in loss of a mechanical barrier preventing ascent. This is compounded by the fact that the bacteriostatic effect of cervical mucus is lowest at the onset of menses, which may explain why up to 75% of cases of PID occur within seven days of menses [5]. Third, retrograde menstruation may favor ascent of microbes to the tubes and peritoneum. Last, individual organisms may have potential virulence factors associated with the pathogenesis of acute chlamydial and gonococcal PID.

Most cases of PID are associated with more than one organism. The proportion of women with PID due to the main inciting agents of *C. trachomatis* and *N. gonorrhoeae* varies widely depending on the population studied. In the United States, *C. trachomatis* has been recovered from the cervix of 5% to 40% of women diagnosed as having PID. *N. gonorrhoeae* has a particularly wide range of recovery rates among women with PID, with isolation rates from the cervix reported from 27% to 80% [6].

Apart from *C. trachomatis* and *N. gonorrhoeae*, a wide variety of anaerobic and aerobic bacteria have been isolated from the upper-genital tract in PID. This has important diagnostic implications because failure to isolate a sexually transmitted agent from the cervix does not rule out PID as the cause for the patient's symptoms. The most common anaerobic bacteria involved in the disease include *Bacteroides*, *Peptostreptococcus*, and *Peptococcus* species. The most common aerobic pathogens include *Gardnerella vaginalis*, *Streptococcus* species, *Escherichia coli*, and *Haemophilus influenzae*. Mycoplasmas have also been recovered from the genital tract, but their role in PID development is less clear. Bacterial vaginosis is more common among women with PID. However, this disease alone has not been shown to be responsible for the development of PID.

Chlamydia trachomatis and *N. gonorrhoeae* are intracellular pathogens that incite characteristic mucosal immune responses by producing various heat-shock proteins (HSPs). Specific HSPs are released when microbes or host mammalian cells are under attack. Chlamydial HSPs incite the patient's cellular and humoral immune responses. Because there is similarity between the bacteria's HSPs and the patient's HSPs, the immune response's attack on the microbes involves fallopian and endometrial epithelial cells. Due to the T-cell and B-cell mediated memory, repeated infections result in dramatically increased inflammatory reactions, resulting in increased tubal destruction. Immune responses focused in the endometrium can adversely affect implantation of the fertilized egg and development of the

Risk Factors for Pelvic Inflammatory Disease

Risk factors for STD acquisition

Age younger than 25 years

Young age at first coitus

New, multiple, or symptomatic partners

History of PID

Factors that have conflicting evidence of PID causality

Low socioeconomic class

Race

Unmarried status

High frequency of sexual intercourse

Coitus during menses

Vaginal douching

Bacterial vaginosis

IUD use

Cigarette smoking

Substance use

Figure 10-1. Risk factors for pelvic inflammatory disease (PID). IUD—intrauterine device; STD—sexually transmitted disease.

trophoblast and placenta. Keys to preventing such dynamic and long-lived immune sequelae include prevention of the initial ascending infection, expedited treatment of cervicitis and PID, and prevention of repeat infections of genital pathogens.

Diagnostic Methods

Pelvic inflammatory disease represents a spectrum of infection, so there is no single diagnostic gold standard and diagnosis is often difficult. The CDC highlighted this fact in their 2002 guidelines, which state that the clinical diagnosis of PID has anywhere from a 65% to 90% positive predictive value [7]. This means that clinicians are wrong when making this diagnosis in up to one in three patients due to the fact that many adjacent organ systems can produce symptoms that overlap with PID. The differential diagnosis includes gastrointestinal processes such as appendicitis, constipation or inflammatory bowel disease, renal disease such as cystitis and pyelonephritis, or other gynecologic etiologies including dysmenorrhea, ectopic pregnancy, or ovarian cysts. The difficult diagnosis is complicated by the fact that many women are found to have subclinical PID, defined as the presence of neutrophils and plasma cells seen histologically in endometrial tissue without clinical symptoms, usually diagnosed during an infertility work-up.

However, given the incidence of PID discussed above and the significant, even dangerous immediate and long-term sequelae of the disease, the index of suspicion for PID should be high, especially in high-risk populations. In recognizing this disease incidence and the low sensitivity of diagnostic measures, the guidelines for making the diagnosis of PID have become more lax. Therefore, empiric diagnosis and treatment is recommended for women with abdominal pain and at least one of the following: cervical, uterine or adnexal tenderness, oral temperature greater then 101°F, peripheral leukocytosis, abnormal cervical or vaginal discharge, presence of white blood cells in vaginal secretions, elevated erythrocyte sedimentation rate, or elevated C-reactive protein (Figure 10-2). The likelihood of PID increases with each additional clinical feature with which a patient presents.

In PID, a thorough patient history most often elicits dull abdominal pain, often greater with intercourse or menstruation and typically present for less then 3 weeks, fevers, and vaginal discharge. Dysuria, irregular vaginal bleeding, and nausea and vomiting are also common features. Classic exam findings include cervical or adnexal tenderness in the presence of elevated temperature, though only 50% of women with PID will have fever. Marked tenderness in the right upper quadrant may represent the 10% of women with PID who have perihepatitis (Fitz-Hugh-Curtis syndrome). Among women with severe clinical signs, more elaborate diagnostic evaluation is warranted to eliminate other diagnoses and prevent further morbidity. Diagnostic testing for PID includes general laboratory studies for signs of pregnancy and infection, culture and microscopy of cervical or vaginal secretions, and imaging studies, particularly transvaginal ultrasound and

pelvic CT. Transvaginal ultrasound is the best tool to assess inflamed or enlarged fallopian tubes, peritoneal fluid or pus, or adnexal masses suspicious for a tubo-ovarian abscess. CT scanning is helpful in assessing other organ systems, including the bowel, to rule out other etiologies of abdominal pain. The patient's sexual partner(s) should also be assessed. Repeat pelvic examination with evaluation of the cervix, uterus, and adnexa should be done within 3 or 4 weeks of completing treatment. Appropriate tests of cure for indicated infections should be obtained at that time in both the patient and her partner(s).

Treatment

Pelvic inflammatory disease is a complex syndrome involving a variety of offending organisms. As there are no reliable signs and symptoms of PID, as discussed above, empirical treatment is common. No single first-line therapeutic regimen exists for all patients with PID. Instead, several treatment options have been designed and studied to provide broad-spectrum antibiotic coverage of likely inciting pathogens, including C. trachomatis, N. gonorrhoeae, anaerobes, and streptococci. Meta-analyses have demonstrated few significant differences between the various regimens [8•,9]. The best regimen remains unproven, and the clinician should choose a treatment option based on the patient, the clinical picture, and the medical environment in which they are practicing. The CDC-recommended treatment options are summarized in Figure 10-3.

There has been a recent trend toward outpatient management for the majority of PID cases. This is due to, in part, improved efficacy of oral antibiotics as well as increased emphasis on cost-efficient medical practice. The CDC recommends that the decision to hospitalize for inpatient PID therapy be at the discretion of the clinician. Patients who are more likely to warrant hospital admission include those who are pregnant, do not respond to or tolerate outpatient therapy, have a surgical abdomen, are at risk for noncompliance of outpatient regimen such as adolescents, have concerning co-morbidities including immunodeficiency, have severe clinical illness, have a pelvic abscess, or patients in whom clinical follow-up within 72 hours of starting antibiotic treatment cannot be arranged [8•]. Should a patient be admitted, a minimum of 24 to 48 hours of hospitalization is necessary to assess response to therapy and to rule out other diagnoses. Parenteral antibiotics should be continued 24 to 48 hours after clinical improvement followed by an outpatient oral antibiotic course as outlined in Figure 10-3.

The safety and efficacy of outpatient PID therapy were validated in the PID Evaluation and Clinical Health (PEACH) study, a randomized trial in 831 women diagnosed with mild to moderate PID [10••,11]. Patients were randomized to receive inpatient therapy with cefoxitin IV for 48 hours and doxycycline orally for 14 days or to receive outpatient treatment with cefoxitin IM and single dose oral probenicid followed by doxycycline orally for 14 days. After a mean follow-up of 35 months, pregnancy rates were nearly equal between the two groups, as were rates of PID recurrence, chronic pelvic pain, and ectopic pregnancy. Ongoing follow-up of this cohort continues to assess the risks, benefits, and costs of inpatient versus outpatient treatment of PID.

In a patient receiving outpatient therapy, reevaluation is necessary within 48 to 72 hours of the initiation of treatment in order to assess the accuracy of the diagnosis and the response to therapy. This is necessary to decrease the occurrence of the long-term sequelae of PID. If no clinical improvement occurs within 72 hours of initial therapy, hospitalization with parenteral antibiotics and further diagnostic evaluation is recommended. Compliance with long courses of antibiotics is problematic for many patients. Therefore, regular outpatient follow-up and education may be necessary to encourage compliance with a full treatment course.

All antibiotic treatment options should be accompanied by sexual education on the acquisition and prevention of sexually transmitted infections, and a full STD work-up and hepatitis B vaccination should be offered at that time. HIV-infected women respond to the same antimicrobial regimens as noninfected patients, but may require surgical intervention more frequently [12]. HIV seropositivity alone is not a criteria requiring inpatient PID treatment. Treatment of the sexual partner(s) of a woman diagnosed with PID is imperative, and a woman's treatment is considered inadequate until her partner(s) is evaluated and treated. Most male partners are asymptomatically infected. If the patient's partner(s) is not treated, she is at risk for recurrent infection and PID sequelae. Furthermore, without proper evaluation and treatment, the sexual partners may unknowingly transmit infection to other women. Therefore, special arrangements should be made to coordinate care for male sexual partners of women with PID. Follow-up should be arranged with the patient within 3 to 4 weeks after completion of therapy to repeat a pelvic exam and to perform test of cure cultures on both the patient and her partner(s).

Complications and Public Health Consequences

The long-term sequelae associated with PID are common, often permanent, and occasionally lethal. These sequelae are related to the scarring and adhesions that result from the bacteria induced tissue damage as well as host inflammatory and immunologic responses to the infection. This scarring results in 10% of women becoming infertile, 30% developing chronic pelvic pain, and 5% developing an ectopic pregnancy after a single episode of PID.

Pelvic inflammatory disease is the leading cause of infertility in the United States, with clinical and subclinical disease resulting in tubal and endometrial dysfunction. Delayed treatment and repeat infections dramatically worsen future infertility from PID. Severity of disease and number of upper genital tract infections also predict pregnancy complications once pregnancy is achieved. A Swedish study found a decreased trend in normal live births as prior PID disease severity worsened and as the number of prior infections increased [13].

Centers for Disease Control and Prevention Recommended Pelvic Inflammatory Disease Diagnosis Criteria

Diagnosis should be made and empirical antibiotic therapy started for women with abdominal pain who have at least one of the following:

Cervical motion tenderness or uterine or adnexal tenderness

Oral temperature > 101°F (> 38°C)

Peripheral leukocytosis or left shift

Abnormal cervical or vaginal mucopurulent discharge

Presence of white blood cells on saline microscopy of vaginal secretions

Elevated erythrocyte sedimentation rate

Elevated C-reactive protein

Patients are considered confirmed cases of PID if they have pelvic pain and at least one of the following:

Acute or chronic endometritis or acute salpingitis on histologic evaluation of biopsy

Demonstration of *Neisseria gonorrhoeae* or *Chlamydia trachomatis* in the genital tract

Gross salpingitis visualized at laparoscopy or laparotomy

Isolation of pathogenic bacteria from a clean specimen from the upper genital tract

Inflammatory/purulent pelvic peritoneal fluid without another source

Figure 10-2. Centers for Disease Control and Prevention recommended pelvic inflammatory disease (PID) diagnosis criteria [8].

Close to one third of women with a history of symptomatic PID develop chronic pelvic pain as a result of adhesion formation and resulting organ tethering or fixation. This pain is often most severe when these fixed organs would otherwise have the freedom of movement, such as during intercourse, physical activity, or ovulation. Similar to tubal infertility, the rate of pelvic pain is proportional to the number and severity of prior PID episodes. Medical therapy with pain medication, oral contraceptives, or tricyclic antidepressants may provide some patients with relief. However, others will need adhesiolysis and even removal of the affected pelvic organs in attempts to alleviate pain.

Almost 100,000 ectopic pregnancies occur annually in the United States, 50 of which result in maternal death. Chow et al. [14] performed a case-control study which indicated that chlamydia-associated PID alone caused one half of these ectopic pregnancies. Furthermore, 10% to 15% of conceptions will be ectopic after laparoscopy proven mild to moderate PID and almost 50% after severe PID. This risk worsened with each recurrence of the upper genital tract infection.

Besides individual adverse outcomes, PID has societal implications as well. Primarily, PID is expensive. Annually PID accounts for 2.5 million outpatient visits, 200,000 hospitalizations, and 100,000 surgical procedures in the United States [1]. It accounts for one in every 60 medical consultations with each episode costing over $1100, leading to an estimated total cost of $1.88 billion for the treatment of PID in 1998 [3•]. Productivity analyses performed to study lifetime productivity losses attributable to PID demonstrate mean weighted productivity losses per case of acute PID at $649 (in year 2001 dollars) [15]. Taken together, the short- and long-term sequelae of PID necessitate prompt accurate diagnosis and appropriate therapy in an attempt to lessen the overall public health and economic consequences of PID.

Special Considerations in Pelvic Inflammatory Disease: Tubo-ovarian Abscess

Tubo-ovarian abscess (TOA) is a serious sequela that occurs in up to 30% of women admitted for PID [16] that is characterized as an inflammatory mass involving the fallopian tube, ovary, and adjacent structures such as the bowel or pelvic peritoneum. TOA also may develop apart from PID, such as after pelvic surgery or as a

Centers for Disease Control and Prevention Recommended Treatment Options for Pelvic Inflammatory Disease

Outpatient Management	Inpatient Management
Preferred treatment	Preferred treatment
Ofloxacin* 400 mg PO twice daily for 14 days or	Cefotetan 2 g IV every 12 hours or
Levofloxacin*† 500 mg PO once daily for 14 days ±	Cefoxitin 2 g IV every 6 hours +
Metronidazole‡ 500 mg PO twice daily for 14 days	Doxycycline* 100 mg IV or PO twice daily for 14 days
Or	Or
Ceftriaxone 250 mg IM once +	Clindamycin 900 mg IV every 8 hours +
Doxycycline* 100 mg PO twice daily for 14 days ±	Gentamicin 2 mg/kg IV once then 1.5 mg/kg IV every 8 hours +
Metronidazole‡ 500 mg PO twice daily for 14 days	Doxycycline* 100 mg PO twice daily for 14 days
Alternative treatment	Alternative treatment
Cefoxitin 2 g IV once + probenecid 1 g PO once ±	Ofloxacin* 400 mg IV every 12 hours or
Doxycycline* 100 mg PO twice daily for 14 days ±	Levofloxacin*† 500 mg IV once ±
Metronidazole‡ 500 mg PO twice daily for 14 days	Metronidazole‡ 500 mg IV every 8 hours until clinically improved +
	Doxycycline* 100 mg PO twice daily for 14 days
	Or
	Ampicillin/sulbactam 3 g IV every 6 hours +
	Doxycycline* 100 mg PO or IV every 12 hours until clinically improved +
	Doxycycline* 100 mg PO twice daily to complete 14 days

*Not recommended in pregnancy.
†Levofloxacin is not approved for patients younger than 18 years of age when effective alternatives are available.
‡The Centers for Disease Control and Prevention has downgraded the importance of anaerobic coverage so the addition of metronidazole is now only an option for regimens containing ofloxacin, ceftriaxone, or cefoxitin. Metronidazole use in patients with TOA is still recommended.

Figure 10-3. Centers for Disease Control and Prevention recommended treatment options for pelvic inflammatory disease [8,9]. IM—intramuscularly; IV—intravenously; PO—orally; TOA—tubo-ovarian abscess.

complication of an intra-abdominal process such as appendicitis or diverticulitis. TOA is an important manifestation of PID as intra-abdominal rupture of a TOA has been associated with mortality rates as high as 9%. Furthermore, long-term sequelae of TOA, which include infertility, pelvic pain, ectopic pregnancy, pelvic adhesive disease, sexual dysfunction, salpingitis isthmic nodosum, and chronic TOAs may develop in up to 25% of patients [17].

The microbiology of TOAs is similar to that of PID infections, as they are typically polymicrobial with a mixture of anaerobic, aerobic, and facultative bacteria. Usually this infection is caused by ascension from the vagina of STDs, particularly *N. gonorrhoeae* and *C. trachomatis*. These organisms enter the fallopian tube and destroy the epithelial tissues, resulting in purulent material that extrudes from the fimbriated ends of the tube. This purulent material then results in inflammation of the surrounding structures including the ovary, bowel, bladder, and pelvic sidewalls, resulting in adhesed tissues and abscess formation.

Patients classically present with fever, pelvic pain, and a pelvic mass. Pelvic imaging, particularly pelvic ultrasound or CT, aids in the diagnosis. The improvements in diagnostic imaging, broad-spectrum antibiotics, and minimally invasive surgical management have evolved treatment options away from major surgical debridement performed historically. Currently, in stable patients without evidence of abscess rupture, antibiotic therapy with inpatient PID regimens is appropriate (Figure 10-3). However, it should be noted that TOAs are slow to respond to antibiotic therapy and should be given 72 hours to demonstrate clinical improvement before the treatment is considered a failure. Percutaneous drainage through the help of interventional radiology is frequently being used to increase effectiveness of antibiotic therapy, either at the time of initiation or after 72 hours of failed therapy.

Special Considerations in Pelvic Inflammatory Disease: Intrauterine Contraceptive Device Use

The modern IUD is a highly effective contraceptive with a pregnancy prevention profile similar to that of tubal sterilization. Furthermore, levonorgestrel-releasing IUDs are proving to be successful alternative treatment options for gynecologic conditions such as menometrorrhagia, endometrial hyperplasias, endometriosis, adenomyosis, and primary dysmenorrhea. Despite the clear effective benefit of IUDs, these devices are underutilized, primarily because of concerns about increased PID risk in IUD users.

In a recent study, Grimes [18••], a leading epidemiologist in the field of obstetrics and gynecology, critically reviewed past and current research on IUDs and their resulting risk of PID (Figure 10-4). Based on his exhaustive review, Grimes concluded that until recently, most IUD research has been flawed by using inappropriate comparison groups, by overdiagnosis of PID in IUD users, and by inability of these studies to control for confounding effects of sexual behavior. Furthermore, in light of the variability of PID definitions researchers have had inconsistent findings and

conclusions about IUDs as a risk factor for PID [19]. Given these methodologic flaws, the clinician should be skeptical about the findings and conclusions drawn based on past studies, many of which strongly connect IUDs with an increased risk of PID.

Fortunately, in the same comprehensive review of the literature, Grimes explored the quality of evidence and strength of the recommendations from past IUD research (Figure 10-4), which allows clinicians to make important conclusions regarding realistic PID risk in IUD users. These conclusions mirror the recommended practice guidelines put forth by the American College of Obstetricians and Gynecologists [20].

In summary, there is a slight increase in PID risk at the time of insertion only, and there is good evidence that any risk of PID after the first three weeks following insertion is minimal. Prophylactic antibiotic therapy at the time of insertion does not seem to decrease the PID risk with insertion. From studies of IUDs with and without strings, investigators are able to conclude that modern monofilament tail strings do not facilitate ascending infection that would extend the risk of infection beyond the first few weeks after insertion. Inserting an IUD in the presence of asymptomatic gonorrhea or chlamydia infections is appropriate as long as a culture is performed at the time of insertion and treatment is provided for positive cultures. Stated alternatively, women with asymptomatic STDs are not at increased risk of developing PID if an IUD is inserted, and IUD insertion should not be delayed to wait for culture results. Furthermore, if cervical gonorrhea or chlamydia or upper genital tract PID are diagnosed while an IUD is in place, the IUD may be left in place, as an IUD in-situ does not affect antibiotic response. However, the IUD should be removed if there is no improvement after 72 hours of antibiotic therapy or based on the judgment of the clinician. Lastly, while further studies are needed, the best designed studies to date do not indicate increased tubal infertility following IUD discontinuation, even in nulliparous patients [18••].

Due to this reassuring research, the candidate selection for IUDs is becoming more lax to include nulliparous and non-monogamous women. The clinician, as always, must balance the risks and benefits of IUDs. The benefits are numerous and expanding. Unlike barrier contraceptives, IUDs do not protect women against STDs. Unlike oral contraceptives, most IUDs do not protect against PID requiring hospital admission. However, protection against infection is not the role of this contraception. Candidate selection remains the most prudent method for risk reduction, as is proper aseptic insertion technique immediately following gonorrhea and chlamydia cervical culture sampling. Scheduling the first follow-up visit within a week of insertion may allow earlier detection of infection.

Special Considerations in Pelvic Inflammatory Disease: High Risk in Adolescent Women

Sexually active adolescent women are at high risk for acquiring and suffering the most severe sequelae of PID. Young women have dramatically increased risk for PID because of biologic, microbiologic, epidemiologic, sociologic, and behavioral factors. Sexually active young women have 1) little acquired mucosal immunity to STDs, 2) relatively advanced endocervical epithelium (ectroplon) on the face of the cervix, 3) partners with a high prevalence of chlamydia and gonococcal infection, and 4) decreased economic resources and psychologic independence to seek out STD screening and early diagnostic and treatment services. Overall, it is about 10 times more likely that a sexually active adolescent woman will develop PID than will an older woman. Yearly risk for PID has been calculated to be 1:8 for 15-year-olds, 1:10 for 16-year-olds, and 1:80 for 24-year-olds. Those with multiple partners, new partners, inconsistent condom use, or a history of STD are at greatest risk. Because of this increased risk, it is rational and cost effective to ensure that primary prevention (comprehensive sexual education and STD screening services) are focused on sexually active adolescents. The CDC recommends screening all sexually active adolescents whenever they undergo a pelvic examination. Other recent guidelines recommend regular 6 month screenings for all adolescent women at risk [21].

Many adolescents present for evaluation to the emergency department. It is essential that care be expedited, and that emergency and primary care physicians closely follow recommended treatment plans. Hospitalization should be favored to ensure compliance and complete treatment in adolescents. Simultaneously, partners should be identified, treated, and provided tests of cure to reduce risk for recurrence. Counseling, including provisional HIV testing and contraception services, is necessary.

Prevention of Pelvic Inflammatory Disease

Preventing PID can occur as primary, secondary, and tertiary prevention. Primary prevention involves education and barrier methods to avoid the acquisition of inciting sexually transmitted pathogens. Secondary prevention involves preventing a lower genital tract infection from ascending to the upper genital tract due to prompt diagnosis and treatment of symptomatic or asymptomatic infection. Tertiary prevention involves preventing upper genital tract infections from producing long-term sequelae from tubal occlusion. At each of these three levels of prevention, the primary health care provider can play a pivotal role.

The primary goals of PID prevention are to alleviate the pain and systemic discomfort associated with the infection, to prevent tubal damage and its associated sequelae including infertility, chronic pelvic pain, and ectopic pregnancy, and to minimize the spread of infection and its associated morbidity to others. Given improvements in ease of microbial diagnosis, the major effort in PID prevention has been in screening for and treating asymptomatic *C. trachomatis* and *N. gonorrhoeae* cervical infections. In a large randomized controlled trial, the incidence of PID decreased from 18 per 10,000 woman-months to eight per 10,000 woman-months when women 18 to 34 years of age who were at risk of PID were screened for lower genital tract infections [22•]. The US Preventive Services Task Force and the

Summary of Intrauterine Devices in Pelvic Inflammatory Disease Risk Using Quality Measures According to the Method Outlined by the US Preventive Services Task Force Rating System

Issue	Highest Level of Evidence	Strength of Conclusion	Conclusion
IUD as a cause of PID	II-2	A	Risk related to inserting process
Tailstring as a cause of PID	I	A	Monofilament tailstring not a vector for infection
IUD insertion in the presence of gonorrhea or chlamydia	II-2	C	Limited data, but no evidence of increased risk compared with gonorrhea or chlamydia without IUD insertion
Acquisition of chlamydia by IUD user	II-2	B	No increased risk
Acquisition of gonorrhea by IUD user	II-2	C	Limited data
Levonorgestrel-releasing IUD and upper-genital tract infection	II-2	C	Conflicting data on protection against PID
Treatment of PID with IUD in situ	I	B	No impaired response to therapy
Infertility after discontinuation	II-2	B	No substantial increase in risk

Figure 10-4. Summary of intrauterine devices (IUD) in pelvic inflammatory disease (PID) risk using quality measures according to the method outlined by the US Preventive Services Task Force Rating System. Quality of evidence: I—evidence obtained from at least one proper randomized controlled trial; II-1—evidence obtained from well-designed controlled trials without randomization; II-2—evidence obtained from well-designed cohort or case-control analytic studies, preferably from more than one center or research group; II-3—evidence obtained from multiple-time series with or without the intervention. Dramatic results could also be regarded as this type of evidence. Based on the highest level of evidence found in the data recommendations are provided and graded according to the following categories: A—good and consistent scientific evidence to support the recommendation; B—fair scientific evidence to support the recommendation; C—there is insufficient evidence to recommend for or against; D—fair evidence against the recommendation; and E—good evidence against the recommendation. (*Adapted from* Grimes [18].)

CDC consider there to be good evidence to screen all women at risk of PID for gonorrhea and chlamydia [8•,23,24]. As urine sample nucleic acid amplification testing is now equally as sensitive and specific as cervical culture, this screening should become more easily accepted in females and males.

References

Papers of particular interest have been highlighted as follows:
- *Of interest*
- *Of outstanding interest*

1. Washington AE, Katz P: Cost of and payment source for pelvic inflammatory disease: trends and projections, 1983 through 2000. *JAMA* 1991, 266: 2565–2569.

2. Cates W, Rolfs RT, Aral SO: Sexually transmitted diseases, pelvic inflammatory disease, and infertility: an epidemiologic update. *Epidemiol Rev* 1990, 12:199–220.

3.• Rein DB, Kassler WJ, Irwin KL, *et al.*: Direct medical cost of pelvic inflammatory disease and its sequelae: decreasing, but still substantial. *Obstet Gynecol* 2000, 95:397–402.

Though decreasing, the economic burden of PID and it sequelae, as determined from claims data, is substantial. The greatest economic expenditure was incurred within one year of diagnosis, emphasizing the importance of primary prevention.

4. Stamm WE, Guinan ME, Johnson C, *et al.*: Effects of treatment regimens for *Neisseria gonorrhoeae* on simultaneous infection with *Chlamydia trachomatis*. *N Engl J Med* 1984, 310:545–549.

5. Eschenbach DA: Acute pelvic inflammatory disease: etiology, risk factors, and pathogenesis. *Clin Obstet Gynecol* 1976, 19:147–169.

6. Ten leading nationally notifiable infectious diseases—United States. *MMWR Morb Mortal Wkly Rep* 1996, 45:883.

7. Centers for Disease Control and Prevention: Sexually transmitted diseases treatment guidelines 2002. *MMWR Recomm Rep* 2002, 51:1–77.

8.• Workowski KA, Berman SM: Sexually transmitted diseases treatment guidelines, 2006. *MMWR Recomm Rep* 2006, 55:39–51.

Multiple inpatient and outpatient treatment recommendations are provided here, as well as the CDC summary of PID microbiology.

9. Drugs for sexually transmitted infections. *Treatment Guidelines from the Medical Letter* 2004, 2:67–74.

10.•• Ness RB, Soper DE, Holley RL, *et al.*: Effectiveness of inpatient and outpatient treatment strategies for women with pelvic inflammatory disease: results from the pelvic inflammatory disease evaluation and clinical health (peach) randomized trial. *Am J Obstet Gynecol* 2002, 186:929–937.

Randomized study design demonstrates that outpatient management is safe and effective for many patients. This has important implications for decreasing the economic burden of PID.

11. Ness RB, Trautmann G, Richter HE, *et al.*: Effectiveness of treatment strategies of some women with pelvic inflammatory disease: a randomized trial. *Obstet Gynecol* 2005, 106:573–580.

12. Korn AP, Landers DV, Green JR, *et al.*: Pelvic inflammatory disease in human immunodeficiency virus-infected women. *Obstet Gynecol* 1993, 82:765–768.

13. Toth M, Chaudhry A, Ledger WJ, *et al.*: Pregnancy outcome following pelvic infection. *Infect Dis Obstet Gynecol* 1993, 1:12.

14. Chow JM, Yonekura ML, Richwald GA, *et al.*: The association between *Chlamydia trachomatis* and ectopic pregnancy. *JAMA* 1990, 263: 3164–3167.

15. Blandford JM, Gift TL: Productivity losses attributable to untreated chlamydial infection and associated pelvic inflammatory disease in reproductive-aged women. *Sex Transm Dis* 2006, 33S:S117–S121.

16. Beigi RH, Wiesenfeld HC: Pelvic inflammatory disease: new diagnostic criteria and management. *Obstet Gynecol Clin North Am* 2003, 30:777–793.

17. Krivak TC, Cooksey C, Propst AM: Tubo-ovarian abscess: diagnosis, medical and surgical management. *Compr Ther* 2004, 30:93–100.

18.•• Grimes DA: Intrauterine device and upper-genital-tract infection. *Lancet* 2000, 356:1013–1019.

Thorough study and critique of prior research indicates most IUD research is flawed when assessing PID risk. With improved study designs, IUD use appears much safer then previously thought. This has important implications, as the IUD is a highly effective contraceptive that is currently underutilized in the United States due to infectious concerns.

19. International Collaborative Post-Marketing Surveillance of Norplant: Post-marketing surveillance of Norplant contraceptive implants: I. Contraceptive efficacy and reproductive health. *Contraception* 2001, 63:167–186.

20. 2006 Compendium of Selected Publications. ACOG Practice Bulletin, Number 59. Washington, DC; 2005:581–590.

21. Burstein GR, Gaydos CA, Diener-West M, *et al.*: Incident *Chlamydia trachomatis* infections among inner-city adolescent females. *JAMA* 1998, 280:521–526.

22.• Scholes D, Stergachis A, Heidrich FE, *et al.*: Prevention of pelvic inflammatory disease by screening for cervical chlamydial infection. *N Engl J Med* 1996, 334:1362–1366.

Identifying, screening, and treating high-risk populations decreases PID incidence. Screening for cervical infection in certain populations is effective primary prevention.

23. US Preventive Services Task Force: Screening for chlamydial infection: recommendations and rationale. *Am J Prev Med* 2001, 20:90–94.

24. US Preventive Services Task Force. Screening for gonorrhea: Recommendation statement. Rockville, MD: Agency for Healthcare Research and Quality, 2005. Accessed online January 22, 2007. Available at: http://www.ahrq.gov/clinic/uspstf05/gonorrhea/gonrs.htm.

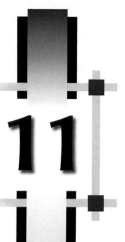

11 Oral Contraceptives

Kelly A. Best and Andrew M. Kaunitz

- Most women who are good pill takers and will benefit from the contraceptive or noncontraceptive benefits of oral contraceptives (OCs) represent appropriate candidates for birth control pills.
- The effectiveness of combination OC use relates to correct and consistent use. Highly compliant women experience one to two pregnancies per 100 woman-years. Teenagers may experience more than 15 pregnancies per 100 woman-years.
- OC use reduces the risk of malignant as well as borderline epithelial ovarian tumors by about 40% in short-term users and by as much as 80% in women who have used OCs for a decade or more.
- Breakthrough spotting and bleeding occur in about one quarter of women during the first 3 months of OC use but become much less common with ongoing use. Counseling patients to anticipate such early breakthrough bleeding and reassuring those who experience this side effect can maximize patients' OC continuation.
- Women who are bothered by hormone withdrawal symptoms or who may benefit from less frequent withdrawal bleeding may benefit from the newer formulations of OCs that shorten or even eliminate the hormone-free interval.
- Women for whom use of combination OCs is contraindicated owing to their high risk of venous thromboembolism can consider using progestin-only methods.
- Many women are concerned that OC use will increase their risk of breast cancer. Overall, the literature is reassuring that OC use does not impact breast cancer risk.
- Perimenopausal women benefit from the regularization of menses, relief from vasomotor symptoms, and positive impact on bone mineral density offered by combination OCs.
- Women with diabetes, controlled hypertension, lupus, or obesity may be candidates for a trial of low-dose OCs provided they are younger than 35 years of age, nonsmokers, and otherwise show no evidence of vascular damage.

Oral contraceptives (OCs) offer women safe, convenient, and reversible fertility regulation. Good pill takers experience high contraceptive efficacy when using OCs. Use of OCs also confers important noncontraceptive health benefits. These positive attributes may explain why OCs are used by over 10 million women in the United States, making them the most widely used hormonal contraceptive method. This chapter describes OCs available in the United States, focusing on education, counseling, and management measures that maximize women's success with the pill.

Composition and Formulations

Since they first became available in the 1960s, the dose of sex steroids in combination OCs has decreased substantially. This decrease has maintained the high contraceptive effectiveness associated with high-dose formulations but with fewer adverse effects. Today, the highest dose formulations marketed in the United States contain 50 μg of estrogen, and almost all OCs prescribed contain 35 μg or less. All modern combination OCs formulated with 35 μg or less of estrogen use the potent estrogen ethinyl estradiol (EE).

Before 1992, combination OCs in the United States contained one of five progestins (norethindrone, norethindrone acetate, ethynodiol diacetate, norgestrel, or levonorgestrel). More recently, formulations containing the less androgenic progestins norgestimate, desogestrel, and drospirenone have become available.

Many OC formulations are marketed in the United States (Figure 11-1). Although there are differences in the laboratory changes associated with various formulations, there is no convincing evidence that important safety or efficacy differences exist between any of the OCs formulated with 35 μg or less of EE. In general contraceptive practice, therefore, the choice of any particular combination OC formulated with 35 μg or less of estrogen can be guided by such factors as physician or patient familiarity and cost. Because some studies have suggested OCs formulated with desogestrel increase the risk of venous thromboembolism more than OCs formulated with other progestins [1], some physicians avoid prescribing desogestrel OCs to patients just starting OC use.

Monophasic OCs have a constant dose of estrogen and progestin in each of the 21 or 24 tablets of active hormones in each cycle pack. Phasic OCs alter the dose of the progestin and (in some formulations) the estrogen component among the active tablets in each pack. In formulating phasic OCs, manufacturers have lowered the total monthly steroid dose with the aim of reducing metabolic effects while maintaining contraceptive efficacy and cycle control.

Reduction of the hormone-free interval (HFI) can be accomplished using newer OC formulations (Figure 11-1). The advantages of such alterations include potentially greater contraceptive success, reduction of hormone withdrawal symptoms, treatment of gynecologic problems such as dysmenorrhea, endometriosis and anemia, as well as accommodation of lifestyle preference [2,3]. A randomized open-label trial with 900 women found that an OC (Loestrin 24 Fe; Warner Chilcott, Rockaway, NJ) with a shorter HFI (4 vs 7 days) was associated with fewer days of withdrawal bleeding as well as less intense withdrawal bleeding [4]. Alteration of the HFI also can be accomplished with OCs that utilize extended cycle regimes of 91 pills. The newest

Oral Contraceptive Formulations Available in the United States (*Continued on next page*)

	Name	Estrogen	Progestin	Progestin Dose, *mg*
EE, 50 μg				
Monophasic	Norlestrin 1/50 (Parke Davis)	EE	Norethindrone acetate	1.0
	Norlestrin 2.5/50	EE	Norethindrone acetate	2.5
	Ovcon 50* (Warner Chilcott)	EE	Norethindrone	1.0
	Ortho-Novum 1/50* (Ortho McNeil)	Mestranol	Norethindrone	1.0
	Norinyl 1 + 50* (Watson Labs)	Mestranol	Norethindrone	1.0
	Demulen (GD Searle)	EE	Ethynodiol diacetate	1.0
	Ovral (Wyeth Pharmaceuticals)	EE	Norgestrel	0.5
EE, 35 μg				
Monophasic	Modicon* (Ortho McNeil)	EE	Norethindrone	0.5
	Brevicon* (Watson Labs)	EE	Norethindrone	0.5
	Ovcon 35*	EE	Norethindrone	0.4
	Ortho-Cyclen* (Johnson RW)	EE	Norgestimate	0.25
	Demulen 1/35*	EE	Ethynodiol diacetate	1.0
	Ortho-Novum 1/35*	EE	Norethindrone	1.0
	Norinyl 1 + 35*	EE	Norethindrone	1.0
EE, 35 μg				
Biphasic	Ortho-Novum 10/11*	EE	Norethindrone	0.5/1.0
Triphasic	Ortho-Novum 7/7/7*	EE	Norethindrone	0.5/0.75/1.0
	Ortho Tri-Cyclen*† (Johnson RW)	EE	Norgestimate	0.18/0.215/0.25
	Tri-Norinyl (Watson Labs)	EE	Norethindrone	0.5/1.0/0.5
	Estrostep† (Warner Chilcott)	EE (20/30/35)	Norethindrone acetate	1.0

*Generic version available.
†Indicated for treatment of acne as well as contraception.
‡Indicated for the treatment of premenstrual dysphoric disorder and acne.

Figure 11-1. (*Continued on the next page*).

product uses an extended 91-day regimen with a 10 μg EE in place of the conventional HFI (Figure 11-1) [5].

Progestin-only OCs (mini-pills) are formulated with doses of progestins even lower than those in low-dose OCs. In contrast to OCs, each cycle of progestin-only pills contains 28 tablets of active hormone. Progestin-only pills can be used by women for whom estrogen is contraindicated (Figure 11-2).

Mechanism of Action, Efficacy, Administration, and Effect on Pregnancy

Combination OCs prevent ovulation by suppressing pituitary gonadotropin release. The progestin component of OCs causes changes in the cervical mucus and the endometrium that enhance the antifertility effect of OCs should ovulation occur. Because failure rates associated with combination OC use relate to individual compliance, they range from less than one per 100 woman-years to greater than 15 per 100 woman-years. Typical first-year combination OC failure rates have been estimated at eight per 100 women [6].

Because progestin-only pills are often prescribed preferentially to lactating women and older women with cardiovascular risk factors, the contraceptive efficacy of progestin-only pills in highly fertile women is hard to assess, but is likely higher than with combination OCs.

Conventionally, OCs are initiated on the first day of the menses or the first Sunday after menses begin. For some patients, starting OCs midcycle using a "quick start" approach, after a negative urine pregnancy test, may facilitate OC initiation [7]. Compliance may be enhanced by advising patients to associate pill taking with a daily ritual (eg, toothbrushing). Compliance is critical to ensure efficacy. If a woman misses one or two combination OC tablets, she should take one tablet as soon as possible. She should then continue to take one tablet twice daily until each of the missed tablets has been taken.

Oral Contraceptive Formulations Available in the United States (Continued)

	Name	Estrogen	Progestin	Progestin Dose, mg
EE, 30 μg				
Monophasic	Loestrin 1.5/30 (Warner Chilcott)	EE	Norethindrone acetate	1.5
	Ortho-Cept* (Ortho McNeil)	EE	Desogestrel	0.15
	Desogen* (Organon USA)	EE	Desogestrel	0.15
	Lo/Ovral* (Wyeth Pharmaceuticals)	EE	Norgestrel	0.15
	Nordette* (Duramed)	EE	Levonorgestrel	0.15
	Levlen* (Bayer Healthcare)	EE	Levonorgestrel	0.15
	Yasmin (Bayer Healthcare)	EE	Drospirenone	3.0
Triphasic	Triphasil* (Wyeth Pharmaceuticals)	EE (30/40/30)	Levonorgestrel	0.05/0.075/0.125
	Tri-Levlen* (Bayer Healthcare)	EE (30/40/30)	Levonorgestrel	0.05/0.075/0.125
Extended cycle	Seasonale* (Duramed)	EE	Levonorgestrel	0.015
	Seasonique (Duramed)	EE	Levonorgestrel	0.015
EE, 25 μg	Cyclessa* (Organon USA)	EE	Desogestrel	0.10/0.125/0.150
	Ortho Tri-Cyclen Lo (Johnson RW)	EE	Norgestimate	0.18/0.215/0.25
EE, 20 μg				
Monophasic	Loestrin 1/20* (Warner Chilcott)	EE	Norethindrone acetate	1.0
	Levlite* (Bayer Healthcare)	EE	Levonorgestrel	0.1
	Alesse* (Wyeth Pharmaceuticals)	EE	Levonorgestrel	0.1
	Mircette* (Duramed)	EE	Desogestrel	0.15
	Yaz‡ (Bayer Healthcare)	EE	Drospirenone	3.0
	Loestrin 24 Fe	EE	Norethindrone acetate	1.0
Progestin-only	Micronor* (Ortho McNeil)		Norethindrone	0.35
	Nor-QD (Watson Labs)		Norethindrone	0.35
	Ovrette (Wyeth Pharmaceuticals)		Norgestrel	0.075

*Generic version available.
†Indicated for treatment of acne as well as contraception.
‡Indicated for the treatment of premenstrual dysphoric disorder and acne.

Figure 11-1. Oral contraceptive formulations available in the United States. EE—ethinyl estradiol.

Women who have missed more than two consecutive tablets should be advised to use an additional form of contraception (eg, condoms) while they complete taking the current pack of pills. Because of the increased risk of accidental pregnancy, women who persistently miss three or more combination OC tablets each cycle should be advised to consider other contraceptive choices that do not require daily compliance. Women who have missed three or more combined OC tablets should also be advised to use postcoital emergency contraception. Because progestin-only pills may be less effective than combination OCs, mini-pill users should use back-up contraception for 48 hours if they are 3 hours or more late in taking a pill [8].

Inadvertent use of OCs during early pregnancy does not increase the risk of fetal anomalies [9]. In conceptions that occur soon after discontinuing OCs, the risk of miscarriage is not increased, but an elevated risk of multiple gestation has been noted [10]. Extending the conventional 7-day hormone-free interval by as few as several days can result in ovulation and unintended pregnancy. Overall, however, return to fertility can be delayed for a number of months after discontinuing OCs compared with women discontinuing use of condoms [11].

Noncontraceptive Health Benefits

Use of OCs is associated with a variety of noncontraceptive health benefits, including quality-of-life benefits, reduction in the risk of common illnesses experienced by women, and protection from certain gynecologic malignancies (Figure 11-3). Educating OC candidates and users regarding these noncon-

traceptive benefits can increase OC compliance and continuation. In addition, physicians are increasingly prescribing OCs specifically for the noncontraceptive benefits they offer, whether or not the patient needs birth control.

Women taking OCs report that menses become more regular and more predictable, the prevalence as well as severity of dysmenorrhea is reduced, and the number of days and amount of flow decline. In addition, iron stores increase in women with iron deficiency associated with menorrhagia. Use of OCs can restore regular menses in women with abnormal bleeding caused by chronic anovulation. Women using OCs also enjoy relative protection from several benign but common conditions that cause morbidity. Benign breast diseases, including fibroadenoma and cystic changes, occur less commonly in women who use OCs. Although earlier higher estrogen OC formulations may have suppressed functional cysts, currently used formulations containing 35 μg or less of estrogen do not appear to suppress functional ovarian cysts [12]. Some clinicians occasionally use OCs formulated with 50 μg of estrogen in women who have had problems related to the occurrence of functional ovarian cysts.

OC use reduces the incidence of pelvic inflammatory disease (PID) [13] and ectopic pregnancy [14], two common and potentially life-threatening conditions. Possible biologic mechanisms for reduced PID incidence include progestational cervical mucus changes, reduced menstrual blood loss, progestin-induced endometrial changes, and less retrograde menstruation associated with OC use. Because OCs prevent ovulation, ectopic pregnancies are rare among users, occurring far less often than among women using no contraception.

Clinical Settings In Which Progestin-only Oral Contraceptives Are More Appropriate Than Combination Oral Contraceptives

Progestin-only contraception in the following settings may be more appropriate than combination oral, transdermal, or vaginal ring contraceptives. Intrauterine devices may also be considered in the following:

Smoking or obesity in women older than 35 years of age

Hypertension in women with vascular disease or older than age 35

Systemic lupus erythematosus with vascular disease, nephritis, or antiphospholipid antibodies

History of thromboembolic disease

Coronary artery disease

Congestive heart failure

Cerebrovascular disease

Migraine headaches

    Migraines with focal neurologic phenomenon

    Migraines that intensify during combination oral contraceptive use

Hypertriglyceridemia

Fully breast-feeding women

When oral contraceptive use causes estrogen-related side effects

Figure 11-2. Clinical settings in which progestin-only oral contraceptives are more appropriate than combination oral contraceptives. (*Adapted from* American College of Obstetricians and Gynecologists [38••].)

Use of OCs appears to maintain bone mineral density. This may be most clinically important in hypoestrogenic women, including those who are perimenopausal [15] or have hypothalamic amenorrhea [16].

Prevention of epithelial ovarian and endometrial cancer represents perhaps the most important noncontraceptive benefit of combination OC use. Epithelial ovarian cancer represents the most lethal gynecologic malignancy in the United States. Worldwide, the literature has consistently found that OC use reduces the risk of malignant as well as borderline epithelial ovarian tumors by approximately 40% in short-term users and by as much as 80% in women who have used OCs for a decade or more [17]. This protection persists for over 15 years after OC discontinuation. Accordingly, a woman in her late 30s or 40s who uses OCs reduces her risk of being diagnosed with ovarian cancer during her 50s or 60s, decades of life when a woman would otherwise experience peak risk of this lethal malignancy. Accordingly, ovarian cancer prophylaxis with OCs may be of particular relevance to high-risk women, including nulliparous women and those with a positive family history [18] or breast cancer gene mutations [19].

Use of OCs is associated with a 50% reduced risk of endometrial adenocarcinoma, the most common gynecologic cancer in women in the United States [17]. Protection occurs for each of the three principal histologic types of endometrial carcinoma and persists for at least 20 years after OC discontinuation [20]. OC use also may decrease the risk of colorectal caner [21].

Physicians have long used OCs to treat a variety of common conditions affecting women of reproductive age (Figure 11-4). Based on the results of well-designed randomized trials [22–25], the US Food and Drug Administration approved three OC formulations (EE/triphasic norgestimate, estrophasic norethindrone acetate and EE/drospirenone [DRSP]) for the treatment of acne in women who are appropriate candidates for OCs. In addition to recognizing a new effective treatment for acne, this US Food and Drug Administration action provides OC candidates concerned about their complexion with an additional reason to initiate and continue OC use. In 2006, the US Food and Drug Administration approved the use of the 24/4 20 μg EE/3 mg DRSP OC formulation for the treatment of the symptoms of premenstrual dysphoric disorder [26].

Side Effects

Side effects of OCs represent an important source of patient dissatisfaction, noncompliance, and discontinuation. Physicians can enhance their patients' contraceptive success by candidly discussing side effects with them before OC initiation.

Nausea and breast tenderness represent common side effects that appear related to the estrogen component of combination OCs. A recent 6-month randomized, double-blind, placebo-controlled trial of EE/triphasic norgestimate found that nausea was reported by 12.7% of OC users compared with 9% of those taking placebos. Breast tenderness was reported by 9.2% of OC users and 4.7% of those taking placebos. Although many physicians and users feel that use of OCs causes weight gain, this same trial observed a nearly identical rate of reported weight gain among the OC and placebo groups (2.2% and 2.1%, respectively) [27].

Menstrual changes during OC use can cause patient anxiety and are a common reason for discontinuation. Intermenstrual or breakthrough spotting and bleeding occur in about

Noncontraceptive Benefits of Oral Contraceptives

Protection against:

Dysmenorrhea and menorrhagia

Menstrual cycle irregularities

Iron deficiency anemia

Ectopic pregnancy

Pelvic inflammatory disease

Ovarian cysts

Benign breast disease

Endometrial cancer

Ovarian cancer

Osteopenia

Figure 11-3. Noncontraceptive benefits of oral contraceptives.

Therapeutic Uses of Oral Contraceptives*

Acne[†]

Premenstrual dysphoric disorder[‡]

Hirsutism

Dysfunctional uterine bleeding

Chronic hyperandrogenic anovulation/polycystic ovary syndrome

Menorrhagia (including when associated with uterine leiomyomas or blood dyscrasias)

Premature ovarian failure

Amenorrhea associated with hyperprolactinemia and hypothalamic disorders

Functional ovarian cysts

Pelvic pain (including secondary dysmenorrhea)

Mittelschmerz

Endometriosis (continuous use preferred)

Perimenopausal symptoms

*Drugs are not approved by the US Food and Drug Administration for these conditions unless otherwise specified.
[†]Triphasic ethinyl estradiol/norgestimate and triphasic ethinyl estradiol/norethindrone acetate are US Food and Drug Administration–approved for the treatment of acne.
[‡]20 ethinyl estradiol/3 drospirenone is US Food and Drug Administration–approved for the relief of symptoms associated with premenstrual dysphoric disorder and the treatment of acne.

Figure 11-4. Therapeutic uses of oral contraceptives.

one quarter of women during the first 3 months of OC use but become much less common with ongoing use. Counseling patients to anticipate such early breakthrough bleeding and reassuring those who experience this side effect can maximize patients' desire to continue OC use. Rates of breakthrough bleeding are higher in OCs formulated with 20 μg than with 30 or 35 μg of EE [28,29]. When intermenstrual bleeding occurs after 3 months of OC use, the patient should be examined for possible causes of bleeding unrelated to OC use, including cervical and endometrial infection and neoplasia. Unscheduled bleeding associated with extended cycle OCs is greater in early cycles and will likely improve with continued use. Women who experience breakthrough bleeding/spotting for more than 7 days during extended use of OCs have been shown to benefit from the institution of a 3-day pill holiday rather than continuation of therapy [30•]. A minimum of 3 weeks of active pills should be taken between pill holidays to ensure inhibition of the pituitary-ovarian axis and adequate suppression of ovulation.

Amenorrhea may occur with OC use, particularly in long-term users. Although such amenorrhea is not medically harmful, it may cause patient anxiety regarding pregnancy. Patients using OCs who are concerned regarding absence of withdrawal bleeding may benefit from counseling that there is no health benefit associated with bleeding among women using hormonal contraception.

Headaches are sometimes reported by women using combination OCs and require appropriate evaluation and management. Tension headaches are not related to OC use and can be treated with over-the-counter analgesics. Some patients with migraines experience worsening of their headaches with low-dose combination OCs, others experience improvement, and still others experience no effect. Women with common migraines, which do not include focal neurologic symptoms, may be allowed a trial of OCs. However, some experts sug-

gest that women with migraines accompanied by aura, which are characterized by symptoms of neurologic dysfunction (eg, scintillating scotomata) preceding or accompanying the attack, should not use combination OCs [31]. Regardless, women who experience increased frequency or intensity of any type of migraine headache should discontinue combination OC use. Such women may be candidates for use of progestin-only contraceptives (see Figure 11-2). Some women using OCs experience migraine headaches only during menses. Elimination of the pill-free interval may be therapeutic in women with such menstrual migraines [32].

Health Risks

Extensive epidemiologic data have evaluated the associations between OC use and the risks of cardiovascular disease and cancer. These data indicate that, for most women, OCs represent a safe contraceptive choice. Contraindications to the use of combination OCs are listed in Figure 11-5.

THROMBOEMBOLISM

The increased risk of thromboembolism observed in women using OCs appears to be related to the estrogenic component. Although low-dose OCs carry less risk than the higher-dose preparations used in the past, they nonetheless increase the risk. However, venous thromboembolism occurs less frequently with use of modern combination OCs than during pregnancy. Women using OCs containing less than 50 mg of EE have a risk of thromboembolism that is some four times higher than nonusers [33]. Physicians and OC candidates need to put this elevated relative risk into perspective by assessing the effect on a woman's absolute risk of experiencing thromboembolism. Although the thromboembolism incidence among low-dose OC users (one to 1.5 per 10,000 woman-years) is about four times greater than in nonpregnant nonusers (0.4 per 10,000 woman-years), the thromboembolism incidence associated with pregnancy (six per 10,000) is several-fold higher than with OC use. This absolute risk should be considered in the context of important contraceptive and noncontraceptive benefits associated with OC use. Fortunately, the case fatality rate for venous thromboembolism is only 1% to 2%. The risk of thromboembolism in women using OCs formulated with 20-mg EE does not appear to be different than that with 30- to 35-mg EE OCs [34]. Women for whom use of combination OCs is contraindicated because of their high risk of venous thrombo-embolism, including obese women older than age 35 years, can consider using progestin-only pills, injectables, implants, or intrauterine contraception (Figure 11-2).

MYOCARDIAL INFARCTION AND THROMBOTIC AND HEMORRHAGIC STROKE

Past use of OCs does not increase the risk of atherosclerosis [35]. Limited evidence, in fact, suggests that OC use may even reduce the risk of coronary artery disease. An angiography-based study of young women suffering myocardial infarctions

---

Contraindications to the Use of Oral Contraceptives*

Smokers older than 35 years of age

Obesity and age older than 35 years

Uncontrolled hypertension

Diabetes with vascular complications

Migraines with aura

Thromboembolic disorders, cerebrovascular disease, or coronary artery disease

Markedly impaired liver function

Known or suspected breast cancer[†]

Undiagnosed abnormal vaginal bleeding

Known or suspected pregnancy

*These contraindications do not apply to progestin-only oral contraceptives.
[†]Progestin-only oral contraceptives are containdicated

Figure 11-5. Contraindications to use of oral contraceptives.

observed that coronary atherosclerosis was less common in OC users than nonusers [36]. Autopsy studies of female monkeys fed an atherogenic diet found less atherosclerosis in animals fed OCs than in those not fed OCs [37]. These studies lead to two insights regarding coronary artery disease and OC use. First, OC use does not cause coronary atherosclerosis, the leading cause of death in women in the United States. Second, in those rare cases in which myocardial infarction occurs in current OC users (most of whom are cigarette smokers), the cause is thrombotic rather than atherosclerotic.

Available evidence suggests that use of modern OCs is associated with little if any increased risk of myocardial infarction or stroke among healthy, nonsmoking women [38••]. In contrast, women older than 35 years who smoke cigarettes are at substantially increased risk of myocardial infarction because smoking and OC use act synergistically to increase risk. Accordingly, women younger than 35 years of age who smoke and desire OCs should be prescribed OCs and be encouraged to stop smoking. Women older than 35 years of age who cannot or will not quit smoking need to choose a contraceptive other than combination OCs (Figure 11-2).

BREAST CANCER

Although many women are concerned that OC use will increase their risk of breast cancer, available data provide reassurance. A pooled analysis of data on breast cancer and OC use has clarified this relationship [39]. This analysis combined data from 54 studies, including more than 53,000 breast cancer patients and more than 100,000 control subjects, with reassuring overall findings. No increased risk of breast cancer was associated with past (10 or more years since OC discontinuation) OC use, regardless of duration of use. The presence or absence of a family history of breast cancer did not affect the above observations, nor did use of OCs formulated with various types or doses of hormones. A slight elevated breast cancer risk was noted with current or recent (within 10 years of stopping) OC use. This excess risk involved tumors less advanced clinically than those diagnosed in OC nonusers. Overall, these observations indicate that OC use does not cause breast cancer. The elevated risk associated with current or recent use is unexplained; some speculate that this reflects surveillance bias; that is, because OC users have more clinical breast examinations and mammograms, tumors are detected earlier [40]. A large case-control study (The Women's Contraceptive and Reproductive Experiences [CARE] Study) funded by the National Institutes of Health and conducted by the Centers for Disease Control found no evidence that OC use (whether long- or short-term) impacted subsequent risk of breast cancer [41]. In the largest study to date of breast cancer risk associated with prior or current OC use in women 35 to 64 years of age with breast cancer gene test (BRCA) 1 and 2 mutations, low-dose OCs did not increase their risk above their own baseline risk. In fact, OC use was associated with a significant reduction in risk for BRCA-1 mutation carriers [42••]. Taken together, available data indicate that women, including those who are high risk, can use OCs with the knowledge that they will not increase their risk of this common and anxiety-provoking disease.

CERVICAL NEOPLASIA

Cervical neoplasia's unique epidemiology, similar to that of a sexually transmitted disease (STD), makes assessing any association with OC use challenging. However, recent studies, which control for potentially confounding factors, including STD risk factors and cytology screening, have clarified our understanding of this subject. Three case-control studies found that the risk of invasive cervical cancer with OC use was not significantly different than that in nonusers [43–45]. Likewise, well-controlled studies have found no association between OC use and cervical intraepithelial neoplasia (CIN) [46,47]. Most studies have found no association between OC use and genital human papillomavirus infection (HPV). Our current understanding of the role HPV plays in cervical neoplasia has provided additional reassurance that use of OC does not increase risk of developing cervical neoplasia. Among women infected with HPV, use of OC does not increase risk of progression to high grade dysplasia [48]. Adenocarcinoma, which accounts for approximately 10% of cervical cancers, may have an epidemiology distinct from that of the more common squamous tumor. Two large and well-controlled studies found that OC use was associated with a significantly increased risk of cervical adenocarcinoma [45,49].

All women at risk for cervical neoplasia, including those who use OCs, should receive regular cytology screening. Women with a history of cervical intraepithelial neoplasia (including those who have had conization, cryotherapy, or laser or loop excision), as well as those being evaluated for CIN, remain appropriate candidates for OCs.

OBESITY

Obesity affects over 25% of reproductive age women and will increasingly impact contraceptive choice. A retrospective analysis that examined OC efficacy and weight suggested that contraceptive failure was increased in women over 70.5 kg (155 lbs) as EE dose decreased [50]. A similar analysis revealed pregnancy rates on OCs for women with a body mass index greater than 27.3 kg/m² were increased [51]. More recent and methodologically superior reports, however, have found no evidence of higher rates of contraceptive failure in obese women [52,53].

Obesity, age over 35, and use of OCs represent independent risk factors for thrombosis. Accordingly, progestin-only and intrauterine contraceptives represent appropriate choices for obese women over age 35 years [38••].

DIABETES

Current evidence suggests that combination OC use in women with type I or type II diabetes has no effect on glycemic control or disease progression. OC use in diabetic women should, however, be limited to otherwise healthy nonsmokers under 35 years of age who show no evidence of hypertension, nephropathy, retinopathy, or other vascular disease [38••].

HYPERTENSION

Oral contraceptive use appears to increase blood pressure. The American College of Obstetricians and Gynecologists suggests that women under the age of 35 with well controlled hypertension are candidates for a trial of low-dose OCs provided they are otherwise healthy with no evidence of end-organ vascular disease and do not smoke. Blood pressure should be closely monitored in these women. In hypertensives over age 35 years, progestin-only contraceptives represent appropriate choices [38••]

SYSTEMIC LUPUS ERYTHEMATOSUS

Older data have suggested that use of combination OCs causes disease flare-ups. Two recently published randomized trials indicate that women with systemic lupus erythematosus can safely use combination OCs if they have stable, mild disease, are seronegative for antiphospholipid antibodies, and have no history of thrombosis [54•,55•].

Use After Abortion, After Birth, or During Lactation

Oral contraceptives may be initiated immediately after induced or spontaneous termination of a first- or second-trimester pregnancy. Women remain at increased risk for thromboembolism for several weeks after childbirth. Women who do not breast feed do not appear to ovulate before 3-weeks postpartum [56]. Based on these observations, some physicians initiate combination OCs in non–breast-feeding women 2 to 3 weeks after childbirth even though package labeling suggests that OCs not be initiated before 4-weeks postpartum. Because progestin-only OCs, injectables, and implants do not contain estrogen, these latter methods may be initiated immediately postpartum (Figure 11-2).

Patient instructions in the package labeling for norethindrone have been updated to indicate that these progestin-only

Hepatic Enzyme-inducing Medications That May Impair Oral Contraceptive Efficacy
Anticonvulsants
Carbamazepine and oxcarbazepine
Felbamate
Barbiturates (including phenobarbital and primidone)
Phenytoin
Topiramate
Vigabatrin
Antibiotic
Rifampin
Herbals
St. John's Wort

Figure 11-6. Hepatic enzyme-inducing medications that may impair oral contraceptive efficacy. (*Adapted from* American College of Obstetricians and Gynecologists [38••].)

OCs can be started within 3-weeks postpartum in women who are not breast-feeding or are breast-feeding with partial formula supplementation, and at 6-weeks postpartum in women who are exclusively breast-feeding.

Use When Estrogen Is Contraindicated

Use of progestin-only OCs, injectables, and implants may be appropriate when contraceptive doses of estrogen are contraindicated. Pregnancy and combination OC use confer an increased risk of morbidity and mortality in women more than 35 years of age who smoke, are obese, or have hypertension, women with coronary artery disease, women at increased risk of thromboembolism, and some women with systemic lupus erythematosus. Progestin-only methods should be considered safe and effective contraceptive choices for such women (Figure 11-2).

A personal history of breast cancer is listed in package labeling as a contraindication to use of all hormonal methods of contraception. The presence of uterine leiomyomas does not contraindicate use of combination OCs, which may improve menorrhagia and dysmenorrhea in women with these tumors (Figure 11-4).

Use of Concomitant Medications

Anticonvulsants and antibiotics that induce hepatic enzymes (Figure 11-6) can reduce the contraceptive efficacy of OCs [57]. The progestin-only contraceptive Depo Provera (Pfizer, Inc., New York, NY), which represents a relatively high-dose method, appears to remain effective in women taking enzyme inducers [58]. Because of the low dose of progestin in progestin-only pill formulations and implants, mini-pills and implants are not a prudent choice in women taking enzyme inducers. Use of the anticonvulsant valproic acid [59] and the antibiotics doxycycline [60], tetracycline [61], metronidazole, and ampicillin [62] does not appear to reduce combination OC efficacy.

Use in Perimenopausal Women

Use of combination OCs is safe in healthy, nonsmoking women of reproductive age. In the United States, women in their 40s are increasingly taking advantage of the effective contraceptive protection offered by OCs. In addition, perimenopausal women benefit from the regularization of menses, relief from vasomotor symptoms, and positive impact on bone mineral density offered by combination OCs (*see* Figures 11-3 and 11-4). Assessment of follicle-stimulating hormone levels to determine when older OC users no longer need contraception is expensive and may be misleading [63]. A preferable approach is for healthy, nonsmoking women who are doing well on combination OCs to continue taking them into their early to middle 50s [64]. At this time, OCs can be arbitrarily stopped, barrier contraception can be offered, and the patient observed. If signs and symptoms of menopause are noted, initiation of hormone replacement can be considered. Otherwise, it may be appropriate to restart OCs and reevaluate in 1 to 2 years.

Use for Postcoital Emergency Contraception

Increased use of OCs for postcoital contraception could substantially reduce the number of unintended pregnancies and induced abortions. Used within 120 hours of unprotected coitus, postcoital contraception prevents pregnancy [65]. Progestin-only emergency contraception (EC) is more effective and causes less nausea than estrogen-progestin EC [65]. With the availability of a marketed formulation containing a two tablet progestin-only EC (Plan B; Duramed Pharmaceuticals, Woodcliff Lake, NJ), estrogen-progestin EC is being used less than previously. Some have suggested that the two tablets in the marketed formulation may be taken immediately following unprotected sex [65], and although labeling indicates tablets should be taken within 72 hours of unprotected sex, EC appears effective for up to 120 hours [65]. Individuals over the age of 17 may currently purchase the two-tablet regimen over the counter; however, to date, women under the age of 18 still require a prescription to obtain EC.

Summary

Oral contraceptives offer women safe, reversible, and convenient birth control, which is highly effective for those who consistently take pills correctly. In many settings, OCs provide important noncontraceptive benefits. By individualizing counseling and follow-up strategies based on relevant behavioral and medical considerations, physicians can maximize their patients' success with OCs.

References

Papers of particular interest have been highlighted as follows:
• Of interest
•• Of outstanding interest

1. Jick SS, Kaye JA, Russmann S, et al.: Risk of nonfatal venous thromboembolism with oral contraceptives containing norgestimate or desogestrel compared with oral contraceptives containing levonorgestrel. *Contraception* 2006, 73:566–570.

2. Spona J, Elstein M, Feichtinger W, et al.: Shorter pill-free interval in combined oral contraceptives decreases follicular development. *Contraception* 1996, 54:71–77.

3. Sulak PJ, Scrow SC, Preece C, et al.: Hormone withdraw symptoms in oral contraceptive users. *Obstet Gynecol* 2000, 95:261–266.

4. Nakajima ST, Archer DF, Ellman H: Efficacy and safety of new 24-day contraceptive regimen of norethindrone acetate 1 mg/ethinyl estradiol 20 μg (Loestrin 24 Fe). *Contraception* 2007, 75:16–22.

5. Anderson FD, Gibbons W, Portman D: Safety and efficacy of an extended-regimen oral contraceptive utilizing continuous low-dose ethinyl estradiol. *Contraception* 2006, 73:229–234.

6. Trussell J: Contraceptive failure in the United States. *Contraception* 2006, 70:89–96.

7. Westhoff C, Kerns J, Morroni C, et al.: Quick start: novel oral contraceptive initiation method. *Contraception* 2002, 66:141–145.

8. Speroff L, Darney P: *A Clinical Guide for Contraception*, edn 2. Baltimore: Williams & Wilkins; 1996.

9. Bracken MB: Oral contraception and congenital malformations in offspring: a review and meta-analysis of the prospective studies. *Obstet Gynecol* 1990, 76:552–557.

10. Rothman KJ: Fetal loss, twinning, and birth weight after oral contraceptive use. *N Engl J Med* 1977, 297:468–471.

11. Hassan MA, Killick SR: Is previous use of hormonal contraception associated with a detrimental effect on subsequent fecundity? *Hum Reprod* 2004, 19:344–351.

12. Kauntiz AM: Noncontraceptive health benefits of oral contraceptives. *Rev Endocr Metab Disord* 2002, 3:277–283.

13. Pasner LA , Phipps WR: Type of oral contraceptive in relation to acute initial episodes of pelvic inflammatory disease. *Contraception* 1991, 43:91–99.

14. Franks AL, Beral V, Cates W, Jr., et al.: Contraception and ectopic pregnancy risk. *Am J Obstet Gynecol* 1990, 163:1120–1123.

15. Gambacciani M, Spinetti A, Taponeco F, et al.: Longitudinal evaluation of perimenopausal vertebral bone loss: effects of low-dose oral contraceptive preparation on bone mineral density and metabolism. *Obstet Gynecol* 1994, 83:392–396.

16. Warren MP, Miller KK, Olson WH, et al.: Effects of an oral contraceptive on bone mineral density in women with hypothalamic amenorrhea and osteopenia: an open-label extension of a double-blind, placebo-controlled study. *Contraception* 2005, 72:206–211.

17. Grimes DA, Economy KE: Primary prevention of gynecologic cancers. *Am J Obstet Gynecol* 1995, 172:227–235.

18. Gross TP, Schlesselman JJ: The estimated effect of oral contraceptive use on the cumulative risk of epithelial ovarian cancer. *Obstet Gynecol* 1994, 83:419–424.

19. Narod SA, Risch H, Moslehi R, et al.: Oral contraceptives and the risk of ovarian cancer. *N Engl J Med* 1998, 339:424–428.

20. Jick SS, Walker AM, Jick H: Oral contraceptives and endometrial cancer. *Obstet Gynecol* 1993, 82:931–935.

21. Fernandez E, Vecchia C, Balducci A, et al.: Oral contraceptives and colorectal cancer risk: a meta-analysis. *Br J Cancer* 2001, 84:722–727.

22. Redmond GP, Olson WH, Lippman JS, et al.: Norgestimate and ethinyl estradiol in the treatment of acne vulgaris: a randomized, placebo-controlled trial. *Obstet Gynecol* 1997, 89:615–622.

23. Lucky AW, Henderson TA, Olson WH, et al.: Effectiveness of norgestimate and ethinyl estradiol in treating moderate acne vulgaris. *J Am Acad Dermatol* 1997, 37:746–754.

24. Gilliam M, Maloney JM, Flack MR, et al.: Acne treatment with a low–does oral contraceptive. *Obstet Gynecol* 2001, 97(Suppl 1):9S.

25. Thorneycroft H, Gollnick H, Schellschmidt I: Superiority of a combined contraceptive containing drosperinone to a triphasic preparation containing norgestimate in acne treatment. *Cutis* 2004, 74:123–130.

26. Freeman EW, Kroll R, Rapkin A, *et al.*: Evaluation of a unique oral contraceptive in the treatment of premenstrual dysphoric disorder. *Gend Based Med* 2001, 10:561–569.

27. Lippman JS, Godwin A, Olson W: The tolerability of a triphasic norgestimate/EE containing OC: results from a double-blind, placebo-controlled trial. *Prim Care Update Ob Gyn* 1998, 5:173–174.

28. Appel TB, Arman KA, Birdsall C, *et al.*: A comparison of a new graduated estrogen formulation with three constant-dosed oral contraceptives. *Contraception* 1987, 35:523–532.

29. Åkerlund M, Røde A, Westergaard J: Comparative profiles of reliability, cycle control and side effects of two oral contraceptive formulations containing 150 µg desogestrel and either 30 µg or 20 µg ethinyl estradiol. *Br J Obstet Gynaecol* 1993, 100:832–838.

30.• Willis S, Kuehl TJ, Spiekerman AM, *et al.*: Greater inhibition of the pituitary-ovarian axis in oral contraceptive regimens with shortened hormone-free interval. *Contraception* 2006, 74:100–103.

This unique study validates a strategy that allows women using OCs in an extended fashion to reduce unscheduled spotting/bleeding.

31. British Association for the Study of Headache: Guidelines for all doctors in the diagnosis and management of migraines and tension–type headache 2nd edition. Available at http://64.227.208.149/NS_BASH/BASH_guideline31Aug05.pdf.

32. Sulak PJ, Cressman BE, Waldrop E, *et al.*: Extending the duration of active oral contraceptive pills to manage hormone withdrawal symptoms. *Obstet Gynecol* 1997, 89:179–183.

33. Sidney S, Petitti DB, Soff GA, *et al*: Venous thromboembolic disease in users of low-estrogen combined estrogen-progestin contraceptives. *Contraception* 2004, 70:3–10.

34. Lidegaard Ø, Edstršm B, Kreiner S: Oral contraceptives and venous thromboembolism: a case-control study. *Contraception* 1998, 57:291–301.

35. Stampfer MJ, Willett WC, Colditz GA, *et al.*: Past use of oral contraceptives and cardiovascular disease: a meta-analysis in the context of the Nurses Health Study. *Am J Obstet Gynecol* 1990, 163:285–291.

36. Engel HJ, Engel E, Lichtlen PR: Coronary atherosclerosis and myocardial infarction in young women: role of oral contraceptives. *Eur Heart J* 1983, 4:1–8.

37. Clarkson TB, Shively CA, Morgan TM, *et al.*: Oral contraceptives and coronary artery atherosclerosis of cynomolgus monkeys. *Obstet Gynecol* 1990, 75:217–222.

38.•• American College of Obstetricians and Gynecologists Committee on Practice Bulletins–Gynecology: ACOG Practice Bulletin. *Use of Hormonal Contraception in Women with Coexisting Medical Conditions*; Washington, DC: American College of Obstetricians and Gynecologists; 2006. Number 73.

An up-to-date authoritative compendium of information to help physicians counsel their patients with medical concerns to make sound contraceptive decisions.

39. Collaborative Group on Hormonal Factors in Breast Cancer: Breast cancer and hormonal contraceptives: collaborative breast cancer reanalysis of individual data on 53,297 women with and 100,239 women without breast cancer from 54 epidemiological studies. *Lancet* 1996, 347:1713–1727.

40. Westhoff CL: Breast cancer risk: perception versus reality. *Contraception* 1999, 59 (Suppl):255–285.

41. Marchbanks PA, McDonald JA, Wilson HG, *et al.*: Oral contraceptives and the risk of breast cancer. *N Engl J Med* 2002, 346(26):2025–2032.

42.•• Milne RL, Knight JA, John EM, *et al.*: Oral contraceptive use and risk of early–onset breast cancer in carriers and non–carriers of BRCA 1 and BRCA 2 mutations. *Cancer Epidemiol Biomarkers* 2005, 14:350–356.

An important multinational case-control study which provides reassuring information regarding the safety of OC use in women with an elevated risk of breast cancer.

43. Parazzini F, La Vecchia C, Negri E, *et al.*: Oral contraceptive use and invasive cervical cancer. *Int J Epidemiol* 1990, 19:259–263.

44. Brinton LA, Reeves WC, Brenes MM, *et al.*: Oral contraceptive use and risk of invasive cervical cancer. *Int J Epidemiol* 1990, 19:4–11.

45. Kjaer SK, Engholm G, Dahl C, *et al.*: Case-control study of risk factors for cervical squamous-cell neoplasia in Denmark, III. Role of oral contraceptive use. *Cancer Causes Control* 1993, 4:513–519.

46. Coker AL, McCann MF, Hulka BS, *et al.*: Oral contraceptive use and cervical intraepithelial neoplasia. *J Clin Epidemiol* 1992, 45:1111–1118.

47. Ley C, Bauer HM, Reingold A, *et al.*: Determinants of genital human papillomavirus infection in young women. *JNCI* 1991, 83:997–1003.

48. Castle PE, Walker JL, Schiffman M, *et al.*: Hormonal contraceptive use, pregnancy and parity, and the risk of cervical intraepithelial neoplasia 3 among oncogenic HPV DNA-positive women with equivocal or mildly abnormal cytology. *Int J Cancer* 2005, 20;117:1007–1012.

49. Ursin G, Peters RK, Henderson BE, *et al.*: Oral contraceptive use and adenocarcinoma of cervix. *Lancet* 1994, 334:1390–1394.

50. Holt VL, Cushing–Haugen KL, Daling JR: Body weight and risk of oral contraceptive failure. *Obstet Gynecol* 2002, 99:820–827.

51. Holt VL, Scholes D, Wicklund KG, *et al.*: Body mass index, weight and oral contraceptive failure. *Obstet Gynecol* 2005, 105:46–52.

52. Zhang HF, LaGuardia KD, Creanga DL: Higher body weight and body mass index are not associated with reduced efficacy in Ortho Tri-Cyclen Lo users. *Obstet Gynecol* 2006, 107:50S.

53. Westhoff CL, Anderson FD: Seasonale (30 µg of ethinyl estradiol/150 µg of levonorgestrel) extended-regimen oral contraceptive efficacy and cycle control by body weight. *Contraception* 2006, 7:181–182.

54.• Petri M, Kim MY, Kalunian KC, *et al.*: Combined oral contraceptives in women with systemic lupus erythematosus. OC–SELENA Trial. *N Engl J Med* 2005, 353:2550–2558.

This study (along with [55•]) represents the first randomized clinical trials of contraceptive use in women with lupus, and indicates that women with mild stable disease and no history of thrombosis, nephritis, or antiphospholipid antibodies can safely use OCs.

55.• Sanchez-Guerrero, Urive AG, Jiminez-Santana L, *et al.*: A trial of contraceptive methods in women with systemic lupus erythematosus. *N Engl J Med* 2005, 353:2539–2549.

This study (along with [54•]) represents the first randomized clinical trials of contraceptive use in women with lupus, and indicates that women with mild stable disease and no history of thrombosis, nephritis, or antiphospholipid antibodies can safely use OCs.

56. Gray RH, Campbell OM, Zacur HA, *et al*.: Postpartum return of ovarian activity in nonbreastfeeding women monitored by urinary assays. *J Clin Endocrinol Metab* 1987, 64:645–651.

57. Crawford P: Interactions between antiepileptic drugs and hormonal contraception. *CNS Drugs* 2002, 16:263–272.

58. Sapire KE: Depo-Provera and carbamazepine. *Br J Fam Plann* 1990, 15:130.

59. Crawford P, Chadwick D, Cleland P, *et al*.: The lack of effect of sodium valproate on the pharmacokinetics of oral contraceptive steroids. *Contraception* 1986, 33:23–29.

60. Neely JL, Abate M, Swinker M, *et al*.: The effect of doxycycline on serum levels of ethinyl estradiol, norethindrone, and endogenous progesterone. *Obstet Gynecol* 1991, 77:416–420.

61. Murphy AA, Zacur HA, Charache P, *et al*.: The effect of tetracycline on levels of oral contraceptives. *Am J Obstet Gynecol* 1991, 164:28–33.

62. Joshi JV, Joshi UM, Sankholi GM, *et al*.: A study of interaction of low-dose combination oral contraceptive with ampicillin and metronidazole. *Contraception* 1980, 22:643–651.

63. Gebbie AE, Glasier A, Sweeting V: Incidence of ovulation in perimenopausal women before and during hormone replacement therapy. *Contraception* 1995, 52:221–222.

64. Kaunitz AM: Oral contraceptive use in perimenopause. *Am J Obstet Gynecol* 2001, 185(Suppl):S32–37.

65. Westhoff CL: Clinical practice: emergency contraception. *N Engl J Med* 2003, 349:1830–1835.

12

Transdermal and Vaginal Ring Estrogen-Progestin Contraception

Andrew M. Kaunitz

- The contraceptive patch (Ortho Evra, Ortho-McNeil Pharmaceuticals, Titusville, NJ) and the contraceptive vaginal ring (NuvaRing, Organon USA, Inc., Roseland, NJ) offer women combination estrogen-progestin contraception without daily pill-taking.
- The patch is applied to the lower abdomen, upper outer arm, the buttock, or the upper torso. A new patch should be applied each week on the same day for 3 weeks, followed by a patch-free week during which withdrawal bleeding is anticipated.
- The ring is inserted in the vagina for 3 weeks and then removed for one week, during which withdrawal bleeding is anticipated. Accordingly, during routine use, a new ring would be inserted on the same day of the week every 4 weeks.
- In consistent users as studied in clinical trials, the contraceptive failure rates with the patch and ring are similar to oral contraceptives (OCs).
- The patch and the ring have not been used extensively enough to assess noncontraceptive benefits; however, they may have a noncontraceptive benefit profile similar to that of OCs.
- The incidence of unscheduled (breakthrough) bleeding and spotting appears somewhat lower with the ring than with OCs.
- Systemic levels of ethinyl estradiol are higher with the patch than with OCs or the ring. The risk of venous thromboembolism is increased with all estrogen-progestin combination contraceptives. The venous thromboembolism risk, however, may be higher with the patch than with OCs.

In 2001, two new estrogen-progestin contraceptives became available in the United States: a 1-week transdermal patch and a 3-week vaginal ring. The patch and the ring release ethinyl estradiol (EE), which is the same potent estrogen contained in modern oral contraceptives (OCs). They offer effective contraception for candidates for combination estrogen-progestin contraception who prefer use of a weekly skin patch or a monthly vaginal ring to taking daily OC tablets (Figure 12-1).

The Transdermal Contraceptive Patch

The patch (Ortho Evra; Ortho-McNeil Pharmaceuticals, Titusville, NJ), a 4.5-cm tan-colored square, releases 20 µg of EE daily along with norelgestromin, which is the biologically active metabolite of the progestin norgestimate found in a number of oral contraceptive formulations (see also Chapter 11). The patch is applied to the lower abdomen, upper outer arm, the buttock, or the upper torso. The patch should not be applied to the breast. A new patch should be applied each week on the same day for 3 weeks, followed by a patch-free week during which withdrawal bleeding is anticipated. Patch application sites should be rotated and free of skin irritation, creams, oils, or lotions. Should a patch become detached for more than 24 hours, the patient should use back up barrier contraception for 1 week and apply a new patch, initiating a new 3-week cycle of patch use (the day of application of the new patch becomes the new patch change day). Serum estrogen and progestin levels maintain contraceptive efficacy even if changing the patch is delayed for as long as 2 days (using the patch for 9 rather than the recommended 7 days) [1]. Sweating associated with vigorous exercise, swimming, and use of a hot tub or sauna have not been found to result in patch detachment or clinically relevant changes in serum hormonal contraceptive levels [2].

Rates of unscheduled (breakthrough) bleeding and spotting are similar with the patch and combination OCs [3•]. Initially, use of the patch is associated with a higher incidence of breast tenderness than with use of OCs [3•]. Although local skin reactions are common, few women in clinical trials have discontinued the patch due to such reaction [3•]. If patch users are concerned regarding the lint ring which forms around the patch during use, mineral ("baby") oil can be used to remove this [4••].

In randomized clinical trials, participants were more likely to use the patch correctly and consistently than OCs [3•], underscoring the advantages of a birth control method that requires weekly rather than daily administration. Unfortunately, however, observational data comparing use of the patch and OCs in a cohort of women considered at high risk for unintended pregnancy noted higher rates of patch discontinuation and contraceptive failure with the patch than with OCs [5].

The Contraceptive Vaginal Ring

The contraceptive vaginal ring (NuvaRing; Organon USA, Inc., Roseland, NJ) is a 54-mm diameter flexible, clear plastic ring that releases EE at 15 µg daily, along with etonogestrel, which is the biologically active metabolite of the progestin desogestrel found in a number of OC formulations (see Chapter 11). The ring is available in one size, which is smaller (and more flexible) than diaphragms. Patients may ask how they can be sure the ring "fits" properly. Such women can be reassured that as long as the ring remains in place and is not causing discomfort, it is in proper position and working appropriately. In clinical trials, some women (fewer than 5%) have discontinued use of the ring due to vaginal discomfort or expulsion. Although couples using the ring report that they are aware of the ring during intercourse, few women discontinue ring use for this reason [6,7]. Some couples leave the ring in during sexual relations, and others remove it for this purpose. If the ring is removed from the vagina for over 3 hours, back up barrier contraception should be used for 1 week.

The ring is inserted in the vagina for 3 weeks and then withdrawn for 1 week, during which withdrawal bleeding is anticipated. Accordingly, during routine use, a new ring would be inserted on the same day of the week every 4 weeks. The ring provides serum steroid levels sufficient to prevent ovulation for at least 4 weeks [8]. Concomitant use of vaginal spermicide, antifungals, and tampons have not been shown to cause clinically meaningful changes in serum levels of contraceptive steroids in women using the vaginal ring [9,10]. Rates of unscheduled (breakthrough) bleeding and spotting are less with the ring than with combination OCs [11•].

Contraceptive Mechanism of Action, Initiation, and Efficacy of the Patch and Ring

As with OCs, the patch and ring provide contraception via suppression of ovulation. When women initiate OCs, peak serum levels of contraceptive steroids are rapidly achieved, meaning that women starting pills on the first Sunday after menses begin do not need to use back up contraception during their first weeks of OC use. In contrast, peak levels of contraceptive steroids are not achieved until several days after initiation of the patch and ring. Accordingly, backup contraception should accompany initiation of the birth control patch or ring unless the first patch is applied/ring inserted on the first day of spontaneous menses (early enough to prevent ovulation in the first cycle of use).

Published reports indicate that in clinical trials, annual failure rates are approximately 1% with use of the patch and ring [3,6,8,12]. Because the patch and ring are new, estimates of contraceptive efficacy with typical use are not available. Therefore, the typical use annual failure rate with the ring and the patch are assumed to be similar to that of OCs (8%) [13•]. Of 15 pregnancies observed in clinical trials of the patch, five occurred in women who weighed 198 pounds (90 kg) or more, suggesting that failure rates for the patch are higher in women above this weight threshold [14]. Physicians should recognize, however, that even in overweight women, the patch represents a method substantially more effective than methods such as condoms and spermicides. When helping women who weigh 198 pounds or more make contraceptive decisions, physicians should weigh the somewhat higher failure rate with the patch against the patient's likelihood of successfully using alternate methods of birth control. Obesity has not been associated with higher failure rates with the vaginal ring [15].

The Contraceptive Patch and Vaginal Ring

Estrogen	Progestin	Schedule	Dimensions
Patch (Ortho Evra; Ortho-McNeil, Raritan, NJ)	Norelgestromin	One patch weekly for 3 weeks, then leave patch off for 1 week	4-cm square
Ring (NuvaRing; Organon USA, Roseland, NJ)	Etonogestrel	One ring for 3 weeks, then remove ring for 1 week	54-mm diameter

Figure 12-1. The contraceptive patch and vaginal ring.

Noncontraceptive Health Benefits and Use When Estrogen is Contraindicated

Because the patch and ring represent new methods of birth control, there are few clinical trials or epidemiologic data on noncontraceptive benefits, which are presumed to be similar to those associated with use of OCs (*see* Chapter 11).

As with estrogen-progestin combination contraceptives, use of the patch is associated with the same contraindications as apply to combination OCs (*see* Chapter 11) [16].

Estrogen Levels with the Patch, Oral Contraceptives, and the Ring: Risk of Venous Thromboembolism

Overall, circulating EE levels are substantially higher with the patch than with combination OCs [17•]. Levels of EE with OC use are higher than with the ring. These observations have led to the question: is the risk of venous thromboembolic disease (VTE) higher with the patch? A case control study found the VTE risks were comparable with use of the patch and OCs [18]. In contrast, a cohort study in which VTE case ascertainment may have been more rigorous than in the case-control study found that use of the patch was associated with a VTE risk some two times higher than with OCs [19•], allowing the conclusion that VTE risk indeed may be higher with the patch than with the pill. Because obesity represents an independent risk factor for VTE, use of the patch may be less appropriate than the ring or OCs in obese women.

References

Papers of particular interest have been highlighted as follows:
• Of interest
•• Of outstanding interest

1. Abrams LS, Skee DM, Wong FA, *et al.*: Pharmacokinetics of norelgestromin and ethinyl estradiol from two consecutive contraceptive patches. *J Clin Pharmacol* 2001, 41:1232–1237.

2. Abrams LS, Skee DM, Natarajan J, *et al.*: Pharmacokinetics of norelgestromin and ethinyl estradiol delivered by a contraceptive patch (Ortho Evra/Evra) under conditions of heat, humidity, and exercise. *J Clin Pharmacol* 2001, 41:1301–1309.

3.• Audet M-C, Moreau M, Koltun WD, *et al.*: For the ORTHO EVRA/EVRA 004 STUDY GROUP. Evaluation of contraceptive efficacy and cycle control of a transdermal contraceptive patch vs an oral contraceptive. A randomized controlled trial. *JAMA* 2001, 285:2347–2354.

Few randomized clinical trials have been conducted comparing one contraceptive with another. This Journal of the American Medical Association report provides valuable comparative data assessing patch versus OCs.

4.•• Speroff L, Darney P: *A Clinical Guide for Contraception*, edn 4. Baltimore: Williams & Wilkins; 2005.

For the practitioner who wishes to dig deeper into the field of contraception, this text represents a masterpiece: easy to read, frequently updated, and written by world experts.

5. Bakhru A, Stanwood N: Performance of contraceptive patch compared with oral contraceptive pill in a high risk population. *Obstet Gynecol* 2006, 108:378–386.

6. Dieben TOM, Roumen FJME, Apter D: Efficacy, cycle control, and user acceptability of a novel combined contraceptive vaginal ring. *Obstet Gynecol* 2002, 100:585–593.

7. Szarewski A: High acceptability and satisfaction with NuvaRing use. *Eur J Contracept Reprod Health Care* 2002, 7(Suppl):31–36.

8. Mulders TM, Dieben TO: Use of the novel combined contraceptive vaginal ring NuvaRing for ovulation inhibition. *Fertil Steril* 2001, 75:865–870.

9. Haring T, Mulders TMT: The combined contraceptive ring NuvaRing and spermicide co-medication. *Contraception* 2003, 67:271–272.

10. Verhoeven CHJ, Dieben TOM: The combined contraceptive vaginal ring, NuvaRing, and tampon co-usage. *Contraception* 2004, 69:197–199.

11.• Bjarnadóttir RI, Tuppurainen M, Killick SR: Comparison of cycle control with a combined vaginal ring and oral levonorgestrel/ethinyl estradiol. *Am J Obstet Gynecol* 2002, 186:389–395.

As with Audet et al. [3], this useful report describes a randomized trial comparing a newer method (vaginal contraceptive ring) with OCs.

12. Roumen FJME, Apter D, Mulders TMS, Dieben TOM: Efficacy, tolerability and acceptability of a novel contraceptive vaginal ring releasing etonogestrel and ethinyl estradiol. *Hum Reprod* 2001, 16:469–475.

13.• Trussell J: Contraceptive failure in the United States. *Contraception* 2004, 70:89–96.

Dr. Trussell is definitely the guru of contraceptive efficacy!

14. Zieman M, Guillebaud J, Weisberg E, *et al.*: Contraceptive efficacy and cycle control with the Ortho Evra/Evra transdermal system: the analysis of polled data. *Fertil Steril* 2002, 77(Suppl 2):S13.

15. O'Connell KJ, Osborne LM, Westhoff C: Measured and reported weight change for women using a vaginal contraceptive ring versus a low-dose oral contraceptive. *Contraception* 2005, 72:323–327.

16. American College of Obstetricians and Gynecologists. Use of hormonal contraception in women with medical problems. Number 73, Washington, D.C., June 2006.

17.• Van den Heuvel MW, van Bragt AJM, Alnabawy A, Kaptein MC: Comparison of ethinyl estradiol pharmacokinetics in three hormonal contraceptive formulations: the vaginal ring, the transdermal patch, and an oral contraceptive. *Contraception* 2005, 72:168–174.

This pharmacokinetic trial provides definitive data comparing EE area under the curve for the contraceptive ring, the patch, and OCs.

18. Jick SS, Kaye JA, Russman S, Jick H: Risk of nonfatal venous thromboembolism in women using a contraceptive transdermal patch and oral contraceptives containing norgestimate and 35 mcg of ethinyl estradiol. *Contraception* 2006, 73:223–228.

19.• Cole JA, Norman H, Doherty M, Walker AM: Venous thromboembolism, myocardial infarction, and stroke among transdermal contraceptive users. *Obstet Gynecol* 2007, 109:339–346.

Because VTE occurs rarely in young women, studying the comparative incidence of VTE in users of the patch and OCs is challenging. This report used national insurance claims data to compare venous thromboembolism risk between the patch and pill.

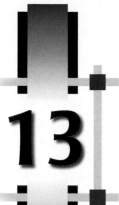

13 Female Tubal Sterilization

Gary H. Lipscomb

- Common female sterilization methods are generally divided into open, laparoscopic, and hysteroscopic methods, and include the Pomeroy (open); Parkland, Uchida, and Irving methods; electrocoagulation (laparoscopic); silastic rings and mechanical clips; and Essure (hysteroscopic [Conceptus, Inc., Mountain View, CA]).
- The isthmic portion of the fallopian tube is the appropriate site for all occlusive techniques.
- Sterilization failures are more common than previously believed, with 10-year cumulative failure rates averaging 1.8% and ranging from 0.37% to over 4.5% depending on method and patient age at the time of sterilization.
- The use of "coag" (modulated) current rather than "cut" (nonmodulated) current during bipolar electrocoagulation is associated with an increased failure rate.
- The use of nonabsorbable or delayed-absorbable suture for Pomeroy type sterilization has historically been one of the more common preventable causes for an increased failure rate in this type of procedure.

This chapter is intended to familiarize the primary care physician with the various aspects of female sterilization. Although surgically oriented, this chapter is also useful for physicians who do not perform sterilizations but wish to provide counseling and advice to patients considering permanent contraception.

Female tubal sterilization procedures are generally grouped into those traditionally performed using open or nonlaparoscopic methods and those performed laparoscopically. However, many laparoscopic techniques have been adapted for use through open incisions, and many of the open techniques can be performed laparoscopically. Additionally, there are now reliable hysteroscopic sterilization methods available.

Open (Nonlaparoscopic) Female Sterilization Procedures

As the name implies, open sterilization methods are performed through an open incision. This is most commonly a subumbilical incision used for postpartum sterilization but may be a suprapubic "minilap" incision, a laparotomy incision, or even a vaginal cul de sac approach. The most common open methods are described below.

MODIFIED POMEROY METHOD

The Pomeroy technique is the most common nonlaparoscopic method of surgical female sterilization (Figure 13-1). Its popularity is primarily because of its simplicity. In this method, the middle portion of the fallopian tube is grasped and elevated with a Babcock clamp. The elevated "knuckle" of the tube is then double-ligated with two #0 plain catgut sutures. The mesosalpinx within the ligated loop is then perforated with scissors, and each limb is individually cut to avoid inadvertently shaving off the top of the tube resulting in an incomplete resection. The excised tubal segment is then sent for pathologic examination. The severed ends are inspected for the presence of a visible tubal lumen as well as for hemostasis. Bleeding is usually minimal, as this method occludes the tubal vasculature before the tubal segment is transected.

The failure rate of the Pomeroy technique will be significantly increased if delayed-absorbable or permanent suture is used for ligation. Originally, chromic catgut was used to allow the tubal ends to rapidly retract away from each other with the belief that this would allow the ends to fibrose and reperitonealize without fistula formation. This is also the rationale for the modification of the Pomeroy in which plain catgut instead of chromic catgut is used. The use of less rapidly absorbed sutures such as polyglycolic acid or a permanent suture such as silk allows the two ends of the tube to be held in close approximation for a greater period of time, thus increasing the probability of fistula formation between the two ends.

PARKLAND METHOD

The Parkland method of tubal ligation is a modification of the Pomeroy technique designed to avoid the initial approximation of the severed tubal ends (Figure 13-2). The initial selection and elevation of a "knuckle" of the tube is identical to the Pomeroy technique. In this method, a hemostat is passed through an avascular portion of the mesosalpinx of the elevated tubal segment. Two, plain catgut sutures are drawn back through this opening and tied on opposite sides of the "knuckle" so that a

segment of tube is isolated. The tubal segment is then removed with scissors. At the conclusion of this procedure, the cut ends remain widely separated. This initial separation may result in a lower failure rate than that of the Pomeroy method. Unfortunately, there are no published studies on the failure rate associated with this sterilization method.

IRVING TECHNIQUE

To perform this type of sterilization, the uterine fundus is delivered into the surgical field and one fallopian tube is identified (Figure 13-3). A hemostat is passed through an avascular portion of the mesosalpinx in the region of the tubal ampullary-isthmic junction in a manner similar to that used at the start of

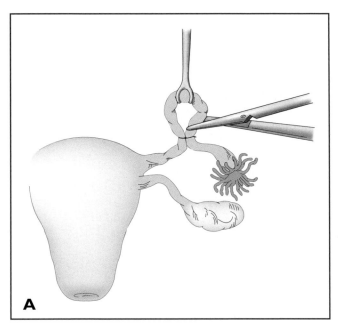

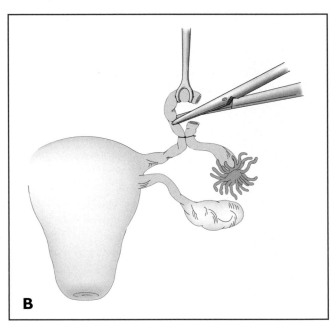

Figure 13-1. Modified Pomeroy method. **A**, Fenestration of mesosalpinx of tubal knuckle. **B**, Excision of tubal segment. (*Adapted from* Peterson *et al.* [5].)

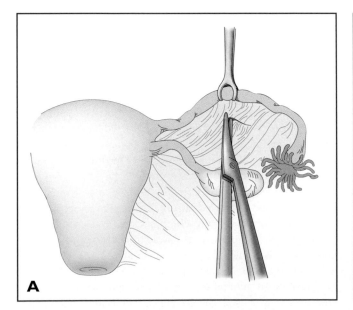

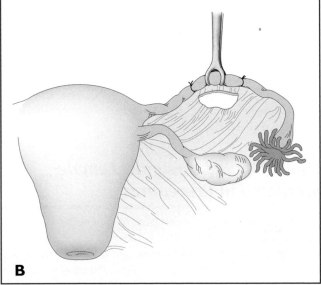

Figure 13-2. Parkland method. **A**, Fenestration of mesosalpinx. **B**, Ligation of tubal segment.
Continued on the next page

the Parkland method. Two #0 absorbable sutures are passed through this opening, a tubal segment double-ligated, and the ends of the suture left long. The tube is now divided between the two ligatures. If desired, the segment of tube between the two ligatures may be completely excised for pathologic examination. An avascular area on the posterior uterus is now pierced with a mosquito hemostat to create a myometrial pocket approximately 1 cm deep. The sutures attached to the proximal tubal segment are now threaded on eyed, curved needles. The needles are then separately passed through the base of the myometrial pocket to exit the uterine surface 1 cm apart. Traction is applied to the sutures, burying the tubal stump in the myometrial pocket and the sutures tied. The original technique not only buried the proximal tubal stump within the myometrium, but also buried the ligated end of the distal tubal segment in the broad ligament. As this step requires additional time and effort but has not been proven to increase effectiveness, it is generally omitted today.

The Irving method has the advantage of an extremely low failure rate, but is associated with increased incidence of

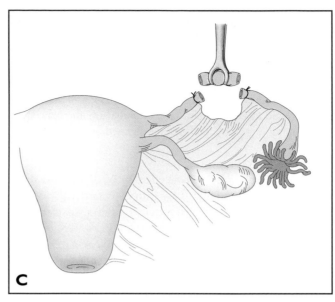

C

Figure 13-2. *(Continued)* **C**, Excision of tubal segment. *(Adapted from* Peterson *et al.* [5].)

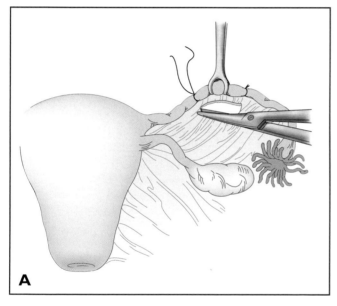

A

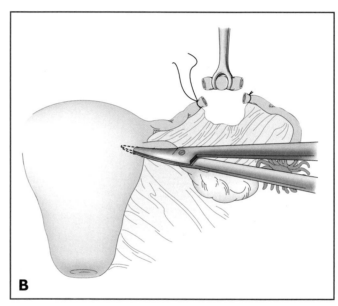

B

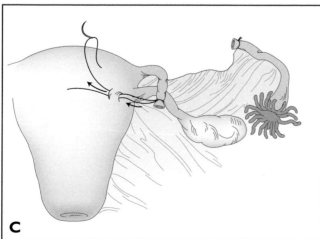

C

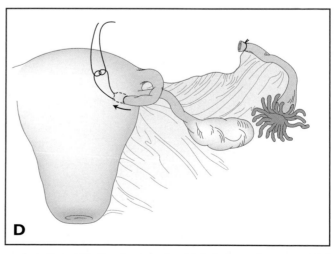

D

Figure 13-3. Irving method. **A**, Fenestration of mesosalpinx. **B**, Ligation of tubal segment and creation of myometrial pocket. **C** and **D**, Burying proximal tubal stump in myometrial pocket. *(Adapted from* Peterson *et al.* [5].)

intraoperative bleeding. Because a relatively large abdominal incision is required for this technique, it is generally only performed when the abdomen has already been entered for other indications such as cesarean section. The Irving procedure is also not recommended for use as an interval sterilization method since the very low failure rate of this method may be partially due to compression and eventual obliteration of the buried tubal lumen by the involuting gravid uterus.

THE UCHIDA METHOD

The Uchida method is the most complex of all the tubal sterilization methods, but failures are extremely rare (Figure 13-4). The disadvantages are that it requires more tubal manipulation and a greater degree of surgical skill to perform than any other methods.

After the fallopian tube is exposed by the chosen operative approach, the tube is grasped with a Babcock clamp and elevated into the surgical field, where the tube is grasped with a second Babcock clamp, and the segment to be operated on is placed on tension. A 25-gauge needle is used to inject saline into the subserosal area of the tube, thus ballooning the serosa away from the tubal muscularis. Alternatively, a solution containing a dilute vasospastic agent such as epinephrine or pitressin may be used for injection. A readily available premixed solution that can be used is lidocaine with epinephrine.

The ballooned serosa is incised longitudinally with a scalpel, and a 2- to 3-cm segment of tube is dissected free of the serosa with a mosquito hemostat. Uchida originally recommended removal of a 5-cm segment, but most surgeons chose to remove a smaller segment to increase the success of any future reanastomosis attempts. Two pieces of plain #0 or 2-0 absorbable suture are passed under the freed segment of tube and tied at opposite ends of the isolated segment of tube. The segment of tube between the two ligatures is excised with scissors and sent for pathologic examination. The ends of the tube are inspected for the presence of a lumen as well as for hemostasis. The suture ligating the proximal tube is cut, allowing this segment to retract back into the mesosalpinx. Traction is applied to the distal tubal segment, elevating it free of the mesosalpinx. A #3-0 synthetic absorbable suture is then used to reapproximate the tubal serosa. At the conclusion of the serosal reapproximation, the suture is used to perform a purse string closure at the base of the distal tubal segment. As a result, the proximal stump is buried within the mesosalpinx while the distal end is exteriorized.

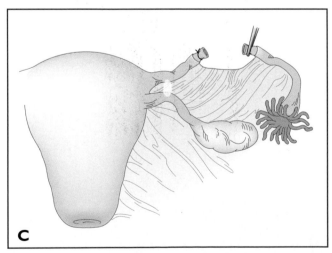
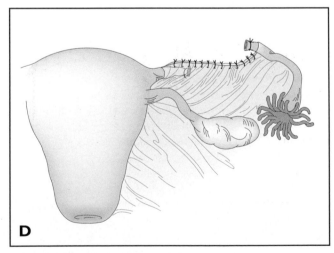
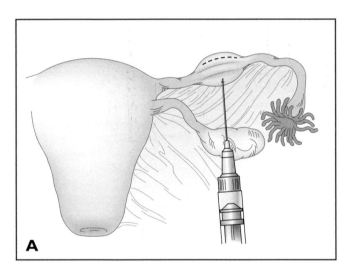
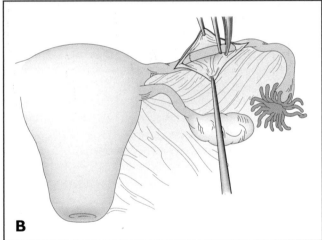
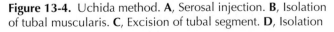

Figure 13-4. Uchida method. **A**, Serosal injection. **B**, Isolation of tubal muscularis. **C**, Excision of tubal segment. **D**, Isolation of proximal segment in mesosalpinx and distal segment in abdominal cavity. (*Adapted from* Peterson *et al.* [5].)

Laparoscopic Female Sterilization Procedures

Multiple laparoscopic methods have been developed for female tubal sterilization. Because of the relative ease and rapidity of tubal occlusion, many of these methods have also been used during open minilap, postpartum, and vaginal sterilization procedures.

ELECTROCOAGULATION

Electrocoagulation is the oldest technique of laparoscopic sterilization. Electrocoagulation utilizing unipolar current gained widespread popularity during the early years of laparoscopic sterilization, but fell into disfavor following reports of increasing numbers of bowel burns resulting from the procedure. Although most bowel injuries were subsequently shown to be trocar injuries and not electrical burns, unipolar electrocoagulation remained unpopular [1]. Today, the inherently safer bipolar electric current has essentially replaced unipolar current for tubal sterilization. Because of the widespread tubal destruction associated with electrocoagulation, this method is less affected by tubal thickness and mobility than many other methods. Thus, electrocoagulation may be preferable when the tube is edematous and thickened or cannot be easily mobilized for mechanical device placement. Conversely, the greater tubal damage associated with electrocoagulation makes tubal reversal more difficult should the patient regret her decision. Electrocoagulation should always be readily available during laparoscopic tubal sterilization both as a back-up method of sterilization and for control of unexpected bleeding.

During sterilization with bipolar electrocoagulation, the fallopian tube is identified and grasped at the mid-isthmus region, approximately 2.5 to 3 cm from the uterotubal junction, with the bipolar forceps (Figure 13-5). The tube is tented up to ensure the forceps are not in contact with any other structure, and the current applied until coagulation is complete. Unlike the widespread coagulation seen during unipolar electrocoagulation, tissue destruction with bipolar current is confined to the area between and immediately adjacent to the bipolar paddles. Therefore, it is generally necessary to repeat the electrocoagulation an additional two times at immediately adjacent sites to duplicate the same amount of coagulation seen with unipolar current. Destruction of a minimum of 2 cm of tube has been suggested as adequate by some authorities, although others advocate coagulation of at least 3 cm to ensure sterilization. Data from the Collaborative Review of Sterilization study appear to indicate that coagulation of three contiguous areas is associated with a significant decrease in failure rates [2].

If unipolar electrocoagulation is used, the initial site of coagulation should be chosen to allow any subsequent application to be closer to the uterus. Unipolar current returns to the return electrode through the path of least resistance. After the initial coagulation of the tube, the desiccated area has increased resistance, thus unipolar current applied distal to this site may flow to the end of tube instead of through the uterus. If the distal end of the tube should touch bowel, a bowel burn could theoretically occur.

Classically, the fallopian tube was cut and divided following coagulation. A segment of tube can also be removed for histologic evaluation as part of this procedure. Because this increases the complexity of the procedure and may lead to hemorrhage from a mesosalpinx tear, it is generally omitted by most laparoscopic surgeons today. Some authorities also believe division of the tube increases the chance of tuboperitoneal fistula and subsequent ectopic pregnancy. Furthermore, any tissue submitted to pathology is often so distorted that an accurate tissue diagnosis cannot be made.

Although gynecologists use electrosurgery on an almost daily basis, many are unfamiliar with the physics involved. The unfortunate designation of current as "cut" and "coag" is especially confusing as "cut" current can coagulate, and "coag" current can cut depending on the manner in which it is used. A more appropriate scientific designation is nonmodulated current for "cut" and modulated current for "coag." When used in a contact mode, nonmodulated (cut) current is a far more efficient desiccator of tissue than modulated (coag) current. In a similar situation, modulated current produces a rapid carbonization of the tubal surface which impedes deeper electrocoagulation.

Electrosurgical units designed solely for tubal electrocoagulation generate only nonmodulated (cut) bipolar current, whereas "Bovie" type electrosurgical generators often permit the selection of either modulated (coag) or nonmodulated (cut) current in the bipolar mode. Unfortunately, many surgeons and operating room nurses automatically select the less efficient "coag" current for tubal sterilization. The result may be a tubal lumen which remains viable despite the visual appearance of complete tubal coagulation. Thus, only nonmodulated current should be used for tubal sterilization.

Many gynecologists use a "blanch, swell, and collapse" visual endpoint to determine complete tubal coagulation. However, it is uncertain whether this method is completely reliable.

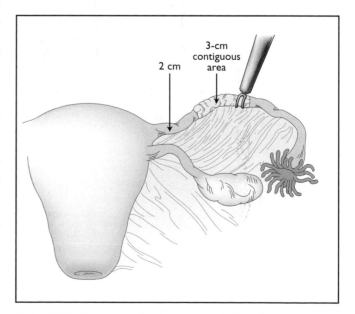

Figure 13-5. Laparoscopic electrocoagulation of 3-cm segment of tube with uncoagulated proximal segment. (*Adapted from* Sammarco *et al.* [6].)

Consistent, adequate coagulation is best achieved by using an ammeter to document cessation of current flow rather than depending on a visual endpoint. Alternatively, a timed coagulation period of at least 10 seconds at 25 W of nonmodulated current will usually assure complete tubal occlusion.

The use of electrosurgical generators with bipolar forceps produced by different manufacturers has been suggested as a cause of insufficient tubal coagulation. However, subsequent research would seem to indicate that complete coagulation is more dependent on selection of the proper waveform and power setting than on generator-forceps mismatch.

The most serious and feared complication occurring with the use of electrocoagulation is thermal injury to the bowel. The use of bipolar current eliminates the majority of risk of this complication. Care to ensure that only the fallopian tube is grasped with the forceps and that the tube is not touching other intra-abdominal structures should further reduce the risk of this complication.

SILASTIC RINGS

Efforts to replace electric current with a safer means of laparoscopic sterilization led to the development of silastic rings for tubal occlusion (Figure 13-6). The silastic ring is a nonreactive, silicone rubber ring with an inner diameter of 1 mm. To permit radiographic identification, 5% barium sulfate is incorporated into the ring. The rings are applied with a specialized applicator device consisting of two concentric cylinders, the inner one of which contains grasping prongs at its distal end. The movement of these cylinders is controlled by a single ring grip. The silastic band is stretched over the inner ring using a conical-shaped applicator. Bands should not be loaded on the application until ready for use to prevent possible loss off elastic memory. Applicators are also available that accommodate two rings so that removal for reloading between banding is not required.

The preloaded silastic ring applicator may be introduced either through a second suprapubic puncture or through the operating channel of an operative laparoscope. The grasping forceps are extended, and the fallopian tube is grasped approximately 2.5 to 3 cm distal to the utero-tubal junction. The tube is drawn into the inner sleeve by retracting the tongs until resistance is felt. The ring is then pushed off the applicator and onto the tube using the sliding mechanism on the applicator. An adequate knuckle of tube should be approximately 1 cm long with an obvious inner loop.

This knuckle of tube then undergoes necrosis from interruption of its blood supply. Complete absorption of the knuckle occurs in 3 to 6 months at which time the proximal and distal stump usually separate completely. The ring itself usually becomes covered with peritoneum and remains near the original occlusion site but may fall free into the abdominal cavity. Occasionally, this characteristic has resulted in lawsuits when uninformed surgeons, operating for an ectopic pregnancy, have assumed that the absence of a ring on the tube indicated incorrect initial ring placement.

Difficulties with silastic ring placement can occur with thickened or adhesed fallopian tubes. These conditions often hinder complete retraction of the tube into the applicator. The end result is often application of the ring to a knuckle containing only serosa, or complete transection of the tube. This complication can generally be prevented by: 1) slow withdrawal of the tube into the sleeve, thus allowing time for the tube to conform to the sleeve diameter, and 2) slightly advancing the entire applicator as the tube is drawn up to avoid countertraction from the fixed uterine end of the tube. In the case of edematous or thickened tubes, using a "milking" action with the tongs will often allow edematous tubes to be drawn into the sleeve. Alternatively, the "Yoon three grasp technique" may be used to allow ring placement on edematous tubes (Figure 13-7). With excessively thick, edematous tubes or scarred tubes, the use of another method such as electrocoagulation should be considered as an alternative to attempted mechanical occlusion.

If the tube is transected, silastic rings may be placed proximal and distal to the transection, interrupting blood supply to the rest. Electrocoagulation of the free ends also may be used to achieve both hemostasis and tubal occlusion.

MECHANICAL CLIPS

Sterilization by mechanical clip is potentially the most reversible of all the laparoscopic methods (Figure 13-8). Originally, mechanical clips for tubal occlusion were essentially identical to the hemostatic clips used to occlude small bleeding vessels

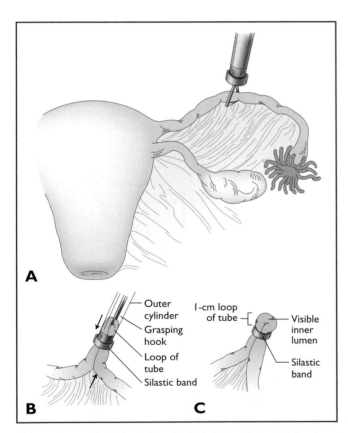

Figure 13-6. Silastic band method. **A**, Forceps grasp isthmic portion of tube 2.5 to 3 cm from cornu. **B**, Tubal loop is drawn into inner cylinder and ring is pushed off. **C**, Adequate knuckle of tube. (*Adapted from* Sammarco *et al.* [6].)

during surgery. These original clips had an unacceptably high failure rate. Such failures occurred when necrosis of the tubal muscularis beneath the clip eliminated the pressure on the deeper endosalpinx and allowed the tubal lumen to reopen. To prevent this complication, modern clips are designed to maintain a constant pressure as the tubal wall undergoes necrosis. When properly placed, only 4 mm of tube and virtually none of the tubal blood supply is destroyed. Thus, elective tubal reanastomosis is more easily accomplished after mechanical clip tubal occlusion. The disadvantage of this limited destruction is that precise and accurate placement is required to achieve acceptable failure rates.

Today, there are primarily two mechanical clips in widespread use, the Hulka-Clemens clip and the Filshie clip. The Hulka-Clemens clip consists of two, toothed jaws of Lexan plastic joined by a metal hinge pin. The lower jaw possesses a distal hook. The stainless steel pin (gold plated to reduce peritoneal irritation) maintains the clip in an open position. When completely advanced, the spring closes and locks the jaws. The Hulka applicator is 7 mm in diameter with a three-ring configuration at the handle. A fixed distal lower jaw cradles the

clip whereas the mobile upper jaw opens and closes the clip. A center piston, when advanced, locks the clip closed. The Filshie clip is made of titanium and silicone. It is technically a simpler device than the Hulka-Clemens clip. A thick silicone coating instead of a metal spring is used to provide constant pressure on the tube.

Application of the Hulka-Clemens clip is described here, but the Filshie clip is applied in a similar manner. The loaded Hulka clip applicator is introduced with the clip in the closed position, and then the clip is opened after the applicator is intra-abdominal. The clip is placed perpendicular to the tube at a site 2.5 to 3 cm from the utero-tubal junction. The clip may be repeatedly opened and repositioned until ideal position is achieved. The center piston is then advanced to permanently lock the clip and unseat it from the applicator. The applicator is withdrawn leaving the clip in place on the tube.

ENDOCOAGULATION

A technique of laparoscopic sterilization using true cautery to coagulate the fallopian tubes has been developed. This system uses direct electric current to heat grasping forceps to 100ºC to 120ºC. Coagulation occurs as a result of heat transfer from the forceps and not by heat generated from the effect of current passing through the tissue. This method, although rarely used in the United States, is popular in many parts of Europe. Proponents believe that endocoagulation is less likely than high frequency electrocoagulation to stimulate tubal recannulization.

During endocoagulation, the tube is grasped 1 to 3 cm from the utero-tubal junction. The tube is then coagulation in two adjacent areas.

Application of Local Anesthesia

The use of mechanical devices for tubal occlusion is often associated with more postoperative discomfort than with electrocoagulation. Electrocoagulation destroys the neural innervation, thus rendering the tube anesthetic. However, mechanical occlusion of the tube may be considered occlusion of a small

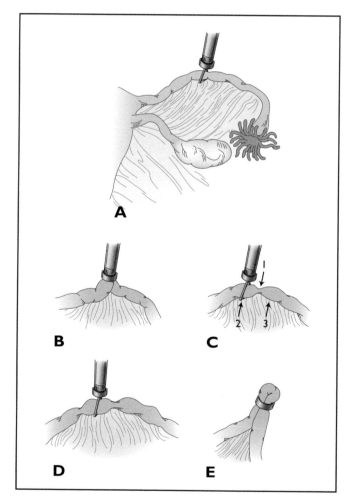

Figure 13-7. Yoon three-grasp technique. **A,** Thickened tube is grasped at the normal position. **B,** Tube is partially retracted into cylinder to squeeze edema from tube and then dropped. **C,** Process is repeated on each side of initial site. **D** and **E,** Tube is regrasped at initial site and band is applied.

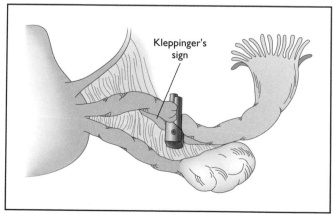

Figure 13-8. Hulka clip. The clip should be perpendicular with the entire tube within the clip.

hollow viscus and produces a similar crampy abdominal pain. Postoperative nausea and vomiting also is reported to be increased with these methods. These side effects can be minimized or eliminated, however, if the fallopian tubes are first anesthetized with a local anesthetic.

Because of its high protein binding and long duration of action, 0.5% bupivacaine is an excellent choice as the local anesthetic. For best results, the local anesthetic should be applied to each tube prior to and not after occlusion. Five milliliters of 0.5% bupivacaine per tube will provide prolonged tubal anesthesia. An aspiration cannula can be used to flow the bupivacaine over all surfaces of the tube. Topical application of bupivacaine has been shown to be equal to tubal injection and is technically much simpler.

Hysteroscopic Sterilization

Hysteroscopic female sterilization has the potential to be simpler, less morbid, and better tolerated than laparoscopic or open methods. Various methods of hysteroscopic sterilization including electrocoagulation, cryocoagulation, injection of various chemicals, mechanical occlusive devices, and plastic formed-in-place plugs have been tried with variable success. Currently, only the Essure (Conceptus, Inc., Mountain View, CA) device is approved by the US Food and Drug Administration for hysteroscopic sterilization in the United States.

This device is a microcoiled device similar in design to interventional radiology stents. When properly placed, the device spans the utero-tubal junction and is held in place by the expanded coils until tubal ingrowth of tissue occurs. This ingrowth is stimulated by the presence of polyethylene terephthalate fibers within the coils. The microinserts are placed using a 5-mm hysteroscope with a 5-French operating channel. In multiparous women, insertion of this size hysteroscope usually does not require cervical dilation but can be accomplished using only hydrodilation.

Essure placement can usually be accomplished in an office setting using only nonsteroidal analgesics and paracervical block. Bilateral placement is achieved in approximately 86% on first attempt with overall placement rising to 90% with a second procedure. Hysteroscopic procedure time averages 15 minutes.

The advertised effectiveness of the Essure device is 99.8%. In the initial studies presented to the US Food and Drug Administration as part of the approval process, no failures were noted with short-term follow-up. More failures would be expected as the follow-up period is extended and as the procedure is performed by more and more physicians.

The procedure cannot be relied on for contraception until tissue ingrowth occludes the tubal lumen. This generally occurs by 3 months after the procedure. Alternative contraception must be used until tubal occlusion is verified. The US Food and Drug Administration requires a follow-up hysterosalpingogram to verify tubal occlusion. The length of time required for Essure to become effective and the need for follow-up hysterosalpingogram have been cited as potential obstacles to patient acceptance for this procedure.

Research continues on other hysteroscopic methods of sterilization that may further simply the procedure or shorten the time to complete tubal occlusion.

Sterilization Failures

Historically, failure rates for sterilization methods have been reported to be one to four per 1000 procedures, with little difference between the various methods. However, much of this data is based on relatively small groups without reliable long-term follow-up. Data from the Collaborative Review of Sterilization have indicated higher failure rates for all methods than previously reported [3••]. Ten-year cumulative failure rates range from 0.54 % to over 3% overall, with failure rates in the more fertile, younger patients ranging from 0.37% to over 4.5%. In the past, it was generally believed that most tubal sterilization failures occurred within the first 1 to 2 years after the sterilization. The Collaborative Review of Sterilization study has shown that failures were evenly divided over the 10-year study period.

Sterilization failures fall into six categories: 1) luteal phase pregnancies, 2) misidentification of the fallopian tube, 3) incomplete occlusion of a properly identified tube, 4) use of inappropriate method or 5) technique for tubal occlusion, and 6) technical failures.

LUTEAL PHASE PREGNANCY

Luteal phase pregnancy is defined as a pregnancy diagnosed after an interval tubal sterilization, but in which contraception occurred before the sterilization procedure. Luteal phase pregnancy has been reported to occur at a rate of one to 15 per 1000 interval sterilizations. Technically speaking, a luteal phase pregnancy is not a true sterilization failure since, by definition, the pregnancy preceded the sterilization. Nevertheless, the result is an undesired pregnancy. A variety of strategies have been suggested to reduce the incidence of luteal phase pregnancies. These include performing sterilization procedures before the date of estimated ovulation, concurrent dilation and curettage, use of effective contraception and/or sexual abstinence before sterilization, and preoperative pregnancy testing. At our institution, we have found that the use of same-day urine pregnancy testing using an enzyme-linked immunosorbent assay has virtually eliminated luteal phase pregnancies [4•].

MISIDENTIFICATION OF THE FALLOPIAN TUBE

On occasion, pelvic structures such as the round ligament, ovarian ligament, infundibulopelvic ligament, or dilated broad ligament blood vessel may be mistaken for a fallopian tube and mistakenly ligated. Poor visualization is generally the primary cause for misidentification of the fallopian tube. Factors which may contribute to poor visualization include inadequate light, poor retraction, and pelvic adhesions. For open procedures, an inadequate incision and a failure to systematically trace the fallopian tube to its fimbriated end can also be contributing factors. For laparoscopic procedures, a failure to adequately elevate the uterus, inadequate pneumoperitoneum, and poor optics are additional confounding factors. With the exception of pelvic adhesions, these factors are easily avoided with the use of proper equipment and technique and should be a rare cause of sterilization failure.

FAILED TUBAL OCCLUSION

A common cause of sterilization failure is the failure to completely occlude the fallopian tube. This is frequently encountered with the use of mechanical occlusive devices during laparoscopy. The mechanical clips are particularly vulnerable to poor placement. Great care must be taken to fully include the tube within the clip. With correct application, the serosa on the surface of the tube is pulled upward to resemble the flat, triangle shape of an envelope flap (Kleppinger's "envelope" sign) (Figure 13-8). A grasper inserted through another abdominal port or the operating laparoscope can be used to place the tube on tension prior to clip application. This decreases the likelihood that the lumen will roll out of the clip during application. The use of mechanical devices on edematous or dilated tubes frequently results in only partial tubal occlusion. When silastic rings are used, the tubal serosa but not tubal lumen may be pulled into the ring. This knuckle of serosa can closely resemble a truly adequate "knuckle." However, close observation will reveal the absence of the vertical crease formed when an entire loop of tube is included in the ring. Some have compared the appearance of an adequate knuckle to that of a baby's buttock and gluteal crease. Incomplete tubal occlusion with electrocoagulation is generally associated with either application of current for too short a time interval or use of modulated (coag) current as discussed previously in this chapter. The use of timed electrocoagulation or ammeter and nonmodulated current should eliminate this cause of tubal sterilization failure.

Attempted occlusion of the wrong segment of a properly identified tube is another cause of failed tubal occlusion. The isthmic portion of the fallopian tube is the proper site for all sterilization procedures that depend on tubal occlusion rather than removal of a tubal segment. The isthmus of the tube has a thick muscularis with a narrow lumen. In contrast, the ampulla has a thin muscularis, wide lumen, and voluminous rugae. Attempted occlusion of the ampulla with mechanical devices may not incorporate all of the tubal lumen, resulting in sterilization failure. Electrocoagulation of the tubal ampulla is more likely to produce complete occlusion, but will not achieve the same failure rate as coagulation of the isthmic portion of the tube. On the other hand, coagulation of the tube too close to the cornu may lead to uteroperitoneal fistula formation. It is believed that the traumatized mucosa proliferates and invades the tubal muscularis, penetrates the serosa, and result in a fistula. The resulting recanalization frequently results in a fistula sufficient to allow passage of sperm but usually not the ovum. This may be one explanation of the high ratio of ectopic to intrauterine pregnancies following failure of sterilization by electrocoagulation.

INAPPROPRIATE TECHNIQUE OR METHOD

The use of an inappropriate technique or method for tubal sterilization is fortunately relatively uncommon today. However, the medical literature reports many such examples in the recent past. One of the more common mistakes was to use the wrong suture for tubal ligation. For example, silk is used for ligation in a Pomeroy tubal ligation. As previously noted, the use of a permanent or delayed absorbable suture prevents the severed ends of the fallopian tube from retracting and increases the failure rate.

Another inappropriate technique was the use of standard hemoclips for tubal ligation. As the tubal serosa and muscularis undergo pressure necrosis, hemoclips are unable to close further, unlike Hulka-Clemens or Filshie clips, which continue to apply pressure to the tube as the wall necrosis occurs. The result is a reopening of the tubal lumen as the surrounding tissue degenerates.

TECHNICAL FAILURES

Technical failures result when a sterilization procedure is performed correctly, but a pregnancy still occurs. Unfortunately, it is difficult to ascertain what proportion of sterilization failures are the result of true technical failures and what proportion are the result of one of the factors previously mentioned.

Conclusions

The surgical techniques presented in this chapter should enable the practitioner to choose an appropriate technique for female tubal sterilization and to employ these techniques in a manner that will minimize morbidity and maximize success.

References

Papers of particular interest have been highlighted as follows:
- Of interest
- • Of outstanding interest

1. Levi BS, Soderstrom RM, Dali DS: Bowel injuries during laparoscopy: gross anatomy and histology. *J Reprod Med* 1985, 30:168.

2. Pregnancy after tubal sterilization with bipolar electrocoagulation. US Collaborative Review of Sterilization Working Group. *Obstet Gynecol* 1999, 94:163–167.

3.•• Peterson HB, Zhisen X, Hughes JM, *et al.*: The risk of pregnancy after tubal sterilization: Findings from the US Collaborative Review of Sterilization. *Am J Obstet Gynecol* 1996, 174:1161–1170.
   A landmark report of a10-year multicenter study that completely changed conventional beliefs regarding the failure rate of sterilization procedures.

4.• Lipscomb GH, Spellman JR, Ling FW: The effect of same-day pregnancy testing on the incidence of luteal phase pregnancy. *Obstet Gynecol* 1993, 82:411–413.
   This study indicated that luteal phase pregnancies were not an uncommon cause of sterilization failures at the study institution. A review of methods for prevention is discussed as well as the use of urine pregnancy testing in detecting very early pregnancies prior to sterilization.

5. Peterson HB, Pollack AE, Warshaw JS: Tubal sterilization. In *TeLinde's Operative Gynecology*, edn 8. Edited by Rock JA, Thompson JD. Philadelphia: Lippincott-Raven; 1997:529.

6. Sammarco MJ, Stovall TG, Steege JF: *Gynecologic Endoscopy: Principles in Practice*. Baltimore: Williams & Wilkins; 1996.

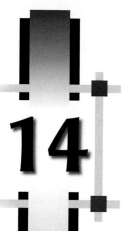

14 | Barrier Methods of Contraception

Deborah L. Nucatola

- These methods provide a physical barrier to sperm, are coitus-dependent, and require consistent and correct use to achieve highest possible efficacy.
- Barrier methods are increasingly used in combination with hormonal methods and other barrier methods to maximize contraception and decrease sexually transmitted disease (STD) risk.
- Barrier methods are the only methods which reduce the risk of transmission and acquisition of HIV and other STDs.
- Eighty-two percent of women of reproductive age have used a condom at some time. Current use is reported by 20% of all contraceptors.
- Latex, rather than natural skin, is recommended for individuals seeking protection from STDs; polyurethane condoms are believed to provide protection similar to latex, although data is scarce.
- Barrier methods have received renewed interest as a vehicle to vaginally deliver microbicides for contraception and STD prevention.
- Future studies will undoubtedly lead to the development of more user-friendly barrier methods.

Barrier methods of contraception provide a physical barrier to sperm. These include male condoms, diaphragms, female condoms, and the sponge. Other than male condoms, these methods have declined in popularity during the past 20 years [1,2••,3]. They are described as coitus-dependent and require consistent and correct use to achieve the highest possible contraceptive efficacy.

Barrier methods are the only methods shown to reduce the risk of transmission and acquisition of HIV and other sexually transmitted diseases (STDs). Recently, they have received interest as a vehicle to vaginally deliver microbicides for contraception and STD prevention. Characteristics of the various barrier methods that differ include availability over the counter, female versus male control of use, use for multiple acts of intercourse, use immediately or longer before intercourse, ease of use, and relative protection against HIV and other STDs [4].

User characteristics determine consistency and correct use. The individual's motivation to avoid pregnancy is one determinant. The capacity to plan intercourse and contraception

is also important. Demographic data indicate that the people most likely to use condoms are young and unmarried. Other barrier methods, such as the diaphragm and sponge, have been used more frequently by older women.

General Issues

General issues related to contraceptive efficacy and STD risk reduction are addressed in this section, but because the specific characteristics of the various barrier methods and barrier users vary, each method is discussed individually later.

Spermicides are an adjunct to the contraceptive efficacy of barrier methods. The extent to which the barrier component or the spermicide contributes to efficacy is not well-established for some methods. Although there is increasing focus on vaginal microbicides (spermicidal and nonspermicidal), from an infectious disease perspective, a discussion of this issue is beyond the scope of this chapter.

Efficacy

CONTRACEPTION

Contraceptive efficacy can be calculated from population-based surveys or from clinical trials and investigations. In general, failure rates derived from population-based surveys are higher than those from clinical trials [5••]. A precise definition of contraceptive effectiveness is the proportional reduction in the monthly probability of conception, a value that is neither observable nor accurately estimated. Thus, contraceptive efficacy is usually assessed by measuring the number of pregnancies that occur during a specified interval of exposure to a given contraceptive method and is reported using either the Pearl index or life-table techniques. The Pearl index is widely used and required by the US Food and Drug Administration (FDA) for approval of a new method of contraception). It is defined as the number of pregnancies per 100 woman-years of exposure. Because failure rates for most methods of contraception decline over time, as women gain experience in using the method, or those most likely to have a failure get pregnant sooner, the life-table analysis calculates a separate failure rate for each month of use.

Contraceptive effectiveness depends on both the inherent effectiveness of a method and correct or perfect usage of the method. The inherent or theoretical efficacy of a method is difficult to ascertain, and even perfect use does not result in zero failures. The failure rates of contraceptive methods during actual use are higher than the estimated rates for perfect use. The failure rate of a method during actual use depends on a number of characteristics of the user including age, experience in method use, and motivation to prevent pregnancy. These factors result in variations in the percentage of users who use a given method incorrectly or inconsistently. Estimates of failure rates among typical married women in the United States are included in Figure 14-1, along with the failure rates given perfect use [3].

In general, failure rates decline with increasing age. The inherent protection of the method, differences in fecundity by age, frequency of intercourse, and exposure to the risk of pregnancy influence these measures [6]. In addition, the gap between the perfect-use failure rate of a given contraceptive method and the failure rate in typical use is a result of differences in the correct and consistent use of the method. The correct and consistent use of barrier methods is determined by a complex set of interactions between the characteristics of the user, characteristics of the method, and the situational context [7]. Characteristics of the method include the extent to which it interferes with sexual spontaneity and enjoyment, the amount of partner cooperation required, and the degree to which the method protects against STDs. User characteristics include the motivation to avoid pregnancy, the ability to plan to use a method, comfort with sexuality, and past use of contraception. Situational influences include the characteristics of the relationship, sexual history, and history of or current physical or sexual abuse [7]. Barrier methods are particularly dependent on correct use, although the component of continuation has been more widely studied for most contraceptive methods.

CONTINUATION

In one study reporting continued contraceptive use, 29% of condom users discontinued the method over the course of 1 year; 30% of diaphragm users did so [8]. Discontinuation rates vary depending on characteristics of the populations studied. Figure 14-2 shows the percentage of women estimated to be continuing to use a given method of contraception at the end of 1 year; continuation rates for barrier methods are lower than those for hormonal contraceptives [3]. Adolescents who begin using a method are more likely than older women to discontinue its use. Of note, in one study, about half of the women who discontinued a method of contraception did not switch to an alternative method and were thus at risk for unintended pregnancy [8].

CORRECT AND CONSISTENT USE

Less study has been devoted to the correct use of the available methods than has been devoted to continuation. Two methods, oral contraceptives and condoms, require that a set of behaviors be performed on a regular basis. One investigator has studied the behaviors around correct contraceptive use and termed them *microbehaviors* [9,10]. These microbehaviors are addressed in the discussion of condom use. Consistent use, that is, use with every episode of intercourse, is likely the most problematic aspect of barrier methods. The 1995 National Survey of Family Growth reported that only about two thirds of individuals using coitus-dependent methods used the method every time they had intercourse in the past 3 months (Figure 14-3) [2••]. The concept of omitting use of a barrier method "just this once" is common. By a similar token, the user may combine "rhythm" or fertility awareness with the barrier method used only during the time of ovulation or perceived risk.

SEXUALLY TRANSMITTED DISEASE RISK REDUCTION

The efficacy of male condoms in decreasing the risk of STD transmission has been well-established. In 2000, the National Institutes of Health, the Centers for Disease Control and Prevention, the FDA, and the US Agency for International Development met to review the evidence regarding the effectiveness of latex male condoms in the prevention of STDs including HIV. They made the following statement:

"Latex condoms, when used consistently and correctly, are highly effective in preventing the transmission of HIV, the virus that causes AIDS. In addition, correct and consistent use of latex condoms can reduce the risk STDs, including discharge and genital ulcer diseases. While the effect of condoms in preventing human papillomavirus (HPV) infection is unknown, condom use has been associated with a lower rate of cervical cancer, an HPV-associated disease" [11].

Since that time, prospective studies have shown that condom use reduces the risk of STDs including chlamydial infection, gonorrhea, herpes simplex virus type-2, and syphilis, and may protect women against trichomonas infection. To date, only one small prospective study has found protection against HPV infection [12,13].

The effectiveness of other barrier methods in decreasing STD risk is less well established. A number of population studies report that users of barrier methods in aggregate have a lower risk of STD acquisition. However, many of these studies do not address specific methods. In addition, patterns of use of barrier methods (such as consistency of use) differ by age and thus may contribute to the lack of benefit seen in some studies [14]. Some reports have suggested that users of the contraceptive sponge and diaphragm experience increased protection against gonorrhea, chlamydial infection, and trichomoniasis compared with condom users [15,16]. The role of spermicides, when used with and without a barrier method, also confounds assessment of the extent to which each method results in a lower risk. Studies to date have yielded conflicting results about the relationships between spermicide use, local vaginal irritation, vaginal flora, and HIV incidence rates [17].

Female-controlled devices and methods are particularly important in decreasing HIV risk, although the impact of sexual and physical abuse, coercion, lack of rights for women, and partner awareness of method choice are important determinants of method use [18–21]. Some

Failure Rates of Barrier Contraceptive Devices

Method	Percentage of Women Experiencing Unwanted Pregnancy within the First Year of Use		Percentage of Women Continuing at 1 Year
	Typical Use	Perfect Use	
Chance	85	85	40
Spermicides	26	6	63
Periodic abstinence	25		
Calendar		9	
Ovulation method		3	
Symptothermal		2	
Postovulation		1	
Cap			
Parous women	40	26	42
Nulliparous women	20	9	56
Sponge			
Parous women	40	20	42
Nulliparous women	20	9	56
Diaphragm	20	6	56
Withdrawal	19	4	
Condom			
Female (Reality)	21	5	56
Male	14	3	61
Pill	5		71
Progestin only		0.5	
Combined		0.1	
Intrauterine device			
Progesterone T	2	1.5	81
Copper T 380A	0.8	0.6	78
LNg 20	0.1	0.1	81
Depo-Provera (Pharmacia & Upjohn, Co., Kalamazoo, MI)	0.3	0.3	70
Norplant and Norplant-2 (Wyeth Pharmaceuticals, Philadelphia, PA)	0.05	0.05	88
Female sterilization	0.5	0.5	100
Male sterilization	0.15	0.1	100

Figure 14-1. Failure rates of barrier contraceptive devices. (*Adapted from* Hatcher *et al.* [3].)

women report that requesting male partners use condoms would create a potentially violent situation in an abusive relationship [22].

Women and men engage in different sexual behaviors with main partners than with other types of partners, such as casual or other frequent (side) partners and thus may report different patterns of contraceptive use and STD protection with different partners [23]. Clinicians should ask patients about sexual behaviors and partner types and tailor prevention messages to the individual patient's risks.

Use of barrier methods has been associated with lower risk of cervical dysplasia and carcinoma, a conclusion that supports the benefits of these methods in lowering the risk of STDs, including HPV [22–26]. This protective effect may differ between the various types of barriers or may have been impacted by the concomitant use of spermicides [27].

Benefits and Positive Aspects of Use of Barrier Methods

In general, and for most barrier methods, benefits include ease of use, personal control, availability without medical examinations or procedures, minimal side effects, and protection against STDs. A cost comparison that factors in the costs of unintended pregnancy, costs of side effects, and costs of the method itself (with costs calculated for a managed payment model) is shown in Figure 14-4. Barrier methods cost relatively little on a unit basis, but in typical use, have higher failure rates than hormonal contraceptives. In addition, they are unlikely to be associated with method-related medical risks. When all of these factors are considered, the costs of barrier methods lie in the middle range of all contraceptive methods.

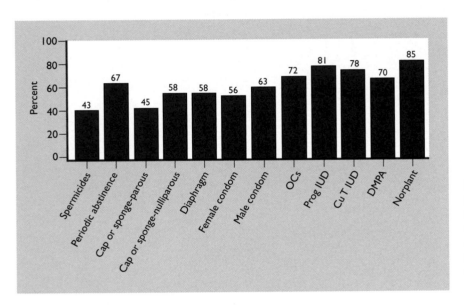

Figure 14-2. Reversible contraceptive methods: percentage of women continuing use after 1 year. OC—oral contraceptives; Prog IUD—progestin-only intrauterine device; Cu T IUD—copper T intrauterine device; DMPA—depomedroxyprogesterone acetate. (*Adapted from* Hatcher *et al.* [3].)

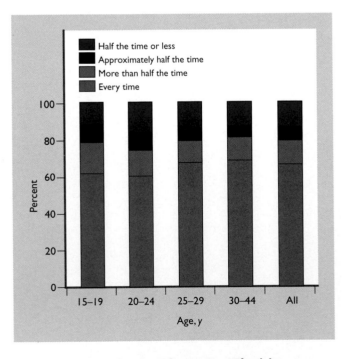

Figure 14-3. Coitus-dependent contraceptive methods used in the previous 3 months. (*Adapted from* Abma *et al.* [2••].)

Risks and Negative Aspects of Use of Barrier Methods

Some of the negative aspects of barrier methods include the facts that irregular or incorrect use increases the risk of failure and that even with perfect use, failure rates tend to be higher than with hormonal methods. The need to plan ahead is important in having the method available for contraception. The possible interruption of love-making is a relative drawback. Failure of the method, such as breakage of a condom, may be a result of manufacturing problems or, more commonly, of incorrect use.

Allergic or chemical reactions can occur in response to latex of condoms or chemical irritation from concomitantly used spermicides. An estimated 1% of patients and 17% of health care workers are allergic to latex [28]. Certain populations, including young women with a history of meningomyelocele, people with repeated exposure to latex-containing medical devices or patients who have undergone multiple urologic procedures have a higher risk of becoming sensitized to latex.

Users of barrier methods (specifically, the sponge and diaphragm) have an increased risk of nonmenstrual toxic shock syndrome than users of nonbarrier methods [29].

Male Condoms

CHARACTERISTICS OF USE AND USERS
National surveys indicate that 82.2% of women of reproductive age (15 to 44 years of age) have used a condom at some time in their lives (Figure 14-5); 93.5% of sexually active ado-lescents report having used a male condom [2••]. Current use is reported by 20.4% of all contraception users and by 36.7% of adolescent contraception users (Figure 14-6) [2••]. Use of a male condom at first intercourse was reported by 29.2% of all women; of women who first had intercourse between 1990 and 1995, 54.3% used a male condom [2••]. Data from the National Survey of Family Growth show that in 1982, 23% used a condom at first intercourse; in 1988, 48% did so; and in 1995, 61% reported use of a condom at first intercourse (Figure 14-7). Youth Risk Behavior Surveys, conducted in 1990, 1991, 1993, and 1995 have shown increasing use of condoms; the percentage of sexually active high school students who used condoms at last intercourse rose from 46% in 1991 to 54% in 1995 [30]. The National Surveys of Adolescent Males found an increase in use of condoms at last intercourse from 57% to 67% from 1988 to 1995 [31]. Data from the National AIDS Behavioral Survey indicate that approximately 8% of women aged 40 to 75 years (4.5 million women) engaged in behaviors that might expose them to HIV [32]. Most women at risk had not used condoms in the previous 6 months, and most did not perceive themselves to be at risk [32].

SKIN, LATEX, AND POLYURETHANE CONDOMS
Most condoms are made of latex; about 5% of condoms are made from lamb intestines [3]. Natural and skin condoms contain pores that may allow passage of virus particles and thus are not recommended for people who require protection from STDs. Polyurethane condoms have been approved for use in the United States; relatively few clinical trials have compared their performance to that of latex condoms. One study reported higher breakage and slippage rates, although in

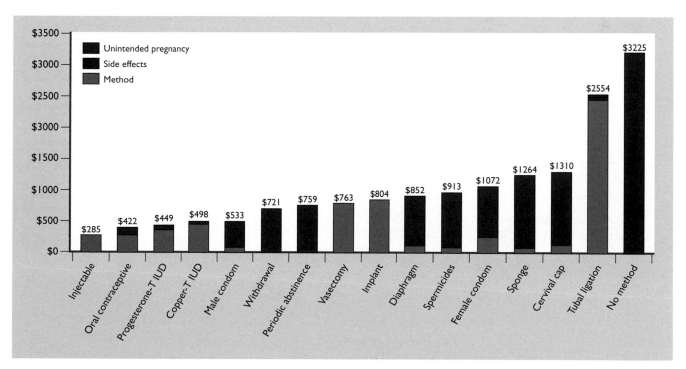

Figure 14-4. One-year costs associated with contraceptive methods in the managed payment model. (*Adapted from* Hatcher *et al.* [3].)

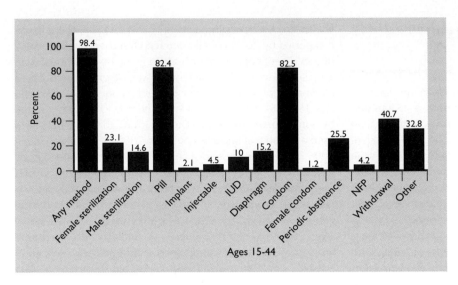

Figure 14-5. Ever use of contraception: all women. IUD—intrauterine device; NFP—natural family planning. (*Adapted from* Abma *et al.* [2••].)

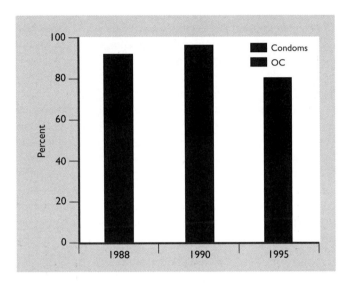

Figure 14-6. Contraceptive method used by young women aged 15 to 19 years. OC—oral contraceptive. (*Adapted from* Abma *et al.* [2••].)

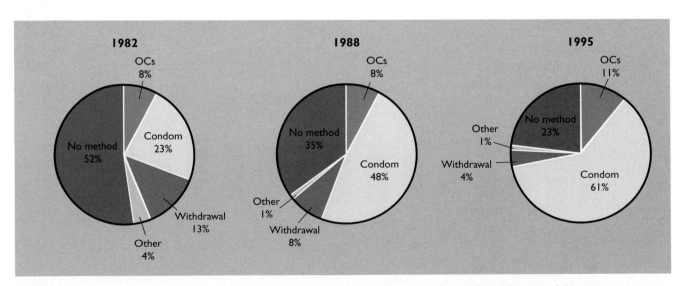

Figure 14-7. Contraceptive method used by adolescents at first intercourse. (*Adapted from* Abma *et al.* [2••].)

this study, male users preferred the sensitivity provided by the polyurethane condoms [33]. Other studies confirm preference for polyurethane over latex in regard to appearance, lack of smell, likelihood of slippage, comfort, sensitivity, natural look, natural feel, and overall characteristics [34]. Polyurethane condoms have not been well studied to confirm STD protection, although they are believed to provide protection similar to that of latex condoms [3]. Currently, several new nonlatex condoms made of synthetic elastomers are in varying stages of research and development.

SIZES AND STYLES

Condoms come in a variety of shapes, sizes, colors, and thicknesses; they are available with and without spermicides and may have a reservoir tip. They may have textured surfaces (ribs) or be smooth-sided. Condom manufacturers have recognized that "one-size-fits-all" condoms may not be appropriate for all users. (See http://www.durex.com/scientific/septforumresult.html) Certain racial and ethnic groups may require different sizing to provide optimal efficacy and comfort.

AVAILABILITY IN SCHOOLS

Several recent reports describe high school condom availability programs. One program in a Los Angeles County high school did not increase sexual activity and did lead to improved condom use among male students [34]. Another study of condom availability in high schools found that availability had a modest but significant effect on condom use and did not increase sexual activity [36•].

DUAL METHODS

The use of two methods of contraception simultaneously, such as a male condom and a spermicide, can increase efficacy [37•]. This is logical, as the spermicide provides back-up if the male condom slips off or breaks. Kestelman and Trussell [37•] also argued that factors contributing to nonuse of a method are not independent. Few studies or surveys have explored the use of condoms plus other methods of contraception.

With an emphasis on the need for STD prevention, public health officials are urging this strategy. The most recent Youth Risk Behavior Survey reported on dual use among young women (14 to 22 years old). The pill and condoms were used by 9.6%, withdrawal and condoms by 13%, and "other" and condoms by 3% (Figure 14-8); condoms alone were used by 37% of women and 52% of men [38]. Condom use was reported by 25% of young men whose partner was using the pill [38]. Significant independent predictors of condom use with the pill among men included younger age, black race, engaging in fewer nonsexual risk behaviors, and having received instruction about HIV in school. Among young women, 21% of those relying on the pill reported also using a condom at last intercourse; for women, independent predictors of dual use included younger age, black race, older age at first sex, fewer nonsexual risk behaviors, having no partners in the previous 3 months, and having talked to parents or other adult relatives about HIV [38]. One study in which reproductive-aged women were encouraged to use condoms for HIV and STD prevention found women were able to increase consistent condom use without discontinuing hormonal contraceptive methods, leading to an overall increase in protection from pregnancy [39].

The Centers for Disease Control and Prevention notes that although latex condoms are highly effective in reducing the risk of HIV infection and other STDs, surgical sterilization or hormonal methods are more effective in preventing pregnancy. In an effort to assess whether encouraging women to use condoms for HIV and STD prevention affects their contraceptive practices, the Centers for Disease Control and Prevention analyzed longitudinal data on contraceptive methods and condom use as part of a randomized trial evaluating HIV counseling methods from 1993 to 1995. Participants' use of condoms and other contraceptive methods was assessed before and 3 months after receiving counseling and education encouraging consistent condom use. In this study, consistent condom use increased among women using each method of contraception; in addition, women using hormonal contraceptive methods continued to use

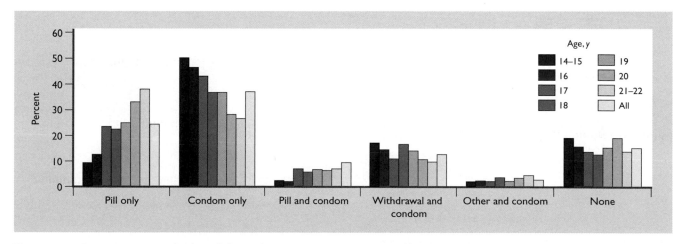

Figure 14-8. Contraceptive method used during last intercourse: women aged 14 to 22 years. OCs—oral contraceptives. (*Adapted from* Santelli *et al.* [38].)

them, and the overall percentage of women who were protected against pregnancy increased.

EFFICACY IN PREGNANCY PREVENTION

In actual use, condoms have higher failure rates than are quoted with perfect use (*see* Figure 14-1) [40]. Reports on the efficacy of male condoms suggest that the failure rate in typical use is about 3% [41••]. However, the failure rate among other subpopulations has been reported to be considerably higher. Use of contraception at the time of first intercourse has increased in the United States from 48% in 1982 to 77% in 1995 (*see* Figure 14-7) [1]. This increase is almost entirely the result of an increase in the use of condoms at the time of first intercourse: from 23% in 1982 to 61% in 1995. Condom failure rate varies by income: from 31% of poor young women aged 20 to 24 years to 10% of higher-income women older than 30 years of age (Figure 14-9) [42••]. This does not suggest that women with higher incomes are able to buy better condoms, rather, that other factors correlating with income and socioeconomic status affect correct and consistent use.

The fact that condom efficacy, like efficacy with other user-dependent methods, is dependent on correct and consistent use is illustrated by a study that examined the microbehaviors of condom use. These included putting a condom on before penetration, holding the condom in place before withdrawal, withdrawing while the penis is still erect, and using a condom during every act of intercourse [43]. This last microbehavior, using a condom during every act of intercourse, is likely the most important behavior in ensuring efficacy of the method; unfortunately, the percentage of condom users who noted that they did so ranged from about one third of adolescents to 56% of women 25 to 29 years old (Figure 14-10) [43].

EFFICACY IN SEXUALLY TRANSMITTED DISEASE PREVENTION

The statement presented earlier by the National Institutes of Health, the Centers for Disease Control and Prevention, the FDA, and the US Agency for Internation Development is clear about the efficacy of latex condoms when used consistently and correctly in reducing the risk of HIV infection and other STDs [11]. Problems with consistent use are highlighted in the discussion of contraceptive efficacy. Data from the National Survey of Family Growth indicate that among women using condoms for disease protection, less than one third of women of all ages used a condom every time they had intercourse in the previous 3 months [2••]. There are somewhat reassuring studies of HIV transmission between serodiscordant heterosexual partners in which consistency of use is assessed. One study reported no seroconversions among partners who used condoms consistently [44]. It is important in counseling patients to discuss the fact that the protective effect of condoms applies to latex but not natural condoms. The efficacy of polyurethane condoms in decreasing STD risk is not well-established.

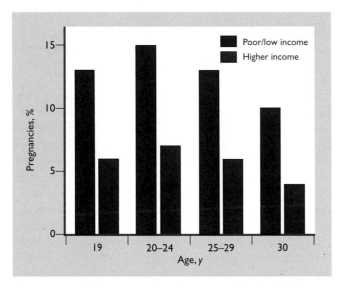

Figure 14-9. Failure rate of oral contraceptives in the first year of use, by age and income. (*Adapted from* The Alan Guttmacher Institute [42].)

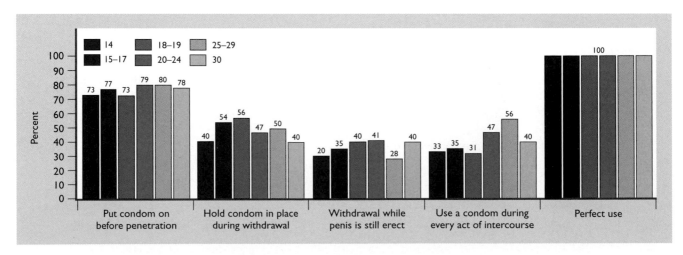

Figure 14-10. Microbehaviors of condom users. (*Adapted from* Oakley *et al.* [43].)

Benefits and Positive Aspects of Use

Condoms are inexpensive, available without a prescription, and easy to use. As noted previously, they decrease the risk of STDs. Their effectiveness, however, depends on consistent and correct use. Male participation in contraception has been described as a benefit of this method. Condoms may help men maintain an erection for a longer period of time and help to prevent premature ejaculation.

Risks and Negative Aspects of Use

Slippage and breakage are infrequent when condoms are used correctly. Slippage has been reported to occur less than 1% of the time, and breakage rates with vaginal intercourse range from 0% to 7% [3]. It appears that condoms are more likely to break with anal intercourse. It has been reported that condoms fall off the penis in up to 5% of acts of vaginal intercourse and slip without coming off in up to 13% [3]. A history of condom breakage and slippage predicts future failure [45]. A recent systematic review of randomized controlled trials comparing the contraceptive efficacy of latex versus nonlatex condoms found that although nonlatex condoms were associated with higher rates of clinical breakage, only three trials actually examined their contraceptive efficacy; more research on efficacy is needed [46].

One disadvantage of condoms is that use involves an interruption in love-making and may be inconvenient. Some men or their partners note a decreased sensation and sensitivity with condom use. Partners may find it difficult to negotiate condom use, and some men may be unwilling to use condoms. Latex allergy may preclude the use of latex condoms.

Female Condoms

Characteristics of Use and Users

Designs for female condoms have been available since the 1920s, but only recently with the arrival of AIDS has there been significant interest and potential for marketing these devices [47]. One design (Reality; The Female Health Company, UK) approved by the FDA in 1993 is available in the United States; other designs are available worldwide. Reality is a polyurethane sheath that is soft and loose fitting within the vagina, measuring 7.8 cm in diameter and 17 cm long. It contains one ring inside the sheath, which anchors the device within the vagina, and a second ring that remains outside the vagina, forming a barrier and offering protection to the labia and base of the penis. The device is manufactured with a nonspermicidal lubricant. It is intended for one-time use, sold over the counter, and can be inserted up to 8 hours before intercourse. Use of the male and female condom concurrently can result in adhesion or slipping and is not advised.

Efficacy in Pregnancy Prevention

The typical-use failure rate of the Reality female condom is based on the results of a clinical trial in which 12.4% of women became pregnant during 6 months of use [48]. In this study, the probability of pregnancy during 6 months of perfect use (according to compliance criteria stipulated in the study protocol) was 2.6%. Extrapolating from this study, assuming that the probability of pregnancy in the second 6 months of perfect use would be the same, the probability of pregnancy during a year of perfect use would be 5.1% (see Figure 14-1).

Contraceptive efficacy of the female condom is comparable to that of other female barrier methods, including the diaphragm, cervical cap, and sponge, when comparisons are made using historical control subjects [49]. Clinical trials in the United States did not include randomization with other methods, and thus no definite conclusions about relative efficacy can be drawn. In addition, meaningful comparisons with the male condom are not possible because of the lack of data from carefully controlled prospective clinical trials [50].

Efficacy in Sexually Transmitted Disease Risk Reduction

Extrapolations from the results of studies on contraceptive efficacy suggest that perfect use of the female condom may reduce the annual risk of acquiring HIV by more than 90% among women who have intercourse twice weekly with an infected male [50]. However, research is limited about this important possible benefit of female condoms. One study reported that female condom users experienced no reinfection with trichomoniasis [51]. Another study using prostate-specific antigen as a biologic marker of semen exposure found that the female condom was less effective than the male condom; however, if this can be related to risk of transmission of STDs remains unclear [52].

Benefits and Positive Aspects of Use

Female condoms are relatively simple to use and can be used intermittently. Unlike other female-controlled barrier methods, the female condom is noticeable to a male partner, and partner acceptability is variable.

Risks and Negative Aspects of Use

Most reports suggest reasonable acceptability, although the available device has been found to make an annoying "snap, crackle, pop" noise during intercourse. Other problems include difficulty inserting the device, concerns from women or their partner about the appearance of the device, slippage, and changes in sensation. One study reported pinholes and tears among 0.6% of female condoms compared with 3.5% of male condoms [49].

Quality control in the United States is good, with few manufacturing errors because condoms have been regulated as medical devices by the FDA since 1976. Every condom manufactured in the United States is electronically tested for holes before it is sold.

The female condom does not alter vaginal flora significantly, nor is it associated with vaginal microtrauma [54].

Diaphragm

CHARACTERISTICS OF USE AND USERS

The contraceptive diaphragm has been used in Europe and the United States since the early 1900s. It has a flexible rim with a dome-shaped cup that fits in the upper vagina, covering the cervix. Rim styles vary, from a flat spring to a coil spring to an arcing spring; the arcing or coil spring styles are also available with a wide seal rim. Sizing is individual and requires fitting by a clinician; sizes range from 50 to 95 mm in diameter. They are composed of latex or silicone. Diaphragms should be used with a spermicide. A plastic inserter can be used to facilitate insertion, although most women are able to insert the diaphragm manually. It can be inserted up to 6 hours before intercourse; additional spermicide should be added if a longer interval elapses. The diaphragm must be left in place for at least 6 hours after intercourse.

Use of the diaphragm is reported by 15.2% of women of reproductive age and 26.5% of women between the ages of 40 and 44 years (see Figure 14-5) [2]. Only 1.2% of women in the United States report current diaphragm use.

Recent clinical trials have focused on three questions: first, if clinician fitting is truly necessary; second, the ability of the diaphragm to prevent STDs, and lastly, the utility of the diaphragm as a delivery vehicle for vaginally applied microbicides. No firm conclusions are available.

EFFICACY IN PREGNANCY PREVENTION

Because use of spermicide is recommended with the diaphragm, efficacy is reported for the diaphragm used in combination with spermicide. The first-year probability of pregnancy has been reported as 20% with typical use and 6% with perfect use (see Figure 14-1) [3]. Approximately half of women experiencing contraceptive failure with barrier methods report inconsistent or incorrect use; the other half experience failure despite perfect use.

EFFICACY IN SEXUALLY TRANSMITTED DISEASE RISK REDUCTION

Studies assessing the efficacy of barrier methods other than male condoms report varying degrees of protection. Because the diaphragm is used with spermicide, some degree of protection may be due to the antimicrobial effect of the spermicide. Diaphragm users have been reported to have a lower risk of pelvic inflammatory disease, cervical dysplasia, and tubal infertility.

BENEFITS AND POSITIVE ASPECTS OF USE

The diaphragm shares characteristics with other vaginal barriers; it is simple to use and can be used with little advance planning. The possible effect in reducing the risk of STDs is of benefit to some women. It can be inserted up to 6 hours before intercourse, and thus its use does not require the interruption of love-making. The diaphragm is a method under female control. Cost is a relative advantage, although a medical visit is necessary for fitting. The life-span of a diaphragm is typically 2 years; the diaphragm costs about $30 to $40. Spermicide is an additional cost: about 25 cents per application.

RISKS AND NEGATIVE ASPECTS OF USE

As with other barrier methods, the efficacy of the diaphragm in preventing pregnancy is dependent on correct and consistent use. Spermicides can be associated with local skin irritation, allergy, or sensitivity. Use of a latex diaphragm should be avoided in patients with latex allergy. The diaphragm has been reported to increase rates of vaginal colonization with uropathogenic bacteria [55] and, thus, to increase the risk of recurrent urinary tract infections [56]. Colonization with *Candida* species has been reported to increase significantly in diaphragm and spermicide users [17,57]. Bacterial vaginosis has been found to be associated with *Escherichia coli* introital colonization and acute symptomatic urinary tract infection in women using diaphragms [58].

Some women are unable to learn to insert or remove the diaphragm successfully. Vaginal relaxation, cystocele, rectocele, significant uterine prolapse, or other abnormalities of vaginal anatomy can preclude appropriate fitting and use. Oil-based lubricants can have a detrimental effect on latex diaphragms although few studies have directly examined this issue.

Sponge

CHARACTERISTICS OF USE AND USERS

Although less than 1% of women reported using the contraceptive sponge in the 1995 National Survey of Family Growth, some women did find the method to be an acceptable contraceptive option [2]. Because of the manufacturer's decision not to modernize manufacturing equipment and reportedly unrelated to the method's popularity or sales, the distribution of the Today Sponge was stopped in the United States in 1995. In 1998, a new manufacturer (Allendale Pharmaceuticals, Allendale, NJ) purchased the rights to the product, and in 2005, the sponge was reintroduced to the American market.

It consists of a soft, small, disposable polyurethane sponge containing nonoxynol-9. One side of the sponge contains an indentation designed to be positioned over the cervix, and the other side holds a woven polyester loop for removal. It was designed as a one-size-fits-all over-the-counter contraceptive device.

The sponge was originally planned to provide contraceptive protection for 2 days (Today), although it was approved for use for only 24 hours. Multiple acts of intercourse can take place during the 24 hours; the sponge should be left in place for 6 hours after intercourse. A similar product, the Protectaid sponge (Axcan Limited, Canada), is available in Canada. It contains benzalkonium chloride, sodium cholate, and nonoxynol-9. The combination of agents may have additional antiviral actions when compared to nonoxynol-9 alone.

EFFICACY IN PREGNANCY PREVENTION

The contraceptive efficacy of the sponge differs depending on whether or not a woman has experienced a birth [59]. The first-year probability of pregnancy using the sponge perfectly has been reported to be 20% for parous women and 9% for nulliparous women (see Figure 14-1) [3]. With typical use, 40% of parous women and 20% of nulliparous women become pregnant within the first year of use.

EFFICACY IN SEXUALLY TRANSMITTED DISEASE RISK REDUCTION

In a study of Thailand prostitutes, users of the sponge were found to have a lower risk of gonorrhea and chlamydial infection than nonusers [17]. Few other studies have addressed this issue, and again, the question remains as to how much of the benefit is due to the presence of the spermicide nonoxynol-9.

BENEFITS AND POSITIVE ASPECTS OF USE

The vaginal contraceptive sponge is a barrier method that enjoyed some popularity because of convenience, availability over the counter, and ease of use. The characteristic of the sponge that contributed to its popularity (its availability without the need for an examination) is likely a factor in the higher failure rate among parous women who typically have larger cervices that may not be well covered by the one-size-fits-all sponge. Due to its recent reintroduction to the United States market, current data on usage are not yet available.

RISKS AND NEGATIVE ASPECTS OF USE

Use for more than 24 to 30 hours is not recommended because of the potential risk of toxic shock syndrome. An association has been reported between use of the sponge and recurrent bacterial vaginosis [60]. In the previously noted study of prostitutes in Thailand, sponge users were found to have an increased risk of vaginal candidiasis [17].

Emerging Methods

Research is ongoing on new barrier methods of contraception, with an additional area of research devoted to barriers to STDs. There is increasing emphasis on barrier methods of birth control that are female-controlled, offering women an option for decreasing STD risk when the male partner is unwilling to use a male condom. Some new methods are undergoing clinical trials, and some methods are newly available in other countries.

New Female-controlled Methods

LEA'S SHIELD
Characteristics of Use and Users
Lea's Shield (Yama, Inc., Millburn, NJ) is a new vaginal barrier device that was approved by the FDA in 2002. It consists of a silicone bowl with a one-way flutter valve and an anterior loop for easier removal. It fills the posterior fornix to remain in place. It can be used with either a spermicidal or nonspermicidal lubricant. Lea's Shield can be used for up to 48 hours and should be left in place for 8 hours after last intercourse.

Efficacy in Pregnancy Prevention
Lea's Shield is reportedly as effective as other available female barrier contraceptives; data are limited. Only one small prospective trial has been published. Women were randomized to Lea's Shield with spermicidal lubricant versus nonspermicidal lubricant. The adjusted six-month life table pregnancy rate was 5.6 for spermicide users and 9.3 for nonspermicide users [61]. This difference was not statistically significant. As with the contraceptive sponge, increasing parity appears to decrease efficacy [61].

Efficacy in Sexually Transmitted Disease Risk Reduction
The efficacy of Lea's Shield and spermicide in reducing the risk of STDs has not been studied.

Benefits and Positive Aspects of Use
Like other vaginal barriers, it is simple to use and can be used with little advance planning. Unlike diaphragms and cervical caps, the device is available in one size only, so fitting should not be a concern. Because Lea's Shield is composed of silicone, latex allergy is also not a concern.

Risks and Negative Aspects of Use
Lea's Shield is available in the United States by prescription only. In addition, like most other vaginal barrier methods, use during menses is not advised due to the potential risk of toxic shock syndrome.

FemCap
Characteristics of Use and Users
FemCap (FemCap, Inc., Del Mar, CA) is a silicone barrier contraceptive which was approved by the FDA in 2003. It is shaped like a sailor's hat, with a dome that covers the cervix, a rim that fits into the fornices, and a brim that conforms to the vaginal walls around the cervix. FemCap is available in three sizes; women are "fitted" based on their obstetrical history. It should be used with spermicide.

Efficacy in Pregnancy Prevention
In a trial comparing FemCap with the contraceptive diaphragm, the adjusted risk of pregnancy among FemCap users was 1.96 times that among diaphragm users [62].

Efficacy in Sexually Transmitted Disease Risk Reduction
The efficacy of FemCap and spermicide in reducing the risk of STDs has not been studied.

Benefits and Positive Aspects of Use
Like the recently discontinued cervical cap and the Lea's Shield, it can be worn up to 48 hours during which time repeated applications of spermicide are not required. Because it must remain in place at least 6 hours following last intercourse, the last act can only occur up to 42 hours following device placement. When compared to the diaphragm, FemCap was associated with significantly fewer urinary tract infections [62].

Risks and Negative Aspects of Use
FemCap is available in the United States by prescription only. In early studies of FemCap, women complained of device

removal difficulties. In response, a removal strap was added to the design; it has not been shown to ease removal and may result in more pain/discomfort and disapproval by both partners [63]. In addition, like most other vaginal barrier methods, use during menses is not advised due to the potential risk of toxic shock syndrome.

Other devices under investigation include those made of polymers that release spermicide, custom-molded barrier devices, and variations on the sponge, with different microbicides or spermicides [3].

Summary

Barrier methods of contraception offer many advantages to users. Although efficacy is extremely variable and dependent on user characteristics as well as consistent and correct use, the potential benefit in decreasing the risks of STDs should not be minimized. Although barrier devices have traditionally been thought of as a contraceptive method, increasingly they are being used in combination with hormonal methods and with other barrier methods in an effort to maximize contraceptive efficacy and decrease the risks of STDs. Increased use of condoms has been noted in the United States and is undoubtedly a factor in declining adolescent pregnancy rates. Future studies will provide more information about the extent to which our current methods provide STD protection (with and without spermicides), and future technologic developments will undoubtedly lead to the development of barrier methods that are more user-friendly. However, efficacy will continue to be dependent on correct and consistent use.

References

Papers of particular interest have been highlighted as follows:
• Of interest
•• Of outstanding interest

1. Piccinino LJ, Mosher WD: Trends in contraceptive use in the US: 1982–1995. *Fam Plann Perspect* 1998, 30:4–10.

2.•• Abma J, Chandra A, Mosher W, *et al.*: Fertility, family planning, and women's health: new data from the 1995 National Survey of Family Growth. National Survey of Family Growth, National Center for Health Statistics. *Vital Health Stat Series* 1997, 23:1–125.
This is a report of the NSFG 1995 and includes the most up–to–date data on pregnancy, contraception, sterilization, abuse, involuntary sexual activity, and partners.

3. Hatcher RA, Trussell J, Stewart F, *et al.*: *Contraceptive Technology.* New York: Ardent Media; 2004:1–871.

4. Beckman LJ, Harvey SM: Factors affecting the consistent use of barrier methods of contraception. *Obstet Gynecol* 1996, 88:65S–71S.

5.•• Trussell J, Hatcher RA, Cates WJ, *et al.*: A guide to interpreting contraceptive efficacy studies. *Obstet Gynecol* 1990, 76:558–567.
This article reviews definitions and measures used to assess contraceptive efficacy, describes and illustrates some flaws that confound interpretation and comparison of studies, and presents a set of recommendations for future studies. A summary table providing comparative failure rates for all methods of contraception is included.

6. Steiner M, Dominik R, Trussell J, *et al.*: Measuring contraceptive effectiveness: a conceptual framework [see comments]. *Obstet Gynecol* 1996, 88:24S–30S.

7. Beckman LJ, Harvey SM: Factors affecting the consistent use of barrier methods of contraception. *Obstet Gynecol* 1996, 88:65S–71S.

8. Grady WR, Hayward MD, Florey FA: Contraceptive discontinuation among married women in the U.S. *Stud Fam Plann* 1988, 19:227–227.

9. Oakley D, Parent J: A scale to measure microbehaviors of oral contraceptive pill use. *Social Biol* 1990, 37:215–222.

10. Oakley D, Sereika O, Bogue E-L: Quality of condom use of reported by female clients of a family planning clinic. *Am J Public Health* 1995, 85:1526–1530.

11.• National Institute of Allergy and Infectious Diseases. Workshop Summary: Scientific Evidence on Condom Effectiveness for Sexually Transmitted Disease (STD) Prevention. July 20, 2001 http://www.niaid.nih.gov/dmid/stds/condomreport.pdf.
This reference contains the official position of the NIH/CDC/FDA/USAID and reviews the most current data on latex condoms and STD prevention.

12. Holmes KK, Levine R, Weaver M: Effectiveness of condoms in preventing sexually transmitted infections. *Bull World Health Organ* 2004, 82:454–461.

13. Winer RL, Hughes JP, Feng Q, *et al.*: Condom use and the risk of genital human papillomavirus infection in young women. *N Engl J Med* 2006, 354:2645–2654.

14. Park BJ, Stergachis A, Scholes D, *et al.*: Contraceptive methods and the risk of *Chlamydia trachomatis* infection in young women. *Am J Epidemiol* 1995, 142:771–778.

15. Rosenberg MJ, Davidson AJ, Chen JH, *et al.*: Barrier contraceptives and sexually transmitted diseases in women: a comparison of female-dependent methods and condoms [see comments]. *Am J Public Health* 1992, 82:669–674.

16. Rosenberg MJ, Rojanapithayakorn W, Feldblum PJ, *et al.*: Effect of the contraceptive sponge on chlamydial infection, gonorrhea, and candidiasis: a comparative clinical trial. *JAMA* 198, 257:2308–2312.

17. Feldblum PJ, Morrison CS, Roddy RE, *et al.*: The effectiveness of barrier methods of contraception in preventing the spread of HIV. *AIDS* 1995, 9(Suppl A):S85–S93.

18. Stein ZA: HIV prevention: the need for methods women can use. *Am J Public Health* 1990, 80:460–462.

19. Elias CJ, Coggins C: Female–controlled methods to prevent sexual transmission of HIV. *AIDS* 1996, 3(Suppl): S43–S51.

20. Cook RJ, Maine D: Spousal veto over family planning services. *Am J Public Health* 1987, 77:339–344.

21. Wingood GM, DiClemente RJ: The effects of an abusive primary partner on the condom use and sexual negotiation practices of African-American women. *Am J Public Health* 1997, 87:1016–1018.

22. Kalichman SC, Williams EA, Cherry C, *et al.*: Sexual coercion, domestic violence, and negotiating condom use among low–income African American women. *J Women's Health* 1998, 7:371–378.

23. Lansky A, Thomas JC, Earp JA: Partner-specific sexual behaviors among persons with both main and other partners. *Fam Plann Perspect* 1998, 30:93–96.

24. Hannaford PC: Cervical cancer and methods of contraception. *Adv Contracept* 1991, 7:317–324.

25. Coker AL, Hulka BS, McCann MF, *et al.*: Barrier methods of contraception and cervical intraepithelial neoplasia. *Contraception* 1992, 45:1–10.

26. Slattery ML, Overall JCJ, Abbott TM, *et al.*: Sexual activity, contraception, genital infections, and cervical cancer: support for a sexually transmitted disease hypothesis. *Am J Epidemiol* 1989, 130:248–258.

27. Hildesheim A, Brinton LA, Mallin K, *et al.*: Barrier and spermicidal contraceptive methods and risk of invasive cervical cancer [see comments]. *Epidemiology* 1990, 1:266–272.

28. Yassin MS, Lierl MB, Fischer TJ, *et al.*: Latex allergy in hospital employees. *Ann Allergy* 1994, 72:245–249.

29. Schwartz B, Gaventa S, Broome CV, *et al.*: Nonmenstrual toxic shock syndrome associated with barrier contraceptives: report of a case-control study. *Rev Infect Dis* 1989, 11(Suppl 1):S43–S48.

30. Warren CW, Santelli JS, Everett SA, *et al.*: Sexual behavior among U.S. high school students, 1990–1995. *Fam Plann Perspect* 1998, 30:170–172.

31. Sonenstein FL, Ku L, Lindberg LD, *et al.*: Changes in sexual behavior and condom use among teenaged males: 1988 to 1995. *Am J Public Health* 1998, 88:956–959.

32. Binson D, Pollack L, Catania JA: AIDS-related risk behaviors and safer sex practices of women in midlife and older in the US: 1990 to 1992. *Health Care Women Int* 1997, 18:343–354.

33. Frezieres RG, Walsh TL, Nelson AL, *et al.*: Breakage and acceptability of a polyurethane condom: a randomized, controlled study. *Fam Plann Perspect* 1998, 40:73–78.

34. Rosenberg MJ, Waugh MS, Solomon HM, *et al.*: The male polyurethane condom: a review of current knowledge. *Contraception* 1996, 53:141–146.

35. Schuster MA, Bell RM, Berry SH, *et al.*: Impact of a high school condom availability program on sexual attitudes and behaviors. *Fam Plann Perspect* 1998, 30:67–72.

36.• Guttmacher S, Lieberman L, Ward D, *et al.*: Condom availability in New York City public high schools: relationships to condom use and sexual behavior. *Am J Public Health* 1997, 87:1427–1433.

This study concludes that "Condom availability has a modest but significant effect on condom use and does not increase rates of sexual activity. These findings suggest that school-based condom availability can lower the risk of HIV and other sexually transmitted diseases for urban teenagers in the US."

37.• Kestelman P, Trussell J: Efficacy of the simultaneous use of condoms and spermicides [see comments]. *Fam Plann Perspect* 1991, 23:226–227.

This paper concludes that the simultaneous use of condoms and spermicides provides greater contraceptive efficacy than either method used alone, and that this efficacy approaches the efficacy of hormonal methods.

38. Santelli J, Warren CW, Lowry R, *et al.*: The use of condoms with other contraceptive methods among young men and women. *Fam Plann Perspect* 1997, 29:261–267.

39. Centers for Disease Control and Prevention: Contraceptive practices before and after an intervention promoting condom use to prevent HIV infection and other sexually transmitted diseases among women-Selected U.S. sites, 1993Ð1994. *MMWR Morb Mortal Wkly Rep* 1997, 46:373–377.

40. Trussell J, Kost K: Contraceptive failure in the US: a critical review of the literature. *Stud Fam Plann* 1987, 18:237–283.

41.•• Trussell J, Hatcher RA, Cates WJ, *et al.*: Contraceptive failure in the US: an update. *Stud Fam Plann* 1990, 21:51–54.

This reference contains the most frequently cited table of contraceptive efficacy of all methods of contraception including estimates of failure rates given typical and perfect use. The concepts of these two methods of reporting failure rates were developed by these authors. The article also includes data about the percentage of women continuing to use each method at the end of 1 year, an important concept regarding contraceptive choices for individuals.

42.•• The Alan Guttmacher Institute: *Sex and America's Teenagers.* New York: The Alan Guttmacher Institute; 1994:1–88.

This report presents a comprehensive picture of sex and America's teenagers. It is eminently readable, including numerous helpful graphs and charts on statistics regarding adolescent contraception.

43. Oakley D, Sereika S, Bogue EL: Oral contraceptive pill use after an initial visit to a family planning clinic. *Fam Plann Perspect* 1991, 23:150–154.

44. de–Vincenzi I: A longitudinal study of human immunodeficiency virus transmission by heterosexual partners. European Study Group on Heterosexual Transmission of HIV. *N Engl J Med* 1994, 331:341–346.

45. Spruyt A, Steiner MJ, Joanis C, *et al.*: Identifying condom users at risk for breakage and slippage: findings from three international sites. *Am J Public Health* 1998, 88:239–244.

46. Gallo MF, Grimes DA, Schulz KF: Nonlatex vs. latex male condoms for contraception: a systematic review of randomized controlled trials. *Contraception* 2003, 68:319–326.

47. Bounds W: Female condoms. *Eur J Contracept Reprod Health Care* 1997, 2:113–116.

48. Trussell J, Sturgen K, Strickler J, *et al.*: Comparative contraceptive efficacy of the female condom and other barrier methods. *Fam Plann Perspect* 1994, 26:66–72.

49. Farr G, Gabelnick H, Sturgen K, *et al.*: Contraceptive efficacy and acceptability of the female condom. *Am J Public Health* 1994, 84:1960–1964.

50. Trussell J, Sturgen K, Strickler J, *et al.*: Comparative contraceptive efficacy of the female condom and other barrier methods. *Fam Plann Perspect* 1994, 26:66–72.

51. Soper DE, Shoupe D, Shangold GA, *et al.*: Prevention of vaginal trichomoniasis by compliant use of the female condom. *Sex Transm Dis* 1993, 20:137–139.

52. Galvão LW, Oliveira LC, Díaz J, *et al*: Effectiveness of female and male condoms in preventing exposure to semen during vaginal intercourse: a randomized trial. *Contraception* 2005, 71:130–136.

53. Leeper MA, Contardy M: Preliminary evaluation of Reality, a condom for women to wear. *Adv Contraception* 1989, 5:229–235.

54. Soper DE, Brockwell NJ, Dalton HP: Evaluation of the effects of a female condom on the female lower genital tract. *Contraception* 1991, 44:21–29.

55. Hooton TM, Roberts PL, Stamm WE: Effects of recent sexual activity and use of a diaphragm on the vaginal microflora. *Clin Infect Dis* 1994, 19:274–278.

56. Stapleton A, Stamm WE: Prevention of urinary tract infection. *Infect Dis Clin North Am* 1997, 11:719–733.

57. Hooton TM, Hillier S, Johnson C, *et al.*: *Escherichia coli* bacteriuria and contraceptive method [see comments]. *JAMA* 1991, 265:64–69.

58. Hooton TM, Fihn SD, Johnson C, *et al.*: Association between bacterial vaginosis and acute cystitis in women using diaphragms. *Arch Intern Med* 1995, 149:1932–1963.

59. Trussell J, Strickler J, Vaughan B: Contraceptive efficacy of the diaphragm, the sponge and the cervical cap. *Fam Plann Perspect* 1993, 25:100–105.

60. Mengel MB, Davis AB: Recurrent bacterial vaginosis: association with vaginal sponge use. *Fam Pract Res J* 1992, 12:283–288.

61. Mauck C, Glover LH, Miller E, *et al.*: Lea's Shield: a study of the safety and efficacy of a new vaginal barrier contraceptive used with and without spermicide. *Contraception* 1996, 53:329–335.

62. Mauck C, Callahan M, Weiner DH, *et al.*: A comparative study of the safety and efficacy of FemCap, a new vaginal barrier contraceptive, and the Ortho All-Flex diaphragm. The FemCap Investigators' Group. *Contraception* 1999, 60:71–80.

63. Mauck C, Weiner D, Crenin M, *et al.*: FemCap with removal strap: ease of removal, safety and acceptability. *Contraception* 2006, 73:59–64.

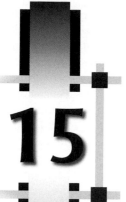

Injectable and Implantable Methods of Contraception

Allison A. Cowett and Jennifer L. Hardman

- Administered every 3 months, depot medroxyprogesterone acetate (DMPA) has a failure rate of 0.3%.
- The etonogestrel implant is a single rod, progesterone-only, subdermal contraceptive implant that provides highly effective contraception for a total of 3 years.
- DMPA and the etonogestrel implant work primarily by inhibiting ovulation.
- Irregular bleeding, amenorrhea, and weight gain are common side effects of DMPA.
- Irregular and unpredictable bleeding patterns are the most common side effect of the etonogestrel implant and the most common reason cited for discontinuation.
- Absolute contraindications for DMPA and the etonogestrel implant include pregnancy, undiagnosed abnormal vaginal bleeding, hormone-dependent cancer, known or suspected breast cancer, coagulation disorder, and active liver disease.

Injectable and implantable steroid preparations are highly effective, convenient, safe, and reversible methods of birth control. For contraceptive use, various dosage regimens have been used throughout the world. Depot medroxyprogesterone acetate (DMPA) is an injectable contraceptive given every 3 months and marketed under the names Depo Provera and depo-subQ provera 104 (Pfizer, New York, NY). For the remainder of this chapter, DMPA will be used to refer to both products; otherwise the brand name will be mentioned specifically. The etonogestrel implant is a single rod, progesterone-only implantable contraceptive marketed under the name Implanon (Organon USA, Roseland, NJ) and is effective for 3 years (Figure 15-1).

Historical Perspective

Depot medroxyprogesterone acetate was developed in 1954 by the Upjohn Company for treatment of endometriosis and habitual or threatened abortions [1]. Contraceptive use of DMPA started in the mid-1960s after the observation that women given DMPA for premature labor experienced a delay in return of fertility. The US Food and Drug Administration (FDA) denied the approval of Depo Provera several times due to concerns about possible carcinogenicity, and it did not receive FDA approval until 1992. FDA approval was granted for Depo-subQ provera 104 in 2004. The etonogestrel implant

has been available in the United States since 2006; however, it has been used abroad in over 30 countries since 1998.

Pharmacology

Medroxyprogesterone acetate (MPA) is a derivative of naturally occurring progesterone, and etonogestrel is a derivative of 19-nortestosterone. Both progestins prevent pregnancy predominantly by inhibiting ovulation through suppressing plasma levels of follicle-stimulating hormone and luteinizing hormone and by eliminating the luteinizing hormone surge [2,3]. They also cause a thickening of cervical mucus and an atrophic endometrium.

Dosing

Depo Provera is given as 150 mg intramuscularly every 11 to 13 weeks [4]. Depo-subQ provera 104 is given as 104 mg subcutaneously every 12 to 14 weeks [5]. It is recommended that the first DMPA injection is given during the first 5 days of a normal menstrual cycle to ensure that the patient is not pregnant. However, the contraceptive injections are often given after the fifth day of menses if the patient has a negative pregnancy test and has not had unprotected intercourse since her last menses. The etonogestrel implant is inserted subdermally in the groove between the bicep and tricep muscle on the inner aspect of the nondominant upper arm [6]. It must be inserted by a health care provider that has been formally trained regarding proper timing of insertion as well as technique for insertion and removal. For women not currently using contraception, it is recommended that the device be inserted between days 1 through 5 of the menstrual cycle. If switching from another method of contraception, Implanon should be inserted before the patient is due to start a new cycle (eg, new pack of pills, next injection, new box of patches). DMPA may be initiated immediately after childbirth, miscarriage, or pregnancy termination. The etonogestrel implant is approved for use after the fourth postpartum week; however, there is no evidence to refute the safety and efficacy of placement in the earlier postpartum period. It also can be placed immediately after miscarriage or pregnancy termination.

Efficacy

The injectable and implantable contraceptives are extremely effective. Depo Provera has a perfect use (ie, patient receives all injections on time) failure rate during the first year of 0.3% [4]. The typical use failure rate, in which a patient may be late occasionally for an injection, is 3%. In studies of over 2000 women receiving depo-subQ provera 104, there were no pregnancies reported [5]. A significant difference in medroxyprogesterone acetate levels in the blood of obese and nonobese women has not been shown, indicating no change in contraceptive efficacy of this method by patient weight [7]. There were only six pregnancies reported in Implanon users after over 20,000 menstrual cycles. The effectiveness of the implant in overweight (> 130% of ideal body weight) women has not been evaluated [6].

Advantages

In addition to the high contraceptive efficacy of DMPA, it confers noncontraceptive and potential therapeutic benefits (Figure 15-2). Because repeated injections of DMPA usually result

in longer cycles, less bleeding, and total amenorrhea, contraception with DMPA is suitable for women with anemia. DMPA also may be an excellent contraceptive choice for women with sickle cell disease. DMPA use among patients with sickle cell disease has been shown to be related to significant increases in fetal hemoglobin, total hemoglobin, red blood cell count, red blood cell survival, and red blood cell mass, as well as reduction in reticulocyte count, irreversible sickle cell count, and total bilirubin [8]. Painful crises also are less frequent during DMPA use than placebo use.

Depot medroxyprogesterone acetate also has been shown to decrease dysmenorrhea as well as midcycle ovulation pain. Depo-subQ provera 104 has been shown to decrease pain from endometriosis and is indicated for the treatment of cyclic pain related to endometriosis in symptomatic women desiring contraception [5].

Other noncontraceptive benefits of DMPA include a reduction in the incidence of vulvovaginal candidiasis and pelvic inflammatory disease (PID) [9–11]. Decrease in the frequency of PID is thought to occur because of increased cervical mucus viscosity and reduced menstrual flow associated with DMPA. Reduction in the incidence of candidiasis has been attributed to the absence of an estrogen component. Also, because DMPA protects against intrauterine and extrauterine pregnancies, a decrease in the incidence of ectopic pregnancies may be expected.

Seizure frequency has been reported to be highest during menstruation, which is when progesterone is low [12–14]. Progestins have been shown to have anticonvulsant properties. In an uncontrolled trial, the addition of DMPA to antiseizure regimens resulted in a significant decrease in the occurrence of seizures among women who became amenorrheic [12]. Furthermore, the contraceptive efficacy of the drug does not appear to be impaired by concurrent use of anticonvulsant medication. Hence, DMPA appears to be an ideal contraceptive option for women with seizure disorder. Other benefits are explained in more detail below.

The major benefit of the etonogestrel implant is that it provides long-term reversible contraception that does not require periodic maintenance. This factor may lead to increased compliance and decreased rates of unintended pregnancy when compared with other methods.

Dosing Regimens of Injectable and Implantable Contraceptives

Generic Name	Brand Name	Dose	Duration of Effectiveness	Common Adverse Effects
Etonogestrel implant	Implanon (Organon, Roseland, NJ)	60 mg etonogestrel subdermally	3 years	Irregular bleeding, weight gain, headache, acne, breast pain, abdominal pain, dizziness, emotional lability
Medroxyprogesterone acetate injectable suspension	Depo Provera (Pfizer, New York, NY)	150 mg IM	11–13 weeks	Irregular bleeding, weight gain, headache, dizziness, asthenia, nervousness
Medroxyprogesterone acetate injectable suspension	Depo-subQ provera 104	104 mg SC	12–14 weeks	Irregular bleeding, weight gain, decreased libido, acne, injection site reactions

Figure 15-1. Dosing regimens of injectable and implantable contraceptives. IM—intramuscularly; SC—subcutaneously.

GYNECOLOGIC CANCERS

Endometrial cancer is one of the most common gynecologic cancers in the United States. Risk factors include advanced age, early menarche, late menopause, chronic anovulation, low parity, and obesity, as well as exposure of the uterus to unopposed estrogens. Progesterone acts as an antiestrogen and thus theoretically protects against the development of endometrial cancer.

Prompted by the lack of sufficient data concerning DMPA use and the risk of endometrial cancer, a multinational hospital-based case control study was undertaken by the World Health Organization [15]. One hundred twenty-two women with endometrial cancer were compared with 939 women admitted to the same hospitals to wards other than obstetrics and gynecology. Overall, DMPA users had a much lower chance of being diagnosed with endometrial cancer than nonusers (odds ratio, 0.21; 95% CI, 0.06 to 0.79). The protective effect of DMPA appeared to be long term and to last at least 8 years after discontinuing use of this contraceptive. There is now consensus that, as for use of combined oral contraceptives, use of DMPA profoundly reduces endometrial cancer risk. There are no data about the risks or benefits of the use of the etonogestrel implant with respect to endometrial cancer. However, endometrial sampling in women using the implant has exhibited primarily inactive or weakly proliferative histology [16].

OVARIAN CANCER

Depot medroxyprogesterone acetate reduces fertility mainly by reducing gonadotropin levels and inhibiting ovulation. Because of the theory that gonadotropin stimulation of the ovary is a risk factor for ovarian cancer, it is believed that DMPA users have a lower risk of ovarian cancer as opposed to nonusers. Although such association is biologically plausible, a protective effect of DMPA has not been shown. To examine the relation between DMPA use and ovarian cancer risk, the World Health Organization conducted a hospital-based case-control study in Mexico and Thailand [17]. Cases were 224 women with histologically confirmed epithelial ovarian cancer. Control subjects were 1781 women matched with cases on age, hospital, and year of interview. The odds ratio for ovarian cancer among women who had ever used DMPA was 1.07 (95% CI, 0.6–1.8), as opposed to the never use of this contraceptive, independent of number of live births and oral contraceptive use. Also, cancer risk did not appear to be related to duration of use, time since first or most recent use, or age at first use of DMPA. Failure to find an expected protective effect in the World Health Organization study has been attributed to the lack of inclusion of subjects who are at highest risk of developing ovarian cancer (nulliparous women) and overall low power of the study. According to the authors, DMPA may not confer any additional protection against ovarian cancer beyond that provided by full-term pregnancies. Based on the existing evidence, DMPA use does not appear to alter risk of ovarian cancer. It is unknown if use of the etonogestrel implant effects the risks of ovarian cancer.

Disadvantages

MENSTRUAL SIDE EFFECTS

Menstrual changes occur in almost all women using DMPA and the etonogestrel implant and are the most common reason for women to discontinue either method. Polymenorrhea, prolonged bleeding, and spotting have been reported to be more frequent after the first injection of DMPA and are gradually replaced by longer cycles, less bleeding, and total amenorrhea after repeated injections [18,19]. More than half (55%) of the women using Depo Provera for 1 year experience amenorrhea, and 68% have amenorrhea after 2 years of use [4,19]. Thirty-nine percent of depo-subQ provera users have experienced amenorrhea at 6 months and 56.5% at 1 year [5]. Bleeding patterns with the etonogestrel implant are irregular and unpredictable and are less likely to exhibit an increase in amenorrhea rates over the duration of implant use. Amenorrhea is reported in 20% of 90 day reference periods over 2 years of use [6].

NONMENSTRUAL SIDE EFFECTS

Weight gain is the most common nonmenstrual side effect associated with the use of DMPA [19–21]. Weight gain of 5.4

Noncontraceptive Benefits of Injectable and Implantable Contraceptives

Etonogestrel Implant	Medroxyprogesterone Acetate Injectable Suspension
Reduces menstrual blood loss and possible amenorrhea	Reduces menstrual blood loss and possible amenorrhea
Reversible	Reversible
Long-term effectiveness	Improves pain from endometriosis (subcutaneous only)
Rapid return of fertility	Reduces risk of endometrial cancer
	Reduces acute sickle cell crises
	Reduces seizure frequency
	Reduces risk of ectopic pregnancy
	Reduces risk of pelvic inflammatory disease
	Possibly reduces risk of ovarian cancer

Figure 15-2. Noncontraceptive benefits of injectable and implantable contraceptives.

and 3.5 pounds has been reported at 1 year and 8.1 and 7.5 at 2 years for Depo Provera and depo-subQ provera 104, respectively [4,5]. Other common reported problems with Depo Provera are abdominal pain or discomfort, dizziness, headache, asthenia, and nervousness. Common side effects of depo-subQ provera 104 are headache and injection site reactions. Side effects reported by more than 5% of etonogestrel implant users include headache, acne, breast pain, abdominal pain, dizziness, and emotional lability [6].

BONE MINERAL DENSITY

Depot medroxyprogesterone acetate is known to decrease bone mineral density (BMD). Although it is likely that the intramuscular and subcutaneous formulations reduce BMD, most of the research on this subject has been done with the intramuscular formulation. The manufacturer of Depo Provera and depo-subQ provera 104 recommends that patients should not use DMPA for more than 2 years unless they are unwilling or unable to use another method [4,5]. Use of long-term DMPA is possibly the most concerning in younger and older users. It is unknown whether DMPA use in younger users will prevent them from reaching their peak bone mass or if older users will not be able to completely recover from the bone loss before menopause.

A systematic review of 39 studies was conducted on articles that evaluated the effects of DMPA on bone loss or fracture risk and were published between 1966 and July 2005 [22••]. Overall, DMPA did cause a reduction in BMD; however, the difference was usually within one standard deviation of the BMD of nonusers. The bone loss was reversible to some extent, but it is unknown if complete recovery of bone density occurs. There are limited data on the future risk of fracture in DMPA users, with only one study finding a nonsignificant increased risk of stress fracture. More recent studies have found that although significant bone loss does occur, the most rapid loss occurs during the first 2 years of use and additional loss with longer use may not be significant [23,24]. This suggests that discontinuing DMPA after 2 years may not be necessary. The Society for Adolescent Medicine suggests no restrictions on the use of DMPA as long as patients are counseled on the risks versus benefits of use [25•]. In addition, patients using DMPA should be counseled regarding the recommended daily allowance of calcium.

Studies of the effects of the etonogestrel implant have not shown similarly concerning results. When compared with subjects using the non–hormone containing intrauterine device, subjects employing the etonogestrel implant exhibited no difference in BMD measurements of the lumbar spine, the proximal femur and the distal radius after 2 years of method use [26]. The fluctuation in BMD over time was minimal and did not reach the clinically significant mean decrease of one standard deviation at any reference point during the 2-year study.

METABOLIC IMPACT

Published studies report inconsistent findings with respect to the influence of DMPA on plasma lipid levels. Some suggest that DMPA use is correlated with lower high-density lipoprotein (HDL) levels with no influence on low-density lipoprotein (LDL), whereas others report lower levels of HDL and higher levels of LDL [27–29]. Overall, these results indicate moderate unfavorable lipid metabolism as a result of long-term DMPA use, which should be considered and for which counseling should be given to women who request this contraceptive method for family planning. Use of DMPA has not been shown to induce clinically significant changes in glucose metabolism, liver function, or coagulation parameters [28,30,31]. Studies of lipid metabolism in etonogestrel implant users reveal a decrease in total cholesterol, LDL levels, and HDL levels over a period of 2 years. A study comparing lipid metabolism in users of Norplant (Wyeth, Madison, NJ) with users of Implanon showed a decrease in HDL of 5.8% from baseline in the later group [32]. As for carbohydrate metabolism, levels of glycosylated hemoglobin A_{1C} are increased in etonogestrel implant users while fasting glucose measurements remain unchanged [33].

IN UTERO EXPOSURE

There is no evidence that DMPA has adverse effects on pregnancy outcome. Specifically, there is no increased risk of miscarriage, multiple pregnancy, preterm labor, stillbirth, or congenital anomalies [34,35]. Also, studies observing DMPA-exposed infants into their teens conclude that DMPA does not impair their long-term growth and pubertal development [36]. However, findings from one study have indicated that fetuses exposed to DMPA may be at an increased risk of low birth weight [37]. Because of the high contraceptive efficacy of DMPA, the impact of such an effect, if valid, would be small. Studies in pregnant animals have not shown any adverse effects with the use of Implanon [6].

EFFECT ON LACTATION

There is a theoretic concern that the administration of progestin-only contraceptives immediately postpartum may result in a decrease in milk production, because the postpartum decline in progesterone is thought to be what initiates lactogenesis [38•]. For this reason, it may be advisable to wait at least 3 days after delivery to administer progestin-only contraceptives. However, although there is no evidence to suggest that DMPA causes any short- or long-term adverse effect in nursing infants exposed to the drug, the World Health Organization recommends waiting 6 weeks after delivery before starting the use of this contraceptive.

Studies examining the effect of DMPA on lactation have shown no significant changes in milk volume or infant growth and only minor shifts occurring in milk composition as a result of DMPA use during breastfeeding [39,40]. Also, DMPA, administered to nursing mothers, has not been shown to influence the hormonal regulation of breast-fed normal male infants [41].

Studies on the concomitant use of the etonogestrel implant and breastfeeding exhibit an estimated 0.2% of the maternal dose is excreted in the breast milk. In a nonrandomized study of breastfeeding women initiating the etonogestrel implant or the copper intrauterine device between 4 and 8 weeks postpartum, there were no differences in infant growth or duration of breastfeeding between the two groups over a 3-year follow-up period [42]. There were no treat-ment-related adverse events in either group for the duration of the study. Use of the etonogestrel implant in breastfeeding women less than 4 weeks postpartum has not been studied.

Drug Interactions

Only one medication has been shown to interact with DMPA. Concurrent use of amino glutethimide with DMPA may significantly depress the serum concentrations of MPA [43]. Therefore, because of a reduction in contraceptive efficacy, use of amino glutethimide with DMPA is inadvisable. Etonogestrel is metabolized by the liver, specifically by the enzyme cytochrome P450 3A4. Medications that increase the activity of this enzyme should be avoided, as they can speed up the metabolism of etonogestrel and reduce contraceptive effectiveness [6]. Examples of cytochrome P450 3A4 inducers include barbiturates, griseofulvin, rifampin, phenytoin, carbamazepine, some protease inhibitors, and possibly St. John's wort.

Acceptability

The continuation rate of DMPA at 1 year in several studies ranges from 23% to 56% [44••,45,46]. The continuation rate of DMPA does not appear to be affected by the users' age, marital status, pregnancy history, clinic site, or proximity of residence to the clinic [20]. However, decision to continue or stop use of this contraceptive appears to be related to the experience of side effects. The most common reasons for stopping the use of DMPA are irregular bleeding and weight gain. Careful patient education and counseling can minimize use of DMPA in inappropriate candidates such as women unwilling to tolerate menstrual changes and weight increases.

Continuation rates for Implanon at 1 year range from 67% to 90% [47–50]. Younger women were more likely to discontinue the implant than older women [48]. Side effects, especially irregular bleeding, and a change of mind about the need for contraception were the most common reasons for discontinuing [47–50].

Return of Fertility

Although DMPA offers maximum contraceptive efficacy during the 3 months after each injection, the drug may inhibit ovulation for some months beyond this period. The median time to conception after a Depo Provera injection is 10 months (range of 4 to 31 months) [4]. In a small group of depo-subQ provera users, the median time to ovulation was 10 months after the last injection [5]. Return to fertility appears to be the same among parous and nonparous women, and there appears to be no correlation between the return to ovulation and the duration of contraceptive use [51,52]. Upon removal of the etonogestrel implant after 3 years of use, the level of etonogestrel falls rapidly to undetectable levels within 1 week [6]. Return to fertility may be faster on average than other forms of contraception with over 90% of users ovulating within 3 months after removal.

Contraindications

Absolute contraindications for DMPA and the etonogestrel implant are known or suspected pregnancy, undiagnosed abnormal vaginal bleeding, sex hormone–dependent cancer such as breast cancer, history of thrombosis or thromboembolic disorder, active liver disease, or hypersensitivity to any component of the product [4–6].

Injectable Contraceptives and Risk of Sexually Transmitted Diseases

Despite the efficacy of DPMA and the etonogestrel implant in preventing pregnancy, it fails to provide protection against sexually transmitted diseases, including HIV. At present, the only available method for preventing sexually transmitted disease transmission among sexually active people is the correct and consistent use of condoms.

Conclusions

Depot medroxyprogesterone acetate and the etonogestrel implant are highly effective, convenient, and safe methods of contraception. These progesterone-only methods of contraception are ideal for women desiring nondaily methods, those unable to use an estrogen containing regimen, or women taking medications that reduce the efficacy of combined contraception. Both methods prevent pregnancy by inhibiting ovulation and confer a number of noncontraceptive health benefits. Menstrual irregularities are common with both methods and may lead to method discontinuation. Because injectable and implantable contraceptives do not protect against sexually transmitted diseases, women should be counseled on the importance of condom use for disease prevention.

References

Papers of particular interest have been highlighted as follows:
• Of interest
•• Of outstanding interest

1. Klitsch M: Injectable hormones and regulatory controversy: an end to the long-running story? *Fam Plann Perspect* 1993, 25:37–40.

2. Fraser IS, Weisberg E: A comprehensive review of injectable contraception with special emphasis on depot medroxyprogesterone acetate. *Med J Aust* 1981, 1:1–20.

3. Mishell DR, Kletzky OA, Brenner PF, *et al.*: The effect of contraceptive steroids on hypothalamic-pituitary function. *Am J Obstet Gynecol* 1977, 128:60–74.

4. Pfizer Inc. Depo Provera [package insert]. New York, NY: Pfizer, Inc.; 2004.

5. Depo-subQ provera 104 [package insert]. New York, NY: Pfizer, Inc.; 2004.

6. Implanon [package insert]. Roseland, NJ; Organon USA Inc.: 2006.

7. Fotherby K, Koetsawang K: Metabolism of injectable formulations of contraceptive steroids in obese and thin women. *Contraception* 1982, 26:51–58.

8. De Ceulaer K, Gruber C, Hayes R, *et al.*: Medroxyprogesterone acetate and homozygous sickle-cell disease. *Lancet* 1982, 2:229–231.

9. Dennerstein GJ: Depo Provera in the treatment of recurrent vulvovaginal candidiasis. *J Reprod Med* 1986, 31:801–803.

10. WHO Task Force of Intrauterine Devices: PID associated with fertility-regulating agents. *Contraception* 1984, 30:1–21.

11. Toppozada M, Onsy FA, Fares E, *et al.*: The protective influence of progestogen only contraception against vaginal moniliasis. *Contraception* 1979, 20:99–103.

12. Mattson RH, Cramer JA, Caldwell BV, *et al.*: Treatment of seizures with medroxyprogesterone acetate: preliminary report. *Neurology* 1984, 34:1255–1258.

13. Backstrome T: Epileptic seizures in women related to plasma estrogen and progesterone during the menstrual cycle. *Acta Neurol Scand* 1976, 54:321–347.

14. Frederiksen MC: Depo medroxyprogesterone acetate contraception in women with medical problems. *J Reprod Med* 1996, 41:414–418.

15. WHO Collaborative Study of Neoplasia and Steroid Contraceptives: Depo-medroxyprogesterone acetate (DMPA) and risk of endometrial cancer. *Int J Cancer* 1991, 49:186–190.

16. Mascarenhas L, van Beek A, Bennink HC, Newton J: A 2-year comparison study of endometrial history and cervical cytology of contraceptive implant users in Birmingham, UK. *Hum Reprod* 1998, 13:3057–3060.

17. WHO Collaborative Study of Neoplasia and Steroid Contraceptives: Depot-medroxyprogesterone acetate (DMPA) and risk of epithelial ovarian cancer. *Int J Cancer* 1991, 49:191–195.

18. WHO Special Programme of Research, Development, and Research Training in Human Reproduction; Task Force on Long-Acting Agents for the Regulation of Fertility: Multinational comparative clinical trial of long-acting injectable contraceptives: norethisterone enanthate given in two dosage regimens and depot-medroxyprogesterone acetate. Final report. *Contraception* 1983, 28:1–20.

19. Sangi-Haghpeykar H, Poindexter AN, Bateman L, *et al.*: Experiences of injectable contraceptive users in an urban setting. *Obstet Gynecol* 1996, 88:227–233.

20. Polaneczky M, Guarnaccia M, Alon J, *et al.*: Early experience with the contraceptive use of depot-medroxyprogesterone acetate in an inner-city clinic population. *Fam Plann Perspect* 1996, 28:174–178.

21. Paul C, Skegg DCG, Williams S: Depot medroxyprogesterone acetate: patterns of use and reasons for discontinuation. *Contraception* 1997, 56:209–214.

22.•• Curtis KM, Martins SL: Progestogen-only contraception and bone mineral density: a systematic review. *Contraception* 2006, 73:470–487.

Review of 39 trials of progestin-only contraception and their effects on bone mass and fracture.

23. Kaunitz AM, Miller PD, Rice VM, *et al.*: Bone mineral density in women aged 25–35 years receiving depot medroxyprogesterone acetate: recovery following discontinuation. *Contraception* 2006, 74:90–99.

24. Clark MK, Sowers M, Levy B, Nichols S: Bone mineral density loss and recovery during 48 months in first-time users of depot medroxyprogesterone acetate. *Fertil Steril* 2006, 86:1466–1474.

25.• Depot medroxyprogesterone acetate and bone mineral density in adolescents: the black box warning: a position paper of the Society for Adolescent Medicine. *J Adol Health* 2006, 39:296–301.

A review of the literature on the effects of DMPA on bone in the adolescent population.

26. Beerthuizen R, van Beek A, Massai R, *et al.*: Bone mineral density during long-term use of the progestogen contraceptive implant Implanon compared to a non-hormonal method of contraception. *Hum Reprod* 2000, 15:118–122.

27. Garza-Flores J, De La Cruz DL, Valles de Bourges V, *et al.*: Long-term effects of depot-medroxyprogesterone acetate on lipoprotein metabolism. *Contraception* 1991, 44:61–71.

28. Fahmy K, Khairy M, Allam G, *et al.*: Effect of depot medroxyprogesterone acetate on coagulation factors and serum lipids in Egyptian women. *Contraception* 1991, 44:431–444.

29. World Health Organization: A multicenter comparative study of serum lipids and apolipoproteins in long-term use of DMPA and a control group of IUD users. *Contraception* 1993, 47:177–191.

30. Kamau RK, Maina FW, Kigundu C, *et al.*: The effect of low estrogen combined pill, progestogen-only pill and medroxyprogesterone acetate on oral glucose tolerance test. *East Afr Med J* 1990, 67:550–555.

31. Virutamasen P, Wongsrichanalai C, Tangkeo P, *et al.*: Metabolic effects of depot-medroxyprogesterone acetate in long-term users: a cross-sectional study. *Int J Obstet Gynecol* 1986, 24:291–296.

32. Biswas A, Viegas OAC, Roy AC: Effect of Implanon and Norplant subdermal contraceptive implants on serum lipids- a randomized comparative study. *Contraception* 2003, 68:189–193.

33. Biswas A, Viegas OAC, Bennink HJT, *et al.*: Implanon contraceptive implants: effects in carbohydrate metabolism. *Contraception* 2001, 63:137–141.

34. Simpson JL: Mutagenicity and teratogenicity of injectable and implantable progestins: probably lack of effect. In *Long Acting Contraceptive Delivery Systems.* Edited by Zatuchni GI, Goldsmith A, Sheldon JD, *et al.* Philadelphia: Harper & Row; 1984:334–361.

35. American College of Obstetricians and Gynecologists: Contraceptives and congenital anomalies. ACOG Committee Opinion 124. Washington, DC: ACOG;1993.

36. Pardthaisong T, Yenchit C, Gray RH: The long-term growth and development of children exposed to Depo-Provera during pregnancy or lactation. *Contraception* 1992, 45:313–324.

37. Gray RH, Pardthaisong T: In utero exposure to steroid contraceptives and survival during infancy. *Am J Epidemiol* 1991, 134:804–811.

38.• Kennedy KI, Short RV, Rose Tully M: Premature introduction of progestin-only contraceptive methods during lactation. *Contraception* 1997, 55:347–350.

A review of the possible and proven effects of progestin-only contraceptives on lactation.

39. Baheiraei A, Ardsetani N, Ghazizadeh SH: Effects of progestogen-only contraceptives on breast-feeding and infant growth. *Int J Gynecol Obstet* 2001, 74:203–205.

40. WHO Task Force on Oral Contraceptives, Special Programme of Research, Development, and Research Training in Human Reproduction: Effects of hormonal contraceptives on breast milk composition and infant growth. *Stud Fam Plann* 1988,19:361–369.

41. Virutamasen P, Leepipatpaiboon S, Kriengsinyot R, *et al.*: Pharmacodynamic effects of depot-medroxyprogesterone acetate (DMPA) administered to lactating women on their male infants. *Contraception* 1996, 54:153–157.

42. Reinprayoon R, Taneepanichskul S, Bunyavejchevin S, *et al.*: Effects of the etonogestrel-releasing contraceptive implant (ImplanonTM) on parameters of breastfeeding compared to those of an intrauterine device. *Contraception* 2000, 62:239–246.

43. Van Deijk WA, Biljham GH, Mellink WAM, *et al.*: Influence of aminoglutethimide on plasma levels of medroxyprogesterone acetate: its correlation with serum cortisol. *Cancer Treat Rep* 1985, 69:85–90.

44.•• Trussell J: Contraceptive failure in the United States. *Contraception* 2004, 70:89–96.

Discusses continuation of all methods of contraception.

45. Westfall JM, Main DS, Barnard L: Continuation rates among injectable contraceptive users. *Fam Plann Perspect* 1996, 78:275–277.

46. Polaneczky M, Guarnaccia M, Alon J, Wiley J: Early experience with the contraceptive use of depot medroxyprogesterone acetate in an inner city clinic population. *Fam Plann Perspect* 1996, 28:174–178.

47. Rai K, Gupta S, Cotter S: Experience with Implanon in a north-east London family planning clinic. *Eur J Contracept Reprod Health Care* 2004, 9:39–46.

48. Smith A, Reuter S: An assessment of the use of Implanon in three community services. *J Fam Plann Reprod Health Care* 2002, 28:193–196.

49. Lakha F, Glasier AF: Continuation rates of Implanon in the UK: data from an observational study in a clinical setting. *Contraception* 2006, 74:287–289.

50. Agrawal A, Robinson C: An assessment of the first 3 years' use of Implanon in Luton. *J Fam Plann Reprod Health Care* 2005, 31:310–312.

51. Pardthaisong T: Return of fertility after use of the injectable contraceptive Depo-Provera: updated analysis. *J Biosoc Sci* 1984, 16:23–34.

52. Garza-Flores J, Cardenas S, Rodriguez V, *et al.*: Return to ovulation following the use of long-acting injectable contraceptives: a comparative study. *Contraception* 1985, 31:361–366.

16 | Intrauterine Devices

Paula H. Bednarek and Jeffrey T. Jensen

- Intrauterine contraceptive devices (IUDs) are safe, highly effective, and underutilized methods of contraception.
- An excess risk of infection associated with current IUDs is low and is seen only associated with insertion.
- The primary mechanism of action of IUDs is not abortifacient.
- IUDs do not increase the risk of ectopic pregnancy.
- IUDs may be used in appropriate nulliparous women.
- Skills needed for routine insertions and removals are well within the scope of primary care providers.
- IUDs are among the most cost effective methods of contraception.
- The Dalkon Shield experience created an unfavorable cultural perception of IUDs in America that persists today.

In the United States, no contraceptive method stirs quite as much debate as the intrauterine contraceptive device (IUD). Worldwide, however, IUDs have a long-standing history as the most popular method of reversible contraception used by nearly 160 million women [1]. A comparative study of five European countries (Italy, Spain, Poland, Germany, and Denmark) estimated that the IUD accounts for 9% to 24% of all contraceptive use [2]. The rate of less than 2% in the United States is the lowest of any developed nation [1]. Interestingly, women physicians in the United States use IUDs at rates between two and five times the rates among age- and income-matched women in the general population [3].

What factors explain the surprisingly low use prevalence in the United States of a safe, highly effective, reversible method of contraception? To help primary care physicians understand the role and place of the IUD as a contraceptive option, this chapter will discuss the background, recent history, and controversy surrounding modern IUDs.

Recent History of Intrauterine Contraception

Although intrauterine contraception has a long and colorful history, widespread use of the method did not begin until the 1960s [4••]. In the decades following World War II,

a renaissance in contraceptive development occurred, fueled by awareness of the global population explosion, improved understanding of reproductive physiology and steroid biochemistry, and more permissive attitudes towards sexuality. By 1970, information regarding the first generation of oral contraceptives was available, and the resulting media attention and U.S. Senate hearings led to growing concern among women regarding the safety of hormonal contraception. Many turned to intrauterine contraceptives.

Because this transition occurred in the midst of the sexual revolution, many women who switched methods were probably not optimal candidates for the IUD because they were at increased risk for sexually transmitted infections (STIs). The introduction of the Dalkon Shield in 1970 needs to be viewed in this historic context. Promoted as a safe, effective alternative to oral contraceptives, well-suited to nulliparous women, it soon became the most popular IUD in America. Concerns regarding safety (an increased risk of septic abortions when the device failed) first surfaced in 1973. By the time sales were discontinued in 1974, over 2.8 million had been sold [5]. A formal call for removal of all Dalkon Shields, however, was not issued until 1980. Prolonged, highly publicized litigation over Shield-related complications followed, as evidence began to mount linking IUDs to pelvic infections and infertility. The public and many health care providers came to believe that all IUDs greatly increased the risk of these complications.

However, there were major methodologic flaws with early case-control studies in the 1970s and 1980s that attributed an increased risk of pelvic inflammatory disease (PID) and infertility to all IUDs. Many of these studies were subsequently reanalyzed, and it was found that most of the increased risk was associated specifically with the Dalkon Shield and with high-risk sexual behavior [6–8]. It was felt that the plastic encased multifilament tail of the Dalkon Shield allowed pathogenic bacteria to ascend into the uterine cavity of Shield users [9]. All other IUDs use monofilament tail strings. In addition, many of the earlier IUD studies failed to control for the reduced risk of PID and infertility in users of hormonal and barrier methods of birth control [10].

Unfortunately, perceptions are more important than science, and by 1986, the damage had been done. Four of the five remaining distributors of IUDs in the United States voluntarily discontinued sales in response to declining market share and increasing legal costs. The use prevalence of IUDs in the United States plummeted from 7.1% of married women of reproductive age in 1982 to 2% in 1988 [11]. Despite the introduction of the copper T380A in 1988, the use prevalence continued to decline to just 0.8% in 1995. The introduction of the levonorgestrel-releasing intrauterine system (LNG-IUS) in 2001 has led to a resurgence of provider and patient interest in IUDs and contributed to an increase in use prevalence to 2% in 2002 [1].

Recent studies have clarified the absence of a strong relationship between IUDs and pelvic infections and reinforce our comfort in recommending this form of contraception to most women. Risk estimates for PID tend to decrease when non-contraceptors are used as controls, and the effect of the Dalkon Shield is isolated. In fact, there is physiologic and clinical evidence that the LNG-IUS may be protective against PID. One of the main physiologic effects of progestin containing contraception is thickening of cervical mucus, which protects against ascending genital tract infection. This is a presumed mechanism of decreased PID in women using combined oral contraceptives, progestin implants, or injectables [12].

Overall, the rates of PID in the few available randomized control trials of IUDs do not exceed estimates for the general population [13]. The small excess risk of PID associated with current IUDs appears to be primarily related to insertion. Combined data from 13 World Health Organization (WHO) clinical trials [9] found that the risk of PID was 1.6 cases per 1000 person-years and was concentrated in the first 20 days after insertion. The polymicrobial nature of these early infections suggests that most occur due to contamination of the uterine cavity with endogenous flora during insertion. In addition, women with pre-existing asymptomatic chlamydia or gonorrhea have a higher risk of PID immediately after IUD insertion. Recommended steps to lower the risk of insertion-related infection include careful screening and the use of multiyear devices (fewer insertions). Randomized trials of women at low risk for sexually transmitted infections have found no benefit of empiric antibiotic prophylaxis in reducing this insertion-associated risk [14]. The role of sexually transmitted pathogens in later infections is independent of the device.

Further reassurance of safety comes from a landmark 2001 case control study in nulliparous women who were seeking treatment for primary infertility that found no association between tubal infertility and past intrauterine contraceptive use [15••]. In this study, 358 women with primary infertility who had documented tubal occlusion were compared with two control groups: 953 nulliparous women with primary infertility and no tubal occlusion (infertile controls) and 584 primigravid women (pregnant controls). Women with tubal occlusion reported prior IUD use at the same rate as infertile women without tubal occlusion or primigravid controls (Figure 16-1). Tubal infertility was associated with past chlamydia infection (as evidenced by chlamydia antibodies) and not with IUD use. This study supports the association between PID and infertility and not IUD use and infertility.

Use of a Copper Intrauterine Device and the Risk of Tubal Occlusion*

IUD Use and the Presence of Antibodies to Chlamydia	Infertile Women with Tubal Occlusion (n = 358), n (%)	Infertile Control Subjects (n = 953), n (%)	OR (95% CI)	Pregnant Control Subjects (n = 584), n (%)	OR (95% CI)†
No use of a copper IUD					
Antibody-negative	203 (56.7)	583 (61.2)	1.0	420 (71.9)	1.0
Antibody-positive	132 (36.9)	313 (32.8)	1.2 (0.9–1.6)	124 (21.2)	2.4 (1.7–3.2)
Use of a copper IUD					
Antibody-negative	18 (5.0)	33 (3.5)	1.5 (0.8–2.8)	32 (5.5)	1.1 (0.6–2.1)
Antibody-positive	5 (1.4)	24 (2.5)	0.6 (0.2–1.5)	8 (1.4)	1.3 (0.4–4.1)

*For infertile women, data represent the use of a copper IUD before they suspected a fertility problem. Antibody titers of 1:256 or greater were considered positive. For all comparisons, women with no use of a copper IUD and no antibodies to chlamydia served as the reference group. The ratios were adjusted for age, income, number of sexual partners, years of education, and history of sexual intercourse during the teenage years.
†The OR are for comparison with the infertile women with tubal occlusion.

Figure 16-1. Use of a copper intrauterine device (IUD) and the risk of tubal occlusion. OR—odds ratio. (*Adapted from* Hubacher *et al.* [15••].)

Types of Intrauterine Conception Devices

Currently only two IUDs are marketed in the United States (Figure 16-2). A variety of other devices are available around the world. Most modern devices are medicated and require replacement at some defined interval. Although some authorities recommend replacing a nonmedicated device with a more effective copper IUD or LNG-IUS [16], there is no evidence to support the routine removal of a well-tolerated inert device (other than the Dalkon Shield) in a patient who desires ongoing contraception.

The copper T380A (ParaGard; Duramed/Barr Pharmaceuticals, Pomona, NY) was approved by the US Food and Drug Administration in 1984 and became available in the United States in 1988. The name comes from the total amount of copper (380 mm^2) wound around the device's stem (314 mm^2 of wire) and arms (two 33 mm^2 copper sleeves). The 36 × 32 mm polyethylene frame contains barium sulfate to make the device radiopaque. A double white monofilament nylon string helps to distinguish the device from the LNG-IUS. The copper T380A is approved for up to 10 years of continuous use.

The LNG-IUS (Mirena; Bayer Health Care Pharmaceuticals, Wayne, NJ) was approved by the US Food and Drug Administration in 2000 for up to 5 years of use. It consists of a 32 × 32 mm, T-shaped polyethylene frame with a steroid reservoir around the vertical stem containing 52 mg of levonorgestrel. The rate of levonorgestrel release decreases progressively from an initial rate of 20 μg/day to 10 μg/day after 5 years. Whereas spotting is common in the first few months of use, this bleeding tapers off. After the first year of use, 70% to 90% of patients experience reduction in monthly bleeding, and approximately 20% of women have no bleeding at all [17].

Mechanism of Contraceptive Action

All IUDs produce a sterile, foreign body reaction within the uterine cavity [18]. A common misconception regarding the IUD is that the primary mechanism of action is confined to the uterus and is abortifacient in nature. As this concern represents a barrier to the use or recommendation of IUDs by some women and health care providers, the issue deserves thorough exploration.

Although interference with implantation plays a role in the postcoital effectiveness of IUDs, the available evidence suggests that this is not the usual mechanism in women using the devices continuously [19••]. Studies on sperm migration suggest reduced numbers of spermatozoa reach the fallopian tubes in IUD users. Copper is spermicidal, and the intrauterine inflammatory response may destroy sperm through phagocytosis [20]. The levonorgestrel-releasing intrauterine system thickens the cervical mucus (interfering with sperm passage) [21], and inhibits sperm motility and function inside the uterus and the fallopian tubes (preventing fertilization) [22]. Studies on the recovery of eggs from women using IUDs compared with women using no method of contraception show that embryos are formed at much lower rates in IUD users, and that almost all of these embryos are abnormal, suggesting parthenogenic activation [19]. Therefore, it can be concluded that when normal fertilization does occur in an IUD user, it is associated with method failure.

Efficacy

Intrauterine contraceptive devices are among the most effective methods of contraception. Typical-use first year pregnancy rates for the LNG-IUS and copper T380A IUD are 0.1% to 0.8%, similar to surgical tubal occlusion [23]. In a large multicenter study with 1124 LNG-IUS users and 1121 copper T380A users,

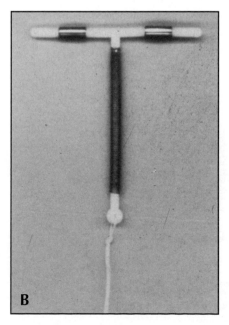

Figure 16-2. Intrauterine devices available in the United States. **A**, The levonorgestrel-releasing intrauterine system. **B**, The copper T380A.

the 5-year pregnancy rates were 1.1% for the LNG-IUS and 1.4% for the copper T380A [24]. Most clinicians believe that proper high position in the uterine fundus is necessary for optimal efficacy. Improper positioning of the device may increase the risk of expulsion and contribute to failure.

Ectopic Pregnancy

Considerable misunderstanding exists over the relationship between IUDs and ectopic pregnancy. Although the predominant mechanism for medicated IUDs is preconceptual, an intrauterine effect discourages implantation when fertilization does occur. For this reason, a disproportionate number of failures resulting in clinical pregnancies will be ectopics. However, the absolute number of ectopic pregnancies is lower among IUD users compared to noncontraceptors because the overall pregnancy rate in IUD users is lower. The 5-year ectopic rate for women using an IUD is 0.02 per 100 woman-years, and 1.2-1.6 per 100 woman-years for a control population of sexually active women not using contraception [25]. Importantly, past or prolonged use of an IUD does not lead to an increased risk of ectopic pregnancy [26,27••].

Although the LNG-IUS package insert continues to list history of ectopic pregnancy as a contraindication to insertion, the copper T380A labeling was updated in 2005 to remove this misperception. Because the evidence shows that copper T380A and LNG-IUS users enjoy a substantial reduction in the overall risk of ectopic and intrauterine pregnancy, these devices should be considered appropriate choices for contraception in women with a history of an ectopic pregnancy (Figure 16-3).

Postcoital Contraception and the Intrauterine Contraceptive Device

Insertion of a copper IUD within 5 days of unprotected intercourse is an effective method of postcoital contraception [28]. In this application, the mechanism of action involves disruption of implantation. Common sense dictates that this application be restricted to women at low risk for sexually transmitted infection who desire ongoing, long-term contraception.

Satisfaction

Discontinuation rates for adverse events such as bleeding, pain, perforation, ectopic pregnancy, and infection correlate significantly with satisfaction. A large multicenter trial in Europe reported continuation rates of 75% for the levonorgestrel-releasing intrauterine system and 78% for the copper T380A 1 year after insertion [29]. As few American women use an IUD, it is perhaps not surprising that only 16% of reproductive age women hold a favorable attitude toward the method [30]. Intrauterine contraceptive device users, however, report higher overall satisfaction than users of other methods. Overall, 99% of IUD users who continue with the method beyond 1 year report being "very satisfied" or "somewhat satisfied" with the method [30]. Thorough counseling about expected changes in bleeding patterns before IUD insertion correlates with satisfaction and continuation rates after 1 year of use [31].

NONCONTRACEPTIVE BENEFITS
Women who use IUDs enjoy a number of noncontraceptive benefits. The LNG-IUS offers many, but not all, of the health benefits seen in users of systemic hormonal contraception: reduction in menstrual blood flow, dysmenorrhea, anemia, and pelvic pain syndromes [32]. Compared with systemic delivery of pills, patches, injections, and rings, the unique local delivery system of the IUD often translates into fewer hormone-related side effects [33].

The marked endometrial suppression of the LNG-IUS results in a significant reduction in menstrual blood loss. This effect has made treatment of idiopathic menorrhagia the leading off-label indication for the LNG-IUS [32]. Evidence from well-designed, randomized controlled and observational studies supports this use as an effective, conservative treatment option for women with menorrhagia that preserves reproductive function and avoids surgical risks and costs [34•].

Emerging evidence also suggests that the LNG-IUS may provide benefit to women with symptomatic leiomyomata, adenomyosis [35], and endometriosis. The LNG-IUS reduces fibroid volume and possibly the development of new fibroids [36,37]. Women randomized to receive a LNG-IUS or gonadotropin-releasing hormone agonist after laparoscopic surgery for endometriosis reported similar benefit, even with Stage III/IV disease [38]. More research is needed to determine whether

Copper T380A and Levonorgestrel-releasing Intrauterine System Event Rates (Per 100 Women 1 Year After Insertion)

Device	Pregnancy*	Expulsion*	Continuation*	Ectopic Rate (During 5 Years of Use)†
Copper T380A	0.3	5.8	75	0.02
LNG-IUS	0.3	6.4	78	0.02

*Data from Sivin et al. [29].
†Data from Sivin [60] and Franks et al. [61].

Figure 16-3. Copper T380A and levonorgestrel-releasing intrauterine system (LNG-IUS) event rates per 100 women 1 year after insertion.

the LNG-IUS actually provides clinically significant protection against the development or worsening of endometriosis.

Emerging evidence also supports a role for the LNG-IUS as endometrial protection during hormone replacement therapy [39,40] and tamoxifen therapy [41] and as treatment for endometrial hyperplasia [42]. A reduction in the risk of endometrial cancer also has been reported in users of inert and copper IUDs [43].

Although these results are encouraging, it must be stressed that treatment of abnormal bleeding currently represents an off-label indication for the LNG-IUS. A clinical trial designed to alter product labeling for this indication is currently enrolling subjects and is expected to yield data by 2009. It is important to keep in mind that the LNG-IUS is not a panacea; undiagnosed genital bleeding remains a contraindication to the use of an IUD.

Return to Fertility

The contraceptive actions of the IUDs reverse soon after removal of the device, and 1-year fertility rates are similar to women who had not been using any form of birth control [44,45]. No delay in conception is seen in former IUD users regardless of duration of use or parity [27••].

Patient Selection

World Health Organization guidelines report few contraindications to IUD use, and suggest most women can safely use an IUD (Figures 16-4 and 16-5) [46•]. Ideal candidates are women in monogamous relationships and at low risk for STIs. Young women are statistically at greater risk of acquiring STIs

because of lifestyle and sexual behavior. Anyone at high risk for STIs should be tested before IUD insertion. Anyone not in a mutually monogamous relationship should utilize condoms for STI prevention in addition to the IUD for contraception.

A history of PID in a woman with no current risk factors for STIs is not a contraindication to IUD use. It is important to point out, however, that a prior episode of PID is associated with a 15% incidence of infertility [47]. Future difficulty with pregnancy should not be attributed to the device. IUD insertion should be postponed for at least 3 months after an episode of PID or cervicitis, and negative cervical screening tests for gonorrhea and chlamydia should be obtained.

Although nulliparity was removed as a contraindication from the US Food and Drug Administration labeling of the copper T380A in 2005, this language persists in the LNG-IUS package insert. However, most experts agree that nulliparity is not a contraindication to use of either device. Nulliparous women may have higher rates of expulsion, bleeding, and pain, probably related to uterine size. Small uterine size and a tight cervical canal may also make insertion more difficult. Still, the advantages of IUD use may make it an appropriate choice for many nulliparous women.

Undiagnosed genital bleeding should be fully worked up before IUD insertion. Anatomic features that distort the uterine cavity, such as leiomyomata or mullerian anomalies, can increase expulsion or bleeding. As copper IUDs may increase bleeding, women with a history of heavy menses or dysmenorrhea should consider the use of the LNG-IUS.

Little is known about the use of IUDs in women who have illnesses that result in a serious immunocompromised state. Therefore these women should be carefully monitored for infection if they choose to use an IUD. The risk of pregnancy should be weighed against the theoretical risk of infection. It is a WHO level 3 recommendation (risk generally outweighs benefits) to insert an IUD in a patient with untreated AIDS [46•].

However, data indicate that the IUD can safely be used in HIV-infected women who have access to medical care. IUD use is a WHO level 2 recommendation (benefit generally outweighs risks) for those at high risk for HIV and for HIV-infected or AIDS patients clinically stable on antiretroviral therapy [46•]. IUD use provides the same general benefits as for immunocompetent women and does not appear to have any drug interactions with antiretroviral therapies. In addition, IUD use in treated HIV patients does not appear to result in an

Contraindications to Intrauterine Contraceptive Device Use

Known or suspected pregnancy

Mucopurulent cervicitis, acute PID, or recent PID (within 3 months)

Abnormalities of the uterus resulting in distortion of the uterine cavity

Uterine cavity sounding < 6 cm or > 10 cm

Known or suspected uterine or cervical malignancy

Unexplained genital bleeding

Postpartum or postabortal endometritis in the past 3 months

Genital actinomycosis

Wilson disease (copper T380A only)

Allergy or hypersensitivity to any component of either IUD

Previously inserted IUD that has not been removed

Figure 16-4. Contraindications to intrauterine contraceptive device (IUD) use. PID—pelvic inflammatory disease.

Selecting an Intrauterine Contraceptive Device

	Copper T380A	LNG-IUS
Menstrual bleeding	Increase	Decrease
Duration of pregnancy	10 years	5 years
Ectopic pregnancy	Decreases risk	Decreases risk

Figure 16-5. Selecting an intrauterine contraceptive device. LNG-IUS— levonorgestrel-releasing intrauterine system.

increased risk in overall complications or infections beyond the insertion interval [48].

Women with diabetes also may safely use an IUD [12]. No increased risk of infection or other complications has been observed. The IUD provides an attractive alternative to systemic hormonal methods, particularly in diabetics with vascular disease, smokers, and women with a history of deep vein clots.

WORK-UP BEFORE INSERTION

A thorough history should identify candidates at high risk for infection or failure of the device. Counseling should include expected changes in bleeding patterns, warning signs of pelvic infection, and other potential problems (Figure 16-6). Although many clinics recommend routine screening for gonorrhea and chlamydia prior to insertion, selective screening of high-risk populations may be preferable. In the absence of obvious infection, antibiotic prophylaxis for bacterial endocarditis is not required during routine IUD insertion or removal [49].

Physical examination should be performed to rule out structural abnormalities or unusual tenderness, and confirm uterine position. Uterine perforation occurs most frequently with an extremely retroverted uterus. Sound the uterine cavity before insertion; ideally, the cavity should range from 6 to 9 cm [12]. Carefully inspect the vagina and cervix for signs of lower genital tract infection. Insertion should not be performed in the presence of mucopurulent cervical discharge or bacterial vaginosis. The presence of a distinct erythema arising from the columnar epithelium of the endocervix (cervical ectropion) or easy bleeding is not necessarily indicative of infection.

INSERTION

In nonpregnant women, IUDs can be inserted during any phase of the menstrual cycle [50]. To avoid an undiagnosed pregnancy, menstrual insertion has traditionally been recommended. Although modern urine human chorionic gonadotropin tests are sensitive enough to detect pregnancy at around the time of the expected menses, a negative test does not exclude an early pregnancy in the late luteal phase. To reduce the risk of luteal phase pregnancy and maximize flexibility in scheduling, it is recommended that insertion of a LNG-IUS occur within 7 days of the onset of menses in women not currently using contraception. Insertion of T-shaped copper IUD during the middle of the menstrual cycle has been shown to be preferable to insertion during

menses. A Centers for Disease Control review of more than 9000 copper T-200 IUD insertions showed that insertion from day 12 to 17 of the menstrual cycle (midcycle) results in higher IUD continuation with fewer removals for expulsion, pain, bleeding, or unintended pregnancy during the first 2 months after IUD insertion [51]. Current users of a hormonal contraceptive method may have an IUD inserted at any time in the cycle.

Immediate insertion after vaginal delivery, cesarean section, or abortion is uncommon in the United States and should not be attempted without special training. Postpartum insertion may be performed any time after 4 weeks. Insertion can be done at any time after a first trimester abortion, but should be delayed until after full uterine involution after a second trimester procedure unless a provider has special training.

As the primary risk of infection appears related to contamination of the uterus during insertion, scrupulous attention to sterile technique and preparation of the cervix and endocervical canal with either chlorhexadine or povidine-iodine must be performed in all patients.

Most patients require no premedication for IUD insertion. Although the administration of a nonsteroidal anti-inflammatory drug such as ibuprofen 600 to 800 mg, 30 to 60 minutes before the procedure is common, a recent well-designed randomized controlled trial found no benefit [52]. Paracervical block may improve comfort, particularly with a closed cervix in a young, nulliparous women. Recognizing that the paracervical block provides no uterine anesthesia, the discomfort of the block may outweigh the benefits, especially in parous women. For this reason, we discourage the routine use of paracervical block. Some women will react to cervical dilation with a vasovagal response. Paracervical block should be used in patients with a history of a vasovagal reaction to cervical manipulation. There is no evidence that the routine use of misprostol is of any benefit.

Health care providers should not attempt to insert an IUD unless they feel extremely comfortable negotiating the cervical canal and sounding the uterus. One should first practice insertions into an inanimate model to gain the required mechanical skills. Clinicians should gain initial experience with patients only under direct supervision. The number of proctored procedures needed to reach proficiency will vary. Experience with other office gynecology procedures such as endometrial biopsy, abortion, and hysteroscopy will decrease the number of supervised IUD insertions needed before a satisfactory level of comfort is reached.

Patient Counseling Before Intrauterine Contraceptive Device Insertion

Contraceptive benefit begins immediately with insertion

Insertion results in temporary, slight increased risk of pelvic infection

Copper devices cause longer, heavier periods

Levonorgestrel-releasing devices cause hypomenorrhea or amenorrhea

The overall risk of ectopic pregnancy is decreased, but when pregnancy occurs, an ectopic must be ruled out

Condoms should always be used if risk of sexually transmitted infections is present

A self examination should be performed monthly to check the IUD strings

Figure 16-6. Patient counseling before intrauterine contraceptive device (IUD) insertion.

The package inserts provides detailed information about insertion. Before insertion, the arms of the copper T380A must be manually folded and tucked into the end of the insertion tube. Preparation is complete with insertion of a solid obturator rod into the bottom of the insertion tube until it comes into contact with the base of the IUD. The LNG-IUS has a system that draws the arms into the insertion tube by pulling on the strings. Meticulous sterile technique must accompany preparation of the device. Thereafter, a no-touch technique should be adopted to ensure that the device remains sterile.

The cervix is prepped and numbing medicine applied to the anterior lip of the cervix. The anterior lip is then grasped with a tenaculum to straighten the cervical canal. With a retroverted uterus, grasping the posterior lip may facilitate this step. Sound the uterine cavity to determine the correct depth for insertion. The copper T380A and LNG-IUS have a small movable guide (flange) to mark correct depth along the insertion tube. While applying firm downward traction on the tenaculum to straighten the canal, pass the insertion tube into the uterine cavity. Take care to position the device so that the arms will lie in the horizontal plan of the uterus with the tips pointing into the cornual regions of the cavity when released.

For the copper T380A, the insertion tube is inserted until the flange contacts the external os of the cervix. At this point, the clinician holds the solid obturator rod to stabilize the IUD while the insertion tube is slowly withdrawn approximately 1 cm. This allows the arms of the T-frame to swing into place. After release of the arms, gently push the insertion tube 1 cm back toward the fundus without moving the obturator. This helps to secure a high fundal placement for the device. Remove the insertion tube and obturator together to expose the IUD's tail.

In contrast, the insertion tube of the LNG-IUS is positioned until the flange is about 1.5 to 2 cm from the external os. At this point, the arms of the device are released from the insertion tube by pulling the slider back to a marked position on the insertion tube. After a slight delay to allow expansion of the arms, the inserter tube is gently pushed into the uterine cavity until the previously set flange guide touches the cervix. The IUD should now be at the fundal position and can be released by pulling the slider down all the way. Confirm that the threads are released (this should occur automatically) and withdraw the insertion tube.

With either device, trim the strings to a length of approximately 3 cm and provide a piece of the string to your patient. This will help her to know what to feel for on her self-examination. Err on the side of extra tail length as the strings may always be trimmed later if they are too long. Long strings usually curl around the cervix into the fornices. Short strings tend to stick out from the os along the long axis of the cervix and may result in dyspareunia for the male partner. Request that your patient follow-up after her next period. This timing allows for identification of expulsion and infection and provides an opportunity to provide additional counseling regarding changes in bleeding or other concerns that may result in premature removal of the device.

Severe pain during insertion may indicate a uterine perforation. Perforation should be suspected if the depth of the sound or insertion tube exceeds that expected based on bimanual examination. Do not insert the device if you feel you may have

perforated. Suspected perforation does not usually require hospitalization, and pain generally resolves promptly. The patient should be counseled regarding the warning signs of peritonitis and provided with instructions to access 24-hour emergency care for progressive symptoms. Alternative contraception should be provided. Most uterine injuries will heal within 4 to 6 weeks.

Problems

BLEEDING

Bleeding changes represent the largest category of concerns of intrauterine contraceptive device (IUD) users. Copper devices often cause increased menstrual bleeding and intermenstrual spotting in the first 3 to 6 months of use that usually decreases over time. Cumulative discontinuation rates for these reasons are 3.6%, 6.1%, and 7.5% at 1, 2, and 3 years, respectively [23]. Remove the device if the patient develops anemia unresponsive to iron therapy. Levonorgestrel-releasing devices frequently cause amenorrhea, usually preceded by progressive hypomenorrhea or irregular spotting during the first year. Rule out pregnancy if amenorrhea occurs at any time in a copper IUD user. Adequate counseling helps women understand and accept the changes in their bleeding pattern, increases satisfaction, and decreases discontinuation for this side effect.

PAIN

Mild cramping and pain are common during insertion and for several days after. Menstrual pain may also increase. These symptoms generally respond to nonsteroidal anti-inflammatory drugs. More intense cramping or pain may indicate partial or complete expulsion. Low-level cramping not associated with menses sometimes persists after insertion. If the uterus is tender on bimanual examination, presumptive treatment for endometritis should be considered and testing for sexually transmitted infections and bacterial vaginosis should be performed.

EXPULSION

Expulsion of an IUD is generally associated with bleeding and cramping, but can occur asymptomatically. Risk factors for expulsion of the copper T380A include young age, heavy menstrual flow, and severe dysmenorrhea before the IUD insertion [53]. Approximately 5% to 6.5% of IUD users will expel the device during the first year of use [29,54]. If expulsion is suspected, the patient should be counseled to use a backup method of contraception and be seen as soon as possible.

Signs of partial expulsion vary from subtle lengthening of the IUD's tail strings to frank visualization of the plastic frame at the external os. If partial expulsion is suspected, the device should be removed. After ruling out pregnancy and infection, patients requesting continuation of the method may have a new device placed.

Complete expulsion may occur asymptomatically or after a prolonged episode of pain or bleeding. Patients should check for the presence of the IUD string after each menses. Missing strings may indicate expulsion, pregnancy, or perforation. Ultrasound and abdominal radiographs can verify the absence of the device. Patients who have expelled an IUD and wish to continue with the method may have a new device inserted.

STRING PROBLEMS

The work-up of missing or shortening strings should include a bimanual exam and pregnancy test. Explore the cervix with a Papanicolaou smear cytobrush to retrieve strings in the canal. Enlargement of the uterus may cause the strings to withdraw. Ultrasound can confirm correct, intrauterine positioning of the device. If ultrasound fails to locate the device, abdominal and pelvic radiographs should be performed to exclude the possibility of uterine perforation and intra-abdominal location of the IUD. Exploration of the uterine cavity with a small forceps or Novak curette to retrieve missing strings should only be attempted if one is comfortable with intrauterine procedures (*see* Removal section).

Short strings may project from the cervical os and create a hazard for male partners. Options include trimming the strings further (accepting the risk that they may become lost) or removing and replacing the device, leaving the strings longer.

PERFORATION

Uterine perforation generally occurs during insertion, but may not be detected until some time later. The risk of perforation is inversely proportional to the experience of the clinician. Overall, perforation occurs in about one in 1000 insertions [55]. Insertion during lactation may increase the risk [27••]. Most patients experience only transient pain with a perforation; the discovery awaits a subsequent examination for missing strings or evaluation for pregnancy. This underscores the importance of a follow-up examination after the first menses.

Most clinicians in the United States will recommend removal of an intra-abdominal IUD. Copper devices seem to stimulate adhesion formation within the abdominal cavity rather quickly. Serious complications rarely occur; however. peritonitis, intestinal perforations, and erosion of adjacent viscera have been reported [17]. Refer patients with an intra-abdominal IUD to a gynecologic surgeon comfortable with operative laparoscopic procedures. If the patient wishes to continue the method, and the perforation site has healed, a new IUD can be placed under direct laparoscopic visualization at the time of removal. Laparoscopic removal can safely be attempted during the first trimester in pregnant, asymptomatic women with intra-abdominal IUDs who desire to continue the pregnancy. Thereafter, the risks of surgical intervention probably outweigh potential benefits.

INFECTION

As discussed earlier, our understanding of the relationship between IUD use and infection has changed considerably since the Dalkon Shield era. The majority of infections occur within the first 20 days of use and is related to insertion. IUD acceptors, like all women, should always use condoms with a new partner or in other situations where the risk of sexually transmitted infection is present.

Usually, insertion-related infections result in a simple endometritis, with uterine tenderness as the sole physical finding. This can be managed without removal of the IUD. Asymptomatic cervical colonization with gonorrhea or chlamydia should be managed in the same way. Remove the IUD promptly if physical findings suggest pelvic inflammatory disease and institute one of the Centers for Disease Control and Prevention recommended treatment protocols (Figure 16-7).

Treatment of Infection in Intrauterine Contraceptive Device Users

Infection	Symptoms/Signs	Treatment
Asymptomatic cervicitis	Cervical cultures show gonorrhea or chlamydia; partner with gonorrhea or chlamydia; abnormal vaginal discharge or spotting, mucopurulent cervicitis, with complete absence of pelvic findings	For gonorrhea: ceftriaxone 125 mg IM × 1; ciprofloxacin 500 mg PO × 1; cefixime 400 mg PO × 1. For chlamydia: doxycycline 100 mg PO bid for 7 days; azithromycin 1 g PO × 1. Counsel regarding risk factors, condom use, and alternative methods
Endometritis	Uterine tenderness without peritoneal signs or adnexal tenderness	Obtain cultures for gonorrhea and chlamydia; doxycycline 100 mg bid for 14 days
PID	Pelvic pain, fever, nausea, abnormal bleeding; peritoneal signs (abdominal rebound tenderness, cervical motion tenderness); adnexal tenderness or mass elevation in WBC	Institute CDC recommended treatment of PID; remove IUD after loading dose of antibiotics
Actinomyces species infection	Asymptomatic; found on Papanicolaou smear	No need for treatment; consider repeat Papanicolaou in 6 weeks
	With uterine tenderness	Remove device; oral antibiotics
	With pelvic mass and fever	Remove device; IV antibiotics; consult

Figure 16-7. Treatment of infection in intrauterine contraceptive device (IUD) users. bid—twice daily; CDC—Centers for Disease Control and Prevention; IM—intramuscular; IV—intravenous; PID—pelvic inflammatory disease; PO—by mouth; WBC—white blood cells.

Actinomyces, a common gram-positive rod that may normally be present in the vagina, becomes an issue when its presence is reported on Papanicolaou smears. Asymptomatic patients do not need to be treated with antibiotics and can be observed without removing the IUD. Removal of the device generally results in clearing of the Papanicolaou smear findings; however, colonization does not predict development of PID or pelvic abscess [56]. If physical findings or symptoms suggest PID, the IUD should be removed and antibiotics should be given.

Vaginitis may occur in women wearing IUDs. Institute standard treatments for yeast and bacterial vaginosis without removing the device. Wet mount examinations of vaginal flora from women wearing IUDs frequently show increased numbers of inflammatory cells, a result of the sterile inflammatory response invoked by the IUD. Do not misinterpret this finding as a problem. The presence of inflammation alone, without an elevation of vaginal pH and clue cells, does not support a diagnosis of bacterial vaginosis. Rule out cervicitis by careful inspection of the cervical mucous and cervical cultures.

Pregnancy

Women with IUDs should be counseled to present immediately if pregnancy is suspected. The initial evaluation must take into account the possibilities of IUD expulsion or perforation as reasons for failure. Ectopic pregnancy must be ruled out by ultrasound or serial measurements of hCG. In the event of an intrauterine pregnancy with an IUD in place, the risk of com-

plications, including spontaneous abortion, septic abortion, and preterm delivery is increased [50]. On diagnosis of pregnancy, if the strings are visible, the IUD should be removed immediately. Although the device may be expelled spontaneously without affecting the pregnancy, waiting may result in a missed opportunity as the enlarging uterus will eventually draw in the strings. The risk of spontaneous abortion decreases from about 50% to 30% with removal of the device. In addition, the risk of preterm delivery increases by a factor of four when the IUD remains in place [57]. Human data about risk of birth defects from copper or intrauterine levonorgestrel exposure are limited. However, studies have not detected a pattern of abnormalities [17]. The patient should be referred to an obstetrician/gynecologist if the strings cannot be seen. Frequently, the device can be retrieved atraumatically using either ultrasound guidance or CO_2 hysteroscopy.

If the patient has signs of pelvic infection or uterine tenderness, antibiotics should be started prior to removal of the device. We recommend inpatient management with appropriate consultation of all pregnant women with pelvic infections. Septic abortion is a serious, life-threatening condition.

Removal

To remove an IUD, simply grasp the tail strings with a Bozeman (uterine packing) or ring forceps. The long, tapered narrow jaws of the Bozeman provide improved visualization and facilitate exploration of the cervical canal should this become necessary. Gentle downward traction on the string will collapse

Situations In Which Consultation or Referral Is Indicated

Infections
  PID
  Pelvic abscess
Pregnancy
  Unable to remove device (strings not visible)
  Continuing pregnancy with device in situ
  Suspected ectopic pregnancy
  Septic abortion
Insertion
  Difficult insertion
  Suspected perforation
Difficult removal
Missing strings
Lost device
  Embedded device
  Need for intrauterine manipulation
  Intra-abdominal device

Figure 16-8. Situations in which consultation or referral is indicated. PID—pelvic inflammatory disease.

the IUD frame and allow it to pass through the cervix. Most patients experience only momentary, mild cramping. Patients who report severe menstrual discomfort may benefit from taking ibuprofen or another nonsteroidal anti-inflammatory drug, 30 minutes before removal. If your patient gives a history of a vasovagal incident with insertion or other gynecologic procedures, consider a paracervical block. Prophylaxis for endocarditis is not warranted for routine IUD removal.

However, it should be considered in the setting of pelvic infection, as bacteremia is theoretically possible [49].

If the strings cannot be seen, exploration of the cervical canal with a Papanicolaou smear cytobrush will often bring them out. Consider reasons for missing strings (pregnancy, expulsion, perforation). Before exploring the uterine cavity, document an intrauterine location of the device with a transvaginal ultrasound. Due to the high risk of perforation, do not

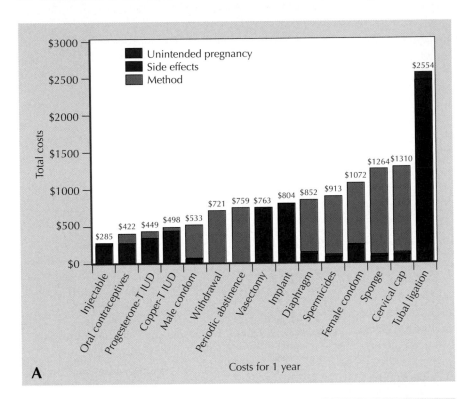

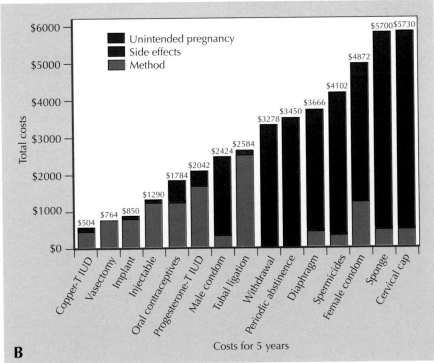

Figure 16-9. One- (**A**) and 5-year (**B**) costs associated with contraceptive methods in a managed payment model. (*Adapted from* Trussell *et al.* [59].)

attempt to explore the cavity unless you are extremely comfortable with this procedure. A narrow, curved flexible plastic cannula, of the type used for suction endometrial biopsies, can be a useful tool to explore the cavity and hook the device. Prior to more vigorous exploration with a Bozeman forceps or Novak curette, a paracervical block should be placed. Real-time abdominal ultrasound can improve safety and guide instruments toward the IUD for removal. Hysteroscopy under general anesthesia may be necessary if the device is embedded or if the cavity is distorted.

As fertility returns to normal rapidly after removal, contraceptive counseling should precede discontinuation of the method. Women who desire to continue with the method may have a new device inserted at the same visit.

When to Refer

The IUD is a safe, effective method of contraception that is currently underutilized. The skills necessary to provide this method are well within the scope of primary care physicians. Situations where consultation with an obstetrician/gynecologist would be desirable include difficulties with insertion or removal, serious infections, pregnancy, and uterine perforation (see Figure 16-8).

Cost Issues

Insurance coverage continues to hinder access to all contraceptives, including IUDs. From a managed care perspective, the IUD should be one of the first methods on the formularies for full coverage, because it is the most cost-effective of all reversible methods [58]. Compared with oral contraception, the cost savings begin to accumulate during the second year of IUD use [59]. Five-year costs associated with the copper T380A are the lowest of any method (Figure 16-9). Savings intensify when copper T380A is used for its full 10-year effective life.

References

Papers of particular interest have been highlighted as follows:
• Of interest
•• Of outstanding interest

1. Mosher WD, Martinez GM, Chandra A, et al.: Use of contraception and use of family planning services in the United States: 1982–2002. Advance data from vital and health statistics. No 350. Hyattsville: National Center for Health Statistics, 2004.

2. Spinelli A, Talamanca IF, Lauria L: Patterns of contraceptive use in 5 European countries. Am J Public Health 2000, 90:1403–1408.

3. Frank E: Contraceptive use by female physicians in the United States. Obstet Gynecol 1999, 94:666–671.

4.•• Speroff L, Darney PD: Intrauterine contraception (the IUD). In A Clinical Guide for Contraception, edn 4. Philadelphia: Lippincott, Williams, & Wilkins; 2005:221–257.
This excellent review of the history of IUDs provides a chart of different IUDs that are available around the world. Extensive references are included.

5. Layde PM: Pelvic inflammatory disease and the Dalkon Shield (editorial). JAMA 1983, 250:796–777.

6. Lee NC, Rubin GL, Ory HW, Burkman RT: Type of intrauterine device and pelvic inflammatory disease revisited: new results from the Women's Health Study. Obstet Gynecol 1988, 72:1–6.

7. Gareen IF, Greenland S, Morgenstern H: Intrauterine devices and pelvic inflammatory disease: meta-analyses of published studies, 1974–1990. Epidemiology 2000, 11:589–597.

8. Farley TM, Rosenberg MJ, Rowe PJ, et al.: Intrauterine devices and pelvic inflammatory disease: an international perspective. Lancet 1992, 339:785–788.

9. Tatum HJ, Schmidt FH, Phillips DM, et al.: The Dalkon Shield controversy: Structural and bacterial studies of IUD tails. JAMA 1975, 231:711–717.

10. Grimes DA: Intrauterine devices and pelvic inflammatory disease: recent developments. Contraception 1987, 36:97–109.

11. Mosher WD, Pratt WF: Use of contraception and family planning services in the United States, 1988. Am J Pub Health 1990, 9:1132–1133.

12. Speroff L, Darney PD: Intrauterine contraception (the IUD). In A Clinical Guide for Contraception, edn 4. Philadelphia: Lippincott, Williams, & Wilkins; 2005:221–527.

13. Mumford SD, Kessel E: Was the Dalkon Shield a safe and effective intrauterine device? The conflict between case-control and clinical trial study findings. Fertil Steril 1992, 57:1151–1176.

14. Grimes DA, Schulz KF: Prophylactic antibiotics for intrauterine device insertion: a meta-analysis of the randomized controlled trials. Contraception 1999, 60:57–63.

15.•• Hubacher D, Lara–Ricalde R, Taylor DJ, et al.: Use of copper intrauterine devices and the risk of tubal infertility among nulligravid women. N Engl J Med 2001, 345:561–567.
Landmark case control study evaluating tubal infertility and past IUD use.

16. McCarthy T, Chew SC, Lim SM, et al.: A prospective randomized comparative trial of the Gravigard, Latex Leaf, Dalkon Shield, and Multiload Cu250 IUDs. Aust N Z J Obstet Gynaecol 1986, 26:228–232.

17. Mirena package insert. Montville, MJ: Berlex Inc; 2006.

18. Sivin I: IUDs are contraceptives, not abortifacient: A comment on research and belief. Stud Fam Plan 1989;20:355–359.

19.•• Ortiz ME, Croxatto HB, Bardin CW. Mechanism of action of intrauterine devices. Obstet Gynecol Survey 1996, 51:S42–S53.
An outstanding review of the literature regarding the mechanism of action of IUDs.

20. Holland MK, White IG: Heavy metals and human spermatozoa. II. The toxicity of copper ions for spermatozoa. Contraception 1988, 38:685–695.

21. Barbosa I, Bakos O, Olsson S–E, et al.: Ovarian function during use of a levornorgestrel-releasing IUD. Contraception 1990, 42:51–66.

22. Munuce MJ, Nascimento JAA, Rosano G, *et al.*: Doses of levonorgestrel comparable to that delivered by the levonorgestrel-releasing intrauterine system can modify the in vitro expression of zona binding sites of human spermatozoa. *Contraception* 2006, 73:97–101.

23. Trussel J: Contraceptive failure in the United States. *Contraception* 2004, 70:89–96.

24. Sivin I, El–Mahgoub S, McCarthy T, *et al.*: Long-term contraception with the levonorgestrel 20 mcg/day (LNg 20) and the Copper T 380Ag intrauterine devices: a five-year randomized study. *Contraception* 1990, 42:361–78.

25. Andersson K, Odlind V, Rybo G: Levonorgestrel-releasing and copper-releasing (Nova T) IUDs during five years of use: a randomized comparative trial. *Contraception* 1994, 49:56–72.

26. Marchbanks PA, Annegers JE, Coulam CB, *et al.*: Risk factors for ectopic pregnancy. A population based study. *JAMA* 1988, 259:1823–1827.

27.•• Grimes DA: Intrauterine devices (IUDs). In *Contraceptive Technology*. 18th ed. New York: Ardent Media, Inc.; 2004:495–530.
An outstanding overview of IUDs with thorough review of the literature.

28. Haspels AA: Emergency contraception: a review. *Contraception* 1994, 50:101–108.

29. Sivin I, Alvarez F, Diaz J, *et al.*: Intrauterine contraception with copper and with levonorgestrel: a randomized study of the Tcu 380Ag and levonorgestrel 20 mcg/day devices. *Contraception* 1984, 30:443–456.

30. Forrest JD: US women's perceptions of and attitudes about the IUD. *Obstet Gynecol Survey* 1996, 51:S30–S34.

31. Costales A, Jensen J, Nelson A, *et al.*: A U.S. multicenter, open-label trial with the levonorgestrel-releasing intrauterine system (LNG_IUS): clinical and device-related experience. *Contraception* 2006, 74:178.

32. Jensen JT: Noncontraceptive applications of the levonorgestrel intrauterine system. *Curr Womens Health Rep* 2002, 2:417–422.

33. Andersson K, Odlind V, Rybo G: Levonorgestrel-releasing and copper-releasing (Nova T) IUDs during five years of use: a randomized comparative trial. *Contraception* 1994, 49:56–72.

34.• Hurskainen R, Teperi J, Rissanen P, *et al.*: Clinical outcomes and costs with the levonorgestrel-releasing intrauterine system or hysterectomy for treatment of menorrhagia: randomized trial 5-year follow-up. *JAMA* 2004, 291:1456–1463.

35. Maia H, Jr., Maltez A, Coelho G, *et al.*: Insertion of Mirena after endometrial resection in patients with adenomyosis. *J Am Assoc Gynecol Laparosc* 2003, 10:512–516.

36. Sivin I, Stern J: Health during prolonged use of levonorgestrel 20 micrograms/d and the Copper Tcu 380Ag intrauterine contraceptive devices: a multicenter study. International Committee for Contraception Research (ICCR). *Fertil Steril* 1994, 61:70–77.

37. Grigorieva V, Chen-Mok M, Tarasova M, Mikhailov A: Use of a levonorgestrel-releasing intrauterine system to treat bleeding related to uterine leiomyomas. *Fertil Steril* 2003, 79:1194–1198.

38. Petta CA, Ferriani RA, Abrao MS, *et al.*: Randomized clinical trial of a levonorgestrel–releasing intrauterine system and a depot GnRH analogue for the treatment of chronic pelvic pain in women with endometriosis. *Hum Reprod* 2005, 20:1993–1998.

39. Varila E, Wahlstrom T, Rauramo I: A 5-year follow-up study on the use of a levonorgestrel intrauterine system in women receiving hormone replacement therapy. *Fertil Steril* 2001, 76:969–973.

40. Suvanto-Luukkonen E, Kauppila A: The levonorgestrel intrauterine system in menopausal hormone replacement therapy: five-year experience. *Fertil Steril* 1999, 72:161–163.

41. Gardner FJ, Konje JC, Abrams KR, *et al.*: Endometrial protection from tamoxifen-stimulated changes by a levonorgestrel-releasing intrauterine system: a randomized controlled trial. *Lancet* 2000, 356:1711–1717.

42. Bahamondes L, Ribeiro-Huguet P, de Andrade KC, *et al.*: Levonorgestrel-releasing intrauterine system as a therapy for endometrial hyperplasia and carcinoma. *Acta Obstet Gynecol Scand* 2003, 82:580–582.

43. Hill DA, Weiss NS, Voigt LF, Beresford SA: Endometrial cancer in relationship to intrauterine device use. *Inter J of Cancer* 1997, 70:278–281.

44. Belhadj H, Sivin I, Diaz S, *et al.*: Recovery of fertility after use of the levonorgestrel 20 mcg/d or copper T 380Ag intrauterine device. *Contraception* 1986, 34:261–267.

45. Sivin I, Stern J, Diaz S, *et al.*: Rates and outcomes of planned pregnancy after use of Norplant capsules, Norplant II rods, or levonorgestrel-releasing or copper Tcu 380Ag intrauterine contraceptive devices. *Am J Obstet Gynecol* 1992, 166:1208–1213.

46.• World Health Organization. Intrauterine devices. In *Medical Eligibility Criteria for Contraceptive Use*, 4th ed. Geneva, Switzerland: World Health Organization; 2004.

47. Weström L: Incidence, prevalence, and trends of acute pelvic inflammatory disease and its consequences in industrialized countries. *Am J Obstet Gynecol* 1980, 138:880–892.

48. Morrision CS, *et al.*: Is the intrauterine device appropriate contraception for HIV-infected women? *BJOG* 2001, 784–790.

49. Dajani AS, Taubert KA, Wilson W, *et al.*: Prevention of bacterial endocarditis. Recommendations by the American Heart Association. *Circulation* 1997, 96:358–366.

50. Trieman K, Liskin L, Kols A, *et al.*: IUDs: an update. In *Pop Rep Series B, No. 6*. Baltimore: Johns Hopkins School of Public Health Population Information Program; 1995.

51. White MK, Ory HW, Rooks JB, *et al.*: Intrauterine device termination rates and the menstrual cycle day of insertion. *Obstet Gynecol* 1980, 55:220–224.

52. Hubacher D, Reyes V, Lillo S, *et al.*: Pain from copper intrauterine device insertion: randomized trial of prophylactic ibuprofen. *Contraception* 2006, 74:181.

53. Zhang J, Chi I–C, Feldblum PJ, Farr MG: Risk factors for copper T expulsion: an epidemiologic analysis. *Contraception* 1992, 46:427–433.

54. Indian Council of Medical Research, Task Force on IUD: Randomized clinical trial with intrauterine devices (levonorgestrel intrauterine device (LNG), CUT 380Ag, CuT 220C and CuT 200B): a 36-month study. *Contraception* 1989, 49:186–188.

55. World Health Organization: Mechanism of action, safety and efficacy of intrauterine devices: technical report series 753. Geneva: World Health Organization; 1987.

56. Lippes J: Pelvic actinomycosis: a review and preliminary look at prevalence. *Am J Obstet Gynecol* 1999, 180:265–269.

57. Chaim W, Mazor M: Pregnancy with an intrauterine device in situ and preterm delivery. *Arch Gynecol Obstet* 1992, 252:21–24.

58. Chiou CF, Trussell J, Reyes E, *et al.*: Economic analysis of contraceptives for women. Contraception 2003;68:3–10.

59. Trussell J, Leveque JA, Koenig JD, *et al.*: The economic value of contraception: a comparison of 15 methods. *Am J Public Health* 1995, 85:494–503.

60. Sivin I: Dose- and age-dependent ectopic pregnancy risks with intrauterine contraception. *Obstet Gynecol* 1991, 78:291–298.

61. Franks AL, Beral V, Cates W, Jr., Hogue CJ: Contraception and ectopic pregnancy risk. *Am J Obstet Gynecol* 1990, 163:1120–1123.

17 | Vaginitis

Lynda Gioia-Flynt

- The vaginal ecosystem is maintained by lactobacilli producing H_2O_2 to keep the pH below 4.5.
- Bacterial vaginosis is an alteration in the normal vaginal flora that is associated with preterm delivery in high-risk women.
- Yeast vaginitis symptoms occur less frequently than does colonization by *Candida* species.
- Systemic metronidazole is necessary for the treatment of trichomoniasis. Topical agents do not deliver adequate dosages.
- Most cases of pediatric vaginitis are thought to be noninfectious in origin.
- There has been no proven benefit for routine screening of vaginitis in low risk, asymptomatic pregnant women to reduce adverse pregnancy outcomes.
- Atrophic vaginitis occurs in postmenopausal women and can cause discharge, irritation, and bleeding.

There is a fine balance between microorganisms that maintain the vaginal ecosystem. When there is a disruption of balance in the vaginal ecosystem, women may experience vulvovaginal symptoms. Although the term *vaginitis* is commonly used as a diagnosis, it is not one specific entity. There are spectrums of diseases that cause vulvovaginal symptoms throughout a woman's lifetime.

Hormonal influences impact the vaginal ecosystem extensively. Estrogen exposure affects the vaginal epithelium, making prepubertal, reproductive age and postmenopausal vaginitis distinct entities with differing, common etiologies. In the prepubertal and postmenopausal age groups, the lack of estrogen causes a thinning of the epithelium and an elevation of the vaginal pH to greater than 4.7. During the reproductive years, lactobacilli are the predominant organism colonized on the vaginal epithelium due to estrogen's effect on increasing the glycogen content in the epithelial cells. The lactobacilli maintain an acidic environment, pH less than 4.5, by the production of hydrogen peroxide (H_2O_2). In this environment, small quantities of yeast and even anaerobes may be asymptomatic. The disruption of the normal vaginal ecosystem can produce symptomatic vulvovaginitis, resulting in one of the most common causes of office visits to gynecologists and accounting for more than 10 million office visits per year [1•].

This chapter discusses the perturbations of the vaginal ecosystem that result in symptomatic vulvovaginitis. Cervical and upper genital tract infections are discussed elsewhere.

Bacterial Vaginosis

Bacterial vaginosis (BV) is the most common cause of vaginitis, accounting for approximately 22% to 50% of vaginitis in reproductive age women. The normal H_2O_2-producing lactobacilli disappear and are replaced by larger numbers of anaerobic bacteria, including *Prevotella, Bacteroides, Mobiluncus, Mycoplasma,* and *Gardnerella* species.

The cause of this vaginal flora shift is not completely understood, but women with multiple sexual partners, those who douche, those who have IUDs for contraception, and those who lack H_2O_2-producing strains of lactobacilli are at increased risk. BV is associated with a higher incidence of preterm labor and delivery, postcesarean section endomyometritis, and postabortal sepsis [2•].

PRESENTATION
Patients often will present with the complaint of abnormal vaginal discharge, typically thin and milky to gray in color, and a fishy odor.

DIAGNOSIS

The diagnosis of bacterial vaginosis can be made clinically (Amsel criteria) or by using Gram stain (Nugent score). Amsel criteria requires three of the four following criteria to be present: 1) abnormal gray discharge, 2) pH of more than 4.5, 3) more than 20% of epithelial cells covered by bacteria (clue cells), 4) a fish-like amine odor when 10% potassium chloride is added to the vaginal discharge. Gram stain diagnosis requires scoring of three morphotypes of bacteria. Quantities of bacteria are measured from 0 to 4+. A score of zero is 4+ lactobacilli, 1+ is less than one morphotype per oil immersion field, 2+ is 1 to 4 morphotypes per field, 3+ is 5 to 30 morphotypes per field, and 4+ is more than 30 morphotypes per field. The morphotypes scored are gram-positive rods (*Lactobacillus* species), small gram-negative or gram-variable rods (*Gardnerella* or *Bacteroides*), and curved gram-negative to gram-variable rods (*Mobiluncus* species). The weighted scores of each bacterial type are summed, and a total score of 7 to 10 is diagnostic of bacterial vaginosis. The sensitivity and specificity of Amsel criteria as compared with Gram's stain are 92% and 77%, respectively [3].

A Papanicolaou test is not reliable to diagnose bacterial vaginosis. When compared with Gram stain, the sensitivity is 49% and the specificity is 93%. Symptomatic women should be seen and evaluated using Amsel criteria.

MANAGEMENT

Oral metronidazole, 500 mg taken twice daily for 7 days; topical clindamycin, 2% vaginal cream applied at bedtime for 7 nights; and topical metronidazole vaginal gel 0.75% applied once daily for 5 days are equally effective regimens.

Acceptable alternative regimens are oral clindamycin, 300 mg taken twice daily for 7 days or clindamycin ovules, 100 mg intravaginally for 3 nights. Treatment is recommended for all nonpregnant patients with and without symptoms. The pregnant population is discussed later in the chapter.

Vaginal Candidiasis

Thirteen million cases of vaginal candidiasis occur annually in the United States. Approximately 75% of women experience at least one episode of vulvovaginal candidiasis during their lifetime. In 85% to 90% of cases, the causative organism is *Candida albicans*.

Factors that favor development of this infection are conditions that predispose women to an overgrowth of yeast, including diabetes mellitus, pregnancy, immunosuppressive therapy, antibiotic usage, HIV infection, and tight-fitting undergarments.

PRESENTATION

Symptoms of vulvovaginal candidiasis include vulvar pruritis, burning, external dysuria, and increased thick, white discharge. Signs may include vulvar edema and erythema, fissures, vaginal erythema, and a thick, white, curdy discharge.

DIAGNOSIS

Accurate diagnosis can not be made on history and physical exam alone. Diagnosis requires microscopic examination of discharge with or without a 10% potassium chloride (KOH) preparation or a positive culture in a symptomatic woman. Microscopic findings include yeast, hyphae, or pseudohyphae. Yeast cultures are the gold standard for diagnosis; however, routine use may overdiagnose asymptomatic women who are colonized with yeast. Therefore, cultures are typically reserved for patients with signs and symptoms of vulvovaginal candidiasis and negative KOH preps or for those women with recurrent infections.

MANAGEMENT

Uncomplicated infections can be treated with multiple topical therapies including 1-, 3-, or 7-day treatments or a single, oral dose of fluconazole 150 mg. One-day vaginal preparations include 2% butoconazole-sustained release, 5 g; miconazole suppository, 1200 mg; or 6.5% tioconazole, 5 g. Three-day treatment regimens include 2% butoconazole, 5 g; clotrimazole, 100 mg or two vaginal tablets; miconazole suppository, 200 mg; 0.8% terconazole, 5 g; or terconazole suppository, 80 mg. Seven-day therapies include 1% clotrimazole, 5 g; clotrimazole vaginal tablet, 100 mg; 2% miconazole, 5 g; miconazole suppository, 100 mg; or 0.4% terconazole, 5 g. These therapies all produce cure rates of approximately 90%. Another acceptable treatment is a 14-day course of nystatin 100,000-U tablets, although the cure rate is slightly lower at approximately 80%.

Complicated vulvovaginal candidiasis cases include recurrent vulvovaginal candidiasis (defined as four or more episodes in a year), severe symptoms or findings, suspected or proven nonalbicans *Candida* species, and cases in women with severe medical illness, diabetes, immunosuppression, or pregnancy. More aggressive therapy may be required to achieve relief of symptoms in complicated cases. Vaginal cultures should be obtained from patients with recurrent vulvovaginal candidiasis to confirm the clinical diagnosis and to identify unusual species. *Candida glabrata* and other nonalbicans *Candida* species are observed in 10% to 20% of patients with recurrent vulvovaginal candidiasis [4••].

Recurrent vulvovaginal candidiasis with *Candida albicans* may require a 7- to 14-day initial course of topical therapy or an every third day dosing of fluconazole (100-, 150-, or 200-mg dose) for a total of three doses on days 1, 4, and 7. After initial remission, a maintenance antifungal regimen is started. Oral fluconazole (100-, 150-, or 200-mg dose) weekly for 6 months is the first line of treatment for maintenance therapy. If this regimen is not possible, topical clotrimazole, 200 mg twice a week, clotrimazole 500-mg suppositories once weekly, or other topical treatments can be used intermittently.

Currently, it is undetermined as to which treatment is optimal for nonalbicans vulvovaginal candidiasis. Treatment with a nonfluconazole azole drug, oral or topical, for 7 to 14 days is first-line therapy. If recurrence occurs, 600 mg of boric acid in a gelatin capsule can be administered vaginally once daily for 2 weeks [5]. If symptoms recur, referral to a specialist is advised.

Trichomonal Vaginitis

Trichomonal vaginitis is a common sexually transmitted disease that accounts for about one fourth of cases of vaginitis. The causative organism, *Trichomonas vaginalis*, is a unicellular, flagellated protozoan parasite that lives in the vagina, periurethral glands, and urethra in women. It survives in anaerobic conditions and is primarily seen in reproductive age women. As a sexually transmitted disease, 70% of exposed men and 85% of exposed women become infected with the disease within 48 hours. Men, however, may clear the infection spontaneously. Infections in women are not only associated with vaginitis but also with preterm delivery, premature rupture of membranes, low birth weight, and increased transmission of HIV [4••]. It is thus an important entity to recognize, diagnose, and treat.

Presentation

Trichomonal infections are asymptomatic in up to half of infected patients. By 6 months, however, one third of the asymptomatic patients develop symptomatic trichomoniasis. The patient typically presents with copious, malodorous discharge, pruritis, or irritation. Dysuria, dyspareunia, or postcoital bleeding also may be noted. Bacterial vaginosis may coexist with trichomonal infection.

Diagnosis

On physical examination, vaginal discharge is commonly seen and may be yellow-green to gray, thin, and foul smelling. Vaginal erythema is present in 75% of patients. The classic "strawberry cervix" with capillary dilation and punctate hemorrhage can be seen in up to 90% of patients on colposcopy but is rarely seen on gross examination.

Microscopic examination of wet mounts may establish the diagnosis by detecting actively motile organisms. This is the most practical and rapid method of diagnosis, which allows for immediate treatment. But wet mount is relatively insensitive; typically 58% when compared with culture and the sensitivity of Papanicolaou smear is only 56% to 78%. FDA-approved tests for trichomoniasis in women include an immunochromatographic assay, which detects trichomonas antigens, OSOM Trichomonas Rapid Test (Genzyme Diagnostics, Cambridge, MA) and a nucleic acid probe test, Affirm VP III (Becton Dickenson, San Jose, CA) [6]. These tests are performed on vaginal secretions and have sensitivity greater than 83% and specificity greater than 97% when compared with culture. Both tests are point-of-care diagnostics. The results of the OSOM Trichomonas Rapid Test are available in approximately 10 minutes, and results of the Affirm VP III, which also tests for *G. vaginalis* and *C. albicans*, are available within 45 minutes. There is currently no US Food and Drug Administration–cleared polymerase chain reaction test for *T. vaginalis*, but such testing may be available from commercial laboratories that have developed their own polymerase chain reaction.

In women in whom trichomoniasis is suspected but not confirmed by microscopy, vaginal secretions should be cultured for *T. vaginalis*. Culture is the most sensitive and specific commercially available method of diagnosis. There are several marketed culture mediums including Diamond's, Trichosel, and InPouch TV culture system (BioMed Diagnostics, Santa Clara, CA). The InPouch TV is less labor intensive, quicker, and is at least as sensitive as Diamond's culture medium. In one study, it was 97.6% sensitive within 24 hours, which is much quicker than results produced by Diamond's or Trichosel.

Management

First-line treatment options include metronidazole, 2 g orally in a single dose or tinidazole, 2 g orally in a single dose. An alternative regimen is metronidazole, 500 mg orally twice a day for 7 days. Patients should be advised to avoid consuming alcohol during treatment with metronidazole or tinidazole. Abstinence from alcohol use should continue for 24 hours after completion of metronidazole or 72 hours after completion of tinidazole.

Metronidazole regimens have resulted in cure rates of approximately 90% to 95%, and the recommended tinidazole regimen has resulted in cure rates of approximately 86% to 100%. Treatment of patients and sex partners results in relief of symptoms, microbiologic cure, and reduction of transmission.

Topically applied antimicrobials are unlikely to achieve therapeutic levels in the urethra or perivaginal glands and are therefore not recommended.

Special Populations

Pediatrics

Children differ from adults with respect to hormonal influences on the vaginal epithelium. There is no pubic hair, and labial fat pads are atrophic; thus, there is less protection of the vagina. The vaginal epithelium is thinner, and the pH is higher. Children play where there may be more irritants, such as sandboxes, and may have poor personal hygiene with wiping and infrequent hand washing. Vulvovaginitis in children needs to be approached as in adults with good history and physical examination. The history should include evaluation of potential sexual abuse; irritant exposure, such as bubble bath, sand, or soap; family history of allergies or eczema; foreign body exposure; and medical and surgical history. Most cases are thought to be noninfectious in origin [7••].

The examination, in compliant patients, should include external inspection and microscopic and aerobic culture of any discharge. Positioning of the patient may be done in the frog-legged or knee chest positions. Examination under anesthesia may be needed for noncompliant patients. Vulvar examination evaluates for a dermatologic condition, pinworm eggs, foreign body, and discharge. Discharge can be obtained with a nonbacteriostatic saline-moistened swab or with a vaginal saline lavage using a small catheter. The discharge should be examined for leukocytosis via microscopy. Leukocytosis is not pathognomonic for an infection, but when leukocytes are absent, such an infection is unlikely. Antibiotic treatment should be based on positive cultures [8•].

Noninfectious etiologies include such entities as atopic or contact dermatitis, seborrhea, psoriasis, lichen sclerosis, atrophic vaginitis, and foreign bodies. Foreign bodies usually produce foul smelling discharge and occasional vaginal bleeding. If a foreign body is suspected, an examination under anesthesia with vaginoscopy can be performed prior to removal of the object. Skin conditions can often be treated with hygiene in regard to cleaning and voiding, sitz baths, protective ointment, and possibly topical steroids or estrogen if indicated by the condition.

Infectious etiologies are often respiratory and enteric organisms as well as sexually transmitted diseases. Common organisms include *Streptococcus pyogenes*, *Haemophilus influenzae*, *Staphylococcus aureus*, *Shigella flexneri*, and *Klebsiella pneumoniae* [9]. Candida is a rare occurrence in prepubertal girls, who are not immunosuppressed or in diapers. When positive cultures are obtained, appropriate antibiotic therapy can be administered.

The possibility of sexual abuse should always be considered when a child presents with genital symptoms. If child abuse is suspected, child protective services should be notified, and the child should be referred to a trained professional that manages such cases [7••].

PREGNANT WOMEN

Vulvovaginal candidiasis frequently occurs during pregnancy. The general prevalence rates are thought to be higher in pregnant women than in the general population. Some of the physiologic changes during pregnancy, including decreased cellular immunity, elevated hormone levels, reduced vaginal pH, and increased vaginal glycogen concentration may be predisposing factors. Currently, only topical azole therapies, applied for 7 days, are recommended for use among pregnant women.

Bacterial vaginosis has been associated with adverse pregnancy outcomes including premature rupture of the membranes, chorioamnionitis, preterm labor, preterm birth, intraamniotic infection, postpartum endometritis, and postcesarean wound infection. Treatment of BV in symptomatic women and asymptomatic pregnant women at high risk for preterm delivery (those who have previously delivered a premature infant) is recommended with an oral regimen of metronidazole, 500 mg orally twice a day for 7 days or metronidazole, 250 mg orally three times a day for 7 days or clindamycin, 300 mg orally twice a day for 7 days. Neither metronidazole nor clindamycin have known teratogenic or mutagenic effects. There is no proven benefit for routine screening or treatment of asymptomatic women in reducing adverse outcomes. Three of four randomized controlled trials [2•] have shown that screening and treating high risk patients may decrease the risk of premature rupture of membranes and preterm delivery.

Vaginal trichomoniasis has also been associated with similar adverse pregnancy outcomes as BV; however, the data do not suggest that metronidazole treatment results in a reduction in perinatal morbidity. Some trials, in fact, suggest the possibility of increased prematurity or low birthweight after metronidazole treatment [10]. Limitations of the studies, including a large percentage of the placebo group receiving treatment outside of protocol and treatment at advanced gestational age, prevent definitive conclusions regarding risks of treatment.

Treatment of *T. vaginalis* may relieve symptoms of vaginal discharge in pregnant women and may prevent further sexual transmission. Patients should be counseled regarding the risks and benefits of treatment. In addition, these pregnant women should be provided careful counseling regarding condom use and the continued risk of sexual transmission.

POSTMENOPAUSAL WOMEN

Atrophic vaginitis may occur in a postmenopausal patient who is receiving no hormone replacement therapy or inadequate replacement therapy. Decreased levels of estrogen result in the thinning of the vaginal epithelium and decreased vaginal lubrication. These factors combine to make the vagina more susceptible to damage from injury during intercourse. Vaginal injury can lead to symptoms of itching, burning, discomfort, dyspareunia, and vaginal bleeding. Microscopic examination can support this diagnosis by findings of elevated vaginal pH with a negative amine test and presence of parabasal or intermediate cells by microscopy. Topical or oral estrogens can be considered for treatment. For those with contraindication or aversion to using estrogens, nonhormonal vaginal moisturizers may be used for symptomatic relief [11]. Rarely, irritation and itching may be associated with vulvar lesions such as vulvar intraepithelial neoplasia, lichen sclerosis, and even carcinoma. Lesions seen upon examination should always be evaluated by biopsy.

Summary

Vaginitis across the life-span should be evaluated with attention to a woman's hormone status, sexual activity that may indicate possible exposure to sexually transmitted diseases, and concomitant medical illnesses and therapies that may alter normal vaginal flora. Treatment should be tailored to the specific cause of the vaginitis.

References

Papers of particular interest have been highlighted as follows:
• Of interest
•• Of outstanding interest

1.• Anderson MR, Klink K, Cohrssen A: Evaluation of vaginal complaints. *JAMA* 2004, 291:1368–1379.
A good article.

2.• Okun N, Gronau K, Hannah M: Antibiotics for bacterial vaginosis or trichomonas vaginalis in pregnancy: a systemic review. *Obstet Gynecol* 2005, 105:857–868.
A good article.

3. Landers DV, Wiesenfeld HC, Heine RP, *et al*.: Predictive value of the clinical diagnosis of lower genital tact infection in women. *Am J Obstet Gynecol* 2004, 190:1004–1010.

4.•• Sexually transmitted diseases treatment guidelines 2006. Centers for Disease Control and Prevention. *MMWR Recomm Rep* 2006, 55(RR-11):1–94.
An outstanding report from the Centers for Disease Control and Prevention.

5.   Sobel JD, Chaim W, Nagappan V, Leaman D: Treatment of vaginitis caused by *Candida glabrata*: use of topical boric acid and flucytosine. *Am J Obstet Gynecol* 2003, 189(5):1297–1300.

6.   Huppert JS, Batteiger BE, Braslins P: Use of immunochromatographic assay for rapid detection of *trichomonas vaginalis* in vaginal specimens. *J Clin Microbiol* 2005, 43:684–687.

7.•• Vaginitis. In *Clinical Management Guidelines for Obstetricians-Gynecologists*. ACOG Practice Bulletin Number 72, May 2006.
An excellent resource.

8.• Kass-Wolff JH, Wilson EE: Pediatric gynecology: assessment strategies and common problems. *Semin Reprod Med* 2003, 21:329–338.
A good article on pediatric gynecologic issues

9.   Stricker T, Navratil F, Sennhauser FH: Vulvovaginitis in prepubertal girls. *Arch Dis Child* 2003, 88:324–326.

10. Klebanoff MA, Carey JC, Hauth JC, *et al.*: Failure of metronidazole to prevent preterm delivery among pregnant women with asymptomatic *Trichomonas vaginalis* infection. *N Engl J Med* 2001, 345:487–493.

11.• American College of Obstetricians and Gynecologists Women's Health Care Physicians: Genitourinary tract changes. *Obstet Gynecol* 2004, 104(Suppl 4):56S–61S.
A nice resource.

12.•• American College of Obstetricians and Gynecologists Women's Health Care Physicians: Genitourinary tract changes. *Obstet Gynecol* 2004, 104(Suppl 4):56S–61S.
An excellent resource.

18 Vulvitis

Frank W. Ling and Ginat W. Mirowski

- Vulvitis is a nonspecific term that describes symptoms; a diagnosis must be pursued to direct treatment.
- Dermatologic, systemic, infectious, and gynecologic conditions should be considered.
- A multidisciplinary approach is advised to maximize treatment success (gynecologists, dermatologists, urologists, neurologists, anesthesiologists, psychologists, and psychiatrists).
- The dermatologist generates a differential diagnosis based on the primary lesion.

Vulvitis is a common but frequently misunderstood condition characterized by pain, burning, itching, or irritation of the female genitalia. A comprehensive physical examination and history are necessary to detect potential etiologic factors. Establishing the diagnosis helps to direct treatment and eliminate precipitating factors.

Chronic vulvitis (primary or secondary) may contribute to sexual dysfunction and psychological disability. Thus, a multidisciplinary approach can maximize treatment success. Although cure is uncommon, some measure of pain relief can be achieved in nearly all patients using a multidisciplinary approach. A specific secondary cause should be investigated in all cases of vulvitis despite the fact that a diagnosis can be made in only a limited number of cases.

Dermatologic Conditions Associated With Vulvodynia

Dermatologists categorize many skin conditions based on the morphology of the primary lesion. Unfortunately, the moist environment of the genitalia and activities of daily living may alter or mask diagnostic clues, such as scales or superficial vesicles. These alterations are called secondary changes and include ulceration, erosions, maceration, and fissures. Thus, it is beneficial to perform a complete mucocutaneous evaluation, including the scalp, glabrous and acral skin, nails, and oral cavity, to observe additional signs when generating a differential diagnosis.

Broad categories of mucocutaneous diseases that may be associated with vulvitis include papulosquamous disorders, eczematous disorders, and vesiculobullous disorders.

PAPULOSQUAMOUS DISORDERS

The papulosquamous disorders are a heterogenous group of disorders characterized by inflammation and scaling. The differential diagnosis of papulosquamous disorders includes lichen planus, seborrheic dermatitis, psoriasis, pityriasis rosea, secondary syphilis, and infestations.

When the mucous membranes or intertriginous areas are affected, scales may be difficult or impossible to appreciate. Rarely, the mucous membranes may appear erosive, as in lichen planus and lichen sclerosus. Because squamous cell carcinoma can arise in areas of chronic inflammation, biopsy should be performed on any area of thickening induration or chronic nonhealing ulcer.

Lichen Planus

Lichen planus is a papulosquamous disorder that affects both the skin and mucous membranes. The cause of lichen planus is unknown. Cellular immune mechanisms appear to be primarily involved. Activated T cells are present in early lesions and appear to target antigenically altered basal cells. In older lesions, suppressor T cells have been shown to predominate.

The onset of cutaneous lesions may occur abruptly, and pruritus is typically severe, although excoriations are rare. The primary skin lesion is a flat-topped, polygonal, purple papule with superficial, fine reticulated white lines (Wickham's striae). Wickham's striae on the mucous membrane (oral, genital, or both) may be the sole manifestation of the disease. The buccal mucosa and the labia minora are typically asymptomatic. Painful erosions and desquamative vaginitis or desquamation of the gingivae are also common.

Vulvar lichen planus may present in several forms: 1) The papulosquamous form usually involves the wrists and ankles and presents with typical pruritic, flat-topped, polygonal, purple papules with fine white scale. Vulvar involvement includes similar findings on the labia and mons pubis and reticulated Wickham's striae on the labia minora and the medial aspect of the labia majora. Similar lesions are noted in the oral cavity.

2) Erosive lichen planus presents with a tender, denuded, red vaginal epithelium and desquamative vaginitis. A similar clinical presentation is noted on the gingivae. In more advanced disease, the vulva may appear eroded or atrophic. End-stage disease is characterized by scarring and adhesions that destroy the vulvar trigone and vagina. This often makes sexual intercourse impossible. A subset of this is the syndrome of chronic erosive lesions of the vulva, vagina, and gingivae, which has been named the vulvovaginal-gingival syndrome. In this syndrome, lichen planus typically presents with pruritus, vulvar pain, burning, and rawness.

3) Hypertrophic lichen planus presents with extensive thickened and hyperkeratotic white plaques of the skin or mucous membranes and is resistant to treatment. On genital mucous membranes, the differential diagnosis includes lichen sclerosus, squamous cell carcinoma, and verruca vulgaris.

The diagnosis of cutaneous lichen planus may be suspected clinically but should be confirmed by biopsy. The slight scaling of each papule suggests a differential diagnosis that includes psoriasis, dermatophyte infection, and neurodermatitis. In lichen planus, a biopsy reveals a characteristic inflammatory reaction pattern. The epidermis exhibits slight dyskeratosis, and an intense bandlike inflammatory infiltrate is evident beneath the epithelium. In contrast, erosive lesions maybe difficult to differentiate clinically from lichen sclerosus, cicatricial pemphigoid, pemphigus vulgaris, and lupus erythematosus. A biopsy with immunofluorescence may be necessary to arrive at the clinical diagnosis.

Seborrheic Dermatitis

Seborrheic dermatitis is a chronic papulosquamous eruption that waxes and wanes. The eruption is bilateral and symmetric, typically affecting the scalp, eyebrows, nasolabial folds, and middle chest. Ill-defined, waxy, erythematous scaling plaques or papules of variable size with diffuse margins are characteristic. Patients of Northern European or Celtic background, children, patients with zinc deficiency, patients receiving hyperalimentation, and those with Parkinson's disease or acquired immunodeficiency syndrome are commonly affected.

In the inverse pattern, moist, pale pink to yellow-red to gray to white patches are noted in intertriginous areas, such as the vulva, gluteal cleft, axillae, groin, and inframammary folds. Secondary fissures along the skin lines are also common. The cause is unknown, but *Pityrosporum orbiculare* appears to play a role.

Psoriasis

Psoriasis is the most common papulosquamous disorder of the skin and occurs in 2% of individuals. It is of unknown etiology but has a strong hereditary influence. Psoriasis appears to be an immunoregulatory disorder in which epidermal changes are related to a defect in the control of keratinocyte proliferation.

The affected epidermis produces a turnover rate that is up to eight times greater than normal. Maturation decreases from the normal 28 days to 3 or 4 days.

Psoriasis occurs at any age but most commonly appears during young adult life. It is a chronic disease that may persist throughout life, with periods of exacerbation and remission. Lesions classically occur on the scalp, elbows, and knees. The intergluteal cleft is another common site. The vulva and intertriginous areas may also be affected. Occasionally, psoriasis may involve the entire skin surface (erythroderma).

Genital involvement may be an isolated reaction or part of widespread psoriasis. Genital psoriasis presents as well-defined erythematous plaques without scale. The presenting complaint is itching or irritation. A family history of psoriasis is positive in about one third of cases. A potassium hydroxide (KOH) preparation of any scale excludes secondary fungal infection or yeast. Biopsies may be helpful in atypical presentations and show characteristic changes, including hyperkeratosis, epidermal hyperplasia, dilated tortuous vessels in the papillary dermis, and an inflammatory infiltrate with neutrophils extending into the epidermis, producing Munro's microabscesses.

Pityriasis Rosea

Pityriasis rosea is an acute, inflammatory dermatosis of unknown etiology. The generalized eruption is preceded by a single lesion, termed the *herald patch* (frequently misdiagnosed as ringworm). The herald patch is followed after several days to weeks by the generalized rash. Pruritus is usually mild. The rash consists of oval, minimally elevated, scaling papules and plaques located mainly on the trunk. The lesions follow the skin lines, creating a chevron pattern on the chest and a fir-tree pattern on the back. A viral cause is suggested by its increased incidence in winter months. Laboratory and biopsy results are not helpful. Therapy is usually not necessary in this self-limited disease.

Secondary Syphilis

Secondary syphilis is an inflammatory response in the skin and mucous membranes to the hematogenously disseminated *Treponema pallidum* spirochete. The secondary phase starts 6 to 12 weeks after the appearance of the primary chancre. The chancre is usually healed by the time the secondary phase begins but may still be remembered by the patient. Systemic symptoms include fever, headache, myalgias, arthralgias, sore throat, and malaise.

Skin lesions are commonly red-brown or yellow-orange. The eruption is often generalized; palms and soles are usually involved. Mucous membrane lesions may be seen in the form of mucous patches or condyloma lata. The serologic test for syphilis is positive in the secondary phase of the disease. Intramuscular benzathine penicillin, 2.4 million units, is the treatment of choice. Tetracycline or erythromycin may be substituted for patients allergic to penicillin.

Infestations

Scabies is an infestation of the skin with the *Sarcoptes scabiei* mite that is acquired by close contact with an infected person. The cardinal symptom is severe unrelenting pruritus, which is frequently more intense at night. Itching begins 1 to 2 months after the initial sensitization to the mite protein. The clinical presentation may be nonspecific, with erythematous papules, rare pustules, vesicles (especially in infants), and inflammatory nodules.

The pathognomonic lesion is the burrow, a thin serpiginous or linear papule rarely longer than 1 cm. Once pruritus develops, excoriations or burrows may be scattered diffusely, although they are typically found on the hands and feet, particularly the interdigital webs, and in the body folds (navel, axillae, groin, and finger webs). Skin scrapings placed in immersion oil and examined microscopically show mites, ova, or fecal concretions. A skin biopsy is rarely necessary.

Topical agents that kill mites and ova include lindane, crotamiton, and sulfur 5% to 10% in petrolatum. All family members and close contacts must be treated. Ivermectin has also been approved by the US Food and Drug Administration for the treatment of crusted or Norwegian scabies. Antihistamines are helpful for pruritus.

The differential diagnosis includes atopic dermatitis, xerosis (dry skin), insect bite reaction, contact dermatitis, and pruritus associated with systemic disease.

ECZEMATOUS DERMATITIS

Eczematous dermatitis is characterized acutely by inflamed, oozing vesicular dermatitis that becomes scaly, crusted, and thickened or lichenified over time. Most patients complain of rawness, burning, soreness, or pruritus. The history of a precipitating contactant may be obvious, or it may be obscure.

On physical examination, erythema with mild edema and tiny superficial vesicles (spongiosis) is noted early. With continued exposure, lichenification, scaling, and erosions become evident. The location and the configuration of the dermatitis may reflect the nature of the exposure. Angular corners, geometric outlines, and sharp margins suggest external exposure. Poison ivy and other plants characteristically cause linear streaks of papulovesicles, whereas contact with feminine hygiene products

or rubber on bike seats spares the folds. The histologic hallmark of this condition is spongiosis or intercellular edema of the epithelium. Figure 18-1 describes the treatment of the aggravating factors of eczematous dermatitis.

Contact dermatitis is an inflammatory reaction of the skin (either irritant or allergic) precipitated by an exogenous chemical. Irritant contact dermatitis is a nonspecific inflammatory reaction caused by toxic injury of the skin. Irritant contact vulvitis occurs after prolonged or repeated exposure to irritating or toxic products, including soaps, perfumes, feminine hygiene products, and some medications. Prolonged skin contact with urine, feces, vaginal secretions, and sweat may also cause irritant contact dermatitis. Skin damage is evident within hours of contact with a strong irritant. Symptoms may occur immediately when the irritant is caustic. Weaker irritants may require multiple applications, and the development of dermatitis may be delayed by several days.

Allergic contact dermatitis also presents with pruritus, burning, and stinging. The most common sensitizers are poison ivy, paraphenylenediamine, nickel, rubber compounds, and ethylenediamine. The symptoms are usually not immediate but occur 24 to 48 hours after exposure. Acute allergic contact dermatitis can present as swelling, vesiculation, erythema, and weeping. Scratching can cause secondary infections, leading to excoriations with crusting. Subacute allergic contact dermatitis can present with erythema, edema, erosions, and crusting. When chronic, the lesions tend to be lichenified, with induration and erythema and altered pigmentation. Hyperpigmentation is common in patients with dark skin. All patients may have marked lichenification.

The clinical presentation and history help to determine this as the cause. If the cause cannot be determined, patch testing can sometimes determine the causative agent. This is often done on the back, but the skin is not as sensitive as the vulva, making false-negative results more likely.

Vehicles for Topical Agents

	Ointments	Creams	Gels	Lotions and Solutions
Potency	Strong	Moderate	Strong	Low
Degree of hydration	Hydrating	Some hydration	Drying	Drying (variable)
Stage of dermatitis	Chronic	Acute to subacute	Acute to subacute	Acute
Sensitization risk	Very low	Significant	Significant	Significant
Irritation risk	Very low	Significant	Relatively high	Moderate
Composition	Water in oil emulsion	Oil in water emulsion	Semisolid emulsion in alcohol base	Powder in water (with some oil)
Heterogeneity among product lines	Relatively low	Very significant	Very significant	Very significant
Patient preference	Dislikes greasiness	High rate of acceptance	Variable	High rate of acceptance
Body sites useful	Nonintertriginous; vulvar	Virtually everywhere on the skin	Oral, scalp	Scalp, intertriginous areas
Body sites to avoid	Face, hands, oral cavity	Oral cavity, mucocutaneous sites with maceration	Fissures, erosions, maceration	Fissures, erosions

Figure 18-1. Vehicles for topical agents. (*Courtesy of* Steve Wolverton, MD; Indiana University.)

TREATMENT OF PAPULOSQUAMOUS AND ECZEMATOUS DISORDERS

Once a definitive diagnosis is made, first-line treatment for any of the inflammatory dermatosis disorders is oral or topical corticosteroids and a variety of symptomatic measures. However, candidal or dermatophyte infections may occur secondary to the use of topical or chronic systemic steroids.

When prescribing topical steroids, the potency of the agent, the various vehicles available, and the affected areas to be treated (Figure 18-2) are important issues to consider. In addition, because genital skin is thin and unintended occlusion increases the potency of steroids, lower-potency steroids are advisable. The least potent corticosteroid that will work should be prescribed. Ultra-high-potency corticosteroid ointment, such as clobetasol propionate 0.05%, can reverse many of the findings in lichen planus, lichen sclerosus, and psoriasis. As the symptoms decrease with treatment, a change should be made to a mid-potency corticosteroid, such as triamcinolone 0.1% ointment or desonide 0.05% ointment. Throughout treatment, the patient must be observed closely for signs of atrophy or maceration.

For nonerosive disease on the skin, a cream-based mid-potency corticosteroid is used, whereas mucosal disease of the vulva is best treated with an ointment base. Oral disease is often most responsive to gels or elixir. In general, erosive mucosal disease is more difficult to control than cutaneous disease. High-potency corticosteroid use must be closely monitored. A cream vehicle minimizes maceration in the inguinal area, but inflammation or pustular disease should be treated with an ointment because the alcohol base in creams causes burning.

As with all topical steroids, high-potency corticosteroids can lead to atrophy, striae, and telangiectasias of the noninvolved adjacent skin and mucosa. Sometimes, particularly in localized disease, intralesional injections with triamcinolone acetonide, 3 mg/mL, can be helpful.

When severe scarring and adhesion formation are anticipated, intermittent oral prednisone, 40 mg daily, may be prescribed. Further development of scars and adhesions can be prevented with the scheduled use of a vaginal dilator. The dilator is coated with corticosteroid and used on a tapering schedule at night. Surgery should not be performed unless the disease is controlled. After surgery, the dilator should be used to prevent new adhesions and scars. The use of oral griseofulvin has not been documented to help with healing or to decrease adhesion formation of lichen planus. Cytotoxic agents may be beneficial, but their harmful side effects limit their use to cases of severe disease.

Recurrences and remissions are characteristic of seborrheic dermatitis. Medicated shampoos that contain zinc pyrithione, tars, selenium sulfide, or ketoconazole are also helpful. Many of these shampoos are available over the counter, but they are also available as prescription shampoos. Low- to mid-potency corticosteroids usually are adequate. The use of both low-potency topical steroids and topical antifungals provides significant benefit. Widespread disease can be best treated with a short course of oral prednisone, 40 mg daily for 5 to 10 days, along with the topical agents.

General treatment for genital psoriasis is to avoid using any irritating substances in that area, such as irritating soaps, lotions, or detergents. Antihistamines help control itching. Cold packs applied to the area or oatmeal solutions can also be used. After bathing, the area should be patted dry, not rubbed. Tar (5% liquor carbonis detergens [LCD] mixed with a topical corticosteroid cream) and anthralin can also be used topically, but they can irritate sensitive genital skin. Tar shampoos remove scale in genital areas.

Although psoriasis responds to systemic steroids, they should be avoided because the disease rebounds after steroids are discontinued. Systemic methotrexate, retinoids, and cyclosporine can be used but are associated with numerous toxicities. The drug or combination of drugs used is dependent on the clinician's training and experience and the patient's response.

Eczematous Dermatitis

Aggravating Factors	Symptomatic Treatment	Pharmacologic Agents	Work-up
Soaps, washes, and cleansers	Identify aggravating factors	Limit topical agents	Fasting glucose, serum iron, folate, vitamin B_6 and B_{12}, magnesium, urinary oxalate, RPR
Medications (topical): antifungals, steroids, hormones, spermicidal agents	Take patient's history Perform biopsy Perform patch tests (delayed hypersensitivity reaction)	Corticosteroids Topical (ointment better than cream) Systemic	Perform a direct cytology examination (potassium hydroxide, cell smear)
Feminine hygiene products	Stop itch-scratch cycle	Use systemic medications	Obtain tissue for histologic evaluation and immunofluorescence
Tampons and pads, vaginal douches and hygiene sprays, suppositories, lubricants	Administer hydroxyzine doxepin Wash with water only Take sitz bath	Antifungal agents Antibiotics Steroids	Culture for fungi: *Candida albicans*, *Candida torulopsis* (*glabrata*) and others; *Chlamydia* species;
Condoms	Pat dry (do not rub)		*Streptococcus epidermidis*; consider viral studies (herpes
Toilet paper	Use only cotton underwear Avoid stockings, tight-fitting pants, and jeans		simplex or human papillomavirus)

Figure 18-2. Eczematous dermatitis. RPR—rapid plasma reagin test.

First-line treatment of contact dermatitis is to stop the use of the causative agent. To alleviate symptoms, a low- to mid-potency topical corticosteroid can be used. In severe reactions, oral prednisone, 40 mg daily for 7 to 10 days, or intramuscular injections of triamcinolone is effective. Antihistamines, tricyclic antidepressants, or benzodiazepines are also appropriate to use. Also, astringent dressings, such as Domeboro solution (Bayer Healthcare, Morristown, NJ) or baths with oatmeal products (Aveeno; Johnson & Johnson Company, New Brunswick, NJ), help decrease the itching.

After the offending agent has been identified, it should be discontinued; if the agent is unknown, all contacts to the area except water should be stopped. Treatment with a topical low-potency steroid helps minimize the inflammation and the pruritus. Steroid use should be monitored carefully because allergens can be present in unrelated products. For more inflamed skin, a mid-potency corticosteroid, such as triamcinolone 0.1%, can be used. An ointment base is better for broken skin. Acute exudative dermatitis is best treated with oral prednisone, 40 mg daily for 7 to 14 days. Also, bedtime sedation is extremely helpful if the patient has severe pruritus and loss of sleep.

Fungal (Dermatophyte) Infections

Infections of the skin caused by fungal organisms that infect keratinous tissues are called *dermatophyte* infections (from the Greek *phyte*, meaning plant). The patient presents with a scaling rash that may be pruritic. A variety of clinical lesions can result, but the most common are scaling, erythematous papules, plaques, and patches, which often have a serpiginous or wormlike border. The dermatophytoses are named according to the body part affected. The word *tinea* (Latin for worm) is followed by a qualifying term that denotes the location of the infection. *Tinea versicolor* is the only exception. Its name derives from the several shades of color that lesions may have in this disease.

Dermatophytes grow on humans and animals and exist in the soil. They are keratinophilic, and produce keratinases, a necessary requirement for their keratinophilic existence. The stratum corneum, hair, and nails are attractive substrates. Dermatophytes rarely invade beyond the epidermis because of their dependence on keratin for nutrition and because of the fungistatic properties of human serum.

The single most important laboratory test for all the fungal infections is the KOH preparation. The finding of hyphae on a KOH preparation is diagnostic of either dermatophytic or candidal infection. Usually, the clinical presentation distinguishes between the two. Scales can also be obtained for fungal culture.

Dermatophyte infections involving only limited areas can be effectively treated with topical antifungal agents. The patient should be instructed to apply the medication once or twice a day to the affected area until the infection is clinically clear and then for an additional 1 to 2 weeks. Extensive cutaneous fungal infections can be treated with systemic agents.

Vesiculobullous, Desquamative, and Erosive Vulvitis

LICHEN SCLEROSUS

Lichen sclerosus is a common disorder that affects the genitalia and less frequently the skin. The cause of lichen sclerosus is unknown, but an autoimmune etiology is hypothesized. Two incidence peaks are noted: it is most common in middle-aged Caucasian and Hispanic women; a smaller peak is noted in prepubertal girls.

Hypopigmented atrophic plaques characterize lichen sclerosus. The underlying vessels are fragile, and ecchymoses are common. Presenting complaints include pruritus, soreness, pain, and dyspareunia. The onset of lichen sclerosus can be insidious and asymptomatic, but with time, pruritus and significant pain are common.

On physical examination, white atrophic patches with a wrinkled epidermis, purpura, telangiectasia, and bullae may be seen, along with secondary erosions. The areas of the labia minora, clitoris, and inner labia majora extending to the posterior fourchette in a figure-8 pattern are frequently involved. Progressive atrophy of the subcutaneous tissue leads to effacement and eventual complete destruction of the clitoris and labia minora. If untreated, extensive scarring occurs, and the introitus narrows and may become stenosed or closed. These late changes are called *kraurosis vulvae*. There is an increased incidence of squamous cell carcinoma in these patients.

BULLOUS PEMPHIGOID

Bullous pemphigoid is an uncommon, self-limiting autoimmune disease characterized by widespread tense blisters accompanied by pruritus. The patient, who is typically between 60 and 80 years of age, presents with a history of gradually progressive, intensely pruritic blisters. Preferred sites of involvement are the groin, axillae, and flexural areas. Up to 33% of patients also have oral lesions. Blisters are large and tense and occur on normal-appearing or erythematous skin. Blisters do not spread laterally when pushed from the top (negative Nikolsky's sign).

Healing occurs without scarring. Bullous drug reactions and severe arthropod bite reactions may resemble pemphigoid. The biopsy of a blister shows a subepidermal bulla with an intact roof. The dermal infiltrate is composed of eosinophils and lymphocytes that are present in the upper dermis. Direct (using the patient's skin) and indirect (using the patient's serum) immunofluorescence studies reveal a linear band of immunoglobulin G (IgG) and C3 cells deposited along the basement membrane zone where blister formation occurs. The IgG autoantibodies are directed against an antigen that is associated with the hemidesmosome of the basement membrane zone. Patients respond to systemic steroids. The addition of tetracycline to the regimen may allow administration of a lower dose of prednisone. The prognosis is excellent, with the disease usually subsiding after months to years.

Pemphigus Vulgaris

Pemphigus vulgaris is a rare autoimmune vesiculobullous disease that affects the skin and mucous membranes. It affects males and females equally and most commonly occurs in middle age. Before the era of systemic steroids, pemphigus vulgaris had a high mortality rate, usually from massive fluid and protein loss or from coexisting secondary infections.

If treated, patients with pemphigus vulgaris do well, but in untreated patients, the mortality rate is 80%. This results from fluid and protein loss, infection, and inability to eat. Even with potent medications, the mortality rate approaches 10%; however, mortality is now usually associated with the complications of therapy.

Patients with pemphigus vulgaris usually present with oral lesions and complain of pain in the mouth and a sore throat. The disease can progress to the scalp and intertriginous areas. The vulvar area is affected in 10% of cases. These patients may be symptom free or present with burning, soreness, and irritation of the genital area.

On physical examination, the vestibule, labia minora, and inner labia majora have ulcers and superficial erosions. The vagina and cervix can also be affected. Secondary infection is common and can often worsen the erosions. As the disease progresses, it can cause erosions and blisters of the hair-bearing areas of the genitalia. Pemphigus vulgaris generally does not cause scarring. However, scarring can result in loss of the labia minora, resorption of the clitoris, and narrowing of the introitus. The end result is indistinguishable from other scarring processes.

Progression is gradual but unremitting. Pruritus is a common complaint. The primary lesion is a flaccid blister that tends to rupture easily and form a crusted erosion. Blisters typically dissect laterally when pressed (Nikolsky's sign). The bulla of pemphigus vulgaris occurs within the epidermis just above the basal layer. It is formed by the loss of cohesion between keratinocytes (acantholysis). Direct and indirect immunofluorescence studies are positive, showing deposits of IgG or C3 cells in the intercellular spaces between keratinocytes.

The differential diagnosis includes many disease processes. The early erosive disease can mimic cicatricial pemphigoid, lichen planus, and erythema multiforme. Later in the disease, the intact bullae of the hair-bearing skin may suggest bullous pemphigoid. The clinical picture of the distribution and appearance of the affected skin and the surrounding skin usually can yield a correct diagnosis, but a biopsy is always necessary because of the seriousness of the disease.

This disease is best treated by a dermatologist, and these cases should be referred. First-line treatment includes systemic corticosteroids. In severe disease, treatment is pulse intravenous methylprednisolone. Mild disease can be treated with oral prednisone, 80 mg daily, with increases of 20 mg daily if new lesions continue to occur. After new lesions cease to appear, the corticosteroids can be carefully and slowly tapered.

Steroid-sparing therapy can be used if the patient cannot tolerate high doses of corticosteroids (up to 200 mg daily). Azathioprine or cyclophosphamide, 2 mg/kg daily, can be used; however, it takes longer for benefits to be seen with these medications. Other treatment options include plasmapheresis, gold sodium thiomalate, and methotrexate.

Local care of the bullae and erosions in the genital area is important. Follow-up of this area is crucial, and any coexisting bacterial, viral, or candidal infections should be treated because disease in this area can be so debilitating. A vaginal dilator, as used with other vaginal scarring diseases, can be used to prevent stenosis.

Patients with primarily vaginal lesions but controlled systemic disease can be treated with high-potency corticosteroids, but close monitoring of the patient is essential. If scarring and stenosis or resorption of genital landmarks occur but the disease is inactive or under control, reparative surgery can performed.

Herpes Simplex Virus Infection

Herpes simplex virus (HSV) infection is an acute, self-limited, intraepidermal vesicular eruption. Primary infection with HSV type 1 (HSV-1) usually occurs in childhood, which is subclinical in 90% of the cases. The remaining 10% of patients have acute gingivostomatitis. In contrast, HSV-2 primary infection usually occurs after sexual contact in postpubertal patients, producing acute vulvovaginitis or progenitalis. Primary infections are often accompanied by systemic symptoms and localized pain.

On physical examination, indurated erythema or grouped vesicles on an erythematous base are detected. The vesicles quickly become pustules, which rupture, weep, and crust. Primary gingivostomatitis or vulvovaginitis is characterized by extensive vesiculation of the mucous membranes. Localized grouped vesicles occurring in the same location characterize recurrent herpes infection. The differential diagnosis includes superficial fungus infections, impetigo, and contact dermatitis.

The diagnosis can be confirmed with a Tzanck smear, which reveals multinucleated giant cells. The organism can also be cultured, although immunofluorescent studies are the most rapid and specific. Acyclovir is the drug most commonly used for HSV infections; famciclovir and Valtrex are also available.

Herpes simplex virus is a highly contagious agent spread by direct contact with infected individuals. The virus penetrates the epidermal cell, undergoes a replicative cycle, and induces protein and DNA synthesis with assembling of intact virions and eventual lysis of the host cell membrane. The destructive effect on epidermal cells results clinically in intraepidermal vesicles.

Latent HSV presumably resides in the dorsal nerve root sensory of autonomic ganglia in a nonreplicative state. Recurrence occurs with reactivation of the replicative cycle, production of new virus, and spread back down the nerve.

Vulvitis

The prevalence of vulvitis is unknown but may be as high as 15% in a general clinical practice. A specific secondary cause should be investigated in all cases of vulvitis. A definitive diagnosis is more likely to be found in cases of desquamative inflammatory vaginitis or acute or chronic vulvar itching than when pain is the only symptom. The diagnosis may be a primary mucocutaneous disease, an infestation, a bacterial or viral infection, or a mucosal reaction to topical or systemic medications. Establishing the diagnosis helps to direct treatment and eliminates precipitating factors.

When mucosal or cutaneous findings do not suggest a cause, the burning sensation may be a manifestation of an infection or of undetected systemic abnormalities. Thus, it is essential to culture for *Candida* species and other fungi, such as *Torulopsis glabrata* and *C. kansasii*, which may be difficult to visualize on a KOH preparation. In addition, viral cultures and serum evaluation to exclude deficiencies of iron, folate, vitamin B_6 and B_{12}, as well as diabetes, are necessary.

Vulvitis is best managed using a multidisciplinary team approach: gynecologists, dermatologists, urologists, neurologists, anesthesiologists, psychologists, and psychiatrists work together to treat this complex problem. Medical management usually employs medication protocols designed to treat neuropathic pain. Pain management techniques, including local treatment regimens, physical therapy such as biofeedback and behavior therapy, and surgical management have been reported to provide positive outcomes. Finally, psychologic support for the patient and her partner should be incorporated in the treatment plan.

When no dermatologic or gynecologic diagnosis is established, a diagnosis of primary vulvodynia is made. Several subtypes of vulvodynia are recognized, including vulvar vestibulitis syndrome, cyclic vulvovaginitis, and dysesthetic vulvodynia. Although burning may be encountered on any or all of the vulvar surfaces, the vestibule is most frequently affected and may be the only site of involvement.

Vulvar vestibulitis syndrome is characterized by severe, chronic pain on vestibular contact or attempted vaginal entry. This is thought to be the most frequent cause of dyspareunia in premenopausal women. The burning may be continuous or intermittent and frequently results in dyspareunia. Empirical treatment options are available when the work-up is negative. Systemic tricyclic antidepressants, such as amitriptyline and desipramine, may be highly effective in the treatment of idiopathic vulvodynia. Antihistamines, such as hydroxyzine, and other tricyclic antidepressants, such as doxepin, may relieve the pruritus. Anticonvulsant medication, including gabapentin, clonazepam, and carbamazepine, should be reserved when a focal trigger area is identified. (Laboratory studies must be followed to avoid adverse effects with these agents.)

Selected Bibliography

Fisher BK, Margesson LJ: *Genital Skin Disorders: Diagnosis and Treatment.* St. Louis: CV Mosby; 1998.

Lynch PJ, Edwards L: *Genital Dermatology.* New York: Churchill Livingstone; 1994.
This is a comprehensive yet concise text with excellent clinical photographs and illustrations. This problem-oriented diagnostic format facilitates rapid and accurate diagnosis of vulvar conditions. Highly recommended for all clinicians involved in caring for women.

Wilkinson EJ, Stone IK: *Atlas of Vulvar Disease.* Baltimore: Williams & Wilkins; 1995.

19 | Delayed Puberty

David Muram

- Puberty is delayed when there are no signs of sexual development by 13 years of age, absence of menarche by 15 years, or a delay in the normal progression of pubertal development.
- Patients with delayed puberty may be classified into one of three major clinical groups according to secondary sexual development.
- The physical examination should include an assessment of growth and pubertal development.
- Patients with adequate pubertal development, normal pelvic examination, and continued estrogen production often have chronic anovulation and should be given a progesterone challenge.
- Follicle-stimulating hormone levels should be determined in all patients with minimal breast development. Levels greater than 60 mIU/L suggest gonadal failure. A karyotype should be obtained when these levels are high. Gonadal extirpation is required when Y chromosome material is identified.
- Androgen levels should be measured in all patients who show signs of virilization.

Normal Pubertal Development

Puberty involves a sequence of physical changes caused by the effect of increased sex steroids produced by the gonads. In females, estradiol plays a primary role in growth during puberty as well as maturation of sexual characteristics. The episodic release of follicle-stimulating hormone (FSH) and luteinizing hormone (LH) represents a reactivation of the hypothalamic-pituitary-ovarian axis that was relatively quiescent during childhood. The trigger that initiates this process is unknown but is related to stimulation or reduced inhibition from the central nervous system. Gonadotropin-releasing hormone (GnRH) stimulates the pituitary, which then produces FSH and LH and these hormones stimulate the ovary to produce sex steroids. The pubertal growth spurt is related to the increased secretion of sex steroids, growth hormone, and somatomedin (insulin-like growth factor-1) [1,2•,3,4•].

Adrenarche, an increase in adrenal androgen secretion, precedes the onset of the gonadal component of puberty. The mechanism of control of adrenarche is unknown. It can be documented by an increase in adrenal dehydroepiandrosterone sulfate levels. Adrenal androgen-stimulated features of puberty include pubic and axillary hair development, oily skin, acne, and body odor. The various features of pubertal development are summarized in Figure 19-1.

The visible physical changes of puberty generally proceed in the following manner: breast development (thelarche), growth acceleration, the appearance of pubic and axillary hair (pubarche or adrenarche), and the onset of menstruation (menarche). Adrenarche may be the first sign of puberty in about 15% of white girls and 50% of African-American girls. The onset of thelarche and pubarche is variable, with a mean of 10.9 and 11.2 years, respectively. Peak growth velocity occurs almost 2.5 years later and precedes the onset of menses (mean age, 12.7 years). After menarche, mean growth is approximately 2 inches. Girls who experience early puberty may have considerable growth (3–5 inches), whereas girls with late menarche may have little or no growth. Growth after 16 years of age ranges from undetectable to 3 inches [5].

The exact age at which menarche occurs cannot be predicted, but in most girls with normal progression of puberty, it follows the onset of puberty by approximately 2 years. Age at menarche depends on genetic and environmental factors and may be associated with body mass or body fat content.

Regular ovulation, 20 months later, marks the completion of the pubertal cycle. The interval between the onset of thelarche and menarche is 2.3 ± 1 year and is independent of the age at which thelarche occurs. Marshall and Tanner [6] recorded the progression of pubertal development, and their classification is useful in following pubertal development in adolescents (Figure 19-2 through 19-4).

Definitions

Delayed sexual development is defined as the absence of normal pubertal events at an age greater than 2.5 SD from the

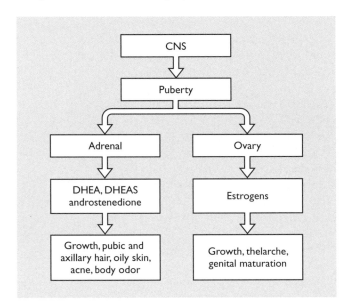

Figure 19-1. Pubertal development. DHEA—dehydroepiandrosterone; DHEAS—dehydroepiandrosterone sulfate.

mean. Thus, puberty is delayed when no signs of sexual development have begun by 13 years of age, absence of menarche by 15 years, or a delay in the normal progression of pubertal development. Because some degree of sexual maturation occurs in more than 30% of patients with gonadal dysgenesis, an investigation is necessary when a girl presents with a delay in progression of pubertal development [7]. The indications are summarized in Figure 19-5.

Differential Diagnosis

Patients presenting with delayed puberty may be classified according to gonadal function. Thus, patients are divided into three major clinical groups according to secondary sexual development:

1. Delayed menarche with adequate secondary sexual development, namely, primary amenorrhea. These disorders have been collectively referred to as eugonadism.

2. Delayed puberty with inadequate or absent secondary sexual development. These disorders have been collectively referred to as hypogonadism. When FSH levels are high, the patient is said to have hypergonadotropic hypogonadism, and when FSH levels are low, the patient is said to have hypogonadotropic hypogonadism.

3. Delayed puberty and heterosexual secondary sexual development, namely, virilization.

The various disorders are listed in Figure 19-6. By using this broad classification, the physician can better direct the diagnostic evaluation. Because the purpose of this chapter is to serve as a guide for the primary care physician, only a brief description of the various disorders is included.

Sexual Development

Breast Development

Stage 1	Preadolescent; elevation of papilla only
Stage 2	Breast bud stage; elevation of breast and papilla as small mound; enlargement of areolar diameter
Stage 3	Further enlargement and elevation of breast and areola with no separation of their contours
Stage 4	Projection of areola and papilla to form a secondary mound above the level of the breast
Stage 5	Mature stage; projection of papilla only caused by recession of the areola to the general contour of the breast

Pubic Hair

Stage 1	Preadolescent; the vellus over the pubes is not more developed than that over the abdominal wall—that is, no pubic hair
Stage 2	Sparse growth of long, slightly pigmented downy hair, straight or curled, chiefly along the labia
Stage 3	Hair considerably darker, coarser, and more curled; the hair spreads sparsely over the junction of the pubes
Stage 4	Hair now adult in type, but area covered is still considerably smaller than in the adult; no spread to the medial surface of the thighs
Stage 5	Adult in quantity and type, with distribution of the horizontal (or classically "feminine") pattern; spread to the medial surface of the thighs, but not up the linea alba or elsewhere above the base of the inverse triangle (spread up the linea alba occurs late and is rated Stage 6)

Figure 19-2. Sexual development.

Patients with Adequate Secondary Sexual Development

Patients with functioning ovaries and delayed sexual maturation usually consult a physician in their mid-teens for primary amenorrhea. They have a well-formed female configuration with appropriately developed breasts. Most of these patients (approximately 80%) suffer from inappropriate LH feedback, anovulatory cycles, and unopposed estrogens, and some have an excess of androgen production. The amenorrhea may persist until the patient is challenged with a progestin, such as medroxyprogesterone (Provera; Pfizer, New York, NY), 10 mg daily for 5 days. After withdrawal bleeding, patients should be monitored for continued menstrual function because in some, anovulation persists.

Congenital anomalies of the müllerian structures are found in approximately 20% of patients with primary amenorrhea. The most common defect is congenital absence of the uterus and vagina. Other anatomic causes of amenorrhea include imperforate hymen, transverse vaginal septa, agenesis of the cervix, and partial or complete agenesis of the vagina. Gynecologic examination supplemented by diagnostic imaging (eg, ultrasonography, magnetic resonance imaging) establishes the diagnosis of these congenital anomalies. Finally, adolescents with complete androgen insensitivity may also present with primary amenorrhea [8–10]. These conditions are discussed in greater detail in Chapter 41.

Patients with Inadequate Secondary Sexual Development

Lack of estrogens may be caused by gonadal failure, lack of ovarian stimulation secondary to hypothalamic-pituitary failure, or constitutional delay. Constitutional delay of puberty is a variant of normal in which pubertal development and biochemical markers are normal for a younger child. Patients with this condition have been labeled as "late bloomers." The lack of signs of puberty (including the pubertal growth spurt) often concerns the patient when her adolescent friends have secondary sexual features and the characteristic increase in height. Excluding other causes of delayed sexual maturation establishes the diagnosis of constitutional delay. However, it is difficult sometimes to distinguish between constitutional delay and hypogonadotropic hypogonadism caused by hypothalamic-pituitary failure. When the diagnosis of constitutional delay is considered, the patient must be kept under observation until she begins normal menstrual cycles. Occasionally, an adolescent requires hormonal replacement therapy because of the emotional distress caused by the delay and the associated immature appearance.

Many patients with delayed sexual development suffer from gonadal failure, which is associated with a marked elevation of serum FSH level. The cause is often a loss of X chromosome material and important ovarian determinant

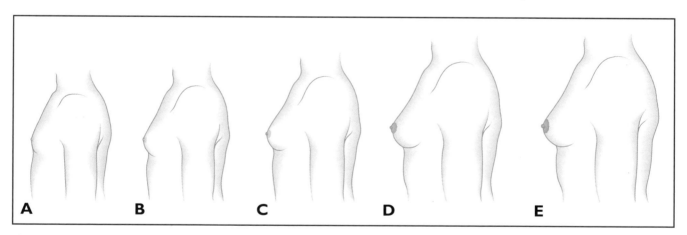

Figure 19-3. Tanner staging: breast development. (*Adapted from* Lee [5].)

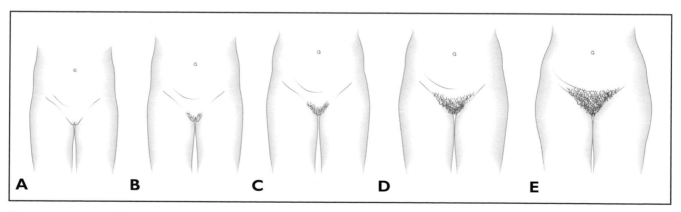

Figure 19-4. Tanner staging: pubic hair development. (*Adapted from* Lee [5].)

genes. Mosaicism with two or more cell lines, one containing an abnormal X chromosome, is probably more common than nonmosaic abnormalities. Certain somatic abnormalities are often seen in patients with gonadal dysgenesis, including short stature, webbing of the neck, shield chest, and coarctation of the aorta. Replacement hormonal therapy given in a cyclic manner is the treatment of choice and prevents long-term complications associated with a hypoestrogenic state, such as cardiovascular disease, osteoporosis, and vaginal dryness. When Y chromosome complement or derivative is discovered, gonadectomy is indicated because a significant percentage of these patients develop a dysgerminoma in the retained gonad [11,12].

Some patients may have ovarian failure with normal sex chromosomes (46,XX). In these patients, ovarian failure may be secondary to causes other than privation of X-chromosome material. An autosomal recessive form of ovarian failure has been determined in some families. Other causes of follicular depletion include chemotherapy, irradiation, infections (eg, mumps), infiltrative disease processes of the ovary, autoimmune diseases, and other known environmental agents. It is also possible, however, that submicroscopic X-chromosome deletions in the ovarian determinant region resulted in ovarian failure. These patients also require long-term hormonal replacement therapy.

The resistant ovary syndrome is characterized by delayed menarche or primary amenorrhea, a 46,XX karyotype, high FSH levels, and ovaries that, despite apparently normal follicle apparatus, do not respond to endogenous gonadotropins. It is assumed that the absence of follicular receptors for gonadotropins is responsible for ovarian failure in these patients. These patients have high FSH levels and a normal chromosome constitution. Estrogen replacement therapy should be initiated to prevent long-term complications, such as vaginal dryness and osteoporosis.

Isolated deficiency of gonadotropin-releasing factor, often associated with intracranial anomalies and anosmia (Kallmann's syndrome), is uncommon. The cause for this disorder is the lack of production of adhesion molecules coded by the KAL gene located on the X chromosome. These patients fail to develop secondary sexual features, and their blood levels of gonadotropins are very low. An increase in gonadotropin levels is normally expected following a GnRH challenge test. Estrogen therapy is used to initiate and later sustain sexual development. When fertility is desired, induction of ovulation may be accomplished with menotropins (Pergonal; Serono, Geneva, Switzerland) or GnRH. A pituitary or parasellar tumor, particularly craniopharyngioma, pituitary adenoma, or prolactinoma, must be considered in the evaluation of a patient with delayed sexual maturation. Weight loss due to severe dieting, marked protein deficiency, and fat loss without notable loss of muscle (often seen in athletes), may also delay or suppress maturation of the hypothalamic-pituitary-ovarian axis [13••].

Delayed Puberty and Heterosexual Secondary Sexual Development

Virilization at puberty is the result of elevated androgen levels from adrenal or gonadal sources. These may be the result of an enzyme deficiency (eg, late-onset congenital adrenal hyperplasia) or a neoplasm (eg, Leydig's cell tumor). A small group of these patients are male pseudohermaphrodites—adolescents who are being reared as girls, have female external genitalia, intra-abdominal or ectopic malfunctioning testes, and a normal 46,XY chromosomal constitution. A thorough investigation is necessary to identify the source of androgenic stimulation. A detailed description of these disorders is beyond the scope of this chapter.

Delayed Puberty

Delayed menarche with adequate secondary sexual development

Inappropriate H-P-O axis feedback mechanism

Anatomic defect

Obstructed outflow tract

Vaginal agenesis

Complete androgen insensitivity syndrome

Delayed puberty (no signs of secondary sexual development)

Gonadal failure (hypergonadotropic hypogonadism)

Constitutional delay

Chronic illness

Weight loss

Gymnasts

Hypothalamic pituitary failure

Delayed puberty with virilization

XY female

Virilizing tumors

Congenital adrenal hyperplasia

Figure 19-6. Delayed puberty. H-P-O—hypothalamic-pituitary-ovarian.

Delayed Sexual Maturation: Indications for a Diagnostic Evaluation

1. Absence of thelarche by age 13 years

2. Absence of menarche by age 15 years

3. Deviation from the normal progression of pubertal development (eg, no menarche 3 or more years after the onset of thelarche)

4. Significant patient or parental anxiety

Figure 19-5. Delayed sexual maturation: indications for a diagnostic evaluation.

Evaluation of Patients with Delayed Sexual Development

Determination of gonadal function for categorization into eugonadal, hypogonadal, or virilized patient groups can be accomplished by obtaining a medical history and performing a physical examination. The history may provide information that may direct the clinician toward the diagnosis. Key elements to be elicited during the history are summarized in Figure 19-7.

The physical examination should include an assessment of growth and pubertal development. The physician should determine the growth velocity. The change in height is converted to centimeters per year and then plotted on a growth velocity chart. Peak height velocity is a discrete physiologic event and can be related to other pubertal milestones (Figure 19-8). The degree of breast development and pubic hair growth is determined based on comparison with the Tanner stages described earlier in this chapter. Presence of breast development signifies prior ovarian function. A vaginal smear can determine whether the gonad is continuing to produce estrogen. Pelvic and rectal examination identifies patients with an obstructed outflow tract as well as patients with congenital absence of the vagina and uterus. Further confirmation of patients with Rokitansky's syndrome is dependent on a karyotype to identify normal 46,XX complement and a pelvic sonogram to confirm uterine absence and ovarian presence. The diagnostic work-up is summarized in Figure 19-9 and Figure 19-10. Although müllerian abnormalities are found in 10% to 15% of girls with adequate secondary sexual features who present with primary amenorrhea, cases in which the müllerian system is absent in girls without sexual development are extremely rare. Therefore, a pelvic examination may be safely deferred in most girls with absent secondary sexual development [14]. Absence of pubic hair is suggestive of the androgen insensitivity syndrome. A karyotype and determination of receptor content and function confirm the diagnosis.

Patients with adequate pubertal development, evidence of continued estrogen production, and normal müllerian systems probably have some hormonal abnormality caused by an inappropriate positive feedback and, hence, chronic anovulation. Progesterone challenge in such patients is helpful; a withdrawal bleed signifies a normal müllerian system and continued estrogen production.

When breast development is minimal, the usual diagnosis is hypogonadism. Serum gonadotropin assays are performed for further elucidation; elevated FSH levels suggest gonadal failure. Other endocrine profiles should be obtained if hypothyroidism, congenital adrenal hyperplasia, or Cushing's syndrome is suspected. Karyotype is necessary in all patients with confirmed gonadal failure. Gonadal extirpation is required when Y-chromosome material is identified.

Low FSH levels suggest an interference with hypothalamic-pituitary maturation and gonadotropin release. Skull films and prolactin assays must be obtained for all patients to rule out the more serious irreversible causes, such as pituitary tumors. Appropriate endocrine evaluation identifies the occasional patient with hypothyroidism or congenital adrenal hyperplasia and the rare patient with Cushing's syndrome. Diagnosis of Kallmann's syndrome is suspected in hypogonadotropic patients who have associated anosmia but is confirmed only after GnRH challenge tests are performed. The presumed diagnosis of physiologic

Elements to Elicit During History Taking

Prenatal and birth history

   Intrauterine abnormalities (*eg*, cystic hygroma, pelvic or abdominal mass)

   Newborn abnormalities (*eg*, lymphedema, small for gestational age)

Family history of disordered puberty

Long-standing vs acute change in growth pattern

   Evidence of masculinization or virilization

Medications, cytotoxic agents, and radiation therapy

Chronic medical illness

   Chronic development disorder

   Endocrine disorder

   Hemoglobinopathies

   Other

Socioeconomic factors

   Nutrition

   Physical and sexual abuse

   Illicit drug use (*eg*, marijuana)

Figure 19-7. Elements to elicit history taking. (*Adapted from* Plouffe [14].)

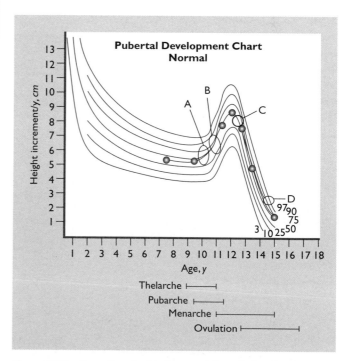

Figure 19-8. Growth velocity chart and the relationship between growth and pubertal milestones. (*Adapted from* Plouffe [14].)

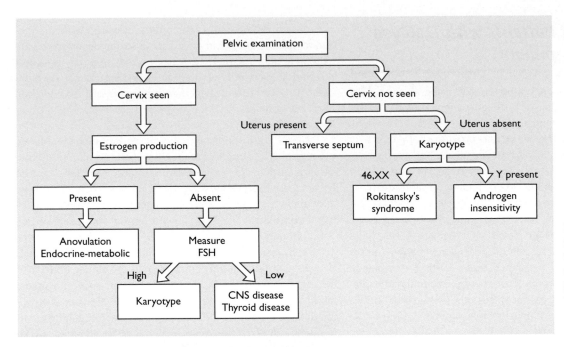

Figure 19-9. A simplified algorithm for the differential diagnosis of delayed puberty. CNS—central nervous system; FSH—follicle-stimulating hormone.

Initial Work-up of the Patient with Delayed Sexual Maturation

History

Physical examination

 Growth status

  Growth velocity charts

  Height

  Predicted adult height calculated from current height and bone age

 Pubertal development using the Tanner staging classification

  Breast development

  Pubic and axillary hair development

 Hormonal status

  Luteinizing hormone, follicle-stimulating hormone, prolactin, thyroid function tests

 Dysmorphic features

  Gonadal dysgenesis, midline fusion defects

 Virilization

  Hirsutism, clitoromegaly, and others

 Uterus

  Present

  Absent

  Obstruction

 Imaging studies

  Bone age

  Other (pelvic ultrasound, MRI of the central nervous system, and so forth)

Figure 19-10. Initial work-up of the patient with delayed sexual maturation. CNS—central nervous system.

delay is made by exclusion of all other causes and by the FSH and LH release patterns following GnRH challenge.

Androgen levels should be measured in patients who show signs of virilization. The source of these elevated androgens should be identified. Adrenal and gonadal neoplasms must be surgically removed. If the patient is an XY female, all testicular tissue must be excised, and the patient should be given estrogen replacement therapy. Patients with congenital adrenal hyperplasia should be treated with the appropriate corticosteroids.

References

Papers of particular interest, have been highlighted as follows:
* Of interest
** Of outstanding interest

1. Sanfilippo J, Muram D, Lee P, *et al.*: *Pediatric and Adolescent Gynecology*. Philadelphia: WB Saunders; 1994.

2.• Emans SJ, Laufer MR, Goldstein DP: *Pediatric and Adolescent Gynecology*, edn 4. Philadelphia: Lippincott-Raven; 1998.
A comprehensive review of pediatric and adolescent gynecology.

3. Carpenter SEK, Rock JA: *Pediatric and Adolescent Gynecology*. New York: Raven; 1992.

4• Goldfarb AF: *Atlas of Clinical Gynecology*. Philadelphia: Current Medicine; 1998.
A pictorial review of the most common disorders leading to delayed puberty.

5. Lee PA: Normal and precocious puberty. In *Atlas of Clinical Gynecology*. Edited by Goldfarb AF. Philadelphia: Current Medicine; 1998.

6. Marshall WA, Tanner JM: Variations in the pattern of pubertal changes in girls. *Arch Dis Child* 1969, 44:91.

7. Dewhurst SJ: *Female Puberty and Its Abnormalities*. Edinburgh, UK: Churchill Livingstone; 1984.

8. Jones HW Jr, Rock JA: *Reparative and Constructive Surgery of the Female Genital Tract*. Baltimore: Williams & Wilkins; 1983.

9. Muram D: Congenital malformations. In: *Textbook of Gynecology*. Edited by C LJ. Philadelphia: WB Saunders; 1993:121–141.

10. Rock JA, Azziz R: Genital anomalies in childhood. *Clin Obstet Gynecol* 1987, 30:682–696.

11. Shulman LP, Elias S: Developmental abnormalities of the female reproductive tract: pathogenesis and nosology. *Adolesc Pediatr Gynecol* 1988, 1:230–238.

12. Simpson JL: *Disorders of Sexual Differentiation: Etiology and Clinical Delineation*. New York: Academic Press; 1976.

13.•• Styne DM: New aspects in the diagnosis and treatment of pubertal disorders. *Pediatr Clin North Am* 1997, 44:505–529.
An excellent review of recent developments in the area of pubertal development.

14. Plouffe L Jr: Delayed sexual maturation. In *Atlas of Clinical Gynecology*. Edited by Goldfarb AF. Philadelphia: Current Medicine; 1998.

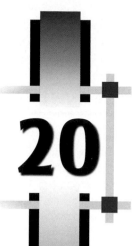

20 Infertility Evaluation

M. Mercedes Sayago and Ringland S. Murray, Jr.

- Infertility is lack of pregnancy after 1 year of adequate unprotected intercourse.
- A five-point work-up will identify the majority of issues.
- Once diagnosed, diminished ovarian reserve predicts poor prognosis, which does not change.
- Timely work-up and referral maintains a patient's positive feelings toward the primary care provider.

Background

Infertility is the absence of pregnancy after 1 year of adequate, unprotected intercourse, affecting 15% of couples at any one time (Figure 20-1). The Centers for Disease Control and Prevention reports male and female factors contribute equally to infertility, and approximately 10% of infertile couples have no identifiable cause [1]. The 1985 World Health Organization task force on female infertility concluded that tubal factors are present in 36% of cases, ovulatory disorders in 33%, 40% unexplained, and 6% due to endometriosis [2].

It is unknown if the prevalence is increasing; however, more couples are seeking evaluation. In 1995, 15% of women reported ever using an infertility service compared with 12% in 1988 [3]. Thus, infertility is commonly encountered by the primary physician. Proper evaluation, counseling, treatment, and referral are critical to the timely delivery of care to these patients.

Fortunately, the evaluation is straightforward. The basic assessment includes 1) evaluation of the presence and quality of ovulation, 2) the quality of the eggs, 3) the identification of any anatomic factors, 4) the evaluation of the male partner, and 5) the adequacy of intercourse.

The entire workup can generally be accomplished within 2 to 6 weeks. Younger women with relatively short duration of infertility, 1 to 2 years, may opt for an incremental workup. Women approaching advanced reproductive age and couples with long-standing infertility should have an aggressive workup.

Normal Fertility

With increasing age, oocytes are depleted and become more frequently genetically abnormal. Thus, normal fecundability (pregnancy rate per month) is largely related to the age of the female partner. Figure 20-2 demonstrates the relationship of age and reproductive performance, and can serve as a useful illustration of what pregnancy rates are to be expected at different ages. Data from in vitro fertilization also show a significant decline in fecundability, most notably in the mid-to-late 30s. The average last spontaneous pregnancy for women not using contraception is in the early 40s.

History

The backbone of the infertility evaluation remains the patient history. A directed and detailed history of the couple can usually identify the likely underlying cause(s) (Figures 20-3 and 20-4). For example, a patient whose cycles have recently shortened from every 28 days to every 24 days is at risk for having diminished ovarian reserve, or possibly a short luteal phase. She will require aggressive workup and possibly a referral to a specialist. Women with secondary dysmenorrhea and infertility have an 80% chance of having endometriosis [4].

A history of sexually transmitted infections is a common cause of infertility. In 2005, nearly one million cases of Chlamydia trachomatis and more than 300,000 cases of Neisseria gonorrhoeae were reported in the United States. These rates have increased yearly and are thought to underestimate the actual disease incidence. The majority of these cases were women, and, even worse, by far the highest infection rates were seen in women younger than 19 years old—before fertility is a significant concern [5]. Fifteen percent of these women can be expected to develop pelvic inflammatory disease. One episode of pelvic inflammatory disease causes infertility in 10% to 15% of women. Two episodes increase the risk to 25%.

Environmental Factors

Tobacco, alcohol, and drugs have been implicated in infertility. Male and female smoking reduces monthly pregnancy rates and success with in vitro fertilization [6–10]. Women who smoke are at increased risk for diminished ovarian reserve [11,12]. Even second-hand smoke decreases fertility [13]. Marijuana has an inhibitory effect on the hypothalamus and recent use is associated with decreased female fertility and in vitro fertilization success [14,15]. Alcohol abuse has been associated with decreased sperm parameters. Environmental toxins such as mercury, lead, pesticides and industrial pollutants also negatively affect sperm parameters. Heat impairs spermato-

genesis. Frequent sauna and hot tub baths are associated with reversible decreased sperm counts [16,17]. Choice of underwear does not affect sperm [18].

Pathophysiology of Female Infertility

For normal pregnancy to occur, a woman must ovulate. Within the 12 to 24 hours, the egg must be fertilized inside the fallopian tube. The resulting embryo enters the uterus on or about post-ovulation day 5. A receptive uterine lining promotes implantation.

The normal menstrual cycle varies from 24 to 35 days, and consists of three phases: the follicular phase, ovulation, and the luteal phase. A cohort of follicles emerges for selection during the late luteal phase of the preceding cycle. These follicles would undergo atresia, but are rescued by follicle-stimulating hormone (FSH), which rises in the early follicular phase. The follicle most responsive to FSH upregulates its own FSH receptors and grows despite the decreasing FSH levels. Other, slightly less-mature, follicles do not survive this decline in FSH. Rising estradiol from the dominant follicle results in a luteinizing hormone (LH) surge. Ovulation occurs approximately 36 hours after the initiation of the surge, and the ovulated follicle forms the corpus

Expected Cumulative Pregnancy Rates in Couples of Reproductive Age	
Months of Unprotected Sex	Pregnant, %
3	57
6	72
12	85
24	93

Figure 20-1. Expected cumulative pregnancy rates in couples of reproductive age. (*Adapted from* Guttmacher [56].)

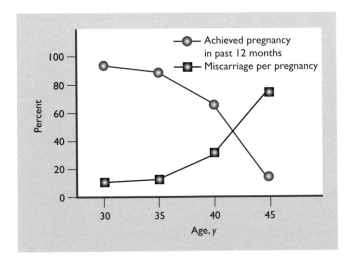

Figure 20-2. Age and fertility. (*Adapted from* Stein [58].)

History and Examination of the Male Partner

Male history
  Past reproductive history
  Sexual dysfunction
  Congenital issues: cryptorchidism, hypospadias, hernia
  Infectious history: mumps after puberty, prostatitis
  Trauma, torsion, testicular pain
  Previous semen analysis
  Previous urologic analysis
  History of frequent saunas, hot tubs, or other toxins
  Smoking, alcohol, or marijuana use
  Medications
  Medical history
  Surgical history (vasectomy/reversal)
Male physical
  Body: rule out eunuchoid habitus
  Rule out anomaly: microphallus, hypospadias
  Testicular size and consistency (should be firm)
  Palpate vas deferens
  Check for masses
  Check for varicocele
  Masculinization (appropriate hair distribution)

Figure 20-3. History and examination of the male partner.

luteum and begins producing large amounts of progesterone to prevent menses.

Conception is possible if intercourse occurred within the 5 days leading up to ovulation; however, intercourse after ovulation rarely results in pregnancy. If pregnancy occurs, human chorionic gonadotrophin is produced by the trophoblast and stimulates the corpus luteum to continue progesterone production. If pregnancy does not occur, if human chorionic gonadotrophin levels are inadequate or if the corpus luteum fails, then progesterone levels drop and menses ensue. In a normal pregnancy, the placenta begins to make progesterone in significant amounts by week 7 and can maintain a pregnancy without a corpus luteum by week 9. Any disruption in these events can result in infertility.

Evaluation of Ovulation

HISTORY

Ovulation is strongly suggested by a history of regular, predictable menses heralded by mid-cycle ovulatory pain (Mittelschmerz) and premenstrual molimina (breast tenderness, mood change, acne, or bloating). However, because some women with regular menses are actually anovulatory, ovulation should be confirmed by another method.

CERVICAL MUCUS

Just before ovulation, estrogen levels rise dramatically and cause an increase in water content of the cervical mucus, making it thin and stretchy. In women with documented ovulation and normal fertility, this can be a useful indicator that ovulation is impending within the next few days. This is a pre-ovulatory event. It does not confirm ovulation. In some anovulatory women, estrogen levels may rise because of a cohort of follicles that starts to develop. Cervical mucus may be thin, but the women fail to ovulate. They have menses when estrogen falls due to atresia of the cohort of follicles.

URINARY OVULATION PREDICTOR KITS

Several kits (OPKs) are produced for home use and they have a high sensitivity for ovulation detection [19–21]. The kit detects urinary levels of LH and turns positive when the hormone level is consistent with the mid-cycle surge. Ovulation generally occurs 0 to 48 hours after detection. To obtain the most accurate results, instruct the patient to discard the first morning urine sample. Women with regular predictable menses should start testing daily at 17 days before the onset of next menses. Women taking an ovulation induction agent should start testing 2 to 3 days after the last pill. Clomiphene raises LH and may result in a false-positive test.

History and Examination of the Female Partner

Female history
  Pregnancy history and complications
  Cycle length and characteristics
  Duration of infertility
  Coital frequency, timing, and sexual difficulties, including dyspareunia
  Gynecologic history: pelvic pain, dysmenorrhea, dyspareunia, sexually transmitted infections
  Prior work-up including ovulation assessment, tubal assessment, sperm assessment
  Past/current medical history
  Past surgical history
  Endocrine: galactorrhea, fatigue, constipation (thyroid symptoms), hirsutism, hot flashes, recent weight changes
  Tobacco, drug, and alcohol use history
  Employment (with focus on environmental exposures)
  Family history of infertility, birth defects, or heritable disorders
  Medicines: including any over-the-counter medicine or herbs
Female examination
  General: height, weight, BMI, blood pressure
  Skin: acanthosis nigricans, hirsutism (insulin or androgen excess)
  EENT: exophthalmos, thyroidomegaly or nodule (thyroid disease)
  Chest: galactorrhea (hyperprolactinemia)
  Pelvic examination: masses, tenderness, vaginal discharge, nodularity
  Reflexes: delayed relaxation associated with thyroid disease

Figure 20-4. History and examination of the female partner. BMI—body mass index; EENT—eyes, ears, nose, and throat.

For anovulatory women not on treatment, OPKs have little value. Monthly use of OPKs is not necessary and has not been shown to achieve pregnancy faster than would be seen with intercourse two to three times per week.

Ovulation prediction kits are useful to 1) plan timing of artificial insemination or 2) to help couples alter incompatible work schedules to allow for intercourse. OPKs also can identify a short luteal phase.

Salivary Ovulation Predictor Kits

Salivary ferning theoretically correlates with the preovulatory rise in estradiol. Pocket microscopes are available to assess salivary ferning. Sadly, the sensitivity and specificity of these OPKs are poor and even predict ovulation in men and postmenopausal women; therefore, they are not recommended [22,23].

Serum progesterone is the most commonly misinterpreted test that confirms ovulation. Progesterone levels peak 7 to 8 days after the LH surge. Levels greater than 3 ng/mL are consistent with ovulation [24]. Many practitioners are under the impression that progesterone levels must be 10 ng/mL to conclude that ovulation has occurred. However, progesterone secretion is pulsatile, and can vary markedly within minutes between 2.3 and 40 ng/dL [25]. Therefore, a single-serum progesterone should not be used to document the quality of ovulation. A more important gauge of ovulatory quality is the duration of the luteal phase.

ULTRASOUND

In rare cases, the LH surge promotes luteinization, but does not induce follicle rupture [19]. Thus, the gold standard for ovulation detection is ultrasound. Serial sonographic examinations detect the presence of a growing follicle, followed by collapse of the follicle. A small amount of fluid around the ovary or in the cul de sac indicates follicular rupture. Unfortunately, this testing is expensive and impractical for most couples.

BASAL BODY TEMPERATURE

Basal body temperature (BBT) is the body's temperature at rest and is best detected on waking, before rising. Before ovulation, BBT generally range between 97°F to 98°F. Progesterone exerts a thermogenic effect on the hypothalamus resulting in an increase of 0.4° to 0.8°. Detecting this change requires a

specialized BBT thermometer. The typical ovulatory cycle is biphasic—uniformly low BBT followed by uniformly elevated BBT (Figure 20-5). Because temperature rises occur 1 to 3 days after ovulation, BBT charting is not useful for planning intercourse in the current cycle. Women with regular predictable menses can use BBT to predict ovulation in upcoming cycles. Aside from documenting probable ovulation, the major advantages to performing BBT are the costs, and that it can help identify a luteal phase that is too short.

ENDOMETRIAL BIOPSY

In the past, the endometrial biopsy was used to diagnose a luteal phase defect; however, convincing literature has debunked the biopsy as a reliable tool for that purpose [26,27]. Biopsy can rule out chronic endometritis and determine if progesterone has transformed the endometrium into a secretory pattern. Given its cost and discomfort, it is not recommended as a test of ovulation.

Some practitioners will perform a timed biopsy to test for αvβ3 integrin, a marker of uterine receptivity. Though aberrations in αvβ3 expression are frequently encountered in women with infertility [28,29], there are few data to guide management of women deficient in this protein.

EVALUATION OF THE LUTEAL PHASE

The luteal phase defect is an elusive diagnosis. For years, the cornerstone of luteal sufficiency was the endometrial biopsy, but it is no longer considered a valid tool [26,27,30]. A single serum progesterone greater than 10 ng/mL obtained 7 days before the onset of menses is frequently used as evidence of adequate ovulation. Unfortunately, given the pulsatile nature of progesterone secretion, a single well-timed sample can be quite variable [25]. Even when using clomiphene, progesterone levels yield little value other than confirming the presence of ovulation, because the progesterone level may be the result of multiple simultaneous ovulations.

The best indicator of luteal sufficiency may be the duration of the luteal phase. An 11-day temperature elevation or 13 days between ovulation detection by an OPK and the onset of menses can be considered adequate [25,31]. If the luteal phase is short, evaluate and correct any thyroid or prolactin disorder. If that fails to restore a normal luteal phase, ovulation enhancement with clomiphene may be indicated.

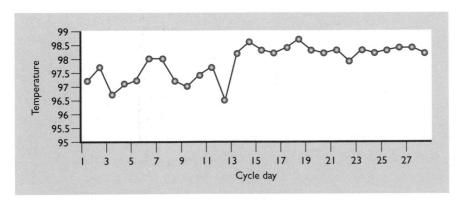

Figure 20-5. Ovulatory basal body temperature chart.

Evaluation of the Anovulatory Patient

If ovulation is not confirmed, one must determine the cause. Usually anovulation is caused by polycystic ovarian syndrome (PCOS), followed by hypogonadotropic hypogonadism, hypergonadotropic hypogonadism, thyroid disorder, or hyperprolactinemia.

Initial testing includes a pregnancy test, a fasting serum prolactin, and thyroid stimulating hormone. Oligo- and amenorrheic patients should receive 10 days of a progestin. Normal menses after the progestin challenge indicates eugonadotropic anovulation and should prompt a work-up for PCOS versus adult-onset congenital adrenal hyperplasia.

Scant menses or a failure to menstruate within 5 to 10 days of the progestin frequently indicates the patient has hypergonadotropic hypogonadism or hypogonadotropic hypogonadism. In rare cases, a severely androgenized woman may also fail to have a withdrawal bleed. FSH, LH, and estradiol levels will lead to the correct diagnosis (Figure 20-6).

Diagnosing Polycystic Ovarian Syndrome

The PCOS diagnosis has confounded physicians ever since it was first identified. Throughout the years, various criteria have been used, altered, and abandoned to establish the diagnosis. The current definition of PCOS has weaknesses and does not satisfy all researchers or practitioners (Figure 20-7).

PCOS is more commonly being recognized as a metabolic disorder—an insulin-resistant state that confers an increased risk of diabetes and heart disease. Careless labeling of patients as having PCOS may have adverse health or life insurance consequences for patients.

The first step in the PCOS diagnosis is to ensure she meets the inclusion criteria. Equally important, one must exclude other causes. Elevated 17-hyrodroxyprogesterone acetate should prompt referral to a reproductive endocrinologist for

Two Strategies to Evaluate Anovulation

1) Check TSH, prolactin, and hCG

  Treat findings accordingly

2) Perform progestin challenge (10 mg medroxyprogesterone acetate for 10 days)

  If patient has normal bleeding, likely anovulatory: PCOS vs congenital adrenal hyperplasia

  If no or light bleeding, patient is likely hypoestrogenic (assuming patient has a normal outflow tract)

3) If hypoestrogenic: measure FSH, LH, and estradiol

  High FSH, LH, and low estradiol—diminished ovarian reserve or ovarian failure is likely

  Low normal (or low) FSH, LH, or low or normal estradiol—likely hypogonadotropic hypogonadism

OR

1) Measure: TSH, prolactin, hCG, FSH, LH, progesterone, estrogen, total testosterone, and DHEAS from the outset

  Treat thyroid and prolactin or pregnancy as indicated

  Elevated progesterone, ovulatory—oligo-ovulation is most likely diagnosis (likely will benefit from ovulation induction agent)

  High FSH, LH, and low estradiol—diminished ovarian reserve or ovarian failure is likely

  Normal or low FSH, LH, with normal or low estradiol and normal testosterone and DHEAS—likely hypogonadotropic hypogonadism

  Normal FSH, normal or slightly elevated LH, normal estradiol, high normal or modestly elevated androgens—PCOS likely

Figure 20-6. Anovulation evaluation: two approaches to the patient with anovulation. DHEAS— dehydroepiandrosterone sulfate; FSH—follicle-stimulating hormone; hCG— human chorionic gonadotrophin; LH—luteinizing hormone; PCOS—polycystic ovarian syndrome; TSH—thyroid-stimulating hormone.

Current Diagnostic Criteria for Polycystic Ovarian Syndrome

Patients must have two of the following:

1. Oligo- or anovulation

2. Clinical (hirsutism) or laboratory evidence of elevated androgens (elevated total testosterone, DHEAS, or free testosterone)

3. Polycystic ovaries (> 12 follicles measuring 2–9 mm on each ovary or ovarian volume > 10 cm³)

Exclusion of other diagnoses

Figure 20-7. Current diagnostic criteria for polycystic ovarian syndrome. DHEAS—dehydroepiandrosterone sulfate. (*Adapted from* Balen et al. [60].)

a confirmatory adrenocorticotropin hormone stimulation test to rule out congenital adrenal hyperplasia.

Androgen assays do not perform well in women. Androgens are most helpful in patients without rapid clinical changes (new onset hirsutism, temporal balding or signs of virilization) or if they have little clinical evidence of hyperandrogenism—as can be the case with Asians and American Indians. In normally cycling women, androgens should be drawn in the follicular phase. In women with oligomenorrhea, laboratory samples can be obtained randomly; however, one also should measure serum progesterone to ensure that the sample was performed at the correct time.

Because of the pulsatile nature of LH, LH:FSH ratios are not in the current diagnosis, but a ratio of 2:1 is consistent with this diagnosis. Because it can be difficult to detect, insulin resistance is not part of the diagnosis. However, if basal insulin levels are elevated, if a patient has acanthosis nigricans or glucose intolerance based on a 2-hour glucose tolerance test, insulin resistance is affirmed and may increase patient compliance with lifestyle changes.

Evaluation of Egg Quality (Ovarian Reserve)

Diminished ovarian reserve (DOR) reflects a decreased number of or quality of oocytes. DOR indicates that all treatments have decreased success rates. Common tests include FSH and estradiol levels, the clomiphene citrate challenge test, and antral follicle counts.

HISTORY
Women who have developed hot flashes or shortened cycles are at increased risk for DOR. Other significant risk factors include: age older than 35 years, unexplained infertility, history of smoking, previous ovarian surgery, family history of premature ovarian failure, and prior chemotherapy or radiation exposure. Yearly testing is recommended for patients with these risk factors.

FOLLICLE-STIMULATING HORMONE
Follicle-stimulating hormone nadirs in the luteal phase, then rises in the early follicular phase. Serum levels should be measured on cycle day 2 or 3. Depending on the laboratory, an FSH level above 10 mIU/mL is considered evidence of DOR, and is an indication for referral to a reproductive endocrinologist [32,33]. Normal FSH levels not paired with estrogen levels or normal FSH levels outside this early window—especially in the luteal phase—have no clinical utility.

ESTRADIOL
Estradiol levels should be low (< 80 pg/mL) in the early follicular phase. A high estradiol is as predictive as a high FSH and should prompt referral to a specialist [34]. Elevated estrogen levels occur because of abnormal FSH levels in the preceding luteal phase [35]. Because high estradiol levels may suppress FSH levels, an isolated normal FSH on cycle day 3 is of little value.

CLOMIPHENE CITRATE CHALLENGE TEST
This stress test for the ovary adds sensitivity to the cycle day 3 laboratory samples. Clomiphene blocks estradiol at the hypothalamus, causing a commensurate release of FSH. A normal ovary responds to the FSH surge by making more estrogen, causing FSH to fall toward the normal range. A patient with DOR will not make enough estradiol to sufficiently suppress FSH. To perform the test, obtain baseline labs on cycle day 2 or 3. The patient then takes clomiphene citrate 100 mg daily for 5 days, beginning on cycle day 5. On cycle day 10 or 11, she returns for a repeat FSH. An FSH > 12 mIU/mL reflects DOR [33].

If any of these tests are abnormal, a patient's prognosis is not changed by subsequent normal testing. Her outcome is not improved by waiting to initiate treatment in a cycle that shows a normal FSH. Finally, age alone is a strong predictor of fertility, that is, normal testing in a 45-year-old woman does not alter her poor prognosis.

ANTRAL FOLLICLE COUNTS
This ultrasonographic test is performed on cycle day 3. Antral follicles are 2 to 5 mm in diameter and reflect the pool of eggs available for ovulation in a given month. Fewer than five total follicles predicts a high cancellation rate with in vitro fertilization [36]. The predictive value of antral follicle counts is unknown for treatments other than in vitro fertilization. However, a timely ultrasound performed by the generalist may result earlier referral to a specialist.

Anatomic Evaluation

HISTORY
The differential diagnosis for anatomic pathology is quite variable. Heavy bleeding, palpable mass, and pelvic pressure suggest the presence of fibroids. Dysmenorrhea combined with infertility strongly suggests endometriosis. Dyspareunia may represent adenomyosis, endometritis, endometriosis, fibroids or even hypoestrogenic states. A history of sexually transmitted disease should prompt evaluation of the tubal anatomy.

POSTCOITAL TEST
Traditionally, the postcoital test is performed within 12 hours of intercourse, which was timed just before ovulation. The woman undergoes a pelvic examination with aspiration of cervical mucus. Thick cervical mucus and immotile or dead sperm indicate a positive test. Lacking sensitivity, specificity, standardization, and reproducibility, the postcoital test has been abandoned by most specialists [37,38].

HYSTEROSALPINGOGRAM
The hysterosalpingogram is commonly used to evaluate tubal anatomy. During the follicular phase, the uterus is instilled

with a radio-opaque dye. Simultaneous fluoroscopic evaluation assesses intracavitary lesions and tubal patency. Rapid filling of the uterus can obscure polyps and fibroids and can result in tubal spasm, which can lead to misdiagnoses.

Proper interpretation is as important as technique. The initial portion of the tube should be thin. Distally, the tube widens. Linear densities suggest normal rugation. The spill pattern should be diffuse. Small spicules in the proximal tube indicate salpingitis isthmic nodosa. Asymmetry and collections of dye may indicate pelvic adhesions from endometriosis or pelvic inflammatory disease.

The overall sensitivity and specificity for hysterosalpingogram are 65% and 83% for tubal patency [39]. Much of the test's low sensitivity comes from incorrectly diagnosing tubal spasm as tubal blockage. Distal and mid-tubal occlusions are more likely to be associated with genuine pathology.

ULTRASOUND AND SONOHYSTOGRAM

Ultrasound can identify conditions associated with infertility, such as fibroids, polyps, endometriomas and on occasion, hydrosalpinges. Submucous myomas and fibroids larger than 4 cm are associated with decreased fertility [40]. The simultaneous injection of sterile water into the uterine cavity at the time of ultrasound increases the sensitivity for intracavitary lesions. Sonohysterography is nearly as sensitive as hysteroscopy and is better tolerated than hysteroscopy and hysterosalpingogram [41,42].

Sonography performed with Doppler or saline mixed with air can detect tubal patency and blockages [43,44]; however, this test fails to detect salpingitis isthmic nodosa and other subtle defects.

ANTICHLAMYDIAL ANTIBODIES

Serum antibodies to *C. trachomatis* help identify women at risk for tubal disease despite a history negative for sexually transmitted disease. In infertile women, *Chlamydia* serology is approximately 70.0% sensitive and 70.0% to 93.0% specific at detecting tubal disease. The positive predictive value is has high as 94% with a negative predictive value of 60% to 70% [39,45–47]. This test is probably best suited for women with unexplained infertility. The presence of such antibodies could justify diagnostic laparoscopy for subtle, occult adhesions.

LAPAROSCOPY AND HYSTEROSCOPY

These are the gold standards by which other diagnostic tests are evaluated. Hysteroscopy and laparoscopy permit direct anatomic visualization and give an opportunity to address underlying pathology.

At laparoscopy, careful systematic inspection of the peritoneal surfaces, tubes, ovaries, ovarian fossa, appendix, and the liver edge can detect endometriosis. Tubes with thickened and stiff isthmic portions may have salpingitis isthmic nodosa. When performing chromopertubation, proper technique minimizes erroneous results. Rapid instillation with indigo carmine can cause tubal spasm, which would falsely be interpreted as tubal blockage. Devices with a balloon (such as a HUMI [Harris-Kronner Uterine Manipulator Injector; Cooper Surgical, Trumbull, CT]) also can result in spasm. Ideally, chromopertubation should be performed under low pressure through a Jarcho cannula.

Neither hysteroscopy nor laparoscopy permits intratubal visualization. Some specialists do perform falloposcopy and salpingoscopy for direct visualization of the proximal and distal tubes. Although these techniques occasionally do find abnormalities not detected by other methods, they have not gained widespread acceptance in the United States.

Differential Diagnosis of Male Factor Infertility

Hypothalamic disease
  Kallmann's syndrome—GnRH neurons
  Anorexia—decreases GnRH
  Tumor
Pituitary disease
  Hyperprolactinemia—decreases GnRH
  Pituitary mass—increases PRL
  Empty sella—hernia into pituitary fossa suppresses FSH, LH
  Isolated LH deficiency
  Isolated FSH deficiency
  Infiltrating diseases (hemochromatosis, sarcoidosis)
Testicular disease (uncorrectable)
  Testicular failure
  Sertoli-only syndrome (germ cell aplasia)
  Y-chromosome microdeletions
  Injury (torsion, orchitis, cryptorchidism, varicocele)
Post-testicular causes
  Congenital blockages
    Congenital bilateral absence of the vas deferens
    Ejaculatory duct obstruction
    Polycystic kidney disease (associated)
    Idiopathic
  Functional obstruction
    Retrograde ejaculation
    Sympathetic nerve damage
  Acquired obstruction
  Vasectomy
  Epididymitis
  Groin surgery
Other
  Exogenous anabolic steroid abuse
  History of radiation to head or testis
  History of chemotherapy

Figure 20-8. Differential diagnosis of male factor infertility. FSH—follicle-stimulating hormone; GnRH—gonadotrophin-releasing hormone; LH—luteinizing hormone; PRL—prolactin.

Pathophysiology of Male Factor Infertility

Approximately 45% of male factor infertility is idiopathic, 35% testicular, 15% post-testicular, and 1% to 2% pre-testicular [48]. The goals of evaluation are to distinguish normal males from men with 1) correctable infertility, 2) uncorrectable factors that can be overcome by using assisted reproductive technologies, versus 3) uncorrectable factors not suitable for assisted reproductive technologies that may require adoption versus donor sperm.

Sperm production is a continuous process beginning during puberty and continuing throughout life. A set number of spermatogonia will give rise to all the sperm. GnRH stimulates pituitary FSH and LH release. FSH promotes spermatogenesis.

When the spermatogonia divides, one cell proceeds through mitotic division and maturation to become sperm, while the other returns to the resting pool. As sperm are produced, Sertoli cells release inhibin, which exerts negative feedback on FSH. (Men with high FSH are unlikely producing sperm, even if testosterone is normal.) LH stimulates the Leydig cells to produce testosterone, which must be available in high local concentrations to promote the development of sperm.

Sperm development requires 72 days. Mature sperm are stored within the epididymis and are ejaculated through the vas deferens and urethra. The prostate gland and seminal vesicles contribute the majority of the ejaculate—the semen. The semen serves as a nutrient supply to the sperm and as a buffer against the acid produced by the vagina. During intercourse, sperm swim out of the semen, into the cervical mucus, and up to the fallopian tube.

Normal Semen Analysis Criteria

Semen Reference Ratings	WHO III	Guzick Fertile Range
Ejaculate volume	2–5 mL	
Concentration	> 20 million/mL	> 13.5 million/mL
Percent motile	> 50%	> 32%
Forward progression (0–4)	> 2	
pH	> 7.2	
Total sperm number	> 40 million	
Normal morphology	> 30%; > 14%*	> 9%

*Kruger (strict) criteria.

Figure 20-9. Normal semen analysis criteria. Azoospermia is defined as the absence of sperm. Asthenozoospermia is defined as poor motility. Oligospermia is defined as less than 200 million sperm per milliliter. Pyospermia is defined as increased white blood cells. Teratozoospermia is poor morphology. WHO—World Health Organization.

Chances of Infertility by Sperm Parameters

Odds Ratio for Infertility for Combination Sperm Parameters

Sperm Parameters			
Morphology	Motility	Concentration	Odds Ratio
Fertile	Fertile	Fertile	1.0
Subfertile	Fertile	Fertile	2.9
Fertile	Subfertile	Fertile	2.5
Fertile	Fertile	Subfertile	2.2
Subfertile	Subfertile	Fertile	7.2
Subfertile	Fertile	Subfertile	6.3
Fertile	Subfertile	Subfertile	5.5
Subfertile	Subfertile	Subfertile	15.8

Figure 20-10. Chances of infertility by sperm parameters. (Adapted from Guzick [49].)

Causes of Specific Sperm Deficits

	Oligospermia	Asthenozoospermia	Teratozoospermia
Varicocele	Associated	Associated	Associated
Antisperm antibodies		Associated	
Genetic abnormalities	Associated		
Hormonal imbalance	Associated		

Figure 20-11. Causes of specific sperm deficits.

Anatomic factors, such as congenital bilateral absence of the vas deferens, or varicocele, or disruptions along the hypothalamic-pituitary-testes axis may result in faulty spermatogenesis, decreased sperm quantity or quality (Figure 20-8).

History
Essential elements of the history include reproductive history, libido, previous infections, injury to the genitalia, hernia, mumps after puberty, and steroid abuse.

Semen Analysis
Not all semen analyses are created equal. Aside from diagnosing severe oligozoospermia or severe asthenospermia many hospital-based analyses have little utility. At a minimum, facilities should follow the World Health Organization III criteria (Figure 20-9). Preferably, men would receive their analyses at a fertility center capable of performing even more advanced analysis. A frequently encountered problem at fertility centers is that the first semen analysis failed to diagnose subtle but significant deficiencies in sperm quality.

The semen analysis is collected between a 2- to 5-day period of abstinence. Patients collect by masturbation without using lubrication. Latex-free condoms are available to collect via intercourse. Samples collected at home should be kept at room temperature and delivered to the lab within the hour. If the first semen analysis is abnormal, a second test should be performed 4 to 8 weeks later. Pyospermia (high white blood cell counts) should be treated with a course of antibiotics for presumed prostatitis or epididymitis.

Except in cases of gonadal failure associated with azoospermia, there is no semen parameter that excludes possible conception. In the absence of extreme abnormalities, the three semen parameters that best predict whether a man's sperm is likely to fertilize an egg are sperm concentration, percent motile, and sperm morphology (Figure 20-10) [49].

Figure 20-11 and the algorithm in Figure 20-12 will delineate most causes. Patients will fall into one of three categories: eugonadal, hypogonadotropic hypogonal, or hypogonadotropic hypogonadal (Figure 20-13). Hypogonadotropic hypogonadal men usually have spermatogonia and simply need the right hormonal stimulus to produce sperm. Injectable gonadotropins such as FSH or human chorionic gonadotrophin generally restore fertility. Hypergonadotropic hypogonadism indicates gonadal failure, which can be confirmed by testicular

biopsy and indicates that donor sperm or adoption is required. Eugonadal (normogonadotropic) men can have quite variable causes—varicocele, functional blockages (retrograde ejaculation), actual blockages (congenital bilateral absence of the vas deferens, or ejaculatory duct obstruction, epididymal obstruction), or genetic abnormalities.

In cases of normogonadotropic azoospermia, sufficient sperm can often be harvested from the testes by means of testicular biopsy, percutaneous epididymal sperm aspiration, microscopic epididymal sperm aspiration, or testicular sperm extraction. In vitro fertilization with intracytoplasmic sperm injection can be accomplished by using sperm or spermatids extracted from the testes [50].

Men with sperm concentrations less than 5 million/mL should be offered genetic testing. Approximately 5% of these men have karyotype abnormalities. Ten percent have a microdeletion of the Y chromosome (MDY) [51]. MDY mutations are not detectable by karyotype and occur in regions of the Y-chromosome that carry DAZ (deleted in azoospermia) genes.

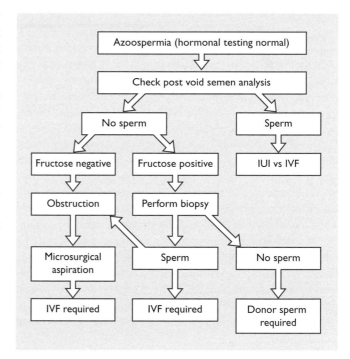

Figure 20-12. Algorithm for evaluating azoospermia. IUI—intrauterine insemination; IVF—in vitro fertilization.

Hormonal Profiles of Normal and Abnormal Spermatogenesis

Condition	FSH	LH	Testosterone	Prolactin
Normal spermatogenesis	Normal	Normal	Normal	Normal
Hypogonadotropic hypogonadism	Low	Low	Low	Normal
Abnormal spermatogenesis	High/normal	Normal	Normal	Normal
Testicular failure	High	High	Normal/low	Normal
Prolactinoma	Normal/low	Normal/low	Low	High

Figure 20-13. Hormonal profiles of normal and abnormal spermatogenesis. (*Adapted from* American Urological Association [59].)

Other Sperm Tests

Antisperm antibodies reduce fecundity, but do not exclude pregnancy. Risk factors include history of obstruction, genital surgery, trauma, or infection. Tests for antisperm antibodies should be obtained when sperm demonstrate agglutination or isolated asthenospermia.

Sperm chromatin structure assay is a test of DNA fragmentation. Up to 8% of infertile men with normal sperm parameters will have abnormal fragmentation [52]. Men with high levels of fragmentation have decreased fertility and increased risk of miscarriage [53,54]. In the largest case series to date, high DNA fragmentation indicates patients have lower success rates with artificial insemination and may benefit from in vitro fertilization with intracytoplasmic sperm injection [55]. Currently, sperm chromatin structure assay is not recommended for routine testing; however, patients should be counseled to avoid gonadotoxins that increase fragmentation (tobacco, hot tubs, and so forth) [52].

Adequacy of Intercourse

Sexual dysfunction, anatomic anomalies, and patient misunderstanding of proper timing and method of intercourse can lead to difficulty conceiving. Erectile or ejaculatory dysfunction may require pharmacologic or psychologic intervention. Hypospadias or microphallus result in sperm not being deposited high inside the vagina.

The physician should inquire about coital frequency, route, timing and use of lubricants. Many lubricants have spermicidal qualities and their use should be discouraged [56]. Optimal intercourse occurs within the 5 days preceding ovulation, with maximum fecundability occurring on the day of ovulation. Intercourse timed to the luteal phase rarely results in pregnancy. Vaginal intercourse two to three times per week should be adequate even without determining the day of ovulation. Young couples who practice infrequent intercourse and have infertility of a short duration may be managed expectantly after proper counseling. If couples have long-standing infertility, 2 or more years, or are of advancing reproductive age, a complete work-up is appropriate.

On occasion, we encounter couples who may have frequent intercourse, but rarely is it vaginal. If you are uncomfortable inquiring about the route of intercourse, you should emphasize this fundamental principle when counseling.

When to Refer

Any couple that requires therapy beyond what is offered in your clinic should be referred to a reproductive endocrinologist. Couples with long-standing unexplained infertility, moderate-to-severe male factor, women of advancing reproductive age or diminished ovarian reserve, or couples who have been adequately treated for 6 months and yet do not conceive should be offered aggressive work-up and referral.

Timely referral reduces patient frustration. In our practice patients who initiated the referral themselves frequently ask for referral to a new primary physician once they are pregnant.

References

1. Centers for Disease Control and Prevention: *2004 Assisted Reproductive Technology Success Rates*. Atlanta: Centers for Disease Control and Prevention; 2006.

2. Cates W, Farley TM, Rowe PJ: Worldwide patterns of infertility: is Africa different? *Lancet* 1985, 2:596–598.

3. Ingram DD PJ, Schenker N, Weed JA, *et al.*: United States Census 2000 population with bridged race categories. National Center for Health Statistics. *Vital Health Stat* 2003, 2:135.

4. Koninckx PR, Meuleman C, Demeyere S, *et al.*: Suggestive evidence that pelvic endometriosis is a progressive disease, whereas deeply infiltrating endometriosis is associated with pelvic pain. *Fertil Steril* 1991, 55:759–765.

5. *Sexually Transmitted Disease Surveillance 2005 Supplement, Chlamydia Prevalence Monitoring Project Annual Report 2005*. Atlanta: US Department of Health and Human Services, Centers for Disease Control and Prevention; 2006.

6. Joesbury KA, Edirisinghe WR, Phillips MR, Yovich JL: Evidence that male smoking affects the likelihood of a pregnancy following IVF treatment: application of the modified cumulative embryo score. *Hum Reprod* 1998, 13:1506–1513.

7. Schmidt F: [Smoking damages male fertility]. *Andrologia* 1986, 18:445–454.

8. Augood C, Duckitt K, Templeton AA: Smoking and female infertility: a systematic review and meta-analysis. *Hum Reprod* 1998, 13:1532–1539.

9. Klonoff-Cohen H: Female and male lifestyle habits and IVF: what is known and unknown. *Hum Reprod Update* 2005, 11:179–203.

10. Soares SR, Simon C, Remohi J, Pellicer A: Cigarette smoking affects uterine receptiveness. *Hum Reprod* 2007, 22:543–547.

11. Sepaniak S, Forges T, Monnier-Barbarino P: [Cigarette smoking and fertility in women and men]. *Gynecol Obstet Fertil* 2006, 34:945–949.

12. Sharara FI, Beatse SN, Leonardi MR, *et al.*: Cigarette smoking accelerates the development of diminished ovarian reserve as evidenced by the clomiphene citrate challenge test. *Fertil Steril* 1994, 62:257–262.

13. Neal MS, Hughes EG, Holloway AC, Foster WG: Side-stream smoking is equally as damaging as mainstream smoking on IVF outcomes. *Hum Reprod* 2005, 20:2531–2535.

14. Mueller BA, Daling JR, Weiss NS, Moore DE: Recreational drug use and the risk of primary infertility. *Epidemiology* 1990, 1:195–200.

15. Klonoff-Cohen HS, Natarajan L, Chen RV: A prospective study of the effects of female and male marijuana use on in vitro fertilization (IVF) and gamete intrafallopian transfer (GIFT) outcomes. *Am J Obstet Gynecol* 2006, 194:369–376.

16. Saikhun J, Kitiyanant Y, Vanadurongwan V, Pavasuthipaisit K: Effects of sauna on sperm movement characteristics of normal men measured by computer-assisted sperm analysis. *Int J Androl* 1998, 21:358–363.

17. Brown-Woodman PD, Post EJ, Gass GC, White IG: The effect of a single sauna exposure on spermatozoa. *Arch Androl* 1984, 12:9–15.

18. Munkelwitz R, Gilbert BR: Are boxer shorts really better? A critical analysis of the role of underwear type in male subfertility. *J Urol* 1998, 160:1329–1333.

19. Crosignani PG, Rubin BL: Optimal use of infertility diagnostic tests and treatments. The ESHRE Capri Workshop Group. *Hum Reprod* 2000, 15:723–732.

20. Behre HM, Kuhlage J, Gassner C, et al.: Prediction of ovulation by urinary hormone measurements with the home use ClearPlan Fertility Monitor: comparison with transvaginal ultrasound scans and serum hormone measurements. *Hum Reprod* 2000, 15:2478–2482.

21. Ghazeeri GS, Vongprachanh P, Kutteh WH: The predictive value of five different urinary LH kits in detecting the LH surge in regularly menstruating women. *Int J Fertil Womens Med* 2000, 45:321–326.

22. Guida M, Tommaselli GA, Palomba S, et al.: Efficacy of methods for determining ovulation in a natural family planning program. *Fertil Steril* 1999, 72:900–904.

23. Braat DD, Smeenk JM, Manger AP, et al.: Saliva test as ovulation predictor. *Lancet* 1998, 352:1283–1284.

24. Wathen NC, Perry L, Lilford RJ, Chard T: Interpretation of single progesterone measurement in diagnosis of anovulation and defective luteal phase: observations on analysis of the normal range. *Br Med J (Clin Res Ed)* 1984, 288:7–9.

25. Filicori M, Butler JP, Crowley WF, Jr.: Neuroendocrine regulation of the corpus luteum in the human: evidence for pulsatile progesterone secretion. *J Clin Invest* 1984, 73:1638–1647.

26. Coutifaris C, Myers ER, Guzick DS, et al.: Histological dating of timed endometrial biopsy tissue is not related to fertility status. *Fertil Steril* 2004, 82:1264–1272.

27. Murray MJ, Meyer WR, Zaino RJ, et al.: A critical analysis of the accuracy, reproducibility, and clinical utility of histologic endometrial dating in fertile women. *Fertil Steril* 2004, 81:1333–1343.

28. Lessey BA, Castelbaum AJ, Sawin SW, et al.: Aberrant integrin expression in the endometrium of women with endometriosis. *J Clin Endocrinol Metab* 1994, 79:643–649.

29. Lessey BA: Endometrial integrins and the establishment of uterine receptivity. *Hum Reprod* 1998, 13(Suppl 3):247–258; discussion 259–261.

30. Myers ER, Silva S, Barnhart K, et al.: Interobserver and intraobserver variability in the histological dating of the endometrium in fertile and infertile women. *Fertil Steril* 2004, 82:1278-1282.

31. Strott CA, Cargille CM, Ross GT, Lipsett MB: The short luteal phase. *J Clin Endocrinol Metab* 1970, 30:246–251.

32. Scott RT, Toner JP, Muasher SJ, et al.: Follicle-stimulating hormone levels on cycle day 3 are predictive of in vitro fertilization outcome. *Fertil Steril* 1989, 51:651–654.

33. Scott RT, Jr., Hofmann GE: Prognostic assessment of ovarian reserve. *Fertil Steril* 1995, 63:1–11.

34. Smotrich DB, Widra EA, Gindoff PR, et al.: Prognostic value of day 3 estradiol on in vitro fertilization outcome. *Fertil Steril* 1995, 64:1136–1140.

35. Sharara FI, Scott RT, Jr., Seifer DB: The detection of diminished ovarian reserve in infertile women. *Am J Obstet Gynecol* 1998, 179:804–812.

36. Frattarelli JL, Levi AJ, Miller BT, Segars JH: A prospective assessment of the predictive value of basal antral follicles in in vitro fertilization cycles. *Fertil Steril* 2003, 80:350–355.

37. De Sutter P: Rational diagnosis and treatment in infertility. *Best Pract Res Clin Obstet Gynaecol* 2006, 20:647–664.

38. Grimes DA: Validity of the postcoital test. *Am J Obstet Gynecol* 1995, 172:1327.

39. Evers JL, Land JA, Mol BW: Evidence-based medicine for diagnostic questions. *Semin Reprod Med* 2003, 21:9–15.

40. Oliveira FG, Abdelmassih VG, Diamond MP, et al.: Impact of subserosal and intramural uterine fibroids that do not distort the endometrial cavity on the outcome of in vitro fertilization-intracytoplasmic sperm injection. *Fertil Steril* 2004, 81:582–587.

41. Guimaraes Filho HA, Mattar R, Pires CR, et al.: Comparison of hysterosalpingography, hysterosonography and hysteroscopy in evaluation of the uterine cavity in patients with recurrent pregnancy losses. *Arch Gynecol Obstet* 2006, 274:284–288.

42. Lopez Navarrete JA, Herrera Otero JM, Quiroga Feuchter G, et al.: [Comparison between hysterosonography and hysterosalpinography in the study of endometrial abnormalities in infertility patients]. *Ginecol Obstet Mex* 2003, 71:277–283.

43. Hoffman L, Chan K, Smith B, Okolo S: The value of saline salpingosonography as a surrogate test of tubal patency in low-resource settings. *Int J Fertil Womens Med* 2005, 50:135–139.

44. Exacoustos C, Zupi E, Carusotti C, et al.: Hysterosalpingo-contrast sonography compared with hysterosalpingography and laparoscopic dye perturbation to evaluate tubal patency. *J Am Assoc Gynecol Laparosc* 2003, 10:367–372.

45. Perquin DA, Beersma MF, de Craen AJ, Helmerhorst FM: The value of *Chlamydia trachomatis*–specific IgG antibody testing and hysterosalpingography for predicting tubal pathology and occurrence of pregnancy. *Fertil Steril* 2007, [Epub].

46. Keltz MD, Gera PS, Moustakis M: *Chlamydia* serology screening in infertility patients. *Fertil Steril* 2006, 85:752–754.

47. den Hartog JE, Land JA, Stassen FR, et al.: The role of chlamydia genus-specific and species-specific IgG antibody testing in predicting tubal disease in subfertile women. *Hum Reprod* 2004, 19:1380–1384.

48. Turek P: *Male Infertility*, edn 16. New York: McGraw-Hill; 2004.

49. Guzick DS, Overstreet JW, Factor-Litvak P, et al.: Sperm morphology, motility, and concentration in fertile and infertile men. *N Engl J Med* 2001, 345:1388–1393.

50. Mansour RT, Fahmy IM, Taha AK, et al.: Intracytoplasmic spermatid injection can result in the delivery of normal offspring. *J Androl* 2003, 24:757–764.

51. Dohle GR, Halley DJ, Van Hemel JO, et al.: Genetic risk factors in infertile men with severe oligozoospermia and azoospermia. *Hum Reprod* 2002, 17:13–16.

52. Committee AP: The clinical utility of sperm DNA integrity testing. *Fertil Steril* 2006, 86(Suppl 4):S35–S37.

53. Evenson DP, Darzynkiewicz Z, Melamed MR: Relation of mammalian sperm chromatin heterogeneity to fertility. *Science* 1980, 210:1131–1133.

54. Carrell DT, Liu L, Peterson CM, *et al.*: Sperm DNA fragmentation is increased in couples with unexplained recurrent pregnancy loss. *Arch Androl* 2003, 49:49–55.

55. Bungum M, Humaidan P, Axmon A, *et al.*: Sperm DNA integrity assessment in prediction of assisted reproduction technology outcome. *Hum Reprod* 2007, 22:174–179.

56. Kutteh WH, Chao CH, Ritter JO, Byrd W: Vaginal lubricants for the infertile couple: effect on sperm activity. *Int J Fertil Menopausal Stud* 1996, 41:400–404.

57. Guttmacher AF: Factors affecting normal expectancy of conception. *JAMA* 1956, 161:855.

58. Stein ZA: A woman's age: childbearing and childrearing. *Am J Epidemiol* 1985, 121:327.

59. American Urological Association: *Report on Optimal Evaluation of the Infertile Male.* Baltimore: American Urological Association; 2001.

60. Balen AH, Laven, JS, Tan ST, Dewailly D: Ultrasound assessment of polycystic ovary: international consensus definitions. *Hum Reprod Update.* 2003, 9:505–514.

21 | Hirsutism

Matthew A. Will

- Hirsutism is more than just a problem of cosmesis.
- The vast majority of patients affected have polycystic ovarian syndrome.
- Women with polycystic ovarian syndrome are at risk for several associated metabolic disorders.
- Differential diagnosis of hirsutism includes tumor or hyperfunctioning of the ovary, adrenals, and pituitary.
- Patients with hirsutism may require an initial work-up to rule out other underlying disorders, but rarely require a lengthy list of laboratory studies.
- Women should be counseled on the benefits of lifestyle modification and weight loss.
- Low-dose oral contraceptives and several adjunct medicines provide relief for hirsutism while also providing other noncontraceptive health benefits.

Epidemiology and Pathogenesis

Hirsutism, or excessive facial and body hair in socially undesirable areas, is a common gynecologic complaint. The incidence varies widely based on ethnicity and family history. Because of the subjective nature of its definition, true prevalence and incidence remain unknown. However, up to 33% to 69% of women 15 to 44 years of age and approximately 75% of women 60 years of age may have excessive facial hair [1,2].

Hirsutism is a complex problem in medicine that confronts not only internal pathology and genetic predispositions, but also cultural expectations and the woman's innate psychologic response. Excessive facial and body hair can be perceived as a threat to one's feminine nature, and still others may go undisturbed. However, regardless of the initial manifestation, appropriate evaluation and further recommendations for possible treatment should be undertaken by a care provider.

Hair growth is largely genetically predetermined. Hair may seem excessive depending on concentration and rate of growth, both of which vary greatly depending on ethnicity (Caucasian more than Asian; Mediterranean more than Nordic) [3]. Excessive hair growth that follows familial trends (or idiopathic hirsutism) is indicative of increased 5-α-reductase activity, the enzyme in skin responsible for peripherally converting testosterone to dihydrotestosterone (DHT). However, other causes such as polycystic ovarian syndrome (PCOS), nonclassical congenital adrenal hyperplasia, and some ovarian tumors associated with overall increased androgen production should be considered.

Rate and type of hair growth are dependent on multiple environmental factors; however, amount is established very early in life. By 22 weeks' gestation, total endowment of hair follicles is present and no new follicles are produced thereafter. Androgens, drugs, and other environmental cues thus influence rate, synchrony, and type of growth. Androgens, adrenal and ovarian, favor a transition from vellus (fine, unpigmented) to terminal hair (course, pigmented). Skin temperature, blood flow, and edema also can have an influence. Hence, in summer, hair grows faster than winter [3]. Certain drugs (cyclosporine, minoxidil, diazoxide, phenytoin) can induce hypertrichosis (generalized increase in fetal lanugo type hair) [4]. Pregnancy can increase the synchrony of hair growth leading to episodic growth or shedding.

As a woman's clinician, not only should one be concerned about excessive hair growth that may be disturbing to the individual but also the implications it may carry in regards to other aspects of their health. Those women with hirsute characteristics associated with polycystic ovarian syndrome who also carry several risk factors for coronary heart disease may be more prone to insulin-resistance and diabetes mellitus and suffer from reduced health-related quality of life [5–7].

Diagnosis

Hirsutism is a common problem among women, and the vast majority that are hyperandrogenic have PCOS. However, when a patient presents with the complaint of excessive hair growth, it is important as the clinician to elucidate characteristics of hair growth (location, shaving habits, past therapies attempted) as well as ask about other manifestations that would cue other underlying pathology. One should inquire about menstrual irregularities, other evidence of hyperandrogenism (acne, skin oiliness, or increased libido), total time of development, and the possible addition of any vitamin supplements or medicines. Other, less common, etiologies require consideration (Figure 21-1); however, unless other components in the clinical history indicate otherwise, expensive testing is usually unnecessary.

Differential Diagnosis for Hirsutism

Adrenal
  Congenital adrenal hyperplasia (21-hydroxylase, 3B-hydoxysteroid dehydrogenase, 11B-hydroxylase deficiencies)
  Cushing syndrome
    Corticotropin-dependent
      Pituitary excess (nontumor or tumor-related)
      Ectopic corticotropin-secreting tumor
    Corticotropin-independent
      Adrenal tumor (adenoma, carcinoma)
      Adrenal nodular hyperplasia
      Adrenal rest tumor of the ovary
      Exogenous corticoid administration
  Adrenal androgen-producing tumors (adenomas, carcinomas)
Thyroid
  Hyperthyroidism
  Hypothyroidism
Ovary
  Polycystic ovarian syndrome
  Androgen-secreting tumor (hilus cell, thecoma, Sertoli-Leydig cell tumor)
Hyperprolactinemia
Pregnancy-related
  Telogen effluvium
  Luteoma
  Theca-lutein cysts
Peripheral tissues
  Excess 5α-reductase and 17-ketosteroid reductase
Drugs and food supplements

Figure 21-1. Differential diagnosis for hirsutism.

A typical presentation for hirsutism is gradual onset. In its mildest forms, hair may present on the upper lip and chin. In more severe cases, it will appear on the cheeks, chest (intermammary), abdomen (superior to the umbilicus), inner aspects of thighs, and lower back and intergluteal areas.

A history of menstrual irregularities, if present, is often sufficient to suggest some endocrinologic disorder. Patients with PCOS are typically oligomenorrheic with onset of hirsutism occurring in their early 20s and may demonstrate physical findings such as central obesity and acanthosis nigricans. Presentation before menarche, most commonly as hypertrichosis, would suggest either PCOS or late-onset congenital adrenal hyperplasia (CAH). Other history components that would lead to the diagnosis of late-onset CAH (most commonly due to 21-hydroxylase enzyme deficiency) would be precocious puberty, hypertension, and some level of virilization [8]. Late-onset CAH is also more common in Native Americans and Ashkenazi Jews and rare in Caucasian and African-American populations [3]. To evaluate for late-onset CAH, an early morning 17-α-hydroxyprogesterone level is a useful laboratory test. If levels are greater than 200 ng/dL, further testing should be undertaken by a reproductive endocrinologist. If less than 200 ng/dL, the diagnosis is very unlikely.

In regards to ruling out an ovarian tumor, the rapidity of onset is the guiding principle. If the patient is over the age of 25 and gives a history of rapid progression of masculinization within a year, the clinician should consider androgen-secreting tumor until proven otherwise [3]. Any addition of medication or supplements within the past several months also warrants investigation into their side effect profile. If a patient gives signs and symptoms concerning for virilization (voice deepening, increase in muscle mass, temporal balding, or clitoromegaly), a total testosterone should be checked. Total testosterone levels greater than 200 ng/mL require evaluation for ovarian tumor. If palpable, surgical exploration is the next step with possible removal. If nonpalpable, imaging with a CT scan or ultrasound to evaluate the ovaries is beneficial. On very rare occasions will noninvasive imaging miss a hilus-cell tumor or very small hormonally-active stromal tissue. However, if no evidence of virilization is present, no laboratory testing is needed to document androgen excess (Figure 21-2).

Other markers for hyperandrogenemia, such as free testosterone, dehydroepiandrosterone (DHEA-S), or ratios of testosterone-to-sex hormone binding globulin (SHBG), are typically not essential or clinically useful in regards to diagnosing and managing hirsutism. More cost effective laboratory testing would include screening for dyslipidemia, glucose intolerance, or frank diabetes mellitus.

When clinical suspicion is high, screening for Cushing syndrome is also indicated. A single-dose overnight dexamethasone test is a good screening test. Dexamethasone (1 mg) is given orally at 11pm and a plasma cortisol level is drawn at 8am the next morning. Values less than 5 µg/dL rule out Cushing syndrome. In patients with intermediate values between 5 and 10 µg/dL, Cushing syndrome is still unlikely. Levels greater than 10 µg/dL are diagnostic of hyperfunctioning adrenals. However, false-positive rates can be up to 13%

in obese patients. If the single-dose dexamethasone test is abnormal, the diagnosis is established with a 24-hour urinary free cortisol with values greater than 250 μg being diagnostic. A low-dose, 2-day suppression test also can provide final confirmation.

Hyperinsulinemia is commonly associated with hyperandrogenemia, often preceding and contributing to the increase in androgens [9]. The increase in insulin results in inhibition of hepatic synthesis of SHBG and insulin-like growth factor binding protein 1, which in turn results in increased levels of free testosterone and insulin growth factor-1 and thus augmented thecal androgen synthesis [10]. Hirsute women who are anovulatory are at increased risk for future noninsulin-dependent diabetes mellitus and cardiovascular disease. As a result, these women should be counseled about the prognosis and interventions that may prevent their development. Obesity seems to be one of the greatest components that pose the largest risk. In studies of women with PCOS, lean women with PCOS, although still hyperinsulinemic, do not seem to have the same risk for future diabetes mellitus [3]. One measure of obesity that has been associated with prognosis is waist circumference. Greater than 90 cm in women is predictive of abnormal endocrinologic function and is associated with increased risk of cardiovascular disease [11]. These women should be screened for insulin resistance as well as monitored periodically. Because fasting glucose-to-insulin ratios vary so much, a modified 2-hour glucose tolerance test with a 75 g load is recommended with checking blood glucose and insulin levels at the 2 hour mark [3]. Glucose levels greater than 140 mg/dL are evidence for impairment, and a level of 200 mg/dL is indicative of diabetes mellitus. Insulin resistance can be defined by 2-hour insulin levels greater than 150 mg/dL. In addition, counseling regarding the positive effects of weight loss and physical activity should be performed, given studies have shown both in combination to be more effective than medicines such as metformin [12••]. Women that continue to be obese and are not overtly diabetic should then continue to be screened annually because of their risk for future disease [3].

Acanthosis nigricans is found in approximately 30% of hyperandrogenic women and about a half of those with PCOS and obesity. HAIR-AN syndrome, referring to hyperandrogenism, insulin resistance, and acanthosis nigricans, was at one point thought to be a distinct syndrome; however, it likely represents a subgroup of women with PCOS [13]. These women in particular are at higher risk for having or developing an associated dyslipidemia. A fasting lipid profile is useful and likely will demonstrate low high-density lipoprotein cholesterol, high low-density lipoprotein cholesterol, and high triglyceride concentrations.

Treatment

Management of hirsutism should be bidirectional, focusing on the patient's concerns, but also keeping in mind their risk for other conditions. First-line recommendations include diet modification, weight loss, and stress management. A second question to ask the patient that allows the physician to tailor therapy to the individual is whether or not the patient wishes to become pregnant. If not, first-line agents to address the androgen excess include low-dose oral contraceptive pills (OCP). OCPs have several mechanisms of action by which they address hirsutism. They suppress luteinizing hormone secretion from the pituitary and subsequent ovarian steroidogenesis and also act to increase SHBG levels, which in turn decreases free androgens. Additionally, OCPs inhibit 5-α-reductase activity in skin, directly affecting the rate of hair growth. If the patient does desire a pregnancy, ovulation can be induced with agents such as clomiphene citrate, which also disrupts the steady state of hyperandrogenemia. Women who are started on OCPs, however, should be counseled not to expect results for at least 6 months before being able to notice a decrease in hair growth. Once the growth cycle is stunted, effective supplemental therapies such as electrolysis (electrocoagulation of the dermal papillae) or laser hair removal can then be employed [3].

Spironolactone, with its antiandrogenic effects, offers a relatively well-tolerated supplement to low dose OCPs. Dosing starts with 200 mg daily but can be reduced to as low as 25 to 50 mg daily for maintenance therapy. Side effects include a brief initial diuresis, hyperkalemia, fatigue, and dysfunctional uterine bleeding. Again, the patient should be informed that most demonstrate response after a 6 month period of treatment. Cyproterone acetate, a potent progestational agent that inhibits ovarian steroidogenesis and androgenic effects at the receptor level, can be given as high dose therapy in combination with estrogen or as combined estrogen-progesterone oral contraceptive. Both have been shown to be effective by the third month of treatment. Effects with the high dose therapy have been seen in studies to be similar to monophasic OCPs and spironolactone [14•].

Other treatment options include flutamide, finasteride, eflornithine, and gonadotropin-releasing hormone (GnRH) agonists. Flutamide, a nonsteroidal antiandrogen, is effective and relatively well-tolerated; however, it requires caution as it has the potential for hepatotoxicity and can interfere with normal male development if the woman is pregnant. Finasteride, a 5-α-reductase

Clinical Manifestations of Androgen Excess

Acne	Hirsutism
Alopecia	Hypertension
Deepening of the voice	Dyslipidemia
Increased muscle mass	Insulin resistance
Increased waist-to-hip ratio	Diabetes
Decreased breast size	Central obesity
Clitoral hypertrophy	Acanthosis nigricans
Vaginal dryness	Cardiovascular disease
Amenorrhea	Psychosocial problems

Figure 21-2. Clinical manifestations of androgen excess.

inhibitor, has minimal daily side effects but can also pose a risk to the development of a male fetus. Randomized controlled trials of finasteride, flutamide, and spironolactone have shown equal efficacy of all three with extended therapy [15]. Eflornithine hydrochloride cream is active at the level of the dermal papilla to inhibit hair growth and has the potential to demonstrate effects within a few weeks; however, patients should be counseled that hair growth will resume on discontinuation. If a woman has hyperandrogenemia derived from the adrenals, suppression with dexamethasone is effective with a lose dose of 0.5 mg nightly; however, this treatment also requires monitoring cortisol levels because of the potential to also suppress the patient's normal stress response. GnRH agonist therapy is an option that is effective; however, it requires injections and subsequent monitoring of hormone levels. Gonadotropin-releasing hormone agonists also have considerable side-effects given the suppression of pituitary gonadotropins. Patients would require add-back estrogen-progestin therapy if continued longer than 6 months due to the potential complications with the induced estrogen deficiency [3].

Medical treatments thus focus on suppressing new hair growth. Temporizing measures until therapy has had enough time to achieve desired effects include shaving, tweezing, and waxing. Measures with more prolonged effects include electrolysis and laser hair removal and generally yield good results if employed after a period of medical therapy. Medical therapy with low dose OCPs, spironolactone, and finasteride can be continued for an undetermined length of time; however, it is not necessary if the patient desires to discontinue. Some reproductive endocrinologists would recommend a trial of stopping medication after 1 to 2 years, followed by a period of observation. Many women will continue to have some suppression for up to 2 years after discontinuing [3].

Prevention

Hirsutism itself can be controlled with medications and alternative therapies. Prevention, however, is difficult as hair growth patterns are established early in life. Once the type of hair follicle growth has been converted to terminal hair, patterns typically persist. Medical therapies thus focus on reducing the rate of growth either peripherally or systemically by decreasing androgen levels.

Preventive medical measures thus focus on preventing long-term sequelae. Diabetes, hypertension, cardiovascular disease, as well as infertility, can all be associated with hirsutism through various disease pathways. Thus, lifestyle modifications that highlight diet changes and weight consciousness become paramount. Periodic monitoring by the physician of blood glucose, lipid profiles, and blood pressure can allow the physician to intervene with medicines when necessary. Metformin therapy, for instance, may help to restore ovulation and achieve a pregnancy, while at the same time treating the hyperinsulinemia and hyperglycemia that pose the future risk of diabetes and cardiovascular disease [16•].

Treatment of hirsutism can be gratifying not only to the patient, but also the physician. Management requires frequent monitoring and stressing compliance to patients with positive feedback from the physician. However difficult, this remains one area in medicine that the clinician continues to play a key role in prevention of sequelae.

References

Papers of particular interest, are highlighted as follows:
•   Of interest
••   Of outstanding interest

1. Givens JK: Hirsutism and hyperandrogenism. *Adv Intern Med* 1976, 21:221–227.

2. Tomas PK, Ferriman DG: Variations in facial and pubic hair in white women. *Am J Physiol Anthropol* 1957, 15:171.

3. Speroff L, Fritz M: Hirsutism. In *Clinical Gynecologic Endocrinology and Infertility*, edn 7. Edited by Speroff L, Fritz MA. Philadelphia: Lippincott Williams & Wilkins; 2005:499–530.

4. Tosi A, Misciali C, Piraccini BM, *et al.*: Drug-induced hair loss and hair growth. Incidence, management and avoidance. *Drug Saf* 1994, 10:310–317.

5. Wild RA, Painter P, Coulson PB, *et al.*: Lipoprotein lipid concentrations and cardiovascular risk in patients with polycystic ovary syndrome. *J Clin Endocrinol Metab* 1985, 61:946–950.

6. Cronin L, Guyatt G, Griffith L, *et al.*: Development of a health related quality of life questionnaire for women with polycystic ovary syndrome. *J Clin Endocrinol Metab* 1998, 83:1976–1986.

7. Nestler J: Role of hyperinsulinemia in the pathogenesis of the polycystic ovary syndrome and its clinical implications. *Semin Reprod Endocrinol* 1997, 15:111–122.

8. Toscano V, Balducci R, Mangiantini A, *et al.*: Hyperandrogenism in the adolescent female. *Steroids* 1998, 63:308–313.

9. Chang RJ, Nakamura RM, Judd HL, Kaplan SA: Insulin resistance in nonobese patients with polycystic ovarian syndrome. *J Clin Endocrinol Metab* 1983, 57:356–369.

10. Nestler JE, Powers LP, Matt DW, *et al.*: A direct effect of hyperinsulinemia on serum sex hormone-binding globulin levels in obese women with the polycystic ovarian syndrome. *J Clin Endocrinol Metab* 1991, 72:83–89.

11. Pouliot MC, Despres JP, Lemieux S, *et al.*: Waist circumference and abdominal sagittal diameter: best simple anthropometric indexes of abdominal visceral adipose tissue accumulation and related cardiovascular risk in men and women. *Am J Cardiol* 1994, 73:460–468.

12.•• Diabetes Prevention Program Research Council: Reduction in the incidence of type 2 diabetes with lifestyle intervention or metformin. *N Eng J Med* 2002, 346:393–403.

This paper still serves as a benchmark in clinical studies performed that can help guide a primary care provider with regard to direction of preventive health care counseling and the importance in the reduction of obesity and type 2 diabetes.

13. Stenchever M, Droegemueller W, Herbst A, Mishell D: Hyperandrogenism. In *Comprehensive Gynecology*, edn 4. Edited by Stenchever MA, Droegemueller W, Herbst A, Mishell D. St. Louis: Mosby; 2001:1143–1168.

14.• Erenus M, Yucelten D, Gurbuz O, *et al*.: Comparison of spironolactone-oral contraceptive versus cyproterone acetate-estrogen regimens in the treatment of hirsutism. *Fertil Steril* 1996, 66:216–219.

This paper is useful in establishing clinically tested treatment regimens for hirsutism as well as helpful in adjusting patient expectations with the commencement of medical therapy.

15. Moghetti P, Tosi F, Tosti A, *et al*.: Comparison of spironolactone, flutamide, and finasteride efficacy in the treatment of hirsutism: a randomized, double blind, placebo-controlled trial. *J Clin Endocrinol Metab* 2000, 85:89–94.

16.• Heard MG, Pierce A, Carson SA, Buster JE: Pregnancies following use of metformin for ovulation induction in patients with polycystic ovary syndrome. *Fertil Steril* 2002, 77:669–673.

This paper highlights the multiple modalities of metformin when concerned about a patient with insulin resistance, as well as the other benefits of medical therapy.

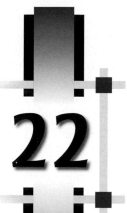

Abnormal Uterine Bleeding

22

Lynn Borgatta and Sarah J. Betstadt

- Irregular menstrual bleeding is a common reason for patients to seek medical care.
- The first objective is to rule out concerning diagnoses in a timely fashion by patient history, age, risk factors, or with pathologic and/or radiologic evaluation.
- The second objective is to try to define the cause of the bleeding and then to offer a solution using hormonal methods, minimally invasive procedures, or surgery.
- Common causes of irregular menstrual bleeding include fibroids, polyps, and dysfunctional uterine bleeding. Dysfunctional uterine bleeding implies there is no anatomic cause of the bleeding; bleeding may be idiopathic, or due to hormonal dysfunction. Systemic medical illness should be considered in the differential of irregular menstrual bleeding.
- Before treating with estrogen, the clinician should be sure the patient has no contraindications.

Abnormal uterine bleeding can present a frustrating situation for clinicians. The many options for treatment—medical and surgical—indicate the diversity of causes of abnormal uterine bleeding. By narrowing the differential diagnosis into categories, it is possible to approach this common patient complaint in a systematic fashion. A systematic approach also assists the clinician in choosing an effective treatment option. The goals of this chapter are to review normal menstrual physiology and bleeding patterns of adult women, present differential diagnoses, and review the roles of medical and surgical treatment options. The following patterns of abnormal bleeding will be considered: intermenstrual bleeding in women with regular cycles, irregular bleeding, and menorrhagia (heavy bleeding) regardless of menstrual pattern, and postmenopausal bleeding.

Menstrual disorders carry the highest annual prevalence rate of all gynecologic conditions [1]. Menstrual problems account for 21% of all gynecology referrals [2]. In one large study, women reporting heavy menses had an odds ratio of 1.45 for use of health care compared with those who did not [3]. Menorrhagia has a reported prevalence worldwide of 19% among women of reproductive age [4].

Uterine leiomyomas or fibroids affect 25% to 50% of women in the United States. Depending on the location and multiplicity of fibroids, as many as two thirds of women with fibroids may have heavy menstrual bleeding [5–8].

Of the coagulation disorders that may contribute to bleeding, von Willebrand's disease has a prevalence of 1% to 3% in the general population, and it is the most common congenital hemostatic disorder [9–11].

Endometrial carcinoma is the most common gynecologic cancer, and it is the fourth most common cancer in white women, following breast, lung, and colorectal cancers. The majority of women with endometrial cancer will present with bleeding [12]. Endometrial cancer is rare in women younger than 35 years of age, but its incidence increases rapidly after the age of 40 years. Two to three percent of women in the United States will develop endometrial cancer [12]. Unopposed estrogen from chronic anovulation, obesity, tamoxifen therapy, or exogenous hormones is one of the strongest predisposing factors for abnormal bleeding and endometrial cancer [13,14].

Menstrual Physiology

The definition of a normal menstrual cycle is an interval of 28 days (± 7 days) and a duration of menses of 4 days (± 2–3 days). The average blood loss per cycle is 30 mL. Blood loss greater than 80 mL is considered heavy menstrual bleeding or menorrhagia [15]. A normal menstrual cycle suggests that the hypothalamic pituitary-ovarian-uterine axis is functioning appropriately. The phases of the menstrual cycle are the follicular and luteal phases (Figure 22-1), separated by ovulation. These phases correspond to the proliferative and secretory phases in the endometrium respectively.

The follicular phase lasts an average of 14 days, but there is substantial variation in length. At the beginning of this phase, estradiol and progesterone levels are low, which signals the pulsatile secretion of gonadotropin-releasing hormone (GnRH). GnRH secretion increases follicle-stimulating hormone (FSH) and luteinizing hormone (LH) levels. LH causes conversion of cholesterol to androgens by ovarian theca cells. These androgens are converted to estrogens within granulosa cells under the stimulation of FSH. This process matures multiple ovarian follicles, and one becomes dominant in preparation for ovulation. The endometrium during this phase responds to increasing levels of estradiol by proliferating glands and stroma. High estradiol levels produced later during the follicular phase (at least 200 pg/mL for at least 36 hours) signal a GnRH surge. The pituitary responds with a large LH and smaller FSH surge, and within 36 hours, ovulation occurs [16].

The third phase of the menstrual cycle, the luteal phase, lasts an average of 14 ± 2 days. After ovulation, the follicle from which the oocyte was released becomes the corpus luteum. Within the corpus luteum, cholesterol is converted to pregnenolone and further to progesterone. The progesterone level peaks on cycle days 20 to 22 of a 28-day cycle, which corresponds to 6 to 8 days after the LH surge. The high levels of progesterone during this phase cause secretory changes in the endometrium associated with increased stromal vascularity. The decline of corpus luteal function begins approximately 10 days after ovulation if fertilization does not take place, resulting in a decrease of estradiol and progesterone. The endometrium then sloughs as blood vessels constrict and the stroma becomes edematous. Local prostaglandins are released, causing myometrial contractions and vasoconstriction [17].

The cycle repeats as low levels of estradiol and progesterone signal a GnRH rise, which initiates an increase in FSH and LH. Any deviation (hormonal or structural) from this process commonly results in irregular uterine bleeding.

Abnormal Uterine Bleeding Patterns

Considerations include the temporal relation of the abnormal bleeding to normal menses, the time period over which bleeding has occurred, the amount of bleeding, the patient's age, and other systemic complaints or observations.

PREGNANCY
Bleeding can be secondary to normal and abnormal pregnancy including ectopic implantation, threatened, spontaneous, incomplete, and missed abortions, gestational trophoblastic disease, or retained placental tissue. A urine or serum human chorionic gonadotropin concentration determination can exclude pregnancy-related causes of abnormal uterine bleeding. A full discussion of pregnancy-related bleeding is beyond the scope of this chapter.

DYSFUNCTIONAL UTERINE BLEEDING
Bleeding in the absence of blood dyscrasias, infection, submucous myomas, endometrial and cervical polyps, uterine carcinoma, and abnormalities of pregnancy is considered dysfunctional uterine bleeding. This type of bleeding is hormonally related, caused by an imbalance or timing abnormality of the sex steroid hormones of the menstrual cycle. It may coexist with other anatomic lesions. It may result from four different processes, classified by Speroff [18] as the following:

1. Estrogen breakthrough bleeding is the abnormal uterine bleeding seen with anovulatory cycles or with the prolonged administration of estrogen.

2. Estrogen withdrawal bleeding is bleeding seen after administration of exogenous estrogen and its subsequent discontinuation in oophorectomized or menopausal women.

3. Progesterone breakthrough bleeding is capillary bleeding due to endometrial atrophy and is commonly seen with the long-term use of oral contraceptive pills and depot medroxyprogesterone acetate (MPA).

4. Progesterone withdrawal bleeding is experienced after the administration and discontinuation of progestin, such as oral MPA.

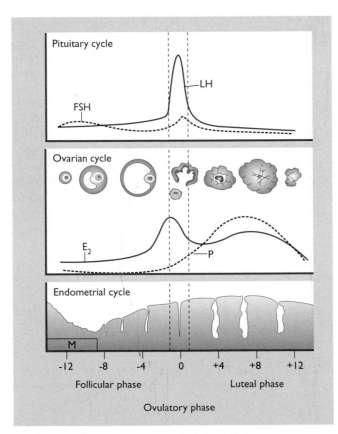

Figure 22-1. Cyclic changes of pituitary hormones, ovarian hormones, the dominant follicle, and the endometrium during reproductive life. Each cycle represents approximately 1 month. FSH—follicle-stimulating hormone; LH—luteinizing hormone. (*Adapted from* Hertweck [17].)

Van Look et al. [19] suggested that the basic defect in chronic anovulation is a relative insensitivity of the hypothalamic-pituitary system to the positive feedback of estrogen. Anovulatory cycles result in continuous estrogen exposure without the periodic modulating effect of progesterone, because progesterone is produced only with ovulation. This exposure to unopposed estrogen results in endometrial proliferation. The proliferation continues, outgrowing its blood supply, and endometrium randomly breaks off as a result of lack of stromal support, resulting in abnormal uterine bleeding [18,19]. Endometritis and micro-erosions may cause and result from bleeding [20].

As women reach menopause, ovulatory cycles become less frequent, although a pattern of regular menses may persist. Menopause occurs between ages 45 and 55 for most women. During the menopausal period ovulatory cycles may alternate with anovulatory periods and menstrual irregularity may occur. The most common cause of abnormal uterine bleeding from the perimenarchal to the perimenopausal years is anovulatory bleeding [18]. Anovulatory bleeding is seen in many perimenopausal women 3 to 5 years before complete ovarian failure and it is also common in the first years after menarche [21]. This type of bleeding is also common in patients with obesity.

POSTMENOPAUSAL BLEEDING

Bleeding occurring more than a year after the last menses is considered postmenopausal bleeding; however, some follicle development is common in postmenopausal women for several years after menopause. Postmenopausal bleeding is usually benign; 60% to 80% of postmenopausal bleeding is related to atrophy, and another 15% to 25% is related to hormone replacement therapy. Fifteen to thirty percent of women with bleeding will have a polyp, fibroid, hyperplasia, or endometrial cancer [22].

ATROPHY

Atrophic endometrium can be seen in postmenopausal women with very little estrogen production. It may been seen in women on prolonged progestational medication, such as combination oral contraceptives, or progestin-only contraceptives. Chronic infection or bleeding also may result in an atrophic pattern.

IDIOPATHIC BLEEDING

Bleeding in ovulatory women who have an apparently normal uterus is termed idiopathic bleeding. It is a diagnosis of exclusion once anovulation and anatomic lesions have been deemed unlikely. Idiopathic bleeding or idiopathic menorrhagia may be recurrent and profuse. Idiopathic bleeding may occur because of, or be exacerbated by, a coexisting medical problem, particularly coagulopathies.

ANATOMIC CAUSES

Pathology of the cervix, uterus, and ovary may present as abnormal uterine bleeding. Infection, abnormalities of pregnancy, leiomyomas, endometrial and cervical polyps, and benign tumors and malignancies of the uterus and cervix are all considered in the differential diagnosis. Fibroids are discussed in more detail in Chapter 36. Bleeding from leiomyomas depends

on the location of the leiomyoma to the uterine cavity and, to a lesser extent, size and multiplicity. In a cross-sectional study by Wegienka et al. [8] 67% of women with submucous fibroids has heavy bleeding compared with 30% to 50% of women with fibroids in other locations, and 28% of women without fibroids. Endometrial polyps are generally benign and may be completely asymptomatic. They seldom cause extensive bleeding, although on occasion they may become as large as several centimeters. The diagnosis is made by hysterosalpingogram, sonohysterogram, or hysteroscopy. Depending on the situation, asymptomatic polyps may be left alone provided endometrial sampling has been done. They should be removed if they are bleeding or if the woman is postmenopausal, or if she is at high risk for carcinoma. On occasion, endometrial carcinoma may arise in a polyp. Polyps may be removed by suction curettage or more reliably by hysteroscopy.

There are several types of endometrial hyperplasia. Simple hyperplasia is the overgrowth of histologically benign cells, and has a benign outcome. Fewer than 1% of women with simple hyperplasia will progress to carcinoma. Complex hyperplasia, atypical hyperplasia, or adenomatous hyperplasia may be precursors to endometrial cancer and require consultation; these types of hyperplasia may warrant aggressive treatment such as hysterectomy [12,23]. Complex atypical hyperplasia is associated with a risk of progression to carcinoma of 29% [24].

COEXISTING MEDICAL DISORDERS AND CHRONIC DISEASE

Secondary disruption of ovarian function, resulting in anovulation, may also be seen with states leading to abnormal endocrine influence on the hypothalamic pituitary axis. These situations may include polycystic ovaries, hypothyroidism and hyperthyroidism, hyperprolactinemia, congenital and acquired adrenal hyperplasia, Cushing syndrome, adrenal insufficiency, strenuous physical exercise, and medications [25]. In many of these situations, the presenting symptom is likely to be amenorrhea; however, breakthrough bleeding from endometrial atrophy or from unopposed estrogen may result in irregular bleeding. If possible, the medical condition should be treated first. Treatment may resolve the bleeding issue. However, with acute bleeding, diagnosis and treatment may have to proceed even if the underlying illness is not stabilized.

Blood Dyscrasias

Defects in hemostasis may result in menorrhagia with ovulatory or anovulatory cycles, and should be considered when the woman gives a history of heavy menstrual bleeding since menarche. Defects in hemostasis may be primary (platelet defects) or secondary (plasma protein defects) [26,27]. Primary hemostatic disorders may result from a quantitative or qualitative platelet disorder.

Vital to primary hemostasis is platelet adherence, which is stabilized by von Willebrand's factor (vWF). Secondary hemostasis is the fibrin deposition that occurs as a result of the coagulation system. Multiple coagulation proteins are required; increased menstrual blood loss may be seen if the coagulation system is deficient in platelets or fibrin [25]. Some of the more common coagulation disorders include von Willebrand's disease, idiopathic thrombocytopenic purpura, Glanzmann's disease, and thalassemia major. Abnormal uterine bleeding associated with von Willebrand's disease and different types of hemophilia responded to the use of desmopressin, a synthetic analog of the neurohypothalamic nonapeptide arginine vasopressin, which causes the release of autologous vWF [26].

A partial thromboplastin time obtained for assessing the secondary hemostatic system evaluates the intrinsic limb of the coagulation cascade and specifically factors XII, HMWK, PK, XI, IX, and VIII. The extrinsic limb is assessed with the prothrombin time. Both tests evaluate the pathway after the activation of factor X. A fibrinogen level can be obtained if the prothrombin time and partial thromboplastin time are prolonged. These can be further evaluated by ordering specific factor assays to evaluate the disorder more extensively [26–28].

Liver Disease

The liver, by producing coagulation proteins, plays a primary role in hemostasis. Severe liver disease may result in decreased production of fibrinogen, prothrombin, and factors V, VII, IX, X, and XI. In addition, the liver is responsible for storing vitamin K, a critical cofactor in the coagulation cascade, and hepatocellular disease may result in deficiency of this compound. Factors II (prothrombin), IX, and X require vitamin K for biologic activity [29]. In addition, the liver is crucial to the metabolic clearance of sex steroid hormones, particularly estrogen. Liver disease interferes with this process, upsetting the hormonal balance of the menstrual cycle and resulting commonly in abnormal bleeding.

Thyroid Disease

Disorders of thyroid function, including hypothyroidism, hyperthyroidism, neoplastic disease, and infectious disease, may present with abnormal uterine bleeding as an associated symptom [30]. Although the mechanism remains obscure, it has been suggested that thyroid abnormalities may interfere with the metabolic clearance of estrogen.

Renal Failure

Abnormal bleeding is often seen in patients with chronic renal failure. In patients with severe renal disease, clotting dysfunction may be the result of prolongation of bleeding time, decreased activity of platelet factor III, abnormal platelet aggregation and adhesiveness, and impaired prothrombin consumption [31,32]. Many patients with menstrual disturbances revert to normal cycles during dialysis or after renal transplantation [33]. During dialysis, levels of LH, FSH, estradiol, and progesterone remain essentially normal, suggesting that other factors, such as uremic toxins, abnormal trace element metabolism, and malnutrition, may be involved [33]. Intravenous conjugated estrogens have been effective in shortening the bleeding time in uremic patients.

Diabetes

Menstrual disturbances are common in women with insulin-dependent diabetes mellitus. A prevalence of 32% has been reported [34]. It has been suggested that insulin affects the hypothalamic-pituitary-ovarian axis at different levels and affects ovarian androgen biosynthesis [34]. Griffin *et al.* [35] reviewed the prevailing views regarding how insulin-dependent diabetes

mellitus affects this axis and concluded that the menstrual dysfunction in these patients results from an abnormality of the GnRH pulse generator. The exact mechanism of this abnormality is not known but may be related to enhanced hypothalamic dopamine tone, decreased metabolic fuels, or neuronal glucose deprivation. Strict glycemic control may improve menstrual irregularities in patients with insulin-dependent diabetes mellitus [34]. Poorly controlled diabetes mellitus may result in diabetic nephropathy and hepatic dysfunction secondary to macrovesicular fatty liver, which may then lead to bleeding abnormalities

Polycystic Ovary Syndrome

Polycystic ovary syndrome is generally defined as chronic anovulation and hyperandrogenism in the absence of other causes, such as adrenal neoplasia. Women with polycystic ovary syndrome typically have impaired glucose tolerance and hyperandrogenemia. Typically ultrasound examination shows multiple follicle cysts; these may be arrayed as a "string of pearls" with multiple small cysts along the ovarian cortex, or one or several dominant cysts. Large cysts may be symptomatic. The presence of ovarian cysts, however, is not sufficient in itself to make the diagnosis of polycystic ovary syndrome. Unopposed estrogen stimulation of the uterus may lead to overgrowth of endometrium in follicular phase with irregular breakthrough bleeding, similar to other women who are anovulatory with prolonged estrogen effect [24,36].

Primary treatment may be insulin-sensitizing agents, such as metformin, which may result in ovulation. Clomiphene, alone or in combination with other agents, is the alternative method of inducing ovulation. If pregnancy is not desired, endometrial proliferation can be controlled with progestins or oral contraceptives [24,36].

Making the Diagnosis

Abnormal bleeding coexisting with ovulation may occur with regular cycles, with intermittent intermenstrual bleeding. The pattern of a small amount of bleeding at the time of ovulation, often associated with *mittelschmerz* (midcycle pain), can be excluded by history. Abnormal and irregular bleeding patterns during ovulation can occur because of an anatomic abnormality such as polyp or fibroid, but may be idiopathic. Idiopathic bleeding by definition occurs in women with regular menses and without evidence of an anatomic lesion. Generally, idiopathic bleeding may be manifest by irregular bleeding, heavy menses, or menorrhagia. If the cycle history of abnormal bleeding suggests anovulation of short duration in a young woman, empiric treatment may be therapeutic and support the diagnosis of anovulation. If an anovulatory pattern has persisted for months, it is reasonable to begin with ordering thyroid-stimulating hormone and prolactin. In cases in which hirsutism is present, evaluation should include total testosterone, dehydroepiandrosterone sulfate, LH, FSH, and ovarian imaging. A more complete discussion of hirsutism is found in Chapter 21. Once underlying disease is considered likely, and irregular bleeding persists despite medical treatment, further diagnostic testing is warranted.

Diagnostic testing is always indicated in women who have perimenopausal or postmenopausal bleeding. The purpose of further diagnostic testing is to identify anatomic lesions, hyperplasia, and malignancy. The primary methods used include dilation and curettage (D & C), endometrial biopsy or aspiration, ultrasonography, saline sonohysterography (SHG), and hysteroscopy.

OVULATORY VERSUS ANOVULATORY CYCLES

The first step in making the diagnosis of abnormal uterine bleeding is to take a history with a detailed description of the timing, amount, and character of bleeding. A distinction between ovulatory and anovulatory cycles is helpful to direct further evaluation and treatment. Ovulatory cycles are predictable and regular, with a mean interval of 28 days (± 7 days), and they are often associated with symptoms such as lower abdominal cramping, midcycle pain, breast tenderness, and bloating [38]. Abnormalities associated with ovulatory cycles include prolonged periods of bleeding (greater than 4 ± 2 to 3 days), as well as bleeding between regular episodes. Anovulatory cycles are more unpredictable and irregular, with variations in quantity of blood loss and length of bleeding period.

Determination of the presence of ovulation is helpful in the initial evaluation of abnormal uterine bleeding. If history alone does not clarify ovulatory versus anovulatory bleeding, the physician may choose one of the described methods [39].

SERUM PROGESTERONE

Within 6 hours of the LH surge, progesterone levels begin to rise; they plateau during the peak of the LH surge, and then rapidly rise approximately 36 hours after the onset of the LH surge until reaching luteal phase levels [40]. Ilesanmi [41] found a serum progesterone level of 11.3 nmol/L (3.55 ng/mL) or higher to be consistent with ovulation. This study was performed using secretory endometrium from biopsies as confirmation. If the reported progesterone level is low and the patient's history supports ovulatory cycles, it may be that the sample was drawn in the proliferative phase. In this situation, it is advisable to obtain another serum progesterone level 1 to 2 weeks later.

ENDOMETRIAL BIOPSY

Secretory endometrium seen histologically from an endometrial biopsy may also serve as a useful indirect detection of ovulation. Noyes et al. [42] established the histologic criteria by which the endometrium is dated. Although there is some disagreement regarding the accuracy in detecting day of ovulation with this method, it remains a useful test to confirm that ovulation has taken place. Pregnancy should be ruled out as a cause of irregular bleeding before performing endometrial biopsy.

ULTRASONOGRAPHY

Direct visualization of follicular growth and collapse after ovulation is possible with ultrasonography. Ultrasound has been used to follow follicular development and predict ovulation knowing that the mean follicular growth rate is approximately 2 mm over the last 6 days of development and that the average

follicular size is 20 mm at the time of ovulation [39,43]. Ultrasonographic findings of ovulation include a disappearance of the follicle or a decrease in mean diameter of the follicle associated with an irregular shape or increased echogenicity [39]. Queenan et al. [43] performed ultrasound studies on patients with regular ovulatory function, infertile patients, patients receiving clomiphene citrate, and women taking oral contraceptive pills to detect ovulation. Their results suggest ovulation is best determined by changes in follicular appearance over serial scans and not by a particular follicular size.

ENDOMETRIAL SAMPLING

In the past, D & C was initially used as a therapeutic modality for treating abnormal uterine bleeding, but studies did not support its use. It gradually became a diagnostic procedure and the standard method of evaluating the endometrium for pathology. D & C has been shown to have high false-negative rates [44]. In response to a need for a cost effective, outpatient, safer method of evaluating the endometrium for malignancy, the endometrial biopsy or endometrial aspiration was developed.

The adequacy of endometrial biopsy has been evaluated, and it was found to be consistently above 87% in premenopausal patients and above 72% in postmenopausal patients [45]. Stovall et al. [46] found that Pipelle (Unimar, Wilton, CT) and hysterectomy specimens sent for pathologic evaluation agreed 96% of the time. The Pipelle had a sensitivity of 97.5% and agreement of the histologic grade in 74.4% of specimens. Two prospective, randomized trials comparing the Pipelle with the Novak curette (Miltex Surgical Instruments, Lake Success, NY) and to the Tis-U-Trap (Milex Products, Chicago, IL) found the devices similar in adequacy and quality [47,48]. In a meta-analysis of several samplers used to detect endometrial hyperplasia, Dijkhuizen et al. [49] found overall sensitivity of 81% and very high specificity; however, they concluded that the Pipelle, with sensitivity over 90%, was the best of the devices evaluated. However, Clark et al. [50] found a sensitivity of 65% and specificity of 95% for the diagnosis of endometrial hyperplasia; they cautioned against sole reliance on a negative endometrial aspiration to rule out hyperplasia.

No cases of perforation with excessive bleeding have been reported with the Pipelle biopsy. Only rare cases of infection have been reported [48]. Because of its safety, accuracy, adequacy, and usefulness in an outpatient setting, endometrial biopsy has in most cases replaced the more invasive, expensive D & C procedure [44].

TRANSVAGINAL ULTRASONOGRAPHY

Transvaginal ultrasonography (TVU) is a noninvasive, accurate, and safe method of evaluating abnormal bleeding. Although TVU can screen for ovarian masses, uterine fibroids, and other abnormalities, the measurement of endometrial thickness has become an integral part of evaluation of women with abnormal bleeding. A thickened endometrium may indicate hyperplasia or neoplasia, or anatomic lesions such as polyps. The endometrium is measured at the widest part (Figure 22-2). The range of normal is wide in premenopausal women; normal women at ovulation may have an endometrial "stripe" of 7 to 12 mm [51,52] However, when evaluating women with abnormal bleeding, a threshold is set to provide very high sensitivity, which results in some false-positive readings and lowered specificity. Postmenopausal women typically have thinner endometrial stripe and fewer false-positive results [53].

Dueholm et al. [54] arranged the results from 355 premenopausal women by endometrial thickness and found that when the endometrium was less than 6 mm, the probability of polyps or hyperplasia was 7.6%. At a thickness of 10 mm, the probability of polyps or hyperplasia was 13% and, with a thickness of 20 mm, 20%.

Transvaginal ultrasound has high sensitivity to detect endometrial cancer. In a prospective study, all cases of endometrial carcinoma were detected by TVU when 5 mm was used as the thickness cutoff [55]. Multiple studies [56–61] have shown sensitivity ranging from 83% to100% (Figure 22-3). Specificity is not quite as high, resulting in positive predictive values (PPV) varying from 40% to nearly 90%. Negative predictive value (NPV) is quite high.

Transvaginal ultrasound is an effective method of evaluating uterine bleeding in postmenopausal women on hormone replacement therapy. Maia et al. [62] performed TVU on 41 patients with abnormal bleeding taking four different hormone

replacement therapy regimens. Atrophic endometrium and lack of structural pathology were confirmed by hysteroscopy and endometrial biopsy when the endometrial thickness was less than 4 mm. Hanggi et al. [59] also demonstrated atrophic endometrium by biopsy when the endometrial thickness was less than 5 mm (sensitivity, specificity, PPV, and NPV are 83%, 95%, 94%, and 86%, respectively).

Although the results of TVU are promising, it has been suggested that TVU not be used as the sole method of evaluating the endometrium for pathology, and it should be combined with endometrial sampling when there is a high suspicion of pathology [62,63].

SONOHYSTEROGRAPHY

Sonohysterography (SHG) is especially useful in evaluating the intrauterine cavity when baseline ultrasonography suggests an abnormality. The procedure is performed by instilling 10 to 40 mL of sterile saline into the uterine cavity through a 5F catheter, while imaging the uterus with abdominal or vaginal ultrasound [64–66].

With SHG, the ultrasonographic appearances of submucosal fibroids and endometrial polyps are distinctive and provide a high degree of accuracy. Fibroids have mixed echogenicity consistent with that of the myometrium. Intramural myomas do not distort the cavity, whereas submucosal myomas result in a cavity with an irregular contour and a sessile attachment to the myometrium (Figure 22-4) [67,68]. Polyps are usually hyperechogenic, and they are attached to the intrauterine wall by a stalk [68]. It is clinically important to make this distinction because the surgical approach may differ as a result. Goldstein et al. [68] and Tur-Kaspa et al. [69] found submucous fibroids in 5% and 9% of women undergoing SHG for abnormal bleeding, while polyps were about three times as common.

Bernard et al. [70] performed a prospective study on 159 patients with abnormal uterine bleeding. The sensitivity and specificity for detecting uterine abnormalities were 98.9% and 76.4%, respectively. The accuracy of SHG in detecting hypertrophy, polyps, and submucosal myomas is evidenced by their respective specificities: 95.6%, 90.7%, and 95%. The sensitivities for each of these pathologic findings were somewhat lower at 88.8%, 87.8%, and 89.6%, respectively. Kamel et al. [71] found that sensitivity and specificity for the

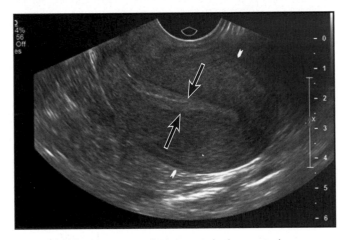

Figure 22-2. Transvaginal ultrasound of a normal premenopausal uterus (*white arrowheads*). The endometrial stripe is 7 mm (*black arrows*). This woman did not have endometrial pathology.

Transvaginal Ultrasound and Screening for Endometrial Malignancy

Participants, *n*	Endometrial Thickness Cutoff, *mm*	Sensitivity, %	Specificity, %	PPV, %	NPV, %	Reference
205	5	100	96	87.3	—	[56]
81	5	95.8	45.5	71.9	88.2	[58]
260	Not defined	96	89	—	—	[60]
80	4	96.7	100	40	—	[53]
80	8	100	62.3	45.25	100	[57]

Figure 22-3. Transvaginal ultrasound and screening for endometrial malignancy. NPV—negative predictive value; PPV—positive predictive value.

detection of polyps were higher when TVU and SHG were both used compared with when each test was used alone; the sensitivity and specificity of the combined tests were 93% and 94%, respectively [71].

O'Connell *et al.* [72] found that combining SHG with endometrial biopsy resulted in a combined specificity of 96% and NPV of greater than 94%. Mihm *et al.* [73] reported that SHG and endometrial biopsy had a sensitivity of 97% and a specificity of 70% when compared with hysteroscopy or hysterectomy findings. The results of selected studies showing the sensitivities and specificities of SHG relative to other tests are displayed in Figure 22-5 [54,71,76–79].

The findings of Bernard *et al.* [70] suggest that cancer is not always predicted by SHG alone; three cases were incorrectly diagnosed as endometrial hypertrophy, polyp, and submucosal myoma, although each indicated surgical exploration (hysteroscopy or hysterectomy), which led to the correct diagnosis. Although the sensitivity of SHG for carcinoma is limited, its sensitivity and specificity for detecting benign intrauterine pathology is very good.

DIAGNOSTIC HYSTEROSCOPY

Diagnostic hysteroscopy allows visualization of the endocervical canal and endometrial cavity and direct visualization of myomas, polyps, and focal areas of proliferation (hyperplasia and carcinoma). In many cases, biopsy or surgical treatment can be performed during the same procedure. It is often performed in the operating room, but may be performed in an outpatient office setting [80–82]. Hysteroscopes in use currently include a 3 mm (outside diameter) flexible scope (Figure 22-6), which can often be used without any analgesia, dilatation, or tenaculum. Newer rigid hysteroscopes may have an outside diameter of 5 mm including the fluid channel. They may be used with minimal or no cervical dilatation; analgesia may not be necessary, or oral or intravenous analgesia may be used. Directed endometrial biopsy can be done with a slender (5F) operating channel. Operative hysteroscopes have an outside diameter of 8 to 10 mm because of the larger instruments

and multiple channels and are usually used in an operating room instead of an outpatient office setting.

Hysteroscopy has been shown to be equal to or more informative than other methods of diagnosing endometrial pathology (Figure 22-5). Nagele *et al.* [82] reported 2500 outpatient hysteroscopic procedures. The procedure was completed in 96% of women, and 68% of women had endometrial biopsy as well. Intrauterine lesions were diagnosed in 48% [83]. Another retrospective study [84] reported sensitivity, specificity, PPV, NPV of 100%, 89.4%, 71.4%, and 100%, respectively, using histopathologic findings as the gold standard. Haller *et al.* [85] found rates of 95.3%, 93.9%, 95.3%, and 93.9% for all benign lesions. In contrast, Saidi *et al.* [76] randomized patients to SHG or TVU followed by hysteroscopy and endometrial biopsy and reported a lower sensitivity (78%) and specificity (54%) of diagnostic hysteroscopy when all uterine cavity lesions were included.

Studies show higher accuracy in detecting benign intrauterine lesions than for hyperplasia and carcinoma. Garuti *et al.* [83]

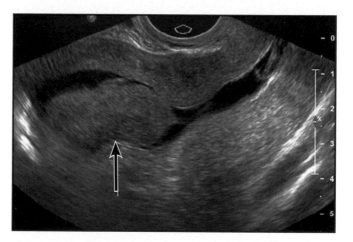

Figure 22-4. This image of a sonohysterogram shows a 2-cm submucous fibroid (*arrow*). The saline appears black as it distends the cavity, allowing the delineation of the fibroid from the rest of the uterus.

Comparison of Sensitivity and Specificity Among Diagnostic Methods

Partici-pants, *n*	Endometrial Abnormality	Transvaginal Ultrasound		Sonohysterography		Hysteroscopy		Author
		Sensitiv-ity, %	Specific-ity, %	Sensitiv-ity, %	Specific-ity, %	Sensitiv-ity, %	Specific-ity, %	
149	Polyp/myoma	54	90			79	90	Towbin *et al.* [75]
104	All	67	89	87	91	90	91	Schwarzler *et al.* [77]
106	All	65	75	93	94			Kamel *et al.* [71]
105	Polyp/myoma	49	81	79	76	81	94	Epstein *et al.* [78]
	Malignancy	60	90	44	96	84	95	
144	Polyp, premenopausal	72	51	92	61	94	59	Cepni *et al.* [79]
	Polyp, postmenopausal	60	33	71	27	100	46	

Figure 22-5. Comparison of sensitivity and specificity among diagnostic methods.

showed sensitivity, specificity, PPV, and NPV of 95%, 95%, 82%, and 99%, respectively, for endometrial polyps, and 70%, 92%, 61%, and 94%, respectively, for endometrial hyperplasia. Epstein *et al.* [78] reported a similar pattern. Haller *et al.* [85] reported a high sensitivity (96.9%) and specificity (100%) for detecting endometrial polyps, but a reduced sensitivity of 50% for endometrial hyperplasia and cancer; however, Loerro *et al.* [86] reported sensitivity and specificity of 98% and 95% for the diagnosis of hyperplasia in a series of 980 women. The hysteroscopic impression of hyperplasia or cancer should be confirmed by focal tissue sampling and directed biopsy.

COMPARISON AMONG DIAGNOSTIC METHODS

Curettage is being replaced by easier, safer, and less expensive office-based methods. TVU and SHG have the advantages of accuracy, noninvasiveness, and quickness, but they are depen-

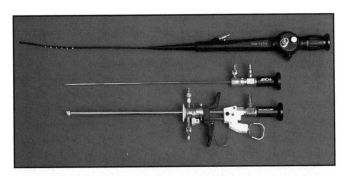

Figure 22-6. Three hysteroscopes. The flexible hysteroscope (*top*) has a 3-mm outside diameter (OD). The rigid hysteroscope (*middle*) has a 3-mm hysteroscope inside a fluid channel, resulting in a 4-mm OD. An operating hysteroscope (*bottom*) typically has an OD of 8 to 9 mm.

dent on the skill of the technician. Pipelle endometrial biopsy is sensitive for endometrial hyperplasia and carcinoma and it is minimally invasive, but it can miss myomas and polyps. Hysteroscopy remains the gold standard, but it is invasive and expensive, and it may not be as accurate at diagnosing hyperplasia. However, the increasing use of office hysteroscopy may change the balance.

Saidi *et al.* [76] reported in 1997 that the average charge of each procedure at their institution was $195 for TVU and SHG, $650 for diagnostic hysteroscopy performed in the office, and $1500 for diagnostic hysteroscopy performed in the ambulatory surgical center. Towbin *et al.* [75] also looked at this issue in 1996 and found similar results: TVU was least expensive, and SHG and office hysteroscopy were similar ($700 and $800, respectively). In the same year, Hidlebaugh [87] reported that office hysteroscopy had higher yield and fewer complications than hospital hysteroscopy; hospital hysteroscopy was more than 10 times the cost of office hysteroscopy.

Triage Algorithms

Distinguishing among polyps, fibroids, hyperplasia, and malignancies can be done in a systematic fashion. A triage paradigm for perimenopausal patients with abnormal uterine bleeding presented by Goldstein *et al.* [88,89] is suggested here (Figure 22-7). TVU is performed, ideally on day 4, 5, or 6 of a bleeding episode, when the endometrium is likely to be thin. If the maximal bilayer thickness of the endometrium is less than 5 mm, it is highly unlikely [55] that any intrauterine pathology exists, and the abnormal bleeding is more likely due to another cause, such as dysfunctional bleeding. If a thickness of 5 mm or more is noted, a saline-infused SHG is performed to evaluate further the endometrial cavity contour. A thin endometrium (unilayer thickness < 3 mm) with no focal abnormalities sug-

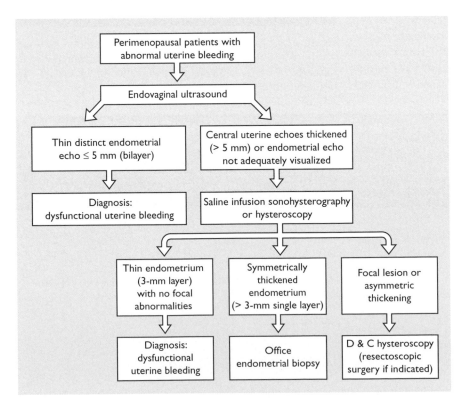

Figure 22-7. Flow chart for the treatment of perimenopausal women with abnormal uterine bleeding, starting with ultrasonography. D&C—dilation and curettage. (*Data from* Goldstein *et al.* [88].)

gests a cause other than anatomic. A uniformly thickened endometrium (unilayer thickness > 5 mm) suggests a global process such as hyperplasia or malignancy, and an endometrial biopsy is indicated. If a focal lesion (polyp or fibroid) or localized area of thickening is seen, then a hysteroscopy with focal biopsy and resection is performed [88].

A slightly different algorithm is suggested for postmenopausal bleeding (Figure 22-8). Initially, TVU and endometrial biopsy should be performed (as suggested earlier by Gupta *et al.* [63] and O'Connell *et al.* [72]). If the endometrial biopsy reveals hyperplasia or carcinoma, then the patient is treated accordingly. In this situation, an abnormal endometrial sampling alone is sufficient for diagnosis. If the endometrial thickness is less than 5 mm and the endometrial biopsy reveals no evidence of hyperplasia or carcinoma, then no further evaluation is necessary. If the endometrial thickness is greater than 5 mm and the endometrial biopsy reveals benign histology, then an SHG or hysteroscopy should be performed next to evaluate the intrauterine cavity for polyps and myomas. TVU also permits evaluation of ovarian pathology.

Treatment of Abnormal Uterine Bleeding

There can be an orderly method to deciding on a treatment based on the most likely cause and severity of the bleeding. Iron therapy should always be included in the treatment regimen when bleeding is moderate to severe. Most bleeding can be classified into three categories. First, dysfunctional bleeding is almost always related to anovulation. Treatment is predominantly hormonal, to counteract the changes in the endometrium caused by hormonal imbalance. The second category, idiopathic bleeding, occurs in women who have an ovulatory pattern. Depending on the severity, it may be treated with suppression of ovulation, suppression of the endometrium, or endometrial destruction. The third category consists of women with anatomic lesions, which are treated by removal or destruction. In addition to these categories, there are women with endometrial hyperplasia, which may be treated hormonally or surgically depending on the type of hyperplasia. There are also women with postmenopausal bleeding resulting from atrophy, who might be treated with local or systemic hormone replacement therapy

DYSFUNCTIONAL UTERINE BLEEDING

There are many variations on the use of hormonal treatment of dysfunctional bleeding; several review articles provide more detail. Although the types of bleeding are classified into four categories, women may have mixed endometrial types and may not always respond as expected. Figure 22-9 provides options for treating the patient with dysfunctional uterine bleeding [18,90–92].

Estrogen Breakthrough Bleeding (Anovulatory Bleeding): Mild or Moderate

For women who do not have contraindications to combined hormonal therapy (*eg*, smoking, over age 35, history of deep vein thrombosis, history of estrogen-dependent neoplasm, classic migraine with aura, severe hypertension, or liver dysfunction), the most commonly used hormonal therapy to treat mild anovulatory bleeding (hemoglobin > 10 mg/dL) is low-dose oral contraceptive pills (OCPs). The combined estrogen and progestogen prevents ovarian response by inhibiting pituitary production of gonadotropins. The result is a discontinuation of endogenous production of estrogen, resulting in only minimal growth of the endometrium and cessation of bleeding [16]. Monophasic and triphasic OCPs are effective [93]. Although 30 to 35 µg pills are frequently used, a 20 µg or 25 µg OCP may also be used; however, the incidence of spotting may be higher.

Although the evidence to support the use of other combined hormonal contraceptives (transdermal patch and vaginal ring) has not yet accumulated, it seems reasonable to use them

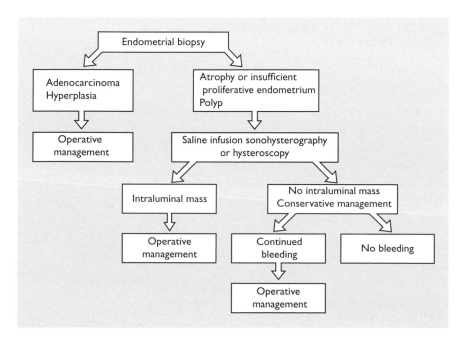

Figure 22-8. Flow chart for the evaluation of postmenopausal women with abnormal uterine bleeding, starting with endometrial sampling. (*Data from* O'Connell *et al.* [72].)

in place of OCPs as serum hormonal levels are similar to oral contraceptives. The transdermal patch may have slightly higher estradiol levels than OCPs [94].

Treatment can begin by inducing a progesterone withdrawal bleed with MPA at 10 mg daily for 7 to 12 days. After the withdrawal bleed, OCPs are continued for 3 to 6 months, at which time the patient is reevaluated. If bleeding is not heavy, another option is to simply start OCPs on the day of the visit. For women with moderate bleeding, another approach is to use OCPs two or three times daily, tapering over 1 to 2 weeks to daily use.

Dysfunctional Uterine Bleeding Treatment Options

Estrogen breakthrough bleeding (anovulatory): mild

Induce progesterone withdrawal bleed with MPA 10 mg PO daily for 7–12 days, or

Start oral contraceptives on that day regardless of bleeding status (once pregnancy is ruled out)

If contraception desired:

Follow withdrawal bleed with an OCP

If the woman does not desire contraception, but does not desire ovulation induction:

Begin cyclic progestin with MPA 10 mg PO daily or norethindrone acetate 2.5–5 mg PO daily for the first 12 days of each month, or every other month

If ovulation induction for pregnancy desired:

On 5th day of bleeding after progesterone withdrawal as above, begin clomiphene citrate 50 mg PO daily for 5 days (may be increased by 50 mg increments up to 150 mg as needed for evidence of ovulation)

Estrogen breakthrough bleeding (anovulatory): moderate

Begin with progestational agent such as:

MPA 10 mg PO daily for 7–12 days every 1–2 months

Norethindrone acetate 2.5–5 mg PO daily for 7–12 days every 1–2 months

Depot MPA 150 mg IM once a month

Levonorgestrel intrauterine system

An alternative is to administer a 35 μg monophasic estrogen-progestin OCP every 6 hours until bleeding stops

If bleeding stops:

Taper OCP as follows: one pill every 8 hours for 3 days ("3 for 3"); one pill every 12 hours for 2 days ("2 for 2"); then continue with one pill daily to complete a 28-day pack. The patient may then continue on OCPs for 3–6 months and then reevaluate

If bleeding does not stop:

Consider coagulation studies, and if normal, consider diagnostic testing for anatomic etiology

Progesterone breakthrough bleeding: moderate

Raw, denuded areas of endometrium may theoretically be repaired using oral estrogens every 6 hours until bleeding stops, then once daily, adding MPA 10 mg PO daily for 1 week. A withdrawal bleed will follow and the patient may then be started on cyclic hormonal contraception or progestin as above

Conjugated estrogen (Premarin, Wyeth Pharmaceuticals, Philadelphia, PA) 0.625 mg PO

Esterified estrogens (Menest, Monarch Pharmaceuticals, Bristol, TN; Estratab, Solvay, Brussels, Belgium) 0.625 mg PO

Estradiol (Estrace, Bristol-Myers Squibb, New York, NY) 0.5 mg PO

Estropipate (Ogen, Pharmacia and Upjohn, Kalamazoo, MI; Ortho-Est, Sun Pharmaceutical Industries, Andheri, Mumbai) 0.625 mg PO

Estrogen breakthrough bleeding (anovulatory): severe

Administer IV conjugated estrogen (Premarin 25 mg) every 4 hours until bleeding stops. Add MPA 10 mg PO daily toward the end of therapy to avoid an estrogen withdrawal bleed; then begin cyclic OCPs or progestin as above

High-dose MPA protocol:

Administer 5 mg PO every 1–2 hours for a total of 60–120 mg in the first 24 hours; follow with 20 mg PO daily

Consider uterine aspiration or curettage if acute

Figure 22-9. Dysfunctional uterine bleeding treatment options. IM—intramuscular; IV—intravenous; MPA—medroxyprogesterone acetate; OCP—oral contraceptive pill; PO—by mouth.

Prostaglandin synthetase inhibitors have been shown to reduce blood loss by 30% to 50%. Mefenamic acid (250 mg taken four times daily), meclofenamic acid (50 mg taken three or four times daily), and naproxen (250 to 500 mg taken twice daily) have all been used and have been shown to be useful adjuvant therapy [95,96]. A double-blind crossover study with naproxen sodium and mefenamic acid in patients with menorrhagia reported reductions in bleeding by 46% and 47%, respectively [97].

Bleeding from the unstable, thickened endometrium of chronic anovulation responds well to progestin therapy. This may be in the form of oral, intramuscular, or intrauterine progestins or estrogen-progestin OCPs (Figure 22-9). MPA 10 mg or norethisterone 2.5 to 5 mg daily for a minimum of 12 days each month for 3 to 6 months may be prescribed to induce endometrial atrophy. An alternative to cyclic monthly oral MPA is to administer 150 mg intramuscularly every 12 weeks.

An alternative to oral or intramuscular progestational agent therapy is the levonorgestrel intrauterine system (LNG-IUS). This system was compared with norethisterone (5 mg three times daily) in a randomized comparative parallel group study. The levonorgestrel intrauterine system compared favorably with any medical treatment available [98].

Estrogen therapy may be effective after prolonged bleeding resulting in raw, denuded or inflamed endometrium. It may also be helpful in treating atrophy resulting from menopause, or long-term OCP or depot MPA use resulting in atrophic endometrium (as evidenced by minimal tissue obtained by endometrial biopsy or curettage) [17,90–92]. These abnormal uterine bleeding situations should respond to exogenous estrogen administration, such as 7 days of oral conjugated estrogen (2.5 mg), esterified estrogens (2.5 mg), or estropipate [18].

Acute and Severe Estrogen Breakthrough Bleeding (Anovulatory Bleeding)

The anemic patient with acute, severe bleeding should be hospitalized and started on intravenous conjugated estrogen (25 mg) given every 4 hours until bleeding stops [18,99,100]. Conjugated estrogens have an effect on platelet aggregation, increase factors V and IX, increase fibrinogen levels, and decrease the effectiveness of bradykinin [100]. After the bleeding diminishes, a progestational agent should be added to avoid estrogen withdrawal bleeding on discontinuation of the intravenous therapy. Once stabilized, the patient may be prescribed cyclic oral contraceptives or cyclic progestin.

Gonadotropin-releasing Hormone Agonist Therapy

Gonadotropin-releasing hormone agonists have been used for abnormal uterine bleeding in patients with contraindications to sex steroid therapy or in patients who have failed conventional hormonal therapy [101]. GnRH agonist therapy induces amenorrhea and avoids acute bleeding episodes, which may be especially beneficial in patients with bleeding disorders. Ovarian suppression with GnRH agonist therapy may take up to 3 weeks and is therefore not useful in the acute situation. A disadvantage of this therapy is its limited duration of use. Therapy is limited to 6 months because of bone demineralization and adverse lipid profiles. Unwanted side effects, such as hot flushes and vaginal dryness, are common, but can be treated with steroid add-back therapy [102].

If severe bleeding continues and repeat coagulation studies are within normal limits, a D & C may be indicated, but its success as a cure is only temporary. The therapeutic effects of D & C disappear by the second month after the procedure [103].

Bleeding Due To Atrophy

Estrogen therapy may be effective after prolonged bleeding resulting in raw, denuded, or inflamed endometrium. It may also be helpful in treating atrophy resulting from menopause or long-term OCP or depot MPA use resulting in atrophic endometrium (as evidenced by minimal tissue obtained by endometrial biopsy or curettage) [17,90–92]. These abnormal uterine bleeding situations should respond to exogenous estrogen administration, such as 7 days of oral conjugated estrogen (2.5 mg), esterified estrogens (2.5 mg), or estropipate [18].

Hyperplasia

Simple hyperplasia may be treated with progestins; follow-up of endometrial sampling in 3 to 6 months is needed to ensure resolution [23]. In young women, OCPs may be the easiest method of providing a continuous progestogen-dominant medication. For older women, cyclic MPA or depot MPA can be used. Complex hyperplasia or hyperplasia with atypia should be referred for consultation [12], because the probability of malignancy is higher [23,24].

Idiopathic Bleeding

Idiopathic bleeding, if not severe, can be treated with suppression of ovulation by combined hormonal contraception, or by cyclic or continuous progestin. The LNG-IUS also may be used, and it has the advantage of decreasing menses while preserving ovarian function. The LNG-IUS does not suppress ovulation for most women; the progestational effect is largely limited to the uterus [104]. Severe bleeding in association with ovulation may require hormonal suppression or local endometrial destruction

Treatment of Menorrhagia and Anatomic Lesions

When abnormal bleeding persists despite medical treatment, or when side effects limit use of medications, there are treatments that alter or destroy the endometrium directly.

Levonorgestrel Intrauterine System

The LNG-IUS releases 20 µg of levonorgestrel daily. Serum levels are very low, while levels of LNG in the endometrium are much higher than serum levels. Each device can be used for up to 5 years. Serious complications are very rare; perforations occur with fewer than one per 1000 insertions [104].

In the first year after insertion, expulsion rates range from 2% to 10% [104]. However, in one study, when the intrauterine device is inserted for treatment of bleeding, expulsion rates are higher than those seen for contraceptive patients (13% vs 5%). After the first year, expulsion occurs in fewer than 1% per year [105].

When the LNG-IUS is used for contraception, menstrual bleeding is reduced up to 90%, although spotting is common in the first months of use. The LNG-IUS has been used to treat idiopathic menorrhagia [106–108]. In a prospective study, the LNG-IUS was more effective than norethisterone, although both resulted in decreases in blood loss [107]. Advantages of the LNG-IUS include office insertion with standard office instruments and reversibility. Although use of the LNG-IUS may decrease bleeding significantly, it may not stop bleeding completely; only 20% of women are amenorrheic [104]. If amenorrhea is desired, the LNG-IUS may not be satisfactory.

The LNG-IUS has not yet been demonstrated to be as effective at controlling abnormal bleeding from anatomic lesions such as polyps and submucous fibroids. If abnormal bleeding persists despite LNG-IUS, an anatomic lesion may be the cause and other investigation such as SHG, hysterosalpingogram, or hysteroscopy should be considered. At the time of this writing, no intrauterine device has been US Food and Drug Administration approved in the United States for the treatment of menorrhagia, although the LNG-IUS is approved for that indication in other countries.

Levonorgestrel intrauterine devices have also been used for postmenopausal women who have bleeding related to hormone replacement therapy [109]. Other causes of the bleeding, such as polyp or hyperplasia, need to be excluded first. The local delivery of progestin to the endometrium may prevent bleeding in women using hormone replacement therapy or unopposed estrogen. This indication has been approved in several countries, but not in the United States. Wildemeersch and Dhont [110] have used another model of an intrauterine device to treat hyperplasia. An LNG-IUS has also been used to prevent hyperplasia related to tamoxifen use [111].

TREATMENT OF ANATOMIC LESIONS OR INTRACTABLE IDIOPATHIC BLEEDING

Hysteroscopic Resection and Endometrial Ablation

Abnormal uterine bleeding from endometrial polyps or submucous myomas diagnosed using ultrasonography, saline SHG, or hysteroscopy may be managed by hysteroscopic resection [80,81,112–114]. The majority of women have improvement, but repeat procedure is sometimes necessary [114]. Hysteroscopic resection has the advantage of preserving fertility for some women [115].

Global endometrial ablation should be considered for those patients who do not desire aggressive surgery, who are not good surgical candidates, or who have failed or declined medical therapy. Women with polyps or, in some cases, with small fibroids are appropriate candidates. Before performing any endometrial ablation technique, an endometrial biopsy to assess uterine malignancy or premalignant changes should be performed.

Hysteroscopic techniques of global ablation include laser ablation, electrosurgical wire loop resection, and rollerball [116–118]. These were compared in a randomized controlled

Comparison of Nonhysteroscopic Ablation Methods with Rollerball Ablation

Ablation Method	Cervical Dilation Necessary, *mm*	Maximum Uterine Cavity Length, *cm*	Use with Submucosal Myomas	Approximate Treatment Time, *min*	Amenorrhea Rates at 12 mo, %	
					Global Endo Ablation	Rollerball Ablation
ThermaChoice (thermal balloon); ThermaChoice Gynecare, Somerville, NJ	5	4–10	No	8	13.9	24.4
Hydro ThermAblator (circulated hot fluid); Boston Scientific, Natick, MA	8	≤ 10.5s	If < 4 cm	10	35.3	47.1
Her Option (cryotherapy); Her Option American Medical Systems, Minnetonka, MN	5	≤ 10	If < 2 cm	10–18	22.2	46.5
NovaSure (RF electrosurgery); Cytyc, Marlborough, MA	8	6–10*	If < 2 cm	1.5	36	32.2
MEA (microwave energy); Microsulis Americas, Inc., Waltham, MA	8.5	6–14		3.5	55.3	45.8

NSAIDs recommended for all procedures.
*Cavity 4–6.5 cm from internal os.

Figure 22-10. Comparison of nonhysteroscopic ablation methods with rollerball ablation. NSAIDs—nonsteroidal anti-inflammatory drugs; RF—radiofrequency.

trial of 372 patients [119]. There was no difference in symptom relief (bleeding and dysmenorrhea), satisfaction, or psychologic outcomes.

Alternatives to hysteroscopic ablation include the five US Food and Drug Administration–approved global endometrial ablation devices. These include thermal balloon ablation therapy, instillation of hot saline solution, cryotherapy, radiofrequency electrosurgery, and microwave energy [120–127]. These are shown in Figure 22-10.

Uterine artery embolization is a treatment option for intractable uterine bleeding. Usually performed by an interventional radiologist under fluoroscopy, a small catheter is placed into the common femoral artery. The catheter is advanced and the uterine arteries are embolized with tiny polyvinyl alcohol particles or trisacryl gelatin microspheres. This procedure can be done as an outpatient or overnight procedure [128]. Spies et al. [129] followed 1797 patients 1 year after uterine artery embolization. They found that 95% of patients had symptomatic improvement, 7% developed amenorrhea, and only 2.9% underwent a hysterectomy [129]. A review by David and Ebert [130] found hysterectomy rates of 1% to 12%. Uterine artery embolization has comparable risks to hysterectomy including febrile morbidity (2%), hemorrhage (0.75%), performance of unintended procedure (3.5%), and life-threatening events (0.5%) [131].

Magnetic resonance–guided focused ultrasonographic myolysis was approved by the US Food and Drug Administration in 2006 as a nonoperative procedure that uses targeted ultrasound to destroy fibroids.

Hysterectomy

If medical or surgical treatment of bleeding has been unacceptable or unsuccessful, a hysterectomy may be considered. There are many different methods of performing a hysterectomy, including the following: abdominal supracervical or total hysterectomy; total vaginal hysterectomy; laparoscopic supracervical or total hysterectomy; and long-term outcome of treatment for menorrhagia.

When considering surgical therapy, long-term results and patient satisfaction must be considered. Learman et al. [132] randomized women with menorrhagia, who had already failed medical treatment with cyclic MPA, to receive additional medical treatment with OCPs and a prostaglandin inhibitor, or hysterectomy. After 24 months, 53% of women requested hysterectomy. Women with hysterectomy had better control of symptoms, but had more hospital days and days off from work [132]. Some studies comparing LNG-IUS and hysteroscopic endometrial resection found comparable outcomes [133,134]. In contrast, a Cochrane Database Review of surgical treatment of menorrhagia (hysterectomy or ablative therapy) versus treatment with LNG-IUS found that hysterectomy and conservative surgery were more effective at reducing bleeding than LNG-IUS. However, all were equally effective in improving quality of life [135].

A randomized, controlled trial of 196 participants comparing endometrial resection with abdominal hysterectomy found a significantly higher satisfaction rate with hysterectomy (94%) than with endometrial resection (85%) at 4 months' follow-up [136]. Success, defined as decrease in menses or amenorrhea, occurred in 91% of patients of women having endometrial resection.

Another prospective, randomized controlled trial compared endometrial laser ablation and hysteroscopic endometrial resection to hysterectomy (abdominal and vaginal) in 204 women with dysfunctional uterine bleeding [137]. At 12 months' follow-up, only 22% of those treated conservatively had amenorrhea, but 62% had hypomenorrhea. At this time, 78% of the hysteroscopy group and 89% of the hysterectomy group were very satisfied. A prospective, randomized study (85 participants) by Crosignani et al. [138] compared endometrial resection to vaginal hysterectomy and reported no significant difference in patient satisfaction or sexual functioning between the two groups at 24 months. Tapper and Heinonen [139] compared hysteroscopic endometrial resection with laparoscopically assisted vaginal hysterectomy and confirmed that operating time, blood loss, and recovery time were all less in the hysteroscopy group. The satisfaction rate was high in both groups: 92% in the hysteroscopy group and 97% in the laparoscopically assisted vaginal hysterectomy group. Comparisons of endometrial ablation and hysterectomy are summarized by a Cochran Database review [135].

Endometrial ablations, hysteroscopic removal of a focal lesion, and uterine artery embolization all have reduced cost, morbidity, and hospitalization compared with hysterectomy; however, long-term health care costs may narrow the difference. Ransom et al. [140] performed a retrospective cost analysis of endometrial ablation, abdominal hysterectomy, vaginal hysterectomy, and laparoscopic-assisted vaginal hysterectomy in patients treated for menorrhagia. As expected, endometrial ablation had the lowest average charge ($3765), but charges associated with long-term failures and complications were not included. Of the other three, laparoscopic-assisted vaginal hysterectomy incurred the highest average charge ($11,534), and vaginal hysterectomy incurred the lowest ($7413). Brumstead et al. [141] found that endometrial ablation ($5159) was slightly less than hysteroscopic myomectomy and ablation ($5525); both were considerably less expensive than vaginal or abdominal myomectomy, which were over $8000 each. Hidlebaugh [142] found that endometrial ablation was less expensive even after all follow-up costs were considered.

Conclusions

Abnormal uterine bleeding is a common gynecologic problem that repeatedly confronts physicians. The systematic approach to diagnosing and treating the various causes begins with understanding the characteristics of each patient's bleeding. This understanding permits the physician to identify the category (ie, dysfunctional uterine bleeding, blood dyscrasias, anatomic abnormality, or chronic disease) to which the bleeding likely belongs. Necessary diagnostic tests may then be performed and an effective treatment chosen.

There is still much that we do not know: the most efficient clinical pathway for diagnosis of abnormal uterine bleeding;

the true efficacy of many hormonal treatment regimens; and the comparative value of many treatments, including their direct and indirect costs and levels of patient satisfaction. However, the advances in ultrasound and direct imaging have allowed diagnosis and treatment with minimally invasive procedures. There are currently many options for diagnosis and treatment. Studies of economic implications as well as patient satisfaction and safety are needed so that the best procedures can be selected.

References

1. Kjerulff KH, Erickson BA, Langenberg PW: Chronic gynecological conditions reported by US women: findings from the National Health Interview Survey 1984 to 1992. *Am J Public Health* 1996, 86:195–199.

2. Coulter A, Bradlow J, Agass M, *et al.*: Outcome of referrals to gynaecology clinics for menstrual problems: an audit of general practice records. *Br J Obstet Gynaecol* 1991, 98:789–796.

3. Cote I, Jacobs P, Cumming DC: Use of health services associated with increased menstrual loss in the United States. *Am J Obstet Gynecol* 2003, 188:343–348.

4. Snowden R, Christian B: *Patterns and Perception of Menstruation: A World Health Organization International Study*. London: Croom Helm; 1983.

5. Stewart EA, Strauss JF: Disorders of the uterus: leiomyomas, adenomyosis, endometrial polyps, abnormal uterine bleeding, intrauterine adhesions, and dysmenorrhea. In *Yen and Jaffe's Reproductive Endocrinology*, edn 7. Edited by Strauss JF, Barbieri RL. Philadelphia: Elsevier-Saunders; 2004.

6. Kramer SF, Patel A: The frequency of uterine leiomyomas. *Am J Clin Pathol* 1990, 94:435–438.

7. *ACOG Practice Bulletin Number 16: Surgical Alternatives in the Management of Leiomyomas*. Washington, DC: American College of Obstetricians and Gynecologists; 2000.

8. Wegienka G, Baird DD, Hertz-Picciotto I, *et al.*: Self-reported heavy bleeding associated with uterine leiomyomata. *Obstet Gynecol* 2003, 101:431–437.

9. Rodeghiero F, Castaman G, Dini E: Epidemiological investigation of the prevalence of von Willebrand's disease. *Blood* 1987, 69:454–459.

10. Werner EJ, Broxson EH, Tucker EL, *et al.*: Prevalence of von Willebrand disease in children: a multiethnic study. *J Pediatr* 1993, 123:893–898.

11. Dilley A, Drews C, Miller C, *et al.*: von Willebrand disease and other inherited bleeding disorders in women with diagnosed menorrhagia. *Obstet Gynecol* 2001, 97:630–636.

12. Lurain JR: Uterine cancer. *Bereak and Novak's Gynecology*, edn 4. Edited by Berek JS. Philadelphia: Lippincott Williams & Wilkins; 2007:1349.

13. Brinton LA, Bennan JL, Mortel R, *et al.*: Reproductive, menstrual, and medical risk factors for endometrial cancer: results from a case-control study. *Am J Obstet Gynecol* 1992, 167:1317–1325.

14. *American College of Obstetricians and Gynecologists Committee Opinion Number 232: Tamoxifen and Endometrial Cancer*. Washington, DC: American College of Obstetricians and Gynecologists; 2000.

15. Hallberg L, Hogdahl AM, Nilsson L, *et al.*: Menstrual blood loss-a population study. *Acta Obstet Gynecol Scand* 1966, 45:320–351.

16. Regulation of the menstrual cycle. In *Fritz's Clinical Gynecologic Endocrinology and Infertility*, edn 7. Edited by Speroff L, Fritz M. Philadelphia: Lippincott Williams & Wilkins; 2005.

17. Hertweck SP: Dysfunctional uterine bleeding. *Obstet Gynecol Clin North Am* 1992, 19:129–149.

18. Dysfunctional uterine bleeding. In *Fritz's Clinical Gynecologic Endocrinology and Infertility*, edn 7. Edited by Speroff L, Fritz M. Philadelphia: Lippincott Williams & Wilkins; 2005.

19. VanLook PFA, Hunter WM, Fraser IS, *et al.*: Impaired estrogen induced luteinizing hormonal release in young women with anovulatory dysfunctional uterine bleeding. *J Clin Endocrinol Metab* 1978, 46:816–823.

20. Ferenczy A: Pathophysiology of endometrial bleeding. *Maturitas* 2003, 45:1-14.

21. Venturoli S, Porcu E, Fabbri R, *et al.*: Menstrual irregularities in adolescents: hormonal pattern and ovarian morphology. *Hormone Res* 1986, 24:269–279.

22. Lidor A, Ismajovich B, Confino E, David MP: Histopathological findings in 226 women with post-menopausal uterine bleeding. *Acta Obstet Gynecol Scand* 1986, 65:41–43.

23. Clark JT, Neelakantan D, Gupta JG: The management of endometrial hyperplasia: an evaluation of current practice. *Eur J Obstet Gynecol* 2006, 125:159–63.

24. Kurman RJ, Kaminski PF, Norris HJ: The behavior of endometrial hyperplasia: a long term study of "untreated" hyperplasia in 170 patients. *Cancer* 1985, 56:403–412.

25. Anovulation and the polycystic ovary. In *Clinical Gynecologic Endocrinology and Infertility*, edn 7. Edited by Speroff L, Fritz M. Philadelphia: Lippincott Williams and Wilkins; 2005.

26. Siegel JE: Abnormalities of hemostasis and abnormal uterine bleeding. *Clin Obstet Gynecol* 2005, 48:284–294.

27. Munro MG, Lukes AS, for the Abnormal Uterine Bleeding and Underlying Hemostatic Disorders Consensus Group: Abnormal uterine bleeding and underlying hemostatic disorders: report of a consensus process. *Fertil Steril* 2005, 84:1335–1337.

27. Brenner PF: Differential diagnosis of abnormal uterine bleeding. *Am J Obstet Gynecol* 1996, 1175:766–769.

28. James A. Matchar DB, Myers ER: Testing for von Willebrand disease in women with menorrhagia: A systematic review. *Obstet Gynecol* 2004, 104:381–388.

29. Ghany M, Hoofnagle JH. Approach to the patient with liver disease. In *Harrison's Principles of Internal Medicine*, edn 16. Edited by Kasper DL, Braunwald E, Fauci AS. New York: McGraw-Hill; 2006.

30. Krassas GE, Pontikides N, Kaltsas T, *et al.*: Disturbances of menstruation in hypothyroidism. *Clin Endocrinol* 1999, 50:655–659.

31. Cochrane R, Regan L. Undetected gynecological disorders in women with renal disease. *Hum Repro* 1997, 12:667–670.

32. Morley JE, Distiller LA, Epstein S, *et al.*: Menstrual disturbances in chronic renal failure. *Hormone Metab Res* 1979, 11:68–72.

33. Handelsman DJ, Dong Q: Hypothalamic-pituitary gonadal axis in chronic renal failure. *Endocrinol Metab Clin North Am* 1993, 22:145–161.

34. Yeshaya A, Orvieto R, Dicker D, *et al.*: Menstrual characteristics of women suffering from insulin-dependent diabetes mellitus. *Int J Fertil* 1995, 40:269–273.

35. Griffin ML, South SA, Yankov VI, *et al.*: Insulin-dependent diabetes mellitus and menstrual dysfunction. *Ann Med* 1994, 26:331–340.

36. *ACOG Clinical Management Guidelines of Obstetricians-Gynecologists, Number 41*. Washington, DC: American College of Obstetricians and Gynecologists; 2002.

37. Martinez AR, Zinaman MJ, Jennings VH, *et al.*: Prediction and detection of the fertile period: the markers. *Int J Fertil Menopausal Stud* 1995, 40:139–155.

38. Vermesh M, Kletzky OA, Davajan V, *et al.*: Monitoring techniques to predict and detect ovulation. *Fertil Steril* 1987, 47:259.

39. Pearlstone AC, Surrey ES: The temporal relation between the urine LH surge and sonographic evidence of ovulation: determinants and clinical significance. *Obstet Gynecol* 1994, 83:184–188.

40. Israel R, Mishell DR Jr, Stone SC, *et al.*: Single luteal phase serum progesterone assay as an indicator of ovulation. *Am J Obstet Gynecol* 1972, 112:1043–1046.

41. Ilesanmi AO: Endometrial dating correlated with multiple luteal progesterone levels in confirming ovulation and luteal function in infertile Nigerian women. *West Afr J Med* 1995, 14:152–156.

42. Noyes RW, Hertig AT, Rock J: Dating the endometrial biopsy. *Fertil Steril* 1950, 1:3.

43. Queenan JT, O'Brien GD, Bains LM, *et al.*: Ultrasound scanning of ovaries to detect ovulation in women. *Fertil Steril* 1980, 34:99.

44. Emanuel MH, Wamsteker K, Lammes FB: Is dilatation and curettage obsolete for diagnosing intrauterine disorders in premenopausal patients with persistent abnormal uterine bleeding? *Acta Obstet Gynecol Scand* 1997, 76:65–68.

45. Apgar BS, Newkirk GR: Endometrial biopsy. *Prim Care* 1997, 24:303–326.

46. Stovall TG, Photopulos GJ, Poston WM, *et al.*: Pipelle endometrial sampling in patients with known endometrial carcinoma. *Obstet Gynecol* 1991, 77:945–946.

47. Stovall TG, Ling FW, Morgan PL: A prospective, randomized comparison of the Pipelle endometrial sampling device with the Novak curette. *Am J Obstet Gynecol* 1991, 165:1287–1290.

48. Koonings PP, Moyer DL, Grimes DA: A randomized clinical trial comparing Pipelle and Tis-U-Trap for endometrial biopsy. *Obstet Gynecol* 1990, 75:293–295.

49. Dijkhuizen FP. Mol BW, Brolmann HA, Heintz AP: The accuracy of endometrial sampling in the diagnosis of patients with endometrial carcinoma and hyperplasia: a meta-analysis. *Cancer* 2000, 89:1765–1772.

50. Clark TJ, Mann CH, Shah N, *et al.*: The accuracy of outpatient endometrial biopsy in the diagnosis of endometrial hyperplasia. *Acta Obstet Gynecol Scand* 2001, 80:784–793.

51. Fleischer AC, Kalemeris GC, Eastman SS: Sonographic depiction of the endometrium during normal cycles. *Ultrasound Med Biol* 1986,12:271.

52. DeLange M, Rouse GA: *Ob/Gyn Sonography: An Illustrated Review*. Pasadena: Davies Publishing Inc.; 2004.

53. Varner RE, Sparks JM, Cameron CD, *et al.*: Transvaginal sonography of the endometrium in postmenopausal women. *Obstet Gynecol* 1991, 78:195–199.

54. Dueholm M, Jensen ML, Laurseon H, Kracht P: Can the endometrial thickness as measured by transvaginal sonography be used to exclude polyps or hyperplasia in pre-menopausal patients with abnormal uterine bleeding? *Acta Obstet Gynecol Scand* 2001, 80:645–651.

55. Nasri MN, Shepherd JH, Setchell ME, *et al.*: The role of vaginal scan measurement of endometrial thickness in postmenopausal women. *Br J Obstet Gynaecol* 1991, 98:470–475.

56. Granberg S, Wikland M, Karlsson B, *et al.*: Endometrial thickness as measured by endovaginal ultrasonography for identifying endometrial abnormality. *Am J Obstet Gynecol* 1991, 164:47–52.

57. Giusa-Chiferi MG, Goncalves WJ, Baracat EC, *et al.*: Transvaginal ultrasound, uterine biopsy and hysteroscopy for postmenopausal bleeding. *Int J Gynecol Obstet* 1996, 55:39–44.

58. Haller H, Matejcic N, Rukavina B, *et al.*: Transvaginal sonography and hysteroscopy in women with postmenopausal bleeding. *Int J Gynaecol Obstet* 1996, 54:155–159.

59 . Hanggi W, Bersinger N, Altermatt HJ, *et al.*: Comparison of transvaginal ultrasonography and endometrial biopsy in endometrial surveillance in postmenopausal HRT users. *Maturitas* 1997, 27:133–143.

60. Emanuel MH, Verdel MJ, Warnsteker K, Lammes FB: A prospective comparison of transvaginal ultrasonography and diagnostic hysteroscopy in the evaluation of patients with abnormal uterine bleeding: clinical implications. *Am J Obstet Gynecol* 1995, 172:547–552.

61. Tabor A, Watt HC, Wald NJ: Endometrial thickness as a test for endometrial cancer in women with postmenopausal vaginal bleeding. *Obstet Gynecol* 2002, 99:663–670.

62. Maia H Jr, Barbosa IC, Marques D, *et al.*: Hysteroscopy and transvaginal sonography in menopausal women receiving hormone replacement therapy. *J Am Assoc Gynecol Laparosc* 1996, 4:13–16.

63. Gupta JK, Wilson S, Desai P, *et al.*: How should we investigate women with postmenopausal bleeding? *Acta Obstet Gynecol Scand* 1996, 75:475–479.

64. *ACOG Technology Assessment in Obstetrics and Gynecology: Saline Infusion Sonohysterography Compendium of Selected Publications, Number 3*. Washington, DC: American College of Obstetricians and Gynecologists; 2003.

65. Dessole S, Farina M, Rubattu G, *et al.*: Side effects and complications of sono-hysterosalpingography. *Fertil Steril* 2003, 80:620–624.

66. Cullinan JA, Fleischer AC, Kepple DM, *et al.*: Sonohysterography: a technique for endometrial evaluation. *Radiographics* 1995, 15:501–514.

67. Fedele L, Bianchi S, Dorta M, *et al.*: Transvaginal ultrasonography versus hysteroscopy in the diagnosis of uterine submucous myomas. *Obstet Gynecol* 1991, 77:745–748.

68. Goldstein SR, Zeltser I, Horan CK, *et al.*: Ultrasonography-based triage for perimenopausal patients with abnormal uterine bleeding. *Am J Obstet Gynecol* 1997, 177:102–108.

69. Tur-Kaspa I, Gal M, Hartman M, *et al.*: A prospective evaluation of uterine abnormalities by saline infusion sonohysterography in 1009 women with infertility or abnormal uterine bleeding. *Fertil Steril* 2006, 86:1731–1735.

70. Bernard JP, Lecuru F, Darles C, *et al.*: Saline contrast sonohysterography as first-line investigation for women with uterine bleeding. *Ultrasound Obstet Gynecol* 1997, 10:121–125.

71. Kamel HS, Darwish AM, Mohamed SA: Comparison of transvaginal ultrasonography and vaginal sonohysterography in the detection of endometrial polyps. *Acta Scand Obstet Gynecol* 2000, 79:60–64.

72. O'Connell LP, Fries MH, Zeringue E, *et al.*: Triage of abnormal postmenopausal bleeding: a comparison of endometrial biopsy and transvaginal sonohysterography versus fractional curettage with hysteroscopy. *Am J Obstet Gynecol* 1998, 178:956–961.

73. Mihm LM, Quick VA, Brumfield JA, *et al.*: The accuracy of endometrial biopsy and saline sonohysterography in the determination of the cause of abnormal bleeding. *Am J Obstet Gynecol* 2002, 186:858–860.

74. Dujhuizen AP, de Vries LD, Mol BW, *et al.*: comparison of transvaginal ultrasonography and saline infusion sonography for the detection of intracavitary abnormalities in premenopausal women. *Ultrasound Obstet Gynecol* 2000, 15:372–376.

75. Towbin NA, Gviazda IM, March CM: Office hysteroscopy versus transvaginal ultrasonography in the evaluation of patients with excessive uterine bleeding. *Am J Obstet Gynecol* 1996, 174:1678–1682.

76. Saidi MH, Sadler RK, Theis VD, *et al.*: Comparison of sonography, sonohysterography, and hysteroscopy for evaluation of abnormal uterine bleeding. *J Ultrasound Med* 1997, 16:587–591.

77. Schwarzler P, Concin H, Bosch H, *et al.*: An evaluation of sonohysterography and diagnostic hysterography for the assessment of intrauterine pathology. *Ultrasound Obstet Gynecol* 1998, 11:337–342.

78. Epstein E, Ramirez A, Skoog L, Valentin L: Transvaginal sonography, saline contrast sonohysterography and hysteroscopy for the investigation of women with postmenopausal bleeding and endometrium > 5 mm. *Ultrasound Obstet Gynecol* 2001, 18:157–162.

79. Cepni I, Ocal P, Erkan A, *et al.*: Comparison of transvaginal sonography, saline infusion sonography and hysteroscopy in the evaluation of uterine cavity pathologies. *Aust N Z J Obstet Gynaecol* 2005, 45:30–35.

80. Baggish MD: Operative hysteroscopy. In *TeLinde's Operative Gynecology*. Edited by Rock JA, Jones HW. Philadelphia: Lippincott Williams & Wilkins; 2003:399–411.

81. *ACOG Technology Assessment in Obstetrics and Gynecology, Number 4: Hysteroscopy*. Washington, DC: American College of Obstetricians and Gynecologists; 2005.

82. Nagele F, O'Connor H, Davies A, *et al.*: 2500 Outpatient diagnostic hysteroscopies. *Obstet Gynecol* 1996, 88:87–92.

83. Garuti G, Sambruni I, Colonnelli, Luerti M: Accuracy of hysteroscopy in predicting histopathology of endometrium in 1500 women. *J Am Assoc Gynecol Laparosc* 2001, 8:207–213.

84. Alcazar JL, Laparte C: Comparative study of transvaginal ultrasonography and hysteroscopy in postmenopausal bleeding. *Gynecol Obstet Invest* 1996, 41:47–49.

85. Haller H, Matejcic N, Rukavina B, *et al.*: Transvaginal sonography and hysteroscopy in women with postmenopausal bleeding. *Int J Gynaecol Obstet* 1996, 54:155–159.

86. Loerro G, Bettocchi S, Cormio G, *et al.*: Diagnostic accuracy of hysteroscopy in endometrial hyperplasia. *Maturitas* 1996, 25:187–191.

87. Hidlebaugh D: A comparison of clinical outcomes and cost of office versus hospital hysteroscopy. *J Am Assoc Gynecol Laparosc* 1996, 4:39–45.

88. Goldstein SR, Zeltser I, Horan CK, *et al.*: Ultrasonography based triage for perimenopausal patients with abnormal uterine bleeding. *Am J Obstet Gynecol* 1997, 177:102–108.

89. Goldstein RB, Bree RL, Benson CB, *et al.*: Society of Radiologists in Ultrasound-Sponsored Consensus Statement. Evaluation of the woman with post-menopausal bleeding. *J Ultrasound Med* 2001, 20:1025–1036.

90. Singh RH, Blumenthal P: Hormonal management of abnormal uterine bleeding. *Clin Obstet Gynecol* 2005, 48:337–352.

91. Chuong CJ, Brenner PF: Management of abnormal uterine bleeding. *Am J Obstet Gynecol* 1996, 175:787–92.

92. *ACOG Practice Bulletin, Number 4: Management of Anovulatory Bleeding*. Washington, DC: American College of Obstetricians and Gynecologists; 2000

93. Davis A, Godwin A, Lippman J, *et al.*: Triphasic norgestimate-ethinyl estradiol for treating dysfunctional uterine bleeding. *Obstet Gynecol* 2000, 96:913–920.

94. van den Heuvel MW, van Bragt AJ, Alnabawy A, Kaptein M: Comparison of ethinyl estradiol pharmacokinetics in three hormonal contraceptive formulations: the vaginal ring, the transdermal patch and an oral contraceptive. *Contraception* 2005, 72:168–174.

95. Bonnar J, Sheppard BL: Treatment of menorrhagia during menstruation: randomized controlled trial of ethamsylate, mefenamic acid and tranexamic acid. *Br Med J* 1996, 313:579–582.

96. Lethaby A, Augood C, Duckitt K: Nonsteroidal anti-inflammatory drugs for heavy menstrual bleeding. *Cochrane Database Syst Rev* 2002, 1:CD000400.

97. Nilsson L, Rybo G: Treatment of menorrhagia. *Am J Obstet Gynecol* 1971, 110:713.

98. Irvine GA, Campbell-Brown MB, Lumsden MA, *et al.*: Randomised comparative trial of the levonorgestrel intrauterine system and norethisterone for treatment of idiopathic menorrhagia. *Br J Obstet Gynaecol* 1998, 105:592–598.

99. Devore GR, Owens O, Kase N: Use of intravenous Premarin in the treatment of dysfunctional uterine bleeding: double blind randomized controlled study. *Obstet Gynecol* 1982, 59:285.

100. Livio M, Mannucci PM, Vigano G, *et al.*: Conjugated estrogens for the management of bleeding associated with renal failure. *N Engl J Med* 1986, 315:731.

101. Laufer MR, Rein MS: Treatment of abnormal uterine bleeding with gonadotropin-releasing hormone analogues. *Clin Obstet Gynecol* 1993, 36:668–678.

102. Thomas EJ: Add-back therapy for long-term use in dysfunctional uterine bleeding and uterine fibroids. *Br J Obstet Gynaecol* 1996, 103:18–21.

103. Smith JJ, Schulman H: Current dilation and curettage practice: a need for reversal. *Obstet Gynecol* 1988, 65:16–18.

104. Grimes DA: Intrauterine devices (IUDs). In *Contraceptive Technology*, edn 18. Edited by Hatcher RA, Trussell J, Stewart F, *et al.* New York: Ardent Media, Inc.; 2004.

105. Hildago M, Bahamondes L, Perrotti D, *et al.*: Bleeding patterns and clinical performance of the levo-norgestrel-releasing intrauterine system (Mireno) up to two years. *Contraception* 2002, 65:129–132.

106. Hubacher D, Grimes DA: Noncontraceptive health benefits of intrauterine devices: a systematic review. *Obstet Gynecol Surv* 2002, 57:120–128.

107. Wildemeersch D, Janssens D, Schacht E, *et al.*: Intrauterine levonorgestrel delivered by a frameless system, combined with systemic estrogen: acceptability and endometrial safety after 3 years of use in peri- and postmenopausal women. *Gynecol Endocrinol* 2005, 20:336–342.

108. Rauramo I, Elo I, Istre O: Long-term treatment of menorrhagia with levonorgestrel intrauterine system versus endometrial resection. *Obstet Gynecol* 2004, 104:1314–1321.

109. Crosignani PG, Vercellini P, Mosconi P, *et al.*: Levonorgestrel-releasing intrauterine device versus hysteroscopic endometrial resection in the treatment of dysfunctional uterine bleeding. *Obstet Gynecol* 1997, 90:257–263.

110. Wildemeersch D, Dhont M: Treatment of non-atypical and atypical endometrial hyperplasia with a levonorgestrel-releasing intrauterine system. *Am J Obstet Gynecol* 2003, 188:1297–1298.

111. Gardner FJ, Konje JC, Abrams KR, *et al.*: Endometrial protection from tamoxifen-stimulated changes by a levonorgestrel-releasing intrauterine system: a randomised controlled trial. *Lancet* 2000, 356:1711–1717.

112. Baggish MS: Operative hysteroscopy. In *TeLinde's Operative Gynecology*, edn 9. Edited by Rock JA, Jones HW. Philadelphia: Lippincott Williams & Wilkins; 2003:399–411.

113. Tjarks M, van Voorhis BJ: Treatment of endometrial polyps. *Obstet Gynecol* 2000, 96:866–869.

114. Emanuel MH, Wamsteker K, Hart AM, *et al.*: Long-term results of hysteroscopic myomectomy for abnormal uterine bleeding. *Obstet Gynecol* 1999, 93:743–748.

115. Lo JS, Pickersgill A: Pregnancy after endometrial ablation: English literature review and case report. *J Minim Invasive Gynecol* 2006, 13:88–91.

116. Munro MG: Endometrial ablation for heavy menstrual bleeding. *Curr Opinion Obstet Gynecol* 2005, 17:381–394.

117. Garry R, Shelley-Jones D, Mooney P, *et al.*: Six hundred endometrial laser ablations. *Obstet Gynecol* 1995, 85:24–29.

118. O'Connor H, Magos A: Endometrial resection for the treatment of menorrhagia. *N Engl J Med* 1996, 335:151–156.

119. Vercellini P, Oldani S, Yaylayan L. *et al.*: Randomized comparison of vaporizing electrode and cutting loop for endometrial ablation. *Obstet Gynecol* 1999, 94:521–527.

120. Sharp HT: Assessment of new technology in the treatment of idiopathic menorrhagia and uterine leiomyomata. *Obstet Gynecol* 2006, 108: 990–1003.

121. Amso NN, Stabinsky SA, McFaul P, *et al.*: Uterine thermal balloon therapy for the treatment of menorrhagia: the first 300 patients from a multicentre study. *Br J Obstet Gynaecol* 1998, 105:517–523.

122. Amso NN: Uterine endometrial thermal balloon therapy for the treatment of menorrhagia: long-term multicenter follow-up study. *Hum Reprod* 2003, 18:1082–1087.

123. Corson SL: A multicenter evaluation of endometrial ablation by HydroThermablator and rollerball for treatment of menorrhagia. *J Am Assoc Gynecol Laparosc* 2001, 8:359–367.

124. Goldrath MH: Evaluation of HydroThermAblator and rollerball endometrial ablation for menorrhagia 3 years after treatment. *J Am Assoc Gynecol Laparosc* 2003, 10:505–511.

125. Duleba AJ: A randomized study comparing endometrial cryoablation and rollerball electroablation for treatment of dysfunctional uterine bleeding. *J Am Assoc Gynecol Laparosc* 2003, 10:17–26.

126. Gallinat A: Novasure impedance controlled system for endometrial ablation: three-year follow-up on 107 patients. *Am J Obstet Gynecol* 2004, 191:1585–1590.

127. Cooper JM: Microwave endometrial ablation versus rollerball electro-ablation for menorrhagia: a multi-center randomized trial. *J Am Assoc Gynecol Laparosc* 2004,11:394–403.

128. *ACOG Committee Opinion, Number 293: Uterine Artery Embolization*. Washington, DC: American College of Obstetricians and Gynecologists; 2004.

129. Spies JB, Myers ER, Worthington-Kirsch R, *et al.*: The FIBROID Registry: symptoms and quality-of-life status 1 year after therapy. *Obstet Gynecol* 2005, 106:1309–1318.

130. David M, Ebert AD: Treatment of uterine fibroids by embolization: advantages, disadvantages, and pitfalls. *Eur J Obstet Gynecol* 2005, 123:1131–1138.

131. Spies JB, Spector A, Roth AR, *et al.*: Complications after uterine artery embolization for leiomyomas. *Obstet Gynecol* 2002, 100:873–880.

132. Learman LA, Summitt RL, Varner RE, *et al.*: Hysterectomy versus expanded medical treatment for abnormal uterine bleeding: clinical outcomes in the Medicine or Surgery Trial. *Obstet Gynecol* 2004, 103:824–833.

133. Andersson JK, Rybo G: Levonorgestrel-releasing intrauterine device in the treatment of menorrhagia. *Br J Obstet Gynecol* 1990, 97:690–694.

134. Lethaby AE, Cooke I, Rees M: Progesterone or progestogen-releasing intrauterine system for heavy menstrual bleeding. *Cochrane Database Syst Rev* 2005, 4: CD002126.

135. Lethaby A, Shepperd S, Cooke I, Farquhar C: Endometrial resection and ablation versus hysterectomy for heavy menstrual bleeding. *Cochrane Database Syst Rev* 2005, 4: CD001501.

136. Sculpher MJ, Dwyer N, Byford S, *et al.*: Randomised trial comparing hysterectomy and transcervical endometrial resection: effect on health related quality of life and costs two years after surgery. *Br J Obstet Gynecol* 1996, 103:142–149.

137. Pinion SB, Parkin DE, Abramovich DR, *et al.*: Randomised trial of hysterectomy, endometrial laser ablation, and transcervical endometrial resection for dysfunctional uterine bleeding. *Br Med J* 1994, 309:979–983.

138. Crosignani PG, Vercellini P, Apolone G, *et al.*: Endometrial resection versus vaginal hysterectomy for menorrhagia: long-term clinical and quality-of-life outcomes. *Am J Obstet Gynecol* 1997, 177:95–101.

139. Tapper AM, Heinonen PK: Comparison of hysteroscopic endometrial resection and laparoscopic assisted vaginal hysterectomy for the treatment of menorrhagia. *Acta Obstet Gynecol Scand* 1998, 77:78–82.

140. Ransom SB, McNeeley SG, White C, *et al.*: A cost analysis of endometrial ablation, abdominal hysterectomy, vaginal hysterectomy, and laparoscopic-assisted vaginal hysterectomy in the treatment of primary menorrhagia. *J Am Assoc Gynecol Laparosc* 1996, 4:29–32.

141. Brumstead JR, Blackman JA, Badger GJ, Riddick DH: Hysteroscopy versus hysterectomy for the treatment of abnormal uterine bleeding: a comparison of cost. *Fertil Steril* 1996, 65:310–316.

142. Hidlebaugh DA: Relative costs of gynecologic endoscopy vs traditional surgery of treatment of abnormal uterine bleeding. *Am J Manag Care* 2001, 7:3SP31–SP37.

23 The Treatment of Infertility

Ringland S. Murray, Jr. and Xavier L. Smith

- The primary physician can deliver infertility care to most couples.
- Combating insulin resistance is the first-line therapy in treating polycystic ovarian syndrome.
- Surgery for endometriosis minimally improves fertility.
- Patients with diminished ovarian reserve or multifactor infertility should be referred to a specialist.

Background

Early diagnosis and the appropriate delivery of care are critical in the management of infertility patients. Physicians who do not understand proper testing and treatment can jeopardize a couple's chances of achieving a family. For these reasons, physicians must know 1) how different diagnoses should be managed, 2) the expected success rates of different treatments, 3) when to refer, and 4) how to recognize and manage complications of assisted reproductive technology (ART). With proper management, most infertile couples will achieve pregnancy.

Anovulation

If the only barrier to conception is a lack of ovulation, then restoring ovulation should be adequate to achieve pregnancy. Therefore, the goal of ovulation induction (OI) is to prompt a solitary egg to ovulate.

The first step in the management of anovulation is to identify the cause. Thyroid disorders, hyperprolactinemia, polycystic ovarian syndrome (PCOS), or hypogonadotropic hypogonadism each warrant different treatment.

With hyperprolactinemia, most macroadenomas (greater than 1 cm) and all microadenomas can be managed with dopamine agonists such as bromocriptine or cabergoline. Bromocriptine (starting at 1.25 mg) is titrated to normalize prolactin, without profound suppression. To avoid orthostatic hypotension, therapy is initiated at bedtime. Cabergoline (0.25 mg orally twice a week) is more costly but has a better side effect profile. Side

effects for both drugs are limited by vaginal administration [1,2]. If adequate therapy fails to restore ovulation, an ovulation induction agent such as clomiphene may be added.

PCOS is the most common cause of anovulation, affecting 7% of the population [3]. PCOS could consume an entire text; however, we will limit our discussion here to ovulation induction.

Combating Insulin

The most common dysfunction in PCOS is insulin resistance [4–7]. With just 5% to 10% weight loss, 89% of obese PCOS women may resume ovulation [8,9]. Lean women, or those who are unwilling or unable to lose weight, should consider Glucophage (Bristol-Myers Squibb, New York, NY) as first-line treatment.

Glucophage is the most commonly used drug to combat hyperinsulinemia. Glucophage decreases gluconeogenesis, thus decreasing insulin requirements [10]. Ovulation will resume in 40% to 70% of patients, with a low rate of twins [11,12]. To avoid common gastrointestinal side effects, start with 500 mg daily and titrate weekly to a target dose of 1500 to 2000 mg daily. In lean PCOS women, Glucophage has greater pregnancy rates compared to clomiphene [13].

With rosiglitazone, in uncontrolled studies, this insulin-sensitizing agent induces ovulation in 55% to 77% of PCOS women [14,15]. It may be superior to Glucophage as an adjunct in clomiphene-resistant patients, but it can lead to weight gain [16]. The dose is 2 to 8 mg daily. Liver toxicity is rare [17].

Oral Ovulation Induction Agents

Couples using OI agents should confirm adequate ovulation as described in the previous chapter. Women who cannot detect ovulation may receive an ultrasound on cycle day 13 to 15. When a follicle is greater than 18 mm, exogenous human chorionic gonadotropin (hCG) may be administered to trigger ovulation. The typical dose is 2500 to 10,000 IU for menopausal hCG and 250 μg for recombinant hCG.

Clomiphene citrate is a partial estrogen antagonist and mimics a hypoestrogen state, causing an increase in gonadotropin-releasing hormone (GnRH), follicle-stimulating hormone (FSH), and luteinizing hormone (LH) secretion. Like all oral ovulation induction agents, clomiphene requires an intact hypothalamic-pituitary-ovarian axis and is not suitable treatment for patients with hypogonadotropic hypogonadism, ovarian failure or untreated hyperprolactinemia, and thyroid disorders.

The typical starting dose is 50 mg on cycle days 3 to 7 or 5 to 9. If ovulation does not occur, the dose is increased by 50 mg per cycle to a maximum of 250 mg per treatment day. As many as 80% of patients will ovulate, with as many as 75% achieving pregnancy within 6 to 9 months [18,19]. If ovulation does not occur by 150 mg, it is unlikely that it will occur at higher doses.

Multiple gestations occur in 5% to 10% of clomiphene pregnancies, with the vast majority being twins [20–22]. Twenty percent of women experience side effects, most commonly hot flashes. Cysts are common but rarely undergo torsion. Visual disturbances are self-limited, but are a cause for immediate cessation of this drug. Clomiphene can have a negative impact on the uterine lining and cervical mucus, thus limiting its efficacy. In patients who have not achieved pregnancy within six ovulatory cycles or who have thin uterine linings (less than 7 mm), another agent should be considered [18,23].

Regarding tamoxifen, this partial estrogen antagonist is a US Food and Drug Administration–approved adjunct treatment for breast cancer and is used off-label as an OI agent. Tamoxifen does not inhibit endometrial development. In unselected patients, tamoxifen and clomiphene have equal efficacy [24].

Patients with refractory anovulation or suboptimal endometrial development with clomiphene are candidates for tamoxifen. The typical dose is 20 to 40 mg for 5 days.

Letrozole is an aromatase inhibitor that limits estradiol production by the ovary, resulting in an increased GnRH, FSH, and LH. In typical doses, 2.5 to 5 mg on cycle days 3 to 7 or 5 to 9, letrozole does not impair endometrial development. It induces ovulation in 50% to 90% of PCOS patients and is effective in the majority of clomiphene resistant patients [25–27]. Compared with clomiphene, letrozole has demonstrated a higher pregnancy rate [28].

After an unpublished study reported an increased risk of birth defects in babies conceived on letrozole, the manufacturer warned against using the drug for OI. The major criticism of this study was that controls were improperly selected. A larger study with a more appropriate control group found no increased risk of malformations [29].

Generally the administration of exogenous gonadotropins (Figure 23-1) is the province of subspecialists. To avoid high-order multiple pregnancies and life-threatening ovarian hyperstimulation syndrome (OHSS), careful ultrasonographic and serologic monitoring and interpretation are required [30].

Women with PCOS require only FSH to promote the growth of follicles. A woman with hypogonadotropic hypogonadism, eg, due to exercise, will be deficient in FSH and LH and therefore requires both hormones to ovulate effectively.

The most common treatment strategy is the Step Up protocol. After induction of menses with a progestin, a low dose of gonadotropin is initiated on cycle day 3. A typical daily starting dose is 37.5 IU to 150 IU, with older and heavier patients requiring higher doses. Lean women with PCOS or hypogonadotropic hypogonadism are often very sensitive to gonadotropins and require low doses. After 4 to 7 days, patients return for a serum estradiol level and ultrasound. If there is no appreciable response, the dose may be increased by 37.5 to 75 IU every 4 to 7 days until a response is noted. An estrogen greater than 50 to 75 pg/mL is generally indicative of a response. Follicles measuring 10 mm or more are likely responding. Once a follicle measures approximately 12 mm in diameter, it grows 1 to 3 mm

Gonadotropins

Gonadotropin	Contains	Manufacturer
Bravelle	Urinary FSH	Ferring
Repronex	Urinary FSH and LH*	Ferring
Menopur	Urinary FSH and LH*	Ferring
Follistim/Puregon	Recombinant FSH	Organon
Gonal F	Recombinant FSH	Merck-Serono
Luveris	Recombinant LH	Merck-Serono
Pregnyl	Urinary hCG	Organon
Choragon	Urinary hCG	Ferring
Ovidrel	Recombinant hCG	Merck-Serono

*LH activity augmented by hCG added to the product.

Figure 23-1. Summary of gonadotropins. FSH—follicle-stimulating hormone; hCG—human chorionic gonadotropin; LH—luteinizing hormone.

per day. Patients return to clinic every 1 to 3 days. The dose may be decreased if more than one follicle is developing. Estradiol levels are usually 150 to 400 pg/mL per mature follicle [31,32]. When the lead follicle measures more than 16 to 18 mm, ovulation is induced. Because of its long half-life and homology with LH, hCG is used to trigger ovulation. Ovulation typically occurs within the next 36 to 38 hours.

Follicles 15 mm and greater, rarely smaller, may produce eggs which result in pregnancy [30,33,34]. Approximately 50% of patients will be pregnant at 6 months [30,33].

Sequential Treatment (Combining Oral Agents with Gonadotropins)

Patients who wish to defray the cost of gonadotropins may opt to initiate clomiphene, tamoxifen, or letrozole for 5 days beginning on cycle day 3, then starting gonadotropins on cycle day 7. Monitoring and ovulation triggering is accomplished in the manner described above.

Ovarian diathermy, also known as ovarian drilling, is a technique variation of the wedge resection. Diathermy is accomplished by laparoscopy with an electrosurgical needle. The needle is inserted into the ovary for stromal cauterization at 8 to 20 sites per ovary. The subsequent reduction in androgens permits ovulation in a majority of clomiphene resistant women [35–38]. Though the therapy can be long-lasting, it can result in adhesion formation or infection and is inferior to Glucophage [39,40].

Progesterone is not considered as an OI agent. However, some women do ovulate when given a progestin to induce menses [41]. Therefore, when prescribing a progestin, instruct the couple to have intercourse on the night they initiate the pills.

Short Luteal Phase

A short luteal phase may decrease pregnancy rates [42–44] and may be caused by inadequate follicular phase stimulation due to stress, hyperprolactinemia, hypothyroidism, or for idiopathic reasons [45–47]. In the absence of an obvious cause, clomiphene is generally curative [48]. The goal of treatment is to lengthen the luteal phase to a minimum of 11 days from the detection of ovulation by basal body temperature [49].

Endometriosis

Endometriosis affects up to 80% of women with pain and infertility [50,51]. Most, but not all, studies [52] have shown endometriosis to have a negative impact on uterine receptivity as well as oocyte quality [53–55]. Available fertility treatments for endometriosis include surgery, superovulation, or in vitro fertilization (IVF) (see "Unexplained Infertility" section).

A meta-analysis of two randomized studies concluded surgery improves fertility. Combining these two studies, 12 women need to undergo excision to achieve one additional pregnancy [56]. However, in clinical practice, it is frequently unknown whether a patient has endometriosis, and the number needed to treat is significantly higher. For women undergoing in vitro fertilization (IVF), there is no evidence that surgery improves outcomes [57–59].

Tubal Factor

In vitro fertilization is the preferred therapy for severe tubal disease such as bilateral hydrosalpinges, salpingitis isthmic nodosa, or bipolar disease (proximal and distal occlusion).

Whether IVF should be offered to patients with mild to moderate tubal disease depends on the age of the patient, ovarian reserve, duration of infertility, and the severity of male factor. Patients with multifactor infertility are encouraged to pursue IVF.

Surgical correction of mild hydrosalpinges has variable success [60–62]. With microsurgery, postoperative pregnancy rates can be as high as 50% to 80% for mild disease [62,63]. There is little data on laparoscopic repair. In the hands of skilled surgeons, neosalpingostomy has resulted in an overall success rate of 29% [64]. No patient should undergo surgical correction without evaluation of the male partner.

Because hydrosalpinges have been shown to decrease live birth rates with IVF by 50%, most specialists remove or ligate hydrosalpinges before treatment [65–69].

Proximal tubal disease which is confirmed by laparoscopy may be treated with hysteroscopic or fluoroscopic canalization. Recurrent blockages, or uncorrectable processes, such as salpingitis isthmic nodosa should be treated with IVF.

Unexplained Infertility

Couples with this diagnosis may pick any of the therapies listed in Figure 23-2 [70], with older couples opting for the more aggressive treatments.

Superovulation is the induction of two or more follicles performed with or without intrauterine insemination. Superovulation can be accomplished with an oral agent, but is more effective with exogenous gonadotropins. The two most commonly employed strategies are the Step Up and Step Down protocols.

The Step Up protocol has been described previously. For superovulation, a higher gonadotropin dose is used, between 75 and 225 IU per day. This protocol is preferred for women undergoing their first stimulation cycle.

The Step Down protocol begins at a higher dose to initiate growth of a larger number of follicles. The dose is gradually decreased to promote development of the lead follicles while withdrawing support from smaller follicles. Ovarian response is assessed by ultrasound and serum estradiol after 4 days of stimulation. An initial estradiol goal will be slightly higher than is seen with ovulation induction, typically in the 75 to 125 pg/mL range. The goal of treatment will be two to three follicles by cycle day 9, 10, or 11. More follicles may be desired for women over 40 years of age or with previous failed cycles.

Uterine Factors

Most studies say fibroids impair fertility [71–76]. Hysteroscopic resection of submucous myomas increases pregnancy rates [74,77,78]. Myomas greater than 4 cm or those that distort the uterine cavity are associated with decreased pregnancy rates; however, it is not certain if resection restores expected pregnancy rates [80,81], and one must weigh the benefits of surgery versus the risk of tubal adhesion formation.

The affect of polyps is less certain; however, polypectomy restores fertility in many women with no other identifiable factors [76,81,82].

Asherman's syndrome has been associated with infertility. Case series show that subfertile patients who undergo hysteroscopic resection of adhesions may have subsequent fertility; however, the minimum amount of uterine cavity required to support a pregnancy has not been established [83–85].

Uterine anomalies such as unicornuate uteri are associated with poor reproductive outcome, but are not a cause of infertility [86]. Septate uteri may lead to pregnancy loss and are also associated with infertility [73]. Multiple studies demonstrate that septoplasty dramatically improves reproductive outcomes and restores fertility [73,87,88]. Anomalies with poor prognosis, such as cervical atresia, may prefer to enlist a gestational carrier or undergo gamete intrafallopian transfer (GIFT), as described later.

Male Factor

Most couples with mild to moderate male factor infertility can be treated by artificial insemination (AI) combined with superovulation. With severe male factor or when intrauterine insemination (IUI) and/or other treatments fail, donor sperm or IVF may be indicated.

Artificial insemination encompasses intracervical insemination (ICI) and IUI and is used to overcome male factor,

cervical factor, antisperm antibodies, or unexplained infertility. Sperm are collected from the male partner or from a donor by masturbation.

With ICI, semen is instilled into the cervix via a catheter or it is placed into a cervical cap and allowed to bathe the cervix. For IUI, sperm are "washed" to separate them from semen. The sperm are placed in culture medium and loaded into a catheter, which is guided into the uterus where the sperm are released. IUI is approximately 2.5 times more likely to result in pregnancy than is ICI [89].

For couples undergoing ovulation induction, IUI is performed the morning following detection of an luteinizing hormone surge by ovulation predictor kits. For women who receive hCG to induce ovulation, IUI is performed 36 hours after hCG administration. Only one IUI is needed per cycle. Double insemination (insemination on two consecutive days) does not increase fecundability [90].

With IVF, absolute sperm parameter cut-offs have not been firmly established to determine which couples require IVF for male factor infertility. However, general indications include severe oligospermia (fewer than 1 million motile sperm [91,92]; severe asthenospermia (poor motility) [91,93,94]; or six failed cycles of IUI [95].

Poor morphology, based on strict criteria (less than 4% normal forms), has been associated with decreased pregnancy rates in natural cycles and with IUI [96–98].

In vitro fertilization with ICSI (intracytoplasmic sperm injection) can be performed with ejaculated or harvested sperm [100]. ICSI requires a single sperm per egg. The sperm is injected into a mature oocyte. Fertilization rates are higher with ICSI than with conventional IVF insemination (in which eggs are co-cultured with sperm). The indications for ICSI will vary by center but the procedure is usually performed for severe defects. With the invention of ICSI, severe male factor is no longer deemed a poor prognosis [100].

As described in the previous chapter, some cases of severe oligozoospermia are simply due to low testosterone, and sperm production may be increased with daily clomiphene or hCG injections. Most azoospermic men with normal follicle stimulating hormone and testosterone levels actually do have sperm which can be harvested by the surgical techniques discussed in the previous chapter. These sperm may be used for IVF.

Treatment Efficacy for Unexplained Infertility

Treatment	Pregnant per Month, %	Cost per Pregnancy, $
Expectant management	1.3–4.1	
IUI alone	3.8	
Clomiphene alone	5.6	
Clomiphene and IUI	8.3	10,000
Superovulation alone	7.7	
Superovulation and IUI	17.1	17,000
IVF	20.7*	50,000

*These pooled data are lower than the current average expected pregnancy rate per cycle in most clinics according to current data.

Figure 23-2. Treatment efficacy for unexplained infertility. IUI—intrauterine insemination; IVF—in vitro fertilization.

Cervical Factor

"Cervical hostility" has long been regarded as a cause of infertility. The postcoital test has largely been abandoned because of its poor predictive value [101]. Given the difficulty in establishing the diagnosis, determining which treatments are beneficial, therefore, becomes an impractical matter. The logical treatment for cervical hostility is IUI, which bypasses the cervix. Proving IUI's superiority to timed intercourse has been difficult [102].

Especially in the setting of clomiphene citrate, some physicians will perform postcoital tests and treat thick cervical mucus with guaifenesin [103]. No randomized data supports this therapy, but it has negligible risks.

Assisted Reproductive Technologies

Since the birth of the first baby conceived by IVF in 1978, [104] there has been rapid expansion of ART. Today, one of every 100 babies born in the United States is the product of IVF [51].

Assisted reproductive technology is any technology which manipulates human eggs outside the body: IVF, GIFT, zygote intrafallopian transfer (ZIFT), and tubal embryo transfer (TET). IVF is the most common procedure, and its indications are listed in Figure 23-3.

Prognosis

In vitro fertilization success rates relate to the age, ovarian reserve, and reproductive history of the female partner. Aside from endometriosis, all other diagnoses have similar success rates [51,105]. Smoking and excessive exercise decrease pregnancy rates and should be discouraged [106–108]. Obesity has shown inconsistent effects [109–111].

Assisted Reproductive Technology Techniques

An ART "cycle" encompasses all factors leading up to the anticipated embryo transfer. Key components may include prestimulation pituitary desensitization, ovarian stimulation with exogenous gonadotropins, egg retrieval, and embryo transfer.

Controlled Ovarian Hyperstimulation for In Vitro Fertilization

Controlled ovarian hyperstimulation promotes the development of a large cohort of follicles (4 to 20 oocytes). Premature ovulation is prevented by pituitary down-regulation with a GnRH-agonist, *eg*, leuprolide acetate, prior to cycle initiation or with a GnRH-antagonist during stimulation.

At the commencement of menses, the patient undergoes evaluation to ensure down-regulation, as evidenced by a lack of ovarian cysts on ultrasound and a low serum estradiol. She then begins injections of exogenous gonadotropins. The response to gonadotropins is assessed by ultrasound and serum estradiol. Once the lead oocytes have reached maturity, typically measuring more than 17 mm, with a corresponding estradiol level of 150 to 250 pg/mL per follicle, hCG is used to trigger ovulation.

Thirty-six hours after hCG administration, the patient returns to clinic for oocyte retrieval by ultrasound-guided needle aspiration through the vagina. Rarely, aspiration will occur through the abdomen or by laparoscopy. After aspiration, the woman begins progesterone supplementation which is continued through the 7th week of pregnancy (or up to the 10th week in some centers).

The embryos are fertilized in the lab by the methods described previously. Over the ensuing 2 to 4 days, the embryos are evaluated for viability and their implantation potential based on morphologic and developmental milestones.

Embryo transfer typically occurs on postretrieval day 3 or on day 5. There has been considerable debate over which day is the best for transfer. Each center will have its own standards on when and how many embryos to transfer. The goal of therapy is a singleton pregnancy. Patients should be cautious of centers with higher than average rate of triplets, and this information is available on the Centers for Disease Control and Prevention web site at www.cdc.gov.

Frozen Embryos

Excess embryos may be cryopreserved for later use or for donation. They are usually not the top tier embryos and experience the strain of the freeze-thaw techniques. Frozen embryos have a lower implantation rate. A "frozen" cycle is much less expensive than a stimulated cycle because it does not require extensive monitoring or expensive drugs.

Assisted Hatching

Assisted hatching involves the disruption of the zona pellucida by chemical, laser, or mechanical means to expose the embryo's surface adhesion molecules. It is performed just prior to embryo transfer and is designed to promote implantation. It may increase implantation rates in women 37 years or older or with prior in vitro fertilization failure, if the zona pellucida is abnormally thick.

Indications for In Vitro Fertilization

Tubal factor infertility

Severe male factor infertility

Need for preimplantation

Unexplained infertility

Severe endometriosis

Diminished ovarian reserve*

Advanced maternal age*

Failed prior treatments for other diagnoses

*Often requires donor eggs.

Figure 23-3. Indications for in vitro fertilization.

EGG DONATION

Women with diminished ovarian reserve, repeated in vitro fertilization failure failures, or those who carry a genetic disease, may opt for egg donation. Egg donors can be known or anonymous. Donors undergo extensive medical and psychologic screening and must meet the standards imposed by the American Association of Tissue Banks, the Centers for Disease Control and Prevention, and the US Food and Drug Administration [112]. Preferred donors are younger than age 35 and have no known endometriosis [113].

OTHER ASSISTED REPRODUCTIVE TECHNOLOGIES

Gamete intrafallopian transfer, ZIFT, and TET are laparoscopic techniques reserved for subsets of patients. Some couples may simply prefer for fertilization to occur inside the woman, such as with GIFT. With GIFT, eggs are collected via laparoscopy and placed into the fallopian tube along with sperm collected from the male partner. The Vatican remains staunchly opposed to IVF, but has no position on GIFT [114].

The other indications for GIFT, ZIFT, and TET are limited, but these are viable options for patients without functional vaginas or cervices.

Assisted Reproductive Technologies for Fertility Preservation

EGG FREEZING

Women facing certain forms of cancer are at risk for premature ovarian failure due to chemotherapy and/or radiation. These women may opt to undergo IVF and freeze all of their embryos for later use.

Egg freezing is an option for women without male partners who do not want to or can not use donor sperm. The patient undergoes stimulation and retrieval as with IVF, but the oocytes are frozen. Later, the oocytes are thawed, fertilized, and the subsequent embryos are transferred to the uterus. Oocyte freezing is currently regarded as experimental by the American Society of Clinical Oncology and the American Society for Reproductive Medicine. Birth rates per oocyte retrieval are markedly reduced compared to IVF, and long-term safety has not been established [115,116]. To date, fewer than 200 babies have been born worldwide by egg freezing. The American Society for Reproductive Medicine recommends against egg freezing for women without cancer who simply want to preserve fertility.

OVARIAN TISSUE CRYOPRESERVATION

Cancer patients who do not have the time to pursue IVF or egg freezing often do have time for ovarian tissue harvesting and cryopreservation. This experimental technique removes the ovary or ovarian cortex and freezes it. Later, the tissue can be transplanted back into the woman. The most concerning risk of this technique is the ovarian tissue could harbor tumor cells [117,118]. Two pregnancies have possibly been achieved through this technique. In the first case, the patient still had ovarian function after chemotherapy and radiation, so one can't be completely certain the pregnancy occurred from the transplanted tissue [119]. The second case was more conclusive, but required IVF [120]. This promising technique remains experimental.

SPERM CRYOPRESERVATION

Males facing chemotherapy or surgery that threatens fertility are excellent candidates for sperm freezing. Frozen sperm can be used for IUI or IVF.

Preimplantation Genetic Screening and Diagnosis

Couples known to carry chromosomal translocations or Mendelian disorders such as sickle cell anemia are good candidates for preimplantation genetic diagnosis. Oocytes may undergo polar body biopsy, or more typically, one to two cells are extracted from each embryo [121,122]. The cells are analyzed to determine which embryos are affected by the disease in question. Preimplantation genetic diagnosis is quite reliable; however, conventional antenatal screening is still indicated [123,124].

Preimplantation genetic diagnosis is the technique of evaluating all embryos for aneuploidy in an effort to improve success rates with IVF. Thus far, it has failed to improve the live-birth rate for any indication.

When to Refer

Recognizing when a patient requires treatment outside your comfort level or area of expertise is the key to timely referral. In general, women reaching advanced maternal age, with diminishing ovarian reserve or couples with multifactor infertility or severe endometriosis, tubal factor, or male factor–associated infertility should be referred with haste. When choosing to manage women with unexplained infertility, strongly consider the age of the woman and the chances of success with the various treatments (Figure 23-2).

Risks of Fertility Treatment

OBSTETRICAL OUTCOMES

Whether achieved spontaneously or via ART, pregnancies in infertile couples may be at increased risk for pregnancy complications and malformations [125,126].

Singleton pregnancies achieved by ART are at higher risk for perinatal mortality, preterm delivery, and low birth weight [127]. Although many studies have shown malformation rates comparable to the general population, a Western Australian study described a twofold increased risk of congenital anomalies [128]. A subsequent meta-analysis by the same group said there is up to a 40% increased risk of birth defects. Using number needed to harm (NNTH) analysis, these authors conclude that 25 to 100 couples would have to undergo IVF to result in an additional major birth defect [129].

In general, there seems to be a slight increased risk of neural tube defects, alimentary atresia, and, with ICSI, hypospadias [99,125,126]. With ICSI and with blastocyst culture, there seems to be an overrepresentation of imprinting disorders such as Beckwith-Wiedemann syndrome. This risk seems quite small; however, additional research is needed [100,127,130–132].

To date, it is not clear whether it is the ART techniques themselves that confer these small risks.

MULTIPLE GESTATIONS

To varying degrees, gonadotropins, IVF and oral OI agents all place patients at risk of multiple gestations. Multiple gestations have higher perinatal mortality, preterm birth, low birth weight, gestational hypertension, placental abruption, and placenta previa. The best way to limit multiple gestations is prevention by limiting the number of embryos transferred and by avoiding overaggressive stimulations with gonadotropins. In cases of triplets or more, some couples will pursue selective embryo reduction.

OVARIAN HYPERSTIMULATION SYNDROME

Ovarian hyperstimulation syndrome is rare with clomiphene but fairly common with superovulation and IVF. Risk factors include young age, PCOS diagnosis, lean body mass, estradiol levels greater than 4000 in IVF, or greater than 1000 with superovulation. A high number of follicles (more than 18) at the time of hCG also increase the risk. OHSS does not occur without ovulation and may not occur until pregnancy is established, due to the emergence of hCG. Clinical manifestations are summarized in Figure 23-4.

Severe OHSS can be prevented by canceling the cycle, by avoiding overaggressive stimulations, or by withholding gonadotropins (coasting) until estradiol levels fall into a safer range. Reducing the hCG dose to 2500 IU may reduce risk. Human albumin, 50 g intravenously at time of retrieval, has been shown to decrease OHSS incidence in high-risk patients [133]. Freezing all embryos and performing the transfer at a later date also reduces the risk.

Pathophysiologically, OHSS is a state of capillary permeability causing intravascular hypovoluminemia, ascites, oliguria, electrolyte abnormalities, pericardial and pleural effusions. Hemoconcentration places patients at increased risk for thrombosis and stroke. Ovarian engorgement may cause pain difficult to differentiate from torsion.

Management requires close surveillance. Daily weights and patient history are simple screening tools. Dizziness, oliguria, anorexia, or a 5-lb weight gain in one day should prompt evaluation. Blood pressure, complete blood counts, liver function tests, Prothrombin time and partial thromboplastin time, chemistries, and urine specific gravity are helpful determinants of changes in severity. Due to fears of rupture,

one should avoid palpation of the ovaries. Tense or painful ascites warrants paracentesis. Patients should be encouraged to drink electrolyte rich fluids [134–136].

ECTOPIC/HETEROTOPIC PREGNANCY

The ectopic rate for ART was 0.7% in the United States for 2004 [51]. Any time a woman receives an OI agent or IVF, she could have a multiple gestation. In cases of heterotopic pregnancy or a nonviable twin, the typical "doubling" of hCG may not occur [137,138]. One might not see an intrauterine pregnancy on ultrasound at the same hCG threshold as expected with spontaneous pregnancy, since more than one pregnancy is contributing to the hCG level. Consider the possibility of

Clinical Manifestations of Ovarian Hyperstimulation Syndrome	
Manifestation	**Management**
Mild	Mild
Mild abdominal distention	Manage expectantly
Increased ovarian size, 5–12 cm	Antiemetics as needed
Nausea/vomiting	
Moderate	Moderate
Ascites on ultrasound	Frequent follow-up, daily weights
Ovarian enlargement	Electrolyte-rich fluids
Severe	Severe
Hypovolemia	Consider hospitalization
Large volume ascites	Paracentesis as needed
Oliguria	Replace electrolytes as needed
Electrolyte abnormalities	IV albumin/fluids
Abnormal LFTs	Heparin prophylaxis
Increased creatinine	No diuretics unless normovolemic
White blood cell count > 22,000	Monitor fluid intake and output
Critical	Critical
Dizziness	Intensive care
Anuria	Invasive hemodynamic monitoring
Hematocrit > 55%	Fluid drainage
Pericardial effusion	Consider pregnancy termination
Hydrothorax	IV heparin
Thromboembolism	

Figure 23-4. Clinical manifestations for ovarian hyperstimulation syndrome. IV—intravenous; LFTs—liver function tests.

heterotopic pregnancy before administering methotrexate or performing a dilation and cutterage.

THROMBOEMBOLISM

Pregnancy alone increases the risk of thromboembolism. In the setting of ART, it is more common with OHSS.

OVARIAN TORSION

The stimulated ovary is at risk for twisting upon its pedicle and can be a surgical emergency. Hyperstimulated ovaries are friable. Gentle, atraumatic manipulation is essential. If bleeding occurs, one should resist initial urges to coagulate as this frequently worsens the bleeding. Generally, even fairly brisk bleeding ceases within minutes.

CANCER

Early improperly controlled studies suggested an increased cancer risk with various fertility therapies [139,140]. When controlled for parity, there is no evidence that fertility treatment increases the risk of cancer in women undergoing stimulation with gonadotropins or OI agents such as clomiphene [141,142].

Summary

Figure 23-5 summarizes treatment options for infertility.

References

1. Ginsburg J, Hardiman P, Thomas M: Vaginal bromocriptine: clinical and biochemical effects. *Gynecol Endocrinol* 1992, 6:119–126.

2. Motta T, de Vincentiis S, Marchini M, *et al.*: Vaginal cabergoline in the treatment of hyperprolactinemic patients intolerant to oral dopaminergics. *Fertil Steril* 1996, 65:440–442.

3. Goodarzi MO, Azziz R: Diagnosis, epidemiology, and genetics of the polycystic ovary syndrome. *Best Pract Res Clin Endocrinol Metab* 2006, 20:193–205.

4. DeUgarte CM, Bartolucci AA, Azziz R: Prevalence of insulin resistance in the polycystic ovary syndrome using the homeostasis model assessment. *Fertil Steril* 2005, 83:1454–1460.

5. Corbould A, Kim YB, Youngren JF, *et al.*: Insulin resistance in the skeletal muscle of women with PCOS involves intrinsic and acquired defects in insulin signaling. *Am J Physiol Endocrinol Metab* 2005, 288:E1047–E1054.

6. Palmert MR, Gordon CM, Kartashov AI, *et al.*: Screening for abnormal glucose tolerance in adolescents with polycystic ovary syndrome. *J Clin Endocrinol Metab* 2002, 87:1017–1023.

7. Dunaif A, Wu X, Lee A, Diamanti–Kandarakis E: Defects in insulin receptor signaling in vivo in the polycystic ovary syndrome (PCOS). *Am J Physiol Endocrinol Metab* 2001, 281:E392–E399.

8. Crosignani PG, Colombo M, Vegetti W, *et al.*: Overweight and obese anovulatory patients with polycystic ovaries: parallel improvements in anthropometric indices, ovarian physiology and fertility rate induced by diet. *Hum Reprod* 2003, 18:1928–1932.

9. Saleh AM, Khalil HS: Review of nonsurgical and surgical treatment and the role of insulin-sensitizing agents in the management of infertile women with polycystic ovary syndrome. *Acta Obstet Gynecol Scand* 2004, 83:614–621.

10. Stumvoll M, Nurjhan N, Perriello G, *et al.*: Metabolic effects of metformin in non–insulin-dependent diabetes mellitus. *N Engl J Med* 1995, 333:550–554.

11. Lord JM, Flight IH, Norman RJ: Insulin-sensitizing drugs (metformin, troglitazone, rosiglitazone, pioglitazone, D-chiro-inositol) for polycystic ovary syndrome. *Cochrane Database Syst Rev* 2003, 3:CD003053.

12. Palomba S, Russo T, Orio F, Jr., *et al.*: Uterine effects of metformin administration in anovulatory women with polycystic ovary syndrome. *Hum Reprod* 2006, 21:457–465.

13. Palomba S, Orio F, Jr., Falbo A, *et al.*: Prospective parallel randomized, double-blind, double-dummy controlled clinical trial comparing clomiphene citrate and metformin as the first-line treatment for ovulation induction in nonobese anovulatory women with polycystic ovary syndrome. *J Clin Endocrinol Metab* 2005, 90:4068–4074.

Summary of Treatment Options

Medical Treatment	Appropriate Candidates
Oral ovulation induction agents	Anovulatory patients, eg, PCOS, adult-onset adrenal hyperplasia
Injectable ovulation induction	Hypogonatrophic hypogonadism and anovulatory patients who are refractory to oral agents
Superovulation	Unexplained infertility, mild male factor infertility, or multiple failed rounds of ovulation induction
Procedures	
Intrauterine insemination	Suspected cervical factor, mild male factor, unexplained infertility, or not pregnant despite adequate ovulation induction
In vitro fertilization	See Figure 23-3
GIFT	Those religiously opposed to fertilization outside the body and those without access to the uterus; cervical atresia
ZIFT/TET	Those without access to the uterus
Surgery	
Myomectomy	Submucous myomas; myomas that distort the cavity
Endometriosis	Patients with pain or distorted anatomy
Ovarian diathermy	Patients intolerant of insulin-sensitizing/reducing agents
Polypectomy	Recommended even if symptomatic

Figure 23-5. Summary of treatment options. GIFT—gamete intrafallopian transfer; PCOS—polycystic ovarian syndrome; TET—tubal embryo transfer; ZIFT—zygote intrafallopian transfer.

14. Cataldo NA, Abbasi F, McLaughlin TL, et al.: Metabolic and ovarian effects of rosiglitazone treatment for 12 weeks in insulin–resistant women with polycystic ovary syndrome. *Hum Reprod* 2006, 21:109–120.

15. Dereli D, Dereli T, Bayraktar F, et al.: Endocrine and metabolic effects of rosiglitazone in non–obese women with polycystic ovary disease. *Endocr J* 2005, 52:299–308.

16. Rouzi AA, Ardawi MS: A randomized controlled trial of the efficacy of rosiglitazone and clomiphene citrate versus metformin and clomiphene citrate in women with clomiphene citrate–resistant polycystic ovary syndrome. *Fertil Steril* 2006, 85:428–435.

17. Isley WL: Hepatotoxicity of thiazolidinediones. *Expert Opin Drug Saf* 2003, 2:581–586.

18. Imani B, Eijkemans MJ, te Velde ER, et al.: Predictors of chances to conceive in ovulatory patients during clomiphene citrate induction of ovulation in normogonadotropic oligomenorrheic infertility. *J Clin Endocrinol Metab* 1999, 84:1617–1622.

19. Imani B, Eijkemans MJ, te Velde ER, et al.: Predictors of patients remaining anovulatory during clomiphene citrate induction of ovulation in normogonadotropic oligomenorrheic infertility. *J Clin Endocrinol Metab* 1998, 83:2361–2365.

20. Schenker JG, Yarkoni S, Granat M: Multiple pregnancies following induction of ovulation. *Fertil Steril* 1981, 35:105–123.

21. Schenker JG, Laufer N, Weinstein D, Yarkoni S: Quintuplet pregnancies. *Eur J Obstet Gynecol Reprod Biol* 1980, 10:257–268.

22. Schenker JG, Simha A: Quintuplet pregnancy. *Obstet Gynecol* 1975, 45:590–593.

23. Liu HM, Xing FQ, Chen SL, Li H: [Predictive value of endometrial ultrasonography and age for the outcome of in vitro fertilization–embryo transfer]. *Di Yi Jun Yi Da Xue Xue Bao* 2005, 25:570–572.

24. Steiner AZ, Terplan M, Paulson RJ: Comparison of tamoxifen and clomiphene citrate for ovulation induction: a meta–analysis. *Hum Reprod* 2005, 20:1511–1515.

25. Mitwally MF, Casper RF: Use of an aromatase inhibitor for induction of ovulation in patients with an inadequate response to clomiphene citrate. *Fertil Steril* 2001, 75:305–309.

26. Begum MR, Quadir E, Begum A, et al.: Role of aromatase inhibitor in ovulation induction in patients with poor response to clomiphene citrate. *J Obstet Gynaecol Res* 2006, 32:502–506.

27. Elnashar A, Fouad H, Eldosoky M, Saeid N: Letrozole induction of ovulation in women with clomiphene citrate–resistant polycystic ovary syndrome may not depend on the period of infertility, the body mass index, or the luteinizing hormone/follicle–stimulating hormone ratio. *Fertil Steril* 2006, 85:511–513.

28. Atay V, Cam C, Muhcu M, et al.: Comparison of letrozole and clomiphene citrate in women with polycystic ovaries undergoing ovarian stimulation. *J Int Med Res* 2006, 34:73–76.

29. Tulandi T, Martin J, Al–Fadhli R, et al.: Congenital malformations among 911 newborns conceived after infertility treatment with letrozole or clomiphene citrate. *Fertil Steril* 2006, 85:1761–1765.

30. Gorry A, White DM, Franks S: Infertility in polycystic ovary syndrome: focus on low–dose gonadotropin treatment. *Endocrine* 2006, 30:27–33.

31. van Schouwenburg JA: [Parameters of ovulation in spontaneous ovulatory cycles]. *S Afr Med J* 13 1984, 66:567–572.

32. Haritha S, Rajagopalan G: Follicular growth, endometrial thickness, and serum estradiol levels in spontaneous and clomiphene citrate–induced cycles. *Int J Gynaecol Obstet* 2003, 81:287–292.

33. Homburg R, Howles CM: Low-dose FSH therapy for anovulatory infertility associated with polycystic ovary syndrome: rationale, results, reflections and refinements. *Hum Reprod Update* 1999, 5:493–499.

34. Silverberg KM, Olive DL, Burns WN, et al.: Follicular size at the time of human chorionic gonadotropin administration predicts ovulation outcome in human menopausal gonadotropin–stimulated cycles. *Fertil Steril* 1991, 56:296–300.

35. Farquhar C, Vandekerckhove P, Arnot M, Lilford R: Laparoscopic "drilling" by diathermy or laser for ovulation induction in anovulatory polycystic ovary syndrome. *Cochrane Database Syst Rev* 2000, (2):CD001122.

36. Farquhar CM: An economic evaluation of laparoscopic ovarian diathermy versus gonadotrophin therapy for women with clomiphene citrate–resistant polycystic ovarian syndrome. *Curr Opin Obstet Gynecol* 2005, 17:347–353.

37. Li TC, Saravelos H, Chow MS, et al.: Factors affecting the outcome of laparoscopic ovarian drilling for polycystic ovarian syndrome in women with anovulatory infertility. *Br J Obstet Gynaecol* 1998, 105:338–344.

38. Greenblatt EM, Casper RF: Laparoscopic ovarian drilling in women with polycystic ovarian syndrome. *Prog Clin Biol Res* 1993, 381:129–138.

39. Amer SA, Banu Z, Li TC, Cooke ID: Long-term follow-up of patients with polycystic ovary syndrome after laparoscopic ovarian drilling: endocrine and ultrasonographic outcomes. *Hum Reprod* 2002, 17:2851–2857.

40. Palomba S, Orio F, Jr., Nardo LG, et al.: Metformin administration versus laparoscopic ovarian diathermy in clomiphene citrate-resistant women with polycystic ovary syndrome: a prospective parallel randomized double-blind placebo-controlled trial. *J Clin Endocrinol Metab* 2004, 89:4801–4809.

41. Petsos P, Ratcliffe WA, Anderson DC: Effects of medroxyprogesterone acetate in women with polycystic ovary syndrome. *Clin Endocrinol (Oxf)* 1986, 25:651–660.

42. Strott CA, Cargille CM, Ross GT, Lipsett MB: The short luteal phase. *J Clin Endocrinol Metab* 1970, 30:246–251.

43. Sherman BM, Korenman SG: Measurement of plasma LH, FSH, estradiol and progesterone in disorders of the human menstrual cycle: the short luteal phase. *J Clin Endocrinol Metab* 1974, 38:89–93.

44. Sherman BM, Korenman SG: Measurement of serum LH, FSH, estradiol and progesterone in disorders of the human menstrual cycle: the inadequate luteal phase. *J Clin Endocrinol Metab* 1974, 39:145–149.

45. Seppala M, Ranta T, Hirvonen E: Hyperprolactinemia and luteal insufficiency. *Lancet* 1976, 1:229–230.

46. De Souza MJ: Menstrual disturbances in athletes: a focus on luteal phase defects. *Med Sci Sports Exerc* 2003, 35:1553–1563.

47. Maruo T, Katayama K, Barnea ER, Mochizuki M: A role for thyroid hormone in the induction of ovulation and corpus luteum function. *Horm Res* 1992, 37:12–18.

48. Quagliarello J, Weiss G: Clomiphene citrate in the management of infertility associated with shortened luteal phases. *Fertil Steril* 1979, 31:373–377.

49. Lenton EA, Landgren BM, Sexton L, Harper R: Normal variation in the length of the follicular phase of the menstrual cycle: effect of chronological age. *Br J Obstet Gynaecol* 1984, 91:681–684.

50. Koninckx PR, Meuleman C, Demeyere S, et al.: Suggestive evidence that pelvic endometriosis is a progressive disease, whereas deeply infiltrating endometriosis is associated with pelvic pain. *Fertil Steril* 1991, 55:759–765.

51. Centers for Disease Control 2004 Assisted Reproductive Technology Success Rates. Atlanta: Centers for Disease Control and Prevention; 2006.

52. Katsoff B, Check JH, Davies E, Wilson C: Evaluation of the effect of endometriosis on oocyte quality and endometrial environment by comparison of donor and recipient outcomes following embryo transfer in a shared oocyte program. *Clin Exp Obstet Gynecol* 2006, 33:201–202.

53. Lessey BA: Implantation defects in infertile women with endometriosis. *Ann N Y Acad Sci* 2002, 955:265–280; discussion 293–265, 396–406.

54. Lessey BA, Palomino WA, Apparao K, et al.: Estrogen receptor-alpha (ER-alpha) and defects in uterine receptivity in women. *Reprod Biol Endocrinol* 2006, 4:S9.

55. Pellicer A, Navarro J, Bosch E, et al.: Endometrial quality in infertile women with endometriosis. *Ann N Y Acad Sci* 2001, 943:122–130.

56. Jacobson TZ, Barlow DH, Koninckx PR, et al.: Laparoscopic surgery for subfertility associated with endometriosis. *Cochrane Database Syst Rev* 2002, CD001398.

57. Marconi G, Vilela M, Quintana R, Sueldo C: Laparoscopic ovarian cystectomy of endometriomas does not affect the ovarian response to gonadotropin stimulation. *Fertil Steril* 2002, 78:876–878.

58. Surrey ES, Schoolcraft WB: Does surgical management of endometriosis within 6 months of an in vitro fertilization-embryo transfer cycle improve outcome? *J Assist Reprod Genet* 2003, 20:365–370.

59. Demirol A, Guven S, Baykal C, Gurgan T: Effect of endometrioma cystectomy on IVF outcome: a prospective randomized study. *Reprod Biomed Online* 2006, 12:639–643.

60. Gomel V: Salpingo-ovariolysis by laparoscopy in infertility. *Fertil Steril* 1983, 40:607–611.

61. Donnez J, Casanas-Roux F: Prognostic factors of fimbrial microsurgery. *Fertil Steril* 1986, 46:200–204.

62. Donnez J, Casanas-Roux F: [Microsurgery of distal tubal lesions. Analysis of 270 operated cases]. *J Gynecol Obstet Biol Reprod* (Paris) 1986, 15:339–346.

63. Schlaff WD, Hassiakos DK, Damewood MD, Rock JA: Neosalpingostomy for distal tubal obstruction: prognostic factors and impact of surgical technique. *Fertil Steril* 1990, 54:984–990.

64. Dubuisson JB, Bouquet de Joliniere J, Aubriot FX, et al.: Terminal tuboplasties by laparoscopy: 65 consecutive cases. *Fertil Steril* 1990, 54:401–403.

65. Strandell A, Waldenstrom U, Nilsson L, Hamberger L: Hydrosalpinx reduces in-vitro fertilization/embryo transfer pregnancy rates. *Hum Reprod* 1994, 9:861–863.

66. Vandromme J, Chasse E, Lejeune B, et al.: Hydrosalpinges in in-vitro fertilization: an unfavourable prognostic feature. *Hum Reprod* 1995, 10:576–579.

67. Mardesic T, Muller P, Huttelova R, et al.: [Effect of salpingectomy on the results of IVF in women with tubal sterility—prospective study]. *Ceska Gynekol* 2001, 66:259–264.

68. Murray DL, Sagoskin AW, Widra EA, Levy MJ: The adverse effect of hydrosalpinges on in vitro fertilization pregnancy rates and the benefit of surgical correction. *Fertil Steril* 1998, 69:41–45.

69. de Wit W, Gowrising CJ, Kuik DJ, et al.: Only hydrosalpinges visible on ultrasound are associated with reduced implantation and pregnancy rates after in-vitro fertilization. *Hum Reprod* 1998, 13:1696–1701.

70. Guzick DS, Sullivan MW, Adamson GD, et al.: Efficacy of treatment for unexplained infertility. *Fertil Steril* 1998, 70:207–213.

71. Griffiths A, D'Angelo A, Amso N: Surgical treatment of fibroids for subfertility. *Cochrane Database Syst Rev* 2006, 3:CD003857.

72. Benecke C, Kruger TF, Siebert TI, et al.: Effect of fibroids on fertility in patients undergoing assisted reproduction. A structured literature review. *Gynecol Obstet Invest* 2005, 59:225–230.

73. Sanders B: Uterine factors and infertility. *J Reprod Med* 2006, 51:169–176.

74. Narayan R, Rajat, Goswamy K: Treatment of submucous fibroids, and outcome of assisted conception. *J Am Assoc Gynecol Laparosc* 1994, 1:307–311.

75. Stovall DW, Parrish SB, van Voorhis BJ, et al.: Uterine leiomyomas reduce the efficacy of assisted reproduction cycles: results of a matched follow-up study. *Hum Reprod* 1998, 13:192–197.

76. Ramzy AM, Sattar M, Amin Y, et al.: Uterine myomata and outcome of assisted reproduction. *Hum Reprod* 1998, 13:198–202.

77. Goldenberg M, Sivan E, Sharabi Z, et al.: Outcome of hysteroscopic resection of submucous myomas for infertility. *Fertil Steril* 1995, 64:714–716.

78. Eldar–Geva T, Meagher S, Healy DL, et al.: Effect of intramural, subserosal, and submucosal uterine fibroids on the outcome of assisted reproductive technology treatment. *Fertil Steril* 1998, 70:687–691.

79. Oliveira FG, Abdelmassih VG, Diamond MP, et al.: Impact of subserosal and intramural uterine fibroids that do not distort the endometrial cavity on the outcome of in vitro fertilization-intracytoplasmic sperm injection. *Fertil Steril* 2004, 81:582–587.

80. Farhi J, Ashkenazi J, Feldberg D, et al.: Effect of uterine leiomyomata on the results of in-vitro fertilization treatment. *Hum Reprod* 1995, 10:2576–2578.

81. Shokeir TA, Shalan HM, El–Shafei MM: Significance of endometrial polyps detected hysteroscopically in eumenorrheic infertile women. *J Obstet Gynaecol Res* 2004, 30:84–89.

82. Varasteh NN, Neuwirth RS, Levin B, Keltz MD: Pregnancy rates after hysteroscopic polypectomy and myomectomy in infertile women. *Obstet Gynecol* 1999, 94:168–171.

83. Roge P, d'Ercole C, Cravello L: [Hysteroscopic treatment of uterine synechias. A report of 102 cases]. *J Gynecol Obstet Biol Reprod* (Paris) 1996, 25:33–40.

84. Cronje HS: [The hysteroscopic treatment of Asherman syndrome]. *S Afr Med J* 1988, 73:424–425.

85. Carp HJ, Ben–Shlomo I, Mashiach S: What is the minimal uterine cavity needed for a normal pregnancy? An extreme case of Asherman syndrome. *Fertil Steril* 1992, 58:419–421.

86. Akar ME, Bayar D, Yildiz S, et al.: Reproductive outcome of women with unicornuate uterus. *Aust N Z J Obstet Gynaecol* 2005, 45:148–150.

87. Patton PE, Novy MJ, Lee DM, Hickok LR: The diagnosis and reproductive outcome after surgical treatment of the complete septate uterus, duplicated cervix and vaginal septum. *Am J Obstet Gynecol* 2004, 190:1669–1675; discussion 1675–1668.

88. Papp Z, Mezei G, Gavai M, *et al.*: Reproductive performance after transabdominal metroplasty: a review of 157 consecutive cases. *J Reprod Med* 2006, 51:544–552.

89. Goldberg JM, Mascha E, Falcone T, Attaran M: Comparison of intrauterine and intracervical insemination with frozen donor sperm: a meta-analysis. *Fertil Steril* 1999, 72:792–795.

90. Cantineau AE, Heineman MJ, Cohlen BJ: Single versus double intrauterine insemination in stimulated cycles for subfertile couples: a systematic review based on a Cochrane review. *Hum Reprod* 2003, 18:941–946.

91. Francavilla F, Romano R, Santucci R, Poccia G: Effect of sperm morphology and motile sperm count on outcome of intrauterine insemination in oligozoospermia and/or asthenozoospermia. *Fertil Steril* 1990, 53:892–897.

92. van Weert JM, Repping S, Van Voorhis BJ, *et al.*: Performance of the postwash total motile sperm count as a predictor of pregnancy at the time of intrauterine insemination: a meta-analysis. *Fertil Steril* 2004, 82:612–620.

93. Zhao Y, Vlahos N, Wyncott D, *et al.*: Impact of semen characteristics on the success of intrauterine insemination. *J Assist Reprod Genet* 2004, 21:143–148.

94. Yalti S, Gurbuz B, Sezer H, Celik S: Effects of semen characteristics on IUI combined with mild ovarian stimulation. *Arch Androl* 2004, 50:239–246.

95. Lee RK, Hou JW, Ho HY, *et al.*: Sperm morphology analysis using strict criteria as a prognostic factor in intrauterine insemination. *Int J Androl* 2002, 25:277–280.

96. Grigoriou O, Pantos K, Makrakis E, *et al.*: Impact of isolated teratozoospermia on the outcome of intrauterine insemination. *Fertil Steril* 2005, 83:773–775.

97. Wainer R, Albert M, Dorion A, *et al.*: Influence of the number of motile spermatozoa inseminated and of their morphology on the success of intrauterine insemination. *Hum Reprod* 2004,19:2060–2065.

98. Guzick DS, Overstreet JW, Factor-Litvak P, *et al.*: Sperm morphology, motility, and concentration in fertile and infertile men. *N Engl J Med* 2001, 345:1388–1393.

99. Mansour RT, Fahmy IM, Taha AK, *et al.*: Intracytoplasmic spermatid injection can result in the delivery of normal offspring. *J Androl* 2003, 24:757–764.

100. Devroey P, Van Steirteghem A: A review of ten years experience of ICSI. *Hum Reprod Update* 2004, 10:19–28.

101. Grimes DA: Validity of the postcoital test. *Am J Obstet Gynecol* 1995, 172:1327.

102. Helmerhorst FM, van Vliet HA, Gornas T, *et al.*: Intrauterine insemination versus timed intercourse for cervical hostility in subfertile couples. *Obstet Gynecol Surv* 2006, 61:402–414; quiz 423.

103. Check JH: Diagnosis and treatment of cervical mucus abnormalities. *Clin Exp Obstet Gynecol* 2006, 33:140–142.

104. Steptoe PC, Edwards RG: Birth after the reimplantation of a human embryo. *Lancet* 1978, 2:366.

105. Barnhart K, Dunsmoor-Su R, Coutifaris C: Effect of endometriosis on in vitro fertilization. *Fertil Steril* 2002, 77:1148–1155.

106. Klonoff-Cohen H: Female and male lifestyle habits and IVF: what is known and unknown. *Hum Reprod Update* 2005, 11:179–203.

107. Augood C, Duckitt K, Templeton AA: Smoking and female infertility: a systematic review and meta-analysis. *Hum Reprod* 1998, 13:1532–1539.

108. Morris SN, Missmer SA, Cramer DW, *et al.*: Effects of lifetime exercise on the outcome of in vitro fertilization. *Obstet Gynecol* 2006, 108:938–945.

109. Spandorfer SD, Kump L, Goldschlag D, et al.: Obesity and in vitro fertilization: negative influences on outcome. *J Reprod Med* 2004, 49:973–977.

110. Dechaud H, Anahory T, Reyftmann L, *et al.*: Obesity does not adversely affect results in patients who are undergoing in vitro fertilization and embryo transfer. *Eur J Obstet Gynecol Reprod Biol* 2006, 127:88–93.

111. Lintsen AM, Pasker-de Jong PC, de Boer EJ, *et al.*: Effects of subfertility cause, smoking and body weight on the success rate of IVF. *Hum Reprod* 2005, 20:1867–1875.

112. 2006 Guidelines for gamete and embryo donation. *Fertil Steril* 2006, 86:S38–S50.

113. Shulman A, Frenkel Y, Dor J, *et al.*: The best donor. *Hum Reprod* 1999,14:2493–2496.

114. Carlson JW: Donum Vitae on homologous interventions: is IVF-ET a less acceptable gift than "GIFT"? *J Med Philos* 1989, 14:523–540.

115. Fertility preservation and reproduction in cancer patients. *Fertil Steril* 2005, 83:1622–1628.

116. Lee SJ, Schover LR, Partridge AH, *et al.*: American Society of Clinical Oncology recommendations on fertility preservation in cancer patients. *J Clin Oncol* 2006, 24:2917–2931.

117. Lee MS, Chang KS, Cabanillas F, *et al.*: Detection of minimal residual cells carrying the t(14;18) by DNA sequence amplification. *Science* 1987, 237:175–178.

118. Oktay K, Buyuk E: Ovarian transplantation in humans: indications, techniques and the risk of reseeding cancer. *Eur J Obstet Gynecol Reprod Biol* 2004, 113:S45–S47.

119. Donnez J, Dolmans MM, Demylle D, *et al.*: Livebirth after orthotopic transplantation of cryopreserved ovarian tissue. *Lancet* 2004, 364:1405–1410.

120. Meirow D, Levron J, Eldar–Geva T, *et al.*: Pregnancy after transplantation of cryopreserved ovarian tissue in a patient with ovarian failure after chemotherapy. *N Engl J Med* 2005, 353:318–321.

121. Dawson A, Griesinger G, Diedrich K: Screening oocytes by polar body biopsy. *Reprod Biomed Online* 2006, 13:104–109.

122. Verlinsky Y, Cohen J, Munne S, *et al.*: Over a decade of experience with preimplantation genetic diagnosis: a multicenter report. *Fertil Steril* 2004, 82:292–294.

123. Pickering SJ, McConnell JM, Johnson MH, Braude PR: Reliability of detection by polymerase chain reaction of the sickle cell–containing region of the beta-globin gene in single human blastomeres. *Hum Reprod* 1992, 7:630–636.

124. Traeger–Synodinos J, Vrettou C, Palmer G, *et al.*: An evaluation of PGD in clinical genetic services through 3 years application for prevention of beta-thalassemia major and sickle cell thalassanemia. *Mol Hum Reprod* 2003, 9:301–307.

125. Ericson A, Kallen B: Congenital malformations in infants born after IVF: a population-based study. *Hum Reprod* 2001, 16:504–509.

126. Kallen B, Finnstrom O, Nygren KG, Olausson PO: In vitro fertilization (IVF) in Sweden: risk for congenital malformations after different IVF methods. *Birth Defects Res A Clin Mol Teratol* 2005, 73:162–169.

127. Allen VM, Wilson RD, Cheung A: Pregnancy outcomes after assisted reproductive technology. *J Obstet Gynaecol Can* 2006, 28:220–250.

128. Hansen M, Kurinczuk JJ, Bower C, Webb S: The risk of major birth defects after intracytoplasmic sperm injection and in vitro fertilization. *N Engl J Med* 2002, 346:725–730.

129. Hansen M, Bower C, Milne E, *et al.*: Assisted reproductive technologies and the risk of birth defects: a systematic review. *Hum Reprod* 2005, 20:328–338.

130. Gosden R, Trasler J, Lucifero D, Faddy M: Rare congenital disorders, imprinted genes, and assisted reproductive technology. *Lancet* 2003, 361:1975–1977.

131. Lidegaard O, Pinborg A, Andersen AN: Imprinting diseases and IVF: Danish National IVF cohort study. *Hum Reprod* 2005, 20:950–954.

132. Valenzuela CY: [The risk of congenital malformations and genomic imprinting defects in assisted reproductive technologies and nuclear transfer cloning]. *Rev Med Chil* 2005, 133:1075–1080.

133. Aboulghar M, Evers JH, Al-Inany H: Intravenous albumin for preventing severe ovarian hyperstimulation syndrome: a Cochrane review. *Hum Reprod* 2002,17:3027–3032.

134. Al–Shawaf T, Grudzinskas JG: Prevention and treatment of ovarian hyperstimulation syndrome. *Best Pract Res Clin Obstet Gynaecol* 2003,17:249–261.

135. Beerendonk CC, van Dop PA, Braat DD, Merkus JM: Ovarian hyperstimulation syndrome: facts and fallacies. *Obstet Gynecol Surv* 1998, 53:439–449.

136. Ulug U, Ben–Shlomo I, Bahceci M: Predictors of success during the coasting period in high-responder patients undergoing controlled ovarian stimulation for assisted conception. *Fertil Steril* 2004, 82:338–342.

137. Silva C, Sammel MD, Zhou L, *et al.*: Human chorionic gonadotropin profile for women with ectopic pregnancy. *Obstet Gynecol* 2006, 107:605–610.

138. Chung K, Sammel MD, Coutifaris C, *et al.*: Defining the rise of serum HCG in viable pregnancies achieved through use of IVF. *Hum Reprod* 2006, 21:823–828.

139. Whittemore AS, Harris R, Itnyre J: Characteristics relating to ovarian cancer risk: collaborative analysis of 12 US case-control studies. II. Invasive epithelial ovarian cancers in white women. Collaborative Ovarian Cancer Group. *Am J Epidemiol* 1992, 136:1184–1203.

140. Rossing MA, Daling JR, Weiss NS, *et al.*: Ovarian tumors in a cohort of infertile women. *N Engl J Med* 1994, 331:771–776.

141. Brinton LA, Lamb EJ, Moghissi KS, *et al.*: Ovarian cancer risk after the use of ovulation–stimulating drugs. *Obstet Gynecol* 2004, 103:1194–1203.

142. Kashyap S, Moher D, Fung MF, Rosenwaks Z: Assisted reproductive technology and the incidence of ovarian cancer: a meta–analysis. *Obstet Gynecol* 2004, 103:785–794.

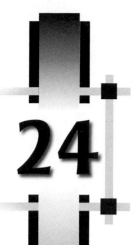

24 Vulvar Cancer

James C. Pavelka and Beth Y. Karlan

- Vulvar cancers constitute 4% of all malignancies of the female genital tract.
- Squamous cell carcinoma is the most common histologic type of vulvar cancer and represents more than 90% of invasive lesions.
- The most common presenting complaints are a vulvar mass and pruritus.
- Vulvar cancer is surgically staged with an overall very good prognosis largely dependent on inguinofemoral lymph node status.
- Treatment primarily consists of surgery, radiation therapy, or a combination of the two. Radiation is increasingly given with concurrent chemotherapy.

Incidence and Epidemiology

Vulvar cancer is a rare neoplasm, accounting fo only 5% of all malignancies of the female genital tract and less than 1% of all malignancies in women. In 2006, an estimated 3740 new cases of vulvar cancer will be diagnosed in the United States, resulting in 880 deaths [1]. Vulvar carcinoma is most frequently encountered in postmenopausal women, with a mean age at diagnosis of 65 years, although some more recent reports have cited a trend toward younger women [2]. Predisposing factors include cigarette smoking, lichen sclerosis, vulvar intraepithelial neoplasia (VIN), condyloma, immunodeficiency (including HIV infection or pharmacologic immunosuppression), and northern European ancestry. Although there appears to be an association of vulvar cancer with obesity, hypertension, and diabetes mellitus, it is not clear whether these are independent risk factors or coexisting medical problems related to increasing age [3–5]. A synchronous secondary malignancy has been reported in up to 22% of patients with a vulvar malignancy, the most common of which is cervical neoplasia [6].

Clinical Presentation

The most common presentation of invasive vulvar carcinoma is a vulvar nodule, plaque, ulcer, or mass with a complaint of pruritus. The pruritus is most often related to coexisting lichen sclerosus or vulvar dysplasia. Dystrophic changes in the adjacent skin have been reported in more than half of patients with vulvar carcinoma [7]. The area may be white, pink, or red in appearance. Most lesions are unifocal and occur on the labia majora (40%), with lesions on the labia minora (20%), clitoris (10%), mons (10%), and perineum (15%) occurring less commonly. Although most patients present with dominant lesions, all vulvar and perianal surfaces should be evaluated because lesions may be multifocal in 5% of cases [8]. In 10% of cases, the lesion may be too extensive to determine the actual site of origin [8].

Diagnosis

The diagnosis of vulvar carcinoma requires histologic evaluation of the epithelium and the underlying dermis. If a lesion exists, a full-thickness biopsy should be obtained from the periphery using a 4- or 5-mm Baker or Keyes punch after dermal infiltration with 1% lidocaine (preferably with epinephrine) using a 25-gauge needle. Sterile tissue forceps and scissors are needed to amputate the specimen. If a punch biopsy is not available, a cervical biopsy forceps (Burke or Tischler) may be used to remove the top of the wheal of tissue raised from the lidocaine injection. The biopsy sample should include the lesion and normal skin if possible. Bleeding from either technique should be minimal and easily controlled with silver nitrite applicators or ferric subsulfate (Monsel's solution). For lesions smaller than 1 cm in diameter, an elliptical excisional biopsy is the treatment of choice. Excisional biopsy often requires a suture for hemostasis. A 3-0 or 4-0

Vicryl suture (Ethicon, Inc., Somerville, NJ), on a cutting needle works well to reapproximate the skin edges.

If a lesion is not grossly evident, colposcopic examination of the vulva should be performed using 5% acetic acid solution. The acetic acid solution must be applied copiously and with prolonged contact to the keratinized vulvar squamous epithelium to dehydrate the cells fully and to define acetowhite lesions and their underlying vascular changes. Alternatively, if a colposcope is not available, 1% toluidine blue stain may aid in the identification of neoplasia. The stain is applied to the vulva with Fuller swabs and left on for 1 minute before being washed off with 3% acetic acid solution. The toluidine blue, a vital dye, is taken up by actively dividing cells and retained in the nucleus. Thus, areas with intense blue discoloration are abnormal and may warrant biopsy. After the diagnosis of invasive squamous cell carcinoma is confirmed, a thorough history and physical examination, including a detailed nodal survey of inguinal, axillary, and supraclavicular areas, is mandatory.

Pathology

A number of histologic variants of vulvar carcinoma exist, but squamous cell carcinoma accounts for more than 85% of cases (Figure 24-1). Two subtypes of vulvar squamous cell carcinoma have been proposed. The first, comprising approximately 40% of vulvar squamous cell carcinomas, is associated with human papillomavirus types 16 and 18 and is more often found in younger women. Other risk factors associated with this subtype include early age at first intercourse, multiple sexual partners, HIV infection, and cigarette smoking. The second and more common subtype occurs in older women and is not related to human papillomavirus infection, but rather is associated with hypertension, obesity, and diabetes. Malignant melanoma of the vulva is the second most common cancer of the vulva, accounting for fewer than 10% of primary vulvar neoplasms [9]. Malignant melanoma occurs predominantly in postmenopausal Caucasian women, with a peak incidence between the sixth and seventh decades. These lesions may arise de novo or from pre-existing junctional or compound nevi [9]. Melanomas of the vulva are more commonly amelanotic than in other regions of

the body [10], underlining the importance of a low threshold for biopsy of suspicious findings.

Carcinomas of the Bartholin's glands are rare, accounting for less than 4% of all vulvar malignancies. The median age at diagnosis for a Bartholin's gland carcinoma is 57 years of age. Up to 20% of Bartholin's carcinomas are associated with lymphatic spread at the time of diagnosis [9]. Therefore, an enlarged Bartholin's gland in a postmenopausal patient should prompt consideration of a malignancy. Bartholin's gland is composed of columnar epithelium, and the ducts are lined by stratified squamous epithelium and transitional cell epithelium. Correspondingly, adenocarcinomas, squamous cell carcinomas, adenoid cystic carcinomas, and rarely transitional cell carcinomas may arise from the gland. Most primary adenocarcinomas of the vulva arise within these glands. In 10% of patients with vulvar cancer, a history of preceding inflammation of Bartholin's gland is obtained.

Vulvar sarcomas constitute 1% to 2% of vulvar malignancies and include leiomyosarcomas, rhabdomyosarcomas, angiosarcomas, neurofibrosarcomas, and epithelioid sarcomas. The prognosis appears to be dependent on three main determinants: lesion size, tumor contour, and mitotic activity. Lesions greater than 5 cm in diameter, those with infiltrating margins, and those demonstrating more than five mitotic figures per 10 high-powered fields (HPF) are most likely to recur.

Treatment Options

Paget's disease of the vulva is an intraepithelial adenocarcinoma that accounts for less than 1% of all vulvar malignancies. Most patients are in their seventh or eighth decade of life when the diagnosis is confirmed. Paget's disease of the vulva is similar in appearance to Paget's disease of the breast. The lesion has slightly raised edges and a red background. In historical series, it has been stated that 20% to 30% of patients with vulvar Paget's disease have a noncontiguous tumor, such as breast, rectal, bladder, urethral, cervical, or ovarian carcinoma. More recent estimates have been significantly lower [11]. Regardless, a patient who has Paget's disease of the vulva should be evaluated for the possibility of synchronous neoplasms.

Histologic Subtypes of Vulvar Cancer and Their Relative Frequencies

Histology	Frequency
Squamous cell carcinoma	86%
Melanoma	5%
Sarcoma	2%
Basal cell	1%
Bartholin's gland	1%
Adenocarcinoma	< 1%
Undifferentiated	4%

Figure 24-1. Histologic subtypes of vulvar cancer and their relative frequencies. (*Adapted from* DiSaia and Creasman [31].)

Basal cell carcinoma represents approximately 2% of vulvar cancers. It usually affects postmenopausal Caucasian women, is locally aggressive, and is almost invariably nonmetastatic. Its common appearance is an ulcer with rolled edges and central ulceration. Wide local excision is the treatment of choice. Basal cell carcinomas are associated with a high incidence of antecedent or concomitant malignancy elsewhere in the body; therefore, a thorough search for other primary malignancies is always warranted [9].

Other tumors appearing in the vulva are exceedingly rare. Malignant schwannomas, endodermal sinus tumors, and adenocarcinomas of the skin appendages resembling breast cancers histologically have all been reported. Metastasis to the vulva from other sites such as the cervix is possible, though in these cases the vulva is almost never the sole metastatic focus.

Staging

A clinical staging system for vulvar cancer, based on the Tumor, Node, Metastasis classification, was adopted by the International Federation of Gynecology and Oncology in 1983. The staging was based on a clinical assessment of the primary tumor and regional lymph nodes. This staging system was inaccurate in predicting groin node metastases in 20% to 30% of cases, which is the most important prognostic indicator for this disease [9]. In light of this inaccuracy, International Federation of Gynecology and Oncology revised the staging for vulvar cancer in 1988 to a surgical staging system. In 1995, International Federation of Gynecology and Oncology once again changed the stage I category to include a microinvasive substage (stage IA) for vulvar tumors with less than 1 mm of invasion in light of the minimal risk of lymph node metastasis, resulting in the staging system now in use (Figure 24-2).

Routes of Spread

Vulvar carcinoma spreads by direct extension to adjacent structures, including the vagina, perineum, clitoris, and anus.

Lymphatic embolization to regional lymph nodes, as well as hematogenous dissemination to distant sites, may occur even with small lesions early in the course of disease. At diagnosis, about 10% of superficially invasive vulvar cancers have already undergone lymph node metastases [12]. Parry-Jones [13] initially mapped the lymphatic drainage of the superficial and deep vulvar lymphatics from the perineal body and labia to the mons pubis and then laterally to the superficial groin nodes. These lymphatics do not ordinarily cross the labial-crural skin crease. The superficial groin nodes (inguinal) drain into the deep groin nodes (femoral) below the cribriform fascia. The deep groin nodes then drain to the pelvic lymphatics.

Hematogenous spread is rare in the absence of inguinofemoral lymph node involvement and usually occurs late in the course of the disease. Patients with fewer than three positive lymph nodes have only a 4% risk of hematogenous spread [14]. By contrast, in patients with three or more positive lymph nodes, the risk of hematogenous spread is 66% [14].

Prognostic Factors

Inguinofemoral nodal metastases are the most important predictor of prognosis in vulvar carcinoma. When stratified for the number of positive nodes, patients with one microscopic positive node have a 5-year survival rate of 94%. By contrast, patients with two and those with three or more positive nodes have 5-year survival rates of about 80% and 15%, respectively [15–19,20••,21–23]. The frequency of lymph node metastases to the inguinofemoral nodes has been shown to be related to lesion size and depth of stromal invasion [12]. For lesions smaller than 2 cm in diameter, Hacker et al. [12] found the incidence to be about 15%. For lesions exceeding 4 cm, the rate of inguinofemoral lymph node metastases is more than 50% (Figure 24-3) [12]. Patients with less than 1 mm stromal invasion have a minimal risk of metastatic disease and do not warrant inguinofemoral node dissection, whereas those with tumors of 1 mm or greater depth of invasion should have evaluation of the inguinofemoral nodes to exclude lymphatic dissemination (see Figure 24-3).

Vulvar Cancer Staging

FIGO	TNM	Description
IA	T1a	Tumor confined to the vulva/perineum; 2 cm or less in diameter; stromal invasion less than or equal to 1 mm
IB	T1B	Tumor confined to the vulva/perineum; 2 cm or less in diameter; stromal invasion greater than 1 mm
II	T2	Tumor confined to the vulva/perineum; over 2 cm in greatest dimension
III	T3 or	Tumor any dimension with extension into vagina, lower urethra, or anus or
	T1-2, N1	FIGO I or II with ipsilateral inguinofemoral lymph node metastasis

Figure 24-2. Vulvar cancer staging. FIGO—International Federation of Gynecology and Obstetrics; TNM—Tumor, Node, Metastasis system.

Treatment

STAGE I

The hallmark of therapy for early-stage vulvar carcinoma is surgery. Recent modifications in the surgical approach to vulvar carcinoma have focused on conservatism and individualization of treatment. In cases with less than 1 mm of stromal invasion (stage IA), in which inguinofemoral lymph node metastases are exceedingly rare, radical local excision is the treatment of choice [17]. A radical local excision involves a wide and deep excision of the lesion with the goal of clearing the lesion by approximately 2 cm at all margins. This is performed by making an elliptical incision parallel to the skin lines down to the inferior fascia of the urogenital diaphragm. This permits primary closure of the incision without undue tension. The surgical defect is then closed in two layers with absorbable sutures. In retrospective series, a margin of 8 mm or more on the final paraffin embedded specimen is sufficient to limit the risk of local recurrence to that seen with wider margins [24].

In cases with more than 1 mm of stromal invasion (stage IB), the risk of inguinofemoral lymph node metastases is about 10%. Therefore, these patients should undergo ipsilateral inguinofemoral lymph node dissection for lateralized lesions and bilateral lymph node dissection for centralized lesions [16].

STAGE II

The management of stage II disease entails modified radical vulvectomy and bilateral inguinofemoral lymphadenectomy using a three-incision technique. The traditional en bloc dissection using a "butterfly" or "longhorn" approach, which removes the entire vulva, the superficial and deep inguinal lymph nodes, and the intervening skin bridge, results in extremely high morbidity with some degree of wound breakdown in more than half of patients [21]. The rationale for the en bloc dissection was based on the concern that leaving tissue between the primary tumor and the regional lymph nodes might leave microscopic foci of tumor in the draining lymphatics. However, squamous carcinoma appears to spread by embolization, not by permeation, and the experience with separate groin incisions has shown that there is little chance of recurrence in the skin bridge in the absence of clinically suspicious groin nodes [15,16]. Thus, the three-incision technique permits radical excision of the primary lesion and groin node evaluation while retaining skin over the groin and is the preferred technique [23••]. Farias-Eisner et al. [17] demonstrated no difference in survival or disease-free interval among patients undergoing a modified radical vulvectomy versus en bloc radical vulvectomy. In addition, the three-incision technique decreased the incidence of wound breakdown from 50% to 20% [16,17]. Skin bridge recurrences have been documented since the widespread adoption of the triple-incision technique. These are relatively rare and have only been reported in the setting of positive groin lymph nodes. If considering primary surgical therapy for a patient with enlarged, fixed pelvic lymph nodes, consideration should be given to the more traditional en bloc radical excision.

Lymphocyst is the most common acute complication of the three-incision technique and occurs in approximately 15% to 20% of cases [16–18]. Other acute complications include urinary tract infection, wound cellulitis, temporary anterior thigh anesthesia from femoral nerve injury, thrombophlebitis, and rarely, pulmonary embolus [15–21].

The most common chronic complications of modified radical vulvectomy and inguinofemoral lymphadenectomy are leg edema and urinary spraying due to anterior anatomic alterations. Again, with the use of separate groin incisions,

Characteristics of Primary Tumor and Risk of Lymphatic Spread

Tumor diameter, cm	Percent with nodal metastasis
< 1.0	18
1.1–2.0	19.4
2.1–3.0	31.4
3.1–4.0	54.3
4.1–5.0	39.6
> 5.0	51.8
Depth of invasion, mm	**Percent with nodal metastasis**
< 1.0	2.6
1.1–2.0	8.9
2.1–3.0	18.6
3.1–4.0	30.9
4.1–5.0	33.3
> 5.0	47.9

Figure 24-3. Characteristics of primary tumor and risk of lymphatic spread. (*Adapted from* Homesley et al. [32].)

the incidence of lymphedema has decreased from 31% to 14% [15–19, 20••, 21,22]; though this increases significantly if adjuvant groin irradiation is required. Other chronic complications include genital prolapse, urinary stress incontinence (10%), temporary weakness of the quadriceps muscle, and introital stenosis. Rare late complications include pubic osteomyelitis, femoral hernia, and rectoperineal fistula [15–19,20••,21]. Farias-Eisner et al. [17] observed a further reduction in acute and chronic morbidity when radical local excision of the primary lesion was used instead of radical total vulvectomy. Sentinel lymph node biopsy, although not yet universally embraced, has been proposed as a means to further limit the morbidity of inguinofemoral lymphadenectomy. Isosulfan blue dye, technetium-99 containing colloid, or preferably both can be injected into the primary tumor bed to indicate the lymph nodes most "at risk" for tumor metastasis. Whereas this has been proven as technically feasible [25], additional data are necessary to endorse its widespread application outside of the setting of clinical trials.

Postoperatively, patients with one microscopically positive groin node require no further treatment. Patients with two or more microscopic positive groin nodes or one or more macroscopically involved lymph node are best treated with ipsilateral pelvic and groin irradiation [19]. Hacker et al. [16,19] observed that no patients with fewer than three positive lymph nodes developed a pelvic recurrence, and all patients with positive pelvic nodes had clinically suspicious groin nodes. For those with positive groin lymph nodes, adjuvant pelvic radiation has been proven superior to pelvic lymphadenectomy for overall survival.

STAGES III AND IV

When advanced squamous cell carcinoma involves the anus, rectum, rectovaginal septum, or proximal urethra, surgical clearance is possible only by radical vulvectomy and bilateral groin dissection combined with pelvic exenteration. In light of the unacceptably high morbidity rate of these procedures, Hacker et al. [19] proposed the use of preoperative teletherapy in patients with advanced vulvar cancer to shrink the primary lesion and permit a more conservative surgical resection. This combined radiosurgical approach is associated with less morbidity and better survival than surgery alone. Metastases to the pelvic lymph nodes nearly always occur in the presence of groin adenopathy, and despite multimodal therapies are nearly always incurable. Treatment in this group of patients should typically be for palliative, rather than curative, intent.

Extrapolating data from squamous cell carcinoma of the cervix, many centers are now using chemotherapy concurrently with external beam radiation as a radiation sensitizer in the treatment of vulvar cancer. Phase II trials have shown significant responses in the neoadjuvant treatment of otherwise unresectable disease in the vulva and lymph nodes [26,27], with surgical resection of the tumor bed to follow. The benefit of this approach has not yet been proven with a phase III, randomized trial. Given the strength of the Phase II and cervical cancer data it may be that such a trial will never be performed, as many centers already consider chemoradiation as the standard of care.

Recurrent Disease

Vulvar recurrences are classified as local, inguinal, or distant. Local recurrences can be successfully treated in up to 75% of cases by re-excision, whereas patients with inguinal recurrences are rarely salvaged by radical resection [9,28••]. Myocutaneous flaps or skin grafts are at times necessary to close the defects created by such treatment and can be made more tenuous in the setting of prior local irradiation. Patients with distant metastases or groin recurrences may be candidates for salvage cytotoxic chemotherapy protocols. Cytotoxic agents that have been used in metastatic squamous cell carcinoma include cisplatin, 5-fluorouracil, doxorubicin, methotrexate, bleomycin, etoposide, piperazinedione, and mitoxantrone. Overall, the response rates are low, and the duration is usually short.

Evolving Therapeutics

Imiquimod has shown some promise as a nonsurgical alternative for VIN 2-3 [29]. Reports additionally detail the successful treatment of individual patients with imiquimod 5% cream for basal cell carcinoma of the vulva, intra-epithelial vulvar melanoma, and extramammary Paget's disease.

With the advent of US Food and Drug Administration approval of prophylactic human papilloma virus vaccines, it is hoped that the incidence of human papilloma virus–related vulvar carcinoma will decrease. Therapeutic vaccines have demonstrated some early efficacy in VIN [30], but have yet to be proven or approved for this indication.

Prevention

Annual pelvic examinations with close inspection of the vulva and perineum are the best methods to prevent vulvar carcinoma. Any suspicious lesions should be excised for biopsy as described previously. In addition, close observation and treatment of VIN with laser ablation or surgical excision is mandatory. In elderly women with extensive VIN, simple vulvectomy may be a reasonable alternative because occult invasion is more likely.

Referral

Primary care physicians who feel uncomfortable in the diagnosis or management of preinvasive vulvar lesions should seek consultation with a gynecologist or a gynecologic oncologist. Patients with unremitting vulvar pruritus or a nonhealing ulcer should have biopsies or get referrals. All women with invasive vulvar carcinoma should be referred to a gynecologic oncologist for further evaluation and treatment planning.

References

Papers of particular interest have been highlighted as follows:
- • Of interest
- •• Of outstanding interest

1. Jemal A, Siegel R, Ward E, *et al.*: Cancer statistics, 2006. *CA Cancer J Clin* 2006, 56:106–130.

2. Messing MJ, Gallup DJ: Carcinoma of the vulva in young women. *Obstet Gynecol* 1995, 86:51–54.

3. Hacker NF, Nieberg RK, Berek JS, *et al.*: Superficially invasive vulvar cancer with nodal metastases. *Gynecol Oncol* 1983, 15:65.

4. Green TH Jr, Ulfelder H, Meigs JV: Epidermoid carcinoma of the vulva: an analysis of 238 cases. Parts I and II. *Am J Obstet Gynecol* 1958, 73:834.

5. Franklin EW, Rutledge FD: Epidemiology of epidermoid carcinoma of the vulva. *Obstet Gynecol* 1972, 39:165.

6. Collins CG, Lee FY, Roman-Lopez JJ: Invasive carcinoma of the vulva with lymph node metastases. *Am J Obstet Gynecol* 1971, 109:446.

7. Buscema J, Woodruff JD: Progressive histobiologic alterations in the development of vulvar cancer. *Am J Obstet Gynecol* 1980, 138:146.

8. Zacur H, Genandery R, Woodruff JD: The patient-at-risk for development of vulvar cancer. *Gynecol Oncol* 1980, 9:199.

9. Hoskins WJ, Perez CA, Young RC, *et al.*: *Principles and Practice of Gynecologic Oncology*, edn 4. Philadelphia: Lippincott Williams & Wilkins; 2005:665–705.

10. Ragnarsson-Olding BK, Kanter-Lewensohn LR, Lagerlof B, *et al.*: Malignant melanoma of the vulva in a nationwide, 25-year study of 219 Swedish females: clinical observations and histopathologic features. *Cancer* 1999, 86:1273–1284.

11. Fanning J, Lambert HC, Hale TM, *et al.*: Paget's disease of the vulva: prevalence of associated vulvar adenocarcinoma, invasive Paget's disease, and recurrence after surgical excision. *Am J Obstet Gynecol* 1999, 180:24–27.

12. Hacker NF, Nieberg RK, Berek JS, *et al.*: Superficially invasive vulvar cancer with nodal metastases. *Gynecol Oncol* 1983, 15:65.

13. Parry-Jones E: Lymphatics of the vulva. *J Obstet Gynecol* 1963, 70:751

14. Hacker NF, Berek JS, Lagasse LD, *et al.*: Management of regional lymph nodes and their prognostic influence in vulvar cancer. *Obstet Gynecol* 1983, 61:408.

15. Dean RE, Taylor ES, Weisbrod DM, *et al.*: The treatment of premalignant and malignant lesions of the vulva. *Am J Obstet Gynecol* 1974, 119:59.

16. Hacker NF, Berek JS, Lagasse LD, *et al.*: Individualization of treatment for stage I squamous cell vulvar carcinoma. *Obstet Gynecol* 1984, 63:155.

17. Farias-Eisner R, Cirisano FD, Grouse D, *et al.*: Conservative and individualized surgery for early squamous carcinoma of the vulva: the treatment of choice for stage I and II (T1-2N0-1M0) disease. *Gynecol Oncol* 1994, 53:55–58.

18. Benedet JL, Turko M, Fairey RN, *et al.*: Squamous carcinoma of the vulva: results of treatment, 1938 to 1976. *Am J Obstet Gynecol* 1979, 134:201.

19. Hacker NF, Berek JS, Julliard GH, *et al.*: Preoperative radiation therapy for locally advanced vulvar cancer. *Cancer* 1984, 54:2056–2059.

20.•• Homesley HD, Bundy BN, Sedlis A, *et al.*: Radiation therapy versus pelvic node resection for carcinoma of the vulva with positive groin nodes. *Obstet Gynecol* 1986, 68:733.

This article continues to direct management of patients today by demonstrating that adjunctive groin and pelvic irradiation is superior to pelvic lymph node dissection.

21. Rutledge F, Smith JP, Franklin EW: Carcinoma of the vulva. *Am J Obstet Gynecol* 1970, 106:1117.

22. Gould N, Kamelle S, Tillmanns T, *et al.*: Predictors of complications after inguinal lymphadenectomy. *Gynecol Oncol* 2001, 82:329–332.

23.•• Hacker NF, Leuchter RS, Berek JS, *et al.*: Radical vulvectomy and bilateral inguinal lymphadenectomy through separate groin incisions. *Obstet Gynecol* 1981, 58:574.

This is one of the initial articles demonstrating that the three-incision technique for vulvectomy reduces morbidity without compromising cure.

24. Heaps JM, Fu YS, Montz FJ, *et al.*: Surgical-pathologic variables predictive of local recurrence in squamous cell carcinoma of the vulva. *Gynecol Oncol* 1990, 38:309.

25. Levenback C, Burke TW, Gershenson DM, *et al.*: Intra-operative lymphatic mapping for vulvar cancer. *Obstet Gynecol* 1994, 84:163.

26. Moore DH, Thomas GM, Montana GS, *et al.*: Preoperative chemoradiation for advanced vulvar cancer: a phase II study of the Gynecologic Oncology Group. *Int J Radiat Oncol Biol Phys* 1998, 42:79–85.

27. Montana GS, Thomas GM, Moore DH, *et al.*: Preoperative chemo-radiation for carcinoma of the vulva with N2/N3 nodes: a gynecologic oncology group study. *Int J Radiat Oncol Biol Phys* 2000, 48:1007–1013.

28.•• Stehman FB, Look KY: Carcinoma of the vulva. *Obstet Gynecol* 2006, 107:719–733.

This excellent contemporary review of the vulvar cancer literature is a "must read" for physicians who may be involved in the diagnosis or management of patients with vulvar cancer.

29. Le T, Hicks W, Menard C, *et al.*: Preliminary results of 5% imiquimod cream in the primary treatment of vulva intraepithelial neoplasia grade 2/3. *Am J Obstet Gynecol* 2006, 194:377–380.

30. Baldwin PJ, van der Burg SH, Boswell CM, *et al.*: Vaccinia-expressed human papillomavirus 16 and 18 e6 and e7 as a therapeutic vaccination for vulval and vaginal intraepithelial neoplasia. *Clin Cancer Res* 2003, 9:5205–5213.

31. DiSaia PJ, Creasman WT, eds: *Clinical Gynecologic Oncology*, edn 6. St. Louis: Mosby, Inc.; 2002.

32. Homesley HD, Bundy BN, Sedlis A, *et al.*: Prognostic factors for groin node metastasis in squamous cell carcinoma of the vulva (a Gynecologic Oncology Group study). *Gynecol Oncol* 1993, 49:279–283.

25 Vaginal Cancer

James C. Pavelka and Beth Y. Karlan

- Primary vaginal cancer constitutes only 3% of malignancies of the female genital tract.
- Most vaginal malignancies are metastatic.
- Squamous cell carcinomas make up roughly 85% of primary vaginal malignancies.
- Most vaginal carcinomas arise in the posterior fornix and present as painless vaginal bleeding.
- The diagnosis of vaginal carcinoma may be made using colposcopy in the setting of an abnormal Papanicolaou smear.
- Vaginal cancer is staged clinically and is based on findings from physical and rectovaginal pelvic examinations, cystoscopy, proctoscopy, and chest radiography.
- Radiation treatment, surgery, or a combination of the two is the treatment of choice. Chemoradiation is an area of evolving interest.

Incidence and Epidemiology

Vaginal cancer is a rare neoplasm that constitutes only 3% of malignant neoplasms of the female genital tract and less than 1% of all malignancies in women. An estimated 2420 new cases of vaginal carcinoma will be diagnosed in 2006 in the United States, with 820 deaths [1]. This small percentage results in part from criteria set forth by the International Federation of Gynecology and Obstetrics for the classification and staging of genital tract malignancies. International Federation of Gynecology and Obstetrics criteria require that any tumor that has extended through the cervix and reached the vagina should be classified as a primary cervical carcinoma, and likewise, any tumor involving the vagina and vulva simultaneously should be classified as vulvar carcinoma. Thus, most malignancies involving the vagina are metastatic and commonly arise from the endometrium, cervix, vulva, ovary, breast, rectum, or kidney [2–5]. Vaginal metastases may occur by direct extension (cervix, vulva, endometrium) or by lymphatic or hematogenous spread (breast, ovary, kidney).

Clinical Presentation

More than half of patients with vaginal carcinomas present with vaginal bleeding. Other symptoms include a watery, blood-tinged, or malodorous vaginal discharge, urinary frequency or pain, and gastrointestinal complaints, such as tenesmus or constipation [6–9]. Pelvic pain is present in 5% of patients and results from disease extension beyond the vagina. Up to 20% of patients are asymptomatic at the time of diagnosis [10–12].

Diagnosis

Diagnosing vaginal carcinoma is often difficult. Twenty percent of tumors are initially detected by Papanicolaou smear [10–12]. The difficulty in diagnosing asymptomatic patients is often secondary to the location of the tumor. The most common site of primary vaginal carcinoma is in the posterior wall of the upper one third of the vagina. Half of vaginal carcinomas arise in the upper vagina, 20% from the middle third, and 30% from the distal third [13]. Furthermore, 57% of the tumors originate in the posterior wall, 27% in the anterior wall, and 16% in the lateral wall. During a pelvic examination, the anterior and posterior blades of the speculum often obscure this area, and the diagnosis is frequently missed on initial examination. To visualize the anterior and posterior vaginal walls, the speculum should always be rotated 90° as it is withdrawn from the vagina.

If no lesion is visualized after an abnormal Papanicolaou smear, colposcopy should be performed following the application of 3% acetic acid solution. The use of Lugol's solution may be particularly helpful in the identification of dysplastic epithelium, as these regions, lacking intracellular glycogen stores, fail to bind the iodine and appear light yellow against the black staining background of normal tissue. Definitive diagnosis is made by biopsy of suspicious nonstaining areas. Care should be taken to inspect all vaginal folds along the full length of the vagina. After hysterectomy and in premenopausal women, this may require the use of a Burke hook or other instrument to expose all vaginal surfaces for inspection. Vaginal biopsy can be performed using "cervical" biopsy forceps (Tischler or Burke). Occasionally, a Burke hook is needed to tent the mucosa to permit biopsy. In some cases, examination under anesthesia during biopsy may be necessary if the patient has significant vaginal stenosis that precludes complete office examination or if cystourethroscopy or proctosigmoidoscopy is contemplated for staging purposes.

Pathology

Primary vaginal tumors compose a heterogeneous group of malignancies, as shown in Figure 25-1. Squamous cell carcinomas are the most common and constitute 80% to 90% of primary vaginal malignancies [8]. The age at diagnosis ranges from 25 to 98 years, with a peak incidence between the fifth and seventh decades of life. Grossly, these tumors may be nodular, ulcerative, indurative, or exophytic plaques of any size. Histologically, they are similar to squamous tumors from other sites. Up to 80% of vaginal carcinomas are in situ, and 60% of invasive vaginal cancers are associated with human papilloma virus infection [14,15]. As a reflection of their human papillomavirus–related etiology, squamous cell carcinomas of the vagina are much more common in women with a history of cervical dysplasia or carcinoma. Women with a history of cervical cytologic abnormality warrant vaginal Papanicolaou surveillance even after total hysterectomy.

Verrucous carcinoma is an uncommon variant of squamous cell carcinoma [16]. Grossly, it presents as a warty, fungating mass. Histologically, it is composed of large papillary fronds covered by dense keratin. Its deep margin creates a pushing border of well-oriented rete ridges. This tumor rarely metastasizes but can extensively infiltrate into surrounding tissues, including the rectum and coccyx.

Adenocarcinomas make up about 10% of primary vaginal neoplasms. The adenocarcinomas occurring in the vagina include papillary, mucinous, adenosquamous, small-cell, and clear-cell variants. The best described of these are the clear-cell malignancies primarily because of their reported occurrence in young women who had been exposed to diethylstilbestrol (DES) in utero [7,17]. The age range of DES-related clear-cell adenocarcinoma is 7 to 42 years [18]. The actual risk of DES-exposed women developing clear-cell adenocarcinoma is only one in 1000, with the highest risk in those women exposed before 12 weeks' gestation [18,19]. Clear-cell carcinomas of the vagina are generally polypoid masses presenting in the vaginal fornices. Histologically, there are well-described patterns: tubulocystic, solid, or papillary. Clear-cell carcinomas are generally diagnosed at an earlier clinical stage than are squamous cell carcinomas. Although the risk of clear-cell carcinoma of the vagina is small in DES-exposed women, 45% of these patients have areas of vaginal adenosis, and 25% have structural abnormalities of the uterus, cervix, or vagina. Thus, it has been recommended that women exposed to DES in utero be initially examined at menarche with careful palpation of the cervix and vagina in addition to cytologic examination. Annual colposcopy is not required unless indicated by the cytology results. The incidence of clear-cell carcinoma of the vagina is now decreasing, as DES has not seen widespread use in pregnancy since being banned by the US Food and Drug Administration in 1971.

Vaginal sarcomas constitute 3% of primary vaginal malignancies [20,21]. Reported vaginal sarcoma types include leiomyosarcomas, endometrial stromal sarcomas (usually arising in the setting of vaginal endometriosis), malignant mixed mullerian tumors, and rhabdomyosarcomas, among others. Embryonal rhabdomyosarcoma (sarcoma botryoides) is a highly malignant tumor that occurs in children up to 6 years of age (mean age 1.8 years). This sarcoma generally presents as soft, grapelike nodules that fill and protrude from the vagina or as abnormal bleeding.

Vaginal melanomas are rare but account for 2% to 4% of vaginal malignancies [21–24]. Three percent of malignant melanomas involve the female genital tract, and the vulva is the most common site of occurrence. Melanomas arising in

Histologies of a Series of Primary Vaginal Malignancies

Histology	Raw Number	Frequency, %
Carcinoma	4486	92
Carcinoma in situ	1242	25
Invasive squamous cell carcinoma	2574	53
Invasive adenocarcinoma	471	10
Other/unknown	194	4
Melanoma	192	4
Sarcoma	135	3
Other/unknown	72	1

Figure 25-1. Histologies of a series of primary vaginal malignancies. (*Adapted from* Creasman *et al.* [21].)

the vagina are thought to originate from in situ melanocytes in areas of melanosis or atypical melanocytic hyperplasia [22]. These malignancies occur at a mean age of 55 years, with an age range of 22 to 83 years. Patients typically present with abnormal vaginal bleeding, discharge, or a mass. These tumors most frequently occur in the lower one third of the vagina on the anterior wall and appear as a blue-black or black-brown mass or plaque.

Staging

Vaginal carcinomas are staged according to criteria set forth by the International Federation of Gynecology and Obstetrics or by the American Joint Committee (Figure 25-2). The staging of vaginal cancers is clinical and is based on the findings on physical and pelvic examination, cystourethroscopy, proctosigmoidoscopy, chest radiography, and skeletal radiography. In addition to vaginal biopsy, cervical cytology and endocervical curettage should be performed to exclude a primary cervical malignancy. Likewise, endometrial sampling should be done to locate an occult uterine primary tumor in patients who present with abnormal bleeding or an enlarged uterus.

Routes of Spread

Vaginal carcinoma may spread by direct extension or by lymphatic or hematogenous dissemination. Direct extension may occur to soft tissue structures such as the paracolpium and parametria, bladder, urethra, rectum, and bony structures of the pelvis. The route of lymphatic dissemination depends on the location of the primary tumor. The lymphatics of the upper vagina communicate with those of the cervix and drain into the pelvic lymph node chain. The lymphatics of the distal third of the vagina drain into the inguinofemoral nodes and secondarily to the pelvic nodes. Hematogenous dissemination usually occurs as a late manifestation of this disease.

Treatment

For in situ carcinomas, multiple therapeutic modalities have been shown to be effective. This is fortunate, as vaginal dysplasia can be multifocal, and at times, difficult to eradicate. Various techniques have been reported, from CO_2 laser vaporization, to local excision with loop electrosurgical excision procedure, or cavitational ultrasonic surgical aspiration to partial colpectomy, to topical treatment with 5% 5-fluorouracil cream, to brachytherapy. Each of these techniques has significant potential for toxicity, and treatment must be individualized for each patient and lesion.

Therapy for invasive vaginal cancers must also be individualized depending on tumor histology, location, size, and clinical stage. Stage I lesions smaller than 2 cm in the upper vagina may be treated with either surgery or radiation thera-

py. The surgical approach may require a radical hysterectomy, partial vaginectomy, and bilateral pelvic lymphadenectomy or a radical upper vaginectomy and bilateral lymphadenectomies, if a hysterectomy had already been performed. The standard treatment of lesions larger than 2 cm and all stage II to IV lesions is radiation therapy using teletherapy and interstitial or intracavitary therapy [9–12,26•]. The exact treatment plan depends on the tumor location, volume, and depth of invasion. External-beam irradiation of 4000 to 5000 cGy to the vagina and pelvis is usually required to shrink the primary tumor and treat the regional lymphatics. Extended-field irradiation that includes the para-aortic lymph nodes may be considered if bulky pelvic or para-aortic disease is seen on CT scan or if metastatic disease has been histologically confirmed. Similarly, treatment of the inguinofemoral lymph nodes is indicated if the primary tumor involves the distal third of the vagina. Chemoradiation is an area of evolving interest, particularly given its proven role in cervical cancer. Though a retrospective study has indicated a good response rate for this treatment [27], no randomized trials specific to vaginal cancer have proven the superiority of radiation with sensitizing chemotherapy to radiation alone. Despite this, chemoradiation has become the standard treatment for advanced vaginal cancer in many institutions. Chemotherapy in these centers, borrowing from cervical cancer data, is typically cisplatin and/or 5-fluorouracil dosed concurrently with external-beam radiation.

Teletherapy is followed by interstitial or intracavitary therapy to a total tumor dose of up to 7500 cGy. For tumors involving the upper third of the vagina, tandem and ovoids may be used, or a vaginal cylinder may be used if the uterus had previously been removed. For carcinomas with more than 0.5 cm of invasion, the use of interstitial implants increases the depth of the radiation penetration without delivering excessive amounts of radiation to the vaginal mucosa [26•].

Staging Vaginal Cancers

FIGO	TNM	Description
0	T0	Carcinoma in situ
I	T1	Tumor limited to vaginal wall
II	T2	Involvement of subvaginal tissue, without invasion to sidewall
III	T3	Extension to pelvic sidewall
IVA	T4	Involvement of rectal or bladder mucosa, or extension out of the true pelvis
IVB	T any, N1 or T any, M1	Palpable adenopathy (typically inguinofemoral) or distant metastases

Figure 25-2. Staging vaginal cancers. FIGO—International Federation of Gynecology and Obstetrics; TNM—Tumor, Node, Metastasis system. (*Adapted from* American Joint Committee on Cancer [25].)

Patients with a central recurrence after previous radiation therapy may be candidates for pelvic exenteration with or without vaginal reconstruction [28–30].

Complications of radiation or surgery occur in 10% to 15% of patients [31••]. The close proximity of the urethra, bladder, and rectum predisposes them to injury. Complications include rectovaginal or vesicovaginal fistulas, radiation cystitis or proctitis, rectal and vaginal strictures, and, rarely, vaginal necrosis.

Survival

Five-year survival rates for all stages of vaginal carcinoma range from 42% to 56% [32–34]. Five-year survival rates according to stage are listed in Figure 25-3 [35].

The lower survival rates for patients with vaginal cancer when compared with those with cervical or vulvar cancer may reflect that a higher proportion of vaginal tumors are of advanced stage when initially diagnosed. For this reason, thorough evaluation of the vagina should be performed with routine examinations, with emphasis not only on the cervix but also on the vaginal tissues. Particular care should be taken in the examination of any patient with a history of vulvar or cervical dysplasia or cancer.

Recurrent Disease

Patients with recurrent vaginal cancer are frequently difficult to treat, largely owing to prior radiation, surgery, or chemotherapy, or all three. For the minority of patients with disease localized to the pelvis who have not undergone pelvic radiation, this can offer some hope of cure. Total pelvic exenteration can be pursued in properly counseled patients with an isolated central pelvic recurrence, though the morbidity of this procedure is such that only well-informed and relatively fit individuals should be considered as candidates. Chemotherapy for vaginal cancer, as is the case for vulvar and cervical cancers, is almost never curative. Owing to a limited number of patients, trials of chemotherapy specifically for metastatic or recurrent vaginal cancer are rare. In one of the few studies of these patients, Thigpen et al. [36] reported a disappointing 6% response rate with single-agent cisplatin.

Five-Year Survival Rates for All Stages of Vaginal Carcinoma

Stage	Relative 5-year Survival Rate, %
0	96
I	73
II	58
III/IV	36

Figure 25-3. Five-year survival rates for all stages of vaginal carcinoma.

References

Papers of particular interest have been highlighted as follows:
• Of interest
•• Of outstanding interest

1. Jemal A, Siegel R, Ward E, et al.: Cancer statistics, 2006. CA Cancer J Clin 2006, 56:106–130.

2. Dunn LJ, Napier JG: Primary carcinoma of the vagina. Am J Obstet Gynecol 1966, 96:1112.

3. Way S: Vaginal metastases of carcinoma of the body of the uterus. Br J Obstet Gynaecol 1951, 58:558.

4. Bergman F: Carcinoma of the ovary: a clinicopathologic study of 86 autopsied cases with special reference to mode of spread. Acta Obstet Gynecol Scand 1966, 45:211–231.

5. Nergrum TA: Vaginal metastases of hypernephroma. Acta Obstet Gynecol Scand 1966, 45:515–524.

6. Choo YC, Anderson DG: Neoplasms of the vagina following cervical carcinoma. Gynecol Oncol 1982, 14:125–132.

7. Herbst AL, Ulfelder H, Poskanzer DC: Adenocarcinoma of the vagina: association of maternal stilbestrol therapy with tumor appearance in young women. N Engl J Med 1971, 284:878–881.

8. Livingston RC: Primary Carcinoma of the Vagina. Springfield, IL: Charles C. Thomas; 1950.

9. Rutledge F: Cancer of the vagina. Am J Obstet Gynecol 1967, 97:635.

10. Underwood RB, Smith RT: Carcinoma of the vagina. JAMA 1971, 217:46–52.

11. Pride GL, Schultz AE, Chuprevich TW, et al.: Primary invasive squamous carcinoma of the vagina. Obstet Gynecol 1979, 53:218–225.

12. Gallup DG, Talledo E, Shah KJ, et al.: Invasive squamous cell carcinoma of the vagina: a 14-year study. Obstet Gynecol 1987, 69:782–785.

13. Plentl AA, Friedman EA: Lymphatic System of the Female Genitalia: The Morphologic Basis of Diagnosis and Therapy. Philadelphia: WB Saunders; 1971.

14. Daling JR, Madeleine MM, Schwartz SM, et al.: A population–based study of squamous cell vaginal cancer: HPV and cofactors. Gynecol Oncol 2002, 84:263–270.

15. Okagaki T, Twiggs LB, Zachow KR, et al.: Identification of human papillomavirus DNA in cervical and vaginal intraepithelial neoplasia with molecularly cloned virus-specific DNA probes. Int J Gynecol Pathol 1983, 2:153–159.

16. Issacs JH: Verrucous carcinoma of the female genital tract. Gynecol Oncol 1976, 4:259–269.

17. Herbst AL, Scully RE: Adenocarcinoma of the vagina in adolescence: a report of 7 cases including 6 clear-cell carcinomas (so-called mesonephromas). Cancer 1970, 25:745–757.

18. Melnick S, Cole P, Anderson D, et al.: Rates and risks of diethylstilbestrol–related clear-cell adenocarcinoma of the vagina and cervix: an update. N Engl J Med 1987, 316:514–516.

19. Herbst AL: Problems of prenatal DES exposure. In Comprehensive Gynecology, edn 2. Edited by Herbst AL, Mishell DR, Stenchever MA, et al. St. Louis: Mosby-Yearbook; 1992.

20. Perez CA, Gersell DJ, McGuire WP, et al.: In Principles and Practice of Gynecology and Oncology, edn 4. Edited by Hoskins WJ, Perez CA, Young RC, et al. Philadelphia: Lippincott Williams & Wilkins; 2005.

21. Creasman WT, Phillips JL, Menck HR: The National Cancer Data Base report on cancer of the vagina. *Cancer* 1998, 83:1033–1040.

22. Lee RB, Buttoni L, Dhru K, *et al.*: Malignant melanoma of the vagina: a case report of progression from preexisting melanosis. *Gynecol Oncol* 1984, 19:238–245.

23. Liu L, Hou Y: Primary malignant melanoma of the vagina: a report of seven cases. *Obstet Gynecol* 1987, 70:569–572.

24. Reid GC, Schmidt RW, Roberts JA, *et al.*: Primary melanoma of the vagina: a clinicopathologic analysis. *Obstet Gynecol* 1989, 74:190–199.

25. American Joint Committee on Cancer: *AJCC Cancer Staging Manual*, edn 6. New York: Springer; 2002:251–257.

26.• Stock RG, Mychalczak B, Armstrong JG, *et al.*: The importance of brachytherapy technique in the management of primary carcinoma of the vagina. *Int J Radiat Oncol Biol Phys* 1992, 24:747.

This reference summarizes the importance of radiation therapy in the treatment of vaginal carcinoma.

27. Dalrymple JL, Russell AH, Lee SW, *et al.*: Chemoradiation for primary invasive squamous carcinoma of the vagina. *Int J Gynecol Cancer* 2004, 14:110–117.

28. Al-Kurdi M, Monaghan JM: Thirty-two years' experience in management of primary tumors of the vagina. *Br J Obstet Gynaecol* 1981; 88:1145–1150.

29. Berek JS, Hacker NF, Lagasse LD: Vaginal reconstruction performed simultaneously with pelvic exenteration. *Obstet Gynecol* 1984, 63:318–323.

30. Benson C, Soisson AP, Carlson J, *et al.*: Neovaginal reconstruction with a rectus abdominis myocutaneous flap. *Obstet Gynecol* 1993, 81:871–875.

31.•• Rubin SC, Young J, Mikuta JJ: Squamous carcinoma of the vagina: treatment, complications and long-term follow-up. *Gynecol Oncol* 1985, 20:346–353.

This reference nicely outlines the treatment options and potential sequelae of vaginal carcinoma.

32. Perez CA, Camel HM: Long-term follow-up in radiation therapy of carcinoma of the vagina. *Cancer* 1982, 49:1308–1315.

33. Nori D, Hilaris BS, Shu F: Radiation therapy of primary vaginal carcinoma. *Int J Radiat Oncol Biol Phys* 1981, 70:20.

34. Puthawala A, Syed AM, Nalick R, *et al.*: Integrated external and interstitial radiation therapy for primary carcinoma of the vagina. *Obstet Gynecol* 1983, 62:367–372.

35. American College of Surgeons National Cancer Data Base. *Cancer* 1998, 83:1033.

36. Thigpen JT, Blessing JA, Howresky HD, *et al.*: Phase II trial of cisplatin in advanced or recurrent cancer of the vagina. *Gynecol Oncol* 1986, 23:101–104.

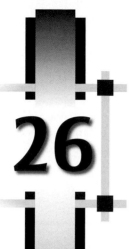

26 | Endometrial Cancer

Aya Sultan and Michael E. Carney

- Endometrial cancer is the most common invasive malignancy of the female genitalia tract, developing in more than 39,000 women a year.
- One quarter of women will be diagnosed with endometrial cancer in the postmenopausal period whereas fully one quarter will be diagnosed in the premenopausal years.
- Three percent of women will develop endometrial cancer at some point in their lives, especially those with risk factors such as obesity, diabetes, unopposed estrogen, atypical endometrial hyperplasia, and hereditary nonpolyposis colon carcinoma.
- Vaginal bleeding in postmenopausal women must always be taken seriously and evaluated completely by a physician who is familiar with the array of potential diagnoses and capable of performing coordinated, logical, accurate, and cost effective investigation.
- The cornerstone of treatment for endometrial cancer is surgery, which should be done in a setting in which the physician is fully capable of performing adequate surgical staging, and the availability for accurate frozen section is present.

Introduction

Endometrial cancer is the most common invasive malignancy of the female genital tract in the United States and the fourth most common malignancy overall, following breast, colon, and lung cancer. It has been estimated that in 2007, 39,080 women will be newly diagnosed with endometrial cancer, whereas 7400 women will die from it [1]. This malignancy has a high cure rate, with an 81% 5-year survival rate when diagnosed at any stage, and it is usually curable if diagnosed and treated in the early stages, with a 96% 5-year survival rate [1].

Epidemiology

INCIDENCE

Endometrial cancer occurs in nearly 3% of American women, usually after menopause. The median age at diagnosis is 61 years, although up to 25% of women develop endometrial cancer before menopause. Up to 5% of patients are diagnosed with the malignancy before the age of 40 years. Endometrial cancer in premenopausal patients is often more difficult to diagnose because of the common occurrence of irregular vaginal bleeding caused by anovulation. The physician must have a heightened sense of suspicion in premenopausal women with abnormal bleeding, particularly when the patient also has identifiable risk factors for the development of endometrial cancer.

RISK FACTORS

Several factors have been identified that increase the risk of developing endometrial cancer (Figure 26-1). Chronic exposure to estrogen achieved either by exogenous sources or endogenous phenomena can lead to the development of excessive endometrial stimulation, hyperplasia, and finally, cancer. Case-controlled cohort studies in the 1970s identified unopposed estrogen intake as a major risk factor for the development of endometrial cancer. Premalignant endometrial changes were 29 times higher, and endometrial cancers were nine times more frequent in patients taking unopposed estrogen. Today, patients rarely are given estrogen without progesterone, a hormone that protects the endometrium and eliminates the increased risk of developing endometrial cancer [2].

One of the most important endogenous risk factors leading to the development of endometrial cancer is obesity. Many obese women have a disruption of the normal hormonal milieu with the conversion of androstenedione, a nonestrogenic steroid, to the weak estrogen, estrone, by aromatase in adipose tissue. The chronically high levels of this estrogen can lead to endometrial hyperplasia and ultimately cancer. It is interesting to note that women living in the wealthier industrialized nations have a much higher incidence of endometrial cancer than is seen in developing nations. Women who are more than 50 pounds over their ideal body weight have 10 times the risk of developing endometrial cancer when compared with their normal-weight counterparts. Even patients who are only 20 to 50 pounds overweight have 3 times the risk of developing endometrial cancer.

Similarly, patients with infertility attributed to chronic anovulation or polycystic ovarian syndrome (PCOS) also have persistently elevated levels of estrogen and are at increased risk for the development of endometrial cancer [3]. Approximately 35% of women with PCOS develop endometrial hyperplasia, and those women who are diabetic in addition to obese are among the highest risk group for the development of uterine cancer. An emerging theory relating these risk factors to endometrial cancer is the hyperinsulin state. It is believed that insulin stimulates cell proliferation, aromatase expression, and enzyme activity, as well as promotes tumor development via angiogenesis and inhibition of apoptosis [4].

Other risk factors have also been identified. When compared with a control population, nulliparous women and women who underwent menopause after age 52 were found to have twice the risk of developing endometrial cancer. Diabetes and hypertension, two medical conditions long considered major risk factors for the development of endometrial cancer, often develop in the obese and are considered to be only minor associated factors even though one in four endometrial cancer patients has hypertension. Women who are diagnosed with a granulosa cell tumor of the ovary develop endometrial cancers in 5% of cases as a result of chronic estrogen overstimulation.

A review of the literature has suggested a racial difference in the development of and death from uterine cancer. In fact, although fewer African Americans presented at earlier stages than whites (54% vs 71%), the 5-year survival rate tended to be lower for African Americans than whites (60% vs 85%) [1].

Endometrial Cancer Risk Factors

Characteristic	Relative Risk
Nulliparity	2–3
Late menopause	2.4
Obesity: 21–50 lb overweight	3
Obesity: > 50 lb overweight	10
Diabetes	2.8
Unopposed estrogen	9
Tamoxifen	2–3
Endometrial hyperplasia	2
Atypical endometrial hyperplasia	8–29
Granulosa cell tumor (ovary)	3
Hereditary nonpolyposis carcinoma	10

Figure 26-1. Endometrial cancer risk factors.

However, a recent report suggests that this discrepancy may be due more to socioeconomic differences rather than race, as lower income levels were associated with advanced disease stage, decreased likelihood in receiving definitive treatment in the form of a hysterectomy, and ultimately contributed to lower rates of survival [5]. Further examination is required before the racial difference can be dismissed. In the meantime, it is important that physicians advocate for improved access to health care to ensure prompt diagnosis and treatment regardless of race and socioeconomic status.

Hormone Replacement

Following the Women's Health Initiative, a significant drop in use of hormone replacement therapy (HRT) was noted. HRT is rarely prescribed despite its well-documented benefits in prevention of osteoporosis, symptomatic relief of vasomotor and genital symptoms, and decrease in the incidence of colon cancer. This is mainly due to the significant detrimental effects on the cardiovascular system and an increased risk of thrombo-embolic events.

The publicity and misinformation surrounding the identification of unopposed estrogen as a cause of endometrial cancer likely lingers today and contributes to the reluctance of many women to initiate estrogen replacement therapy. Unopposed estrogen replacement is certainly a well-documented risk factor for the development of endometrial cancer, but patients should be educated that the addition of either daily low-dose progestin or cyclic monthly higher-dose progestin eliminates the risk of cancer attributable to estrogen alone [6].

TAMOXIFEN AND RALOXIFENE

Randomized trials published in the early and middle 1990s identified tamoxifen as an independent risk factor for the development of endometrial cancer. Patients treated with tamoxifen for 5 years were consistently found to have a threefold to sevenfold increased risk for the development of endometrial cancer. Even so, the small increased risk for developing endometrial cancer was far outweighed by the significant reduction in recurrent breast cancer.

Tamoxifen is a selective estrogen-receptor modulator (SERM) that has become the adjuvant antineoplastic agent of choice after standard surgery, chemotherapy, and radiation therapy for the long-term treatment of most breast cancer patients. Although its anti-estrogenic effects are responsible for its therapeutic actions in breast cancer, it also has moderate pro-estrogenic effects, which may be associated with the increased risk of developing endometrial hyperplasia, polyp formation, invasive carcinoma, and uterine sarcoma. These pathologic changes appear to be more common in the postmenopausal than premenopausal woman [7]. However, ultrasonographic measurements of endometrial thickness do not correlate well with the presence of abnormal pathology since tamoxifen induces subepithelial stromal hypertrophy.

A recent American College of Obstetrics and Gynecology committee opinion suggests that postmenopausal patients being treated for breast cancer with tamoxifen should be monitored closely not only for the development of recurrent breast cancer but also for the development of endometrial cancer by physicians familiar with both diseases. Premenopausal women have no increased risk of uterine cancer, and so endometrial cancer screening is not currently recommended for patients being treated with tamoxifen. Despite this, any vaginal bleeding, pelvic pain, or pelvic pressure necessitates prompt and complete investigation [7].

Newer hormonal antineoplastic agents are being studied for the treatment of breast cancer, such as raloxifene, which appear to have fewer estrogenic effects in the endometrium despite also being SERMs and are being evaluated as alternatives to tamoxifen [8]. In the Study of Tamoxifen and Raloxifene (STAR) trial, a trend towards a decreased incidence of uterine cancer was observed, although this was deemed not to be statistically significant [9]. Furthermore, there was a statistically significant decrease in the incidence of endometrial hyperplasia in raloxifene users [9]. This may prove promising for raloxifene use as primary neoadjuvant treatment for breast cancer, as no difference was seen between raloxifene and tamoxifen in preventing invasive breast cancer, whereas only a small nonstatistically significant decrease in noninvasive cancers was observed in tamoxifen versus raloxifene users [9].

Hereditary Endometrial Cancer

Patients diagnosed with colon cancer attributable to the Lynch syndrome or hereditary nonpolyposis colorectal cancers (HNPCC) are at significantly elevated risk for the development of endometrial cancer. The syndrome was initially described as an autosomal dominant disorder that predisposed the patient to colorectal and other cancers. However, it was subsequently determined that endometrial cancer was the most common cancer seen in HNPCC and developed in 40% to 60% of patients, with a mean age of diagnosis of 50 years [10]. Considering that 2% to 5% of colon cancer patients have HNPCC, endometrial cancer associated with this genetic syndrome is not uncommon.

Current recommendations advocate offering yearly screening for endometrial cancer in HNPCC patients via annual endometrial biopsies (transvaginal ultrasound remains controversial as the premenopausal years are a time when endometrial thickness can vary widely). Studies have shown a reduction in the risk of developing endometrial cancer in patients who have undergone prophylactic hysterectomy and bilateral salpingo-oopherectomy (BSO). Thus, prophylactic hysterectomy with BSO may be offered in lieu of annual screening for women who have completed child-bearing. Hysterectomy is indicated in patients undergoing colon surgery. More than half of HNPCC patients develop a second cancer at some point in their lifetime, so all HNPCC patients should be closely monitored.

Currently, there are no recommendations for screening all women with endometrial cancer for HNPCC as the likelihood of having HNPCC is low [11]. If a patient reveals pertinent factors associated with a high likelihood of having Lynch syndrome, such as a family history of a predisposition to early age of onset for certain cancers, then this patient should be offered genetic counseling and testing.

Endometrial Cancer Screening and Prevention

Endometrial cancer is the most common gynecologic cancer in the western world and thus should be considered as a reasonable candidate for screening. Endometrial biopsy can accurately detect endometrial cancer in more than 90% of symptomatic cases and is the screening method of choice. Ultrasound, Papanicolaou smear, and dilation and curettage with hysteroscopy are not ideal screening methods because of low specificity, low sensitivity, and high cost, respectively. Patients who develop endometrial cancer are generally older, have symptoms early in the disease process, and are ultimately cured. Therefore, the years of life saved by offering screening with available methods to the entire population would be few, and the cost and inconvenience to patients would be enormous [12]. Screening for endometrial cancer is not offered to the general population at this time, but there are subsets of patients who are good candidates for selected screening. Women who have been diagnosed with HNPCC, morbid obesity, or endometrial hyperplasia are reasonable candidates for yearly endometrial cancer screening.

Primary prevention of endometrial cancer in the United States can be accomplished in at least two ways. First, women who are able to maintain an ideal body weight develop endometrial cancer at much lower rates than overweight women. The increased risk of endometrial cancer seen in obese women has been confirmed in no fewer than 19 studies reporting a relative risk as high as 20 times greater than that of the general population [13]. Public health policy should encourage the maintenance of ideal body weight not only for the reduction of endometrial cancer but also for the reduction of many other associated cancers and health problems.

The use of combination oral contraceptives has been documented in several studies to lower the risk substantially of subsequently developing endometrial cancer. Sixteen studies have evaluated oral contraceptives and endometrial cancer, and all but one small study found a reduction in risk as low as 80%. Protection was seen in all of the three major histologic subtypes after 1 year of contraceptive use and lasted up to 15 years after discontinuation.

Clinical Presentation

The most common presenting sign and symptom of endometrial cancer is abnormal vaginal bleeding, which occurs in about 90% of endometrial cancer patients and allows for early diagnosis and treatment. Others complain of pelvic pain and pressure, abdominal pain, shortness of breath, or purulent vaginal discharge. Fewer than 5% of patients diagnosed with endometrial cancer are symptom free. Patients who do not have vaginal bleeding and are subsequently diagnosed with endometrial cancer often have obstruction of the uterine outflow by cervical stenosis.

Any patient who has undergone menopause and presents with a complaint of vaginal bleeding or is found to have blood in the vaginal vault at pelvic examination needs a thorough gynecologic evaluation to exclude an endometrial cancer. Many conditions other than endometrial cancer can cause a postmenopausal patient to have vaginal bleeding. Often, the cause is found to be atrophic vaginal epithelial changes caused by low systemic estrogen levels. Figure 26-2 lists the most common causes of postmenopausal bleeding. Even though most of the conditions listed are benign, endometrial cancer or its precursors are detected in 1 of 10 postmenopausal patients presenting for evaluation of vaginal bleeding.

The diagnosis of endometrial cancer in the premenopausal patient is more difficult. Commonly, these patients have had a long history of irregular menses from chronic anovulation, making the bleeding from a uterine cancer clinically indistinct from that of irregular menses and hence less concerning. However, patients with chronic anovulation are at increased risk for endometrial cancer and need evaluation. Once malignant endometrial pathology is excluded, these women may be considered for hormonal therapy to regulate menses. Nonpregnant women 35 years and older who present with heavy cyclic bleeding (menorrhagia) or prolonged irregular bleeding (metrorrhagia) deserve evaluation for endometrial cancer, particularly if they are obese or anovulatory (Figure 26-3).

Diagnosis

EVALUATION OF ABNORMAL VAGINAL BLEEDING

Vaginal bleeding in a postmenopausal woman must always be taken seriously and evaluated completely by a physician who is both familiar with the array of potential diagnoses and capable of performing a coordinated, logical, accurate, and cost-effective investigation. Referral to a gynecologic specialist is frequently, if not always, indicated.

Evaluation of vaginal bleeding begins with a complete history and physical examination. Questions regarding the onset, timing, quantity, and frequency of the bleeding should be answered. It is important to know if the patient is certain that the bleeding is vaginal and not rectal. A personal history of other cancers, hormone replacement, medical conditions such as diabetes and hypertension, abnormal Papanicolaou smears, weight and appetite changes, infertility, and other questions directed at risk factors should be obtained. The physical examination should be directed at potential sites of metastasis and physical signs that may be associated with other causes of vaginal bleeding. A survey of the lymph nodes, including supraclavicular and inguinal node chains, and an abdominal examination evaluating liver size, ascites, masses, and pain can detect distant metastatic disease. Auscultation of the chest may detect pleural effusions or a large lung mass.

The pelvic examination begins with an evaluation of the external genitalia and rectum for possible alternative sources of the vaginal bleeding. Inspection of the vagina can reveal atrophy or masses that may require biopsy to confirm metastatic disease. The cervix is another possible source of vaginal bleeding and should be evaluated completely. A Papanicolaou smear is always indicated, and colposcopy or biopsies can identify cervical involvement and primary cervical disease. A wet prep or cervical cultures may reveal infection as another potential cause of vaginal bleeding. Size, consistency, contour, and mobility of the uterus and adnexa are evaluated on the bimanual examination. The rectovaginal examination facilitates assessment of the adnexa, parametria, and cul de sac. The rectal mucosa should be palpated for polyps or masses, and a stool guaiac test should be obtained. In most cases of endometrial cancer, the physical examination is completely normal with the exception of vaginal bleeding and possibly a slightly enlarged uterus. Even if vaginal blood is not seen at the time of the examination, the history of vaginal bleeding alone is enough to prompt an investigation of the endometrial cavity.

Indications for Endometrial Cavity Evaluation

Premenopausal women

  Menorrhagia or metrorrhagia in a woman older than 35 years

  Hereditary nonpolyposis colon carcinoma

  Infertility due to chronic anovulation

  Morbid obesity

Postmenopausal women

  Any unexplained vaginal bleeding

  Vaginal bleeding while on tamoxifen

  Endometrial stripe larger than 5 mm (detected on ultrasound)

  Endometrial cavity mass or irregularity detected on radiologic scanning

  Unexplained bleeding after 6 months on hormone replacement therapy

  Noncyclic bleeding on hormone replacement therapy

Figure 26-3. Indications for endometrial cavity evaluation.

Causes of Vaginal Bleeding in Postmenopausal Women

Endometrial cancer	Vaginal cancer
Endometrial hyperplasia	Trauma
Atypical endometrial hyperplasia	Cervicitis
Atrophic vaginitis	Endometrial polyps
Bacterial vaginosis	Uterine leiomyomas
Monilial vaginitis	Bleeding diathesis
Cervical cancer	Estrogen replacement

Figure 26-2. Causes of vaginal bleeding in postmenopausal women.

Papanicolaou Smear

A Papanicolaou smear is an important part of the vaginal bleeding evaluation but is inadequate as a method to detect endometrial cancer; although the Papanicolaou smear is the most accurate way to screen for cervical cancer; only half of patients with a diagnosis of adenocarcinoma of the endometrium have their cancers detected by this method. Moreover, patients whose Papanicolaou test results suggest abnormal endometrial or glandular cells should be evaluated completely, including the procurement of endometrial and endocervical specimens. Endometrial cells reported on the Papanicolaou smear of a postmenopausal patient who is not on hormone replacement therapy are an abnormal finding and require further investigation, including endometrial cavity evaluation.

Endometrial Sampling

The cornerstone of endometrial cancer diagnosis is pathologic evaluation of the endometrium. In the past, most patients were taken to the operating room for a fractional dilation and curettage under general anesthesia to obtain a diagnosis. Now, the diagnosis can usually be made in the office setting with minimal anesthesia and minimal discomfort to the patient.

Several devices are available that can be used to aspirate the contents of the uterine cavity (Figure 26-4). The one most commonly used is the Pipelle uterine aspirator. This device is introduced through the cervical canal, and the stylet is withdrawn to create a negative vacuum so that endometrial cells and tissue are obtained. Frequently, a cervical tenaculum is necessary for countertraction.

Occasionally, a paracervical anesthetic block, a larger curet such as a Novak or Duncan curet, or minor cervical dilation is necessary to gain access to the endometrial cavity in the clinic. The larger curets are more painful for the patient and are infrequently used, although they sample more of the endometrial cavity. Endometrial biopsy causes significant pain in less than 5% of patients.

Office endometrial biopsy is almost always able to detect cancer. The accuracy of office endometrial biopsy is 90% to 98% higher than more extensive surgical evaluation (dilation and curettage) [14]. Even though the procedure is relatively simple, there are several potentially severe complications that can occur with office endometrial sampling, including uterine perforation and hemorrhage. Therefore, the procedure should be performed only by those capable of dealing with these rare but significant sequelae. A diagnosis of cancer requires prompt referral to a gynecologic oncologist. Patients found to have benign pathology can be monitored closely for continued unexplained vaginal bleeding, which often requires further surgical investigation. In addition, patients with cervical stenosis, inadequate or suspicious pathology, or negative pathology but a high index of suspicion should be referred for surgical evaluation.

Surgical Evaluation

Surgical evaluation includes fractional dilation and curettage, a procedure in which the endocervical epithelium is evaluated separately from the endometrial epithelium, and hysteroscopy, in which the endocervix and endometrium can be directly visualized to assist in diagnosis. Both procedures are performed simultaneously while the patient is under regional or general anesthesia. Occasionally, hysteroscopy can be performed in the office.

Dilation and curettage alone is adequate to diagnose endometrial cancer; however, hysteroscopy aids in identifying benign causes of bleeding, such as endometrial polyps or submucous uterine fibroids. Hysteroscopy is also useful for characterizing a cancer with respect to size and location.

Ultrasound and MRI

Transvaginal ultrasound (TVUS) with or without endometrial fluid instillation is the newest way to image the endometrial cavity. The advantages of ultrasound in evaluating a patient with vaginal bleeding are that it causes minimal discomfort to the patient and that additional uterine or adnexal pathology can be seen simultaneously. The major disadvantage of transvaginal ultrasound is that pathologic evaluation is not possible. TVUS cannot consistently differentiate between benign proliferation, hyperplasia, polyps, and cancer.

Studies have consistently found that postmenopausal patients with an endometrial stripe of less than 5 mm are rarely found to have an endometrial cancer [15]. Even so, it is our belief that pathologic evaluation of the endometrial cavity remains the primary and preferred method of evaluating vaginal bleeding. In certain circumstances when a patient either refuses an endometrial biopsy or is a poor medical candidate for surgical evaluation, ultrasound is invaluable as an alternative tool for endometrial cavity evaluation. In most circumstances, however, until studies further evaluate the role of ultrasound in the diagnosis of endometrial cancer, the additional expense of ultrasound is not warranted.

Sometimes, a radiologic scan is obtained for another indication, and an enlarged endometrial cavity is noted. Postmenopausal patients who are not taking hormone replacement and who have irregular endometrial cavities or endometrial stripes greater than 5 mm, require further evaluation, even in the absence of vaginal bleeding.

There is currently no role for CT or MRI in the initial evaluation of unexplained vaginal bleeding. However, a number of

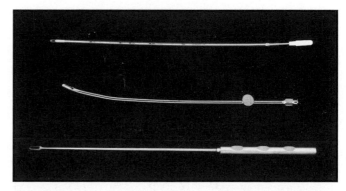

Figure 26-4. Uterine sampling devices. Top, Pipelle uterine aspirator. Middle, Novak uterine curet. Bottom, Duncan uterine curet.

recent reports have reviewed MRI in the staging of endometrial carcinoma [16,17]. Several reports have identified MRI as a promising imaging modality in the preoperative evaluation of endometrial cancer stage in an attempt to guide surgical management and postoperative therapy. The superior soft-tissue contrast resolution of MRI renders it superior to TVUS in the assessment of myometrial invasion [16]. The addition of dynamic contrast-enhanced MRI improves assessment of the premenopausal uterus, as well as suggesting the histology diagnosis of specific types of uterine cancer, namely the commonly misdiagnosed malignant mixed mesodermal tumor [17]. However, MRI is still unable to evaluate microscopic lymph node involvement, although enlargement may be readily seen. A promising modality that may aid in the identification of microscopic lymph node metastases is the use of lymph node-specific contrast agents [18].

ENDOMETRIAL HYPERPLASIA

In some cases, the endometrial biopsy confirms a diagnosis of endometrial hyperplasia. There are three categories of endometrial hyperplasia, each with a different clinical significance (Figure 26-5).

Cystic hyperplasia of the endometrium is a completely benign finding. In general, this reflects atrophy and inactivity of the endometrium. There is no increased malignant potential with cystic hyperplasia, and the condition can be treated with hormone replacement.

The remaining two categories of endometrial hyperplasia are separated based on glandular complexity and on the presence or absence of cytologic atypia. These two categories were proposed by the World Health Organization (WHO) in 1994 to decrease confusion in terminology. Endometrial hyperplasia without atypia is characterized by abnormal proliferation and crowding of the endometrial glands. Endometrial hyperplasia commonly arises in a background of proliferative endometrium reflecting estrogen stimulation and can be subdivided into those cases with simple or complex architecture based on the degree of gland crowding.

The malignant potential of endometrial hyperplasia without atypia is low. One study followed an untreated group of patients with endometrial hyperplasia for a mean of 13.4 years and found that only 1% to 3% developed endometrial cancer [19]. Therefore, these patients can be treated with progesterone cyclically (eg, medroxyprogesterone acetate [Depo-Provera], 10 to 20 mg/day orally for 14 days per month) or continuously (eg, megestrol acetate, 20 to 40 mg/day

orally, or medroxyprogesterone acetate, 200 mg/month intramuscularly). Hyperplasia resolves in most patients after 3 to 6 months of therapy, at which time periodic biopsies can confirm the disappearance of hyperplasia and subsequently monitor for recurrence. Patients at high risk of developing endometrial cancer benefit from long-term treatment with progesterone at least several times a year. Endometrial hyperplasia without atypia is not an indication for hysterectomy; however, high-risk patients, those failing treatment, and those who cannot tolerate progesterone therapy may be considered for definitive surgical therapy.

Endometrial hyperplasia with cellular atypia is a more ominous finding. Atypia refers to specific nuclear abnormalities, including large dark nuclei of variable sizes and shapes, prominent nucleoli, irregularly clumped chromatin, and increased nucleus-to-cytoplasm ratio. Atypical endometrial hyperplasia, or endometrial carcinoma in situ, is a premalignant lesion that requires careful attention. One fourth of patients in whom an outpatient biopsy reveals hyperplasia have associated endometrial carcinoma; therefore, further endometrial cavity evaluation is indicated. In these circumstances, dilation and curettage with a hysteroscopy is the appropriate next step in the evaluation. If endometrial hyperplasia with atypia is confirmed, the patient is an appropriate candidate for hysterectomy. Most patients with atypical hyperplasia will likely eventually progress to endometrial carcinoma without intervention. Current standard care for patients with endometrial hyperplasia with atypia is hysterectomy.

Young patients who desire future fertility are sometimes diagnosed with atypical hyperplasia. With the understanding that many of these cases progress to invasive cancer, most patients choose hysterectomy as their definitive treatment. Despite the risk of neoplasia, patients who have a strong desire for fertility may choose treatment with progestins and close monitoring with at least twice yearly endometrial sampling. If the atypical hyperplasia clears as documented on hysteroscopic evaluation, we suggest that these patients become pregnant sooner rather than later because the risk of progression to cancer may continue even with progesterone treatment. Often the hyperplasia is a result of anovulation; therefore these patients may benefit from an infertility consultation with a reproductive endocrinologist in an effort to achieve pregnancy. Once a patient with a history of atypical endometrial hyperplasia completes childbearing, it is recommended she proceed with a hysterectomy at that time or close monitoring with continued progestin suppression.

Recently, the WHO classification of endometrial hyperplasia has come under attack as not being reproducible nor easily adaptable to management options. A new classification of three categories, using endometrial hyperplasia, endometrial intraepithelial neoplasia (EIN), and adenocarcinoma has been proposed to further standardize these precancerous lesions and aid with the approach for optimal clinical management [20,21]. However, due to its recent inception, the subdivisions of EIN have yet to be delineated and appropriate, standard management options have yet to be defined.

Endometrial Hyperplasia

Type of Hyperplasia	Frequency of Malignancy, %
Cystic hyperplasia	1
Adenomatous hyperplasia	1–3
Atypical adenomatous hyperplasia	30

Figure 26-5. Endometrial hyperplasia type and frequency.

Endometrial Cancer

Pathology

Most endometrial cancers arise from the epithelial lining of the uterine cavity. The endometrium is a glandular structure and therefore gives rise to adenocarcinomas. The adenocarcinomas, termed endometrioid because they resemble normal endometrium, are assigned one of three grades based on the amount of cellular differentiation (Figure 26-6). Well-differentiated (grade 1) cancers can be difficult to distinguish histologically from endometrial hyperplasia with atypia but are distinguished by papillary and squamous cell differentiation, desmoplastic stroma, and "back-to-back" glandular formation without intervening stroma. The malignant potential and ultimate prognosis of endometrial cancers are determined in large part by the grade of the tumor. Grade 3 (poorly differentiated) lesions have the worst prognosis and are most likely to have associated metastatic disease when compared with grade 1 cancers. As would be predicted, grade 2 (moderately differentiated) lesions fall in between (Figure 26-7). Tumors associated with long-term unopposed estrogen stimulation are more frequently grade 1 lesions, whereas patients without clinical characteristics suggestive of elevated estrogen tend to have higher-grade lesions.

Certain, far less common histologic subtypes of endometrial cancer have a poorer prognosis when compared with others. Cancers demonstrating papillary serous and clear-cell histologic differentiation behave more like grade 3 endometrial lesions with a greater likelihood of metastasis and worse long-term prognosis. Tumors that have either benign or malignant squamous differentiation have a prognosis that is determined by the grade of the adenocarcinoma component and, contrary to earlier held beliefs, not by the squamous component. Endometrial cancers are also commonly screened for estrogen and progesterone receptors. These receptors are more likely to be present in lower-grade lesions and have been found to be independent predictors of survival [22].

Molecular Genetics

Endometrial cancers have been classified as type I and II. Type I consists of endometrioid histology, is due to unopposed estrogen, is preceded by malignant disease, and comprises 70% to 80% of newly diagnosed cases. Type II consists of nonendometrioid, papillary serous or clear cell typically, and is more aggressive. Most type II cancers have a mutation in the *p53* tumor suppressor, *Her-2/neu*, and *STK15* genes, whereas type I cancers may result from a number of genetic changes including microsatellite instability (MSI), *PTEN*, K-ras, and β-catenin mutations [23–25]. The use of microarrays has also exposed novel pathways like the downregulation of SOCS2, which suppresses the cytokine signaling family

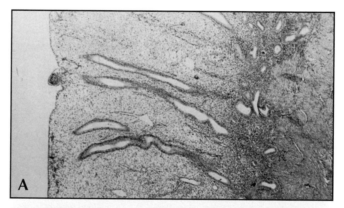

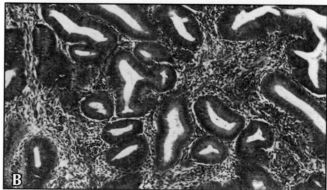

Figure 26-7. Endometrial histology. **A**, Normal endometrium. Early proliferative phase endometrium with straight, pencil-like glands in which mitoses are frequently conspicuous and abundant in the gland epithelium and stroma. **B**, Complex adenomatous hyperplasia without atypia. Crowded irregular glands with little intervening stroma. Glands may be "back to back" or bizarrely shaped. For the diagnosis of atypical hyperplasia, the nuclei should be enlarged, round (instead of oval), pleomorphic, and hyperchromatic with prominent nucleoli.

Continued on the next page

Endometrial Cancer: Histologic Types

Histology	Frequency, %
Endometrial adenocarcinoma	60
Adenocarcinoma with benign squamous differentiation	19
Adenocarcinoma with malignant squamous differentiation	7
Papillary serous	5
Clear cell	3
Secretory	2
Other	4
Mucinous	
Squamous carcinoma	
Undifferentiated carcinoma	
Metastatic	
Grade	
Well differentiated (grade 1)	29
Moderately differentiated (grade 2)	46
Poorly differentiated (grade 3)	25

Figure 26-6. Histologic types of endometrial cancer.

of proteins involved in the negative regulation of cytokine signal transduction [25]. Molecular studies are currently in their infancy but propose to be a boon to the diagnosis and treatment of endometrial cancers. In the future, tumors will be easily distinguished and treatment regimens will be tailor made on the basis of underlying genetic profiles.

PATTERNS OF SPREAD

Beginning in the epithelial lining of the uterus (endometrium), these malignancies initially grow within the endometrial cavity and can fill the space without invading the myometrium. Typically, however, the cancer invades locally into the myometrium and can eventually erode all the way through to the serosa. The cancer can also invade inferiorly by direct extension into the cervix and vagina. Superiorly, the cancer may invade the fallopian tube or ovary. As the tumor grows, it encounters lymphatic channels into which the malignant cells can be shed.

Two main uterine lymphatic drainage routes serve as channels for metastatic spread of endometrial cancer. First, malignant cells from the lower half of the uterus can travel along lymphatic channels, draining the cervix. Cancer may then be found in the obturator, hypogastric, and external iliac lymph node chains. A second route of lymphatic drainage arises from the rich network of lymphatics in the uterine fundus. From

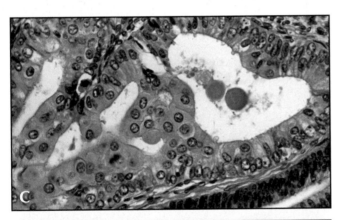

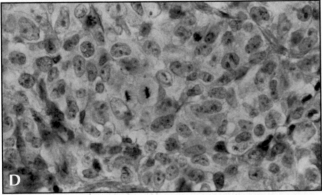

Figure 26-7. *(Continued)* **C**, Well differentiated (grade 1) endometrial adenocarcinoma. Crowded, easily recognizable glands without intervening stroma. **D**, Poorly differentiated (grade 3) endometrial adenocarcinoma. Glands are not recognizable in most of the tumor. Sheets of undifferentiated and abundantly mitotic cells with pleomorphic nuclei predominate. (*From* Stanley J. Robboy, MD and Gyn-Path Associates, Durham, NC.)

this area of the uterus, malignant cells can travel along the ovarian vessels to the aortic and vena caval lymphatic chains. Occasionally, metastatic implants can be found in the peritoneal cavity, lower vagina, vulva, liver, lungs, or brain. Ascites, malignant peritoneal washings, and pleural effusions also represent metastatic disease. The most common site for hematogenous spread is the lung, followed by the liver, brain, and bone (the least common site for spread).

STAGING

The purposes of staging endometrial cancer are to identify the primary location of the malignancy and to evaluate as many sites as possible for the presence of metastatic disease. Staging in endometrial cancer helps not only to give patients a reasonable idea of prognosis but also to direct therapy. Until 1988, clinical staging was used to identify the size of the primary tumor and the location of metastatic disease without surgery (Figure 26-8). Clinical staging is useful for patients who are not candidates for surgical intervention because of poor medical health; however, many studies comparing clinical and surgical staging have found that metastatic sites are frequently missed with clinical staging.

In 1988, the International Federation of Gynecology and Obstetrics (FIGO) adopted a surgical staging system to identify more accurately sites of metastatic spread. This method takes into account the depth of myometrial invasion; cervical, adnexal, and lymphatic spread; vaginal extension; malignant peritoneal cytology; distant spread; and tumor grade. In a study comparing clinical and surgical staging, nearly half of endometrial cancer patients had their clinical stage changed when surgical criteria were applied [26]. The most important factor affecting prognosis in endometrial cancer patients is surgical stage. Therefore, with accurate staging, therapies can be tailored to specific patients, resulting in longer survival times and minimization of unnecessary and potentially harmful additional treatments.

Appropriate staging consists of pelvic washings, bilateral pelvic and para-aortic lymphadenectomy, and complete resection of all disease. Per the recent American College of Gynecology (ACOG) practice bulletin, exceptions to the need for surgical staging include young or perimenopausal women with grade I endometrioid adenocarcinoma associated with atypical endometrial hyperplasia and women at increased risk of mortality secondary to comorbidities [27].

Treatment

PRIMARY SURGICAL THERAPY

Endometrial cancer is primarily a surgically treated disease. In most cases, the cancer is confined to the uterus; therefore, surgical therapy serves as both a diagnostic and therapeutic intervention. Many patients diagnosed with endometrial cancer have significant medical comorbidities, including obesity, hypertension, and diabetes. Even so, more than 90% of these patients can safely undergo an operation. Because of the significant risk of complications related to the frequency of associated medical problems, patients should have a thorough preoperative evaluation before surgery. However, per ACOG practice bulletin recommendations, "only a physical examination and a chest radiograph are required for preoperative staging of the usual clinical stage I patient. All other preoperative testing should be directed toward optimizing the surgical outcome" [27].

A preoperative complete history and physical examination should be undertaken in all patients by the surgical team. Appropriate consultations should be obtained when complicated medical conditions are encountered so that the preoperative performance status can be maximized and potential postoperative complications anticipated and avoided. Abnormal symptoms and findings, such as abdominal pain, bladder discomfort, hematuria, occult fecal blood, and shortness of breath, should be investigated.

A chest radiograph, electrocardiogram, complete blood count, liver chemistries, renal chemistries, and urinalysis are adequate preoperative laboratory investigations for most patients. The serum CA 125 level, a serum marker for ovarian cancer, is commonly elevated in advanced endometrial cancer but is rarely elevated in early endometrial cancer. The CA 125 level may serve as a marker to follow during treatment but is generally not a standard preoperative test in endometrial cancer. Cystoscopy, sigmoidoscopy, upper gastrointestinal series, barium enema, CT scan, MRI scan, ultrasound, and intravenous pyelography are rarely helpful unless patient complaints or findings suggestive of more advanced disease indicate the need for a specifically focused investigation. As described previously, some investigators have reported the ability to evaluate myometrial invasion preoperatively with ultrasound or MRI. Although interesting, these studies do little to change current patient management and simply add to costs. We do not routinely order these studies and prefer to evaluate myometrial invasion at the time of surgery when frozen section can guide us in our decision to proceed with more extensive surgical staging.

Preoperatively, patients are given prophylactic antibiotics, usually cephazolin, 1 g intravenously, to reduce the rate of postoperative infection. In addition, endometrial cancer patients are at increased risk of developing deep vein thrombosis because of increased age or obesity and are routinely given compression boots or low-dose heparin as prophylaxis. Deep venous thromboembolism of the lower extremity leading

Clinical and Surgical Staging of Endometrial Cancer

FIGO Clinical Staging of Endometrial Carcinoma (1971)

Stage I	Carcinoma is confined to the corpus
IA	Length of the uterine cavity is 8 cm or less
IB	Length of the uterine cavity is more than 8 cm
	Stage I cases should be subgrouped with regard to the histologic type of adenocarcinoma as follows:
G1	Highly differentiated adenomatous carcinoma
G2	Differentiated adenomatous carcinoma with partly solid areas
G3	Predominantly solid or entirely undifferentiated carcinoma
Stage II	Carcinoma involves the corpus and cervix
Stage III	Carcinoma extends outside the corpus but not outside the true pelvis (it may involve the vaginal wall or parametrium but not the bladder or rectum)
Stage IV	Carcinoma involves the bladder or rectum or extends outside the pelvis

FIGO Surgical Staging of Endometrial Carcinoma (1988)

Stage IA G123	Tumor limited to endometrium
IB G123	Invasion to less than half of the myometrium
IC G123	Invasion to more than half of the myometrium
Stage IIA G123	Endocervical glandular involvement only
IIB G123	Cervical stromal invasion
Stage IIIA G123	Tumor invading serosa, adnexa, or both; and/or positive peritoneal cytology
IIIB G123	Vaginal metastases
IIIC G123	Metastases to pelvic and/or para-aortic lymph nodes
Stage IVA G123	Tumor invades bladder, bowel, mucosa, or both
IVB G123	Distant metastases, including intra-abdominal and/or inguinal lymph node

Figure 26-8. Clinical and surgical staging of endometrial cancer. Rules related to staging include the following: 1) Because corpus cancer is now surgically staged, procedures previously used for differentiation of stages are no longer applicable, for example, the findings of dilation and curettage to differentiate between stage I and stage II. It is appreciated that there may be a small number of patients with corpus cancer who are treated primarily with radiation therapy. If that is the case, the clinical staging adopted by the International Federation of Gynecology and Obstetrics (FIGO) in 1971 would still apply, but use of that staging system would be noted. 2) Ideally, the width of the myometrium is measured along with the width of tumor invasion.

to pulmonary embolus is the most common cause of immediate postoperative death after surgery for endometrial cancer.

Most patients who undergo surgery for endometrial cancer are explored through a midline abdominal incision to allow for adequate surgical exposure and a complete abdominal survey, although some studies have documented excellent surgical evaluation and treatment via a Pfannenstiel incision. Vaginal hysterectomy with preservation of the ovaries if desired is acceptable for patients found to have atypical endometrial hyperplasia at hysteroscopy. In cases in which abdominal surgery would be associated with excessive morbidity, vaginal hysterectomy may be considered for the treatment of cancer. If vaginal hysterectomy is contemplated for endometrial cancer, it is usually performed with laparoscopic assistance. Laparascopically assisted vaginal hysterectomy (LAVH) permits a reasonable abdominal survey and vaginal removal of the uterus, cervix, fallopian tubes, ovaries, and in some cases, lymph nodes. With LAVH, the uterus can be removed vaginally; if a higher-grade lesion or deep myometrial invasion is found, surgical staging can proceed either laparoscopically or with an open incision. Endometrial cancer patients staged with LAVH have a shorter postoperative hospital stay and more rapid recovery.

In the past, safe laparoscopic surgery tended to be more difficult to perform in these often obese patients, and it was believed that these patients would be commonly served better by an open procedure. Recent reports have indicated that laparoscopic surgery and staging is a viable option when performed by experienced operators, and proper patient selection can minimize complication rates [28–30]. Definitive recommendations are pending following analysis of the Gynecologic Oncology Group (GOG)-LAP2 trial examining laparoscopic surgery versus laparotomy in patients with early-stage endometrial cancer. Furthermore, the common concern of port-site metastases appears to be noncontributory in the decision to

perform laparoscopy as surgical site metastases were seen in 0% to 0.97% of patients with malignant disease [28,30].

All patients who undergo surgical exploration for endometrial carcinoma should initially have peritoneal washings obtained to look for malignant cells. Malignant peritoneal cytology is found in 15% of patients otherwise thought to have early-stage disease. Patients then undergo an extensive abdominal survey to look for gross metastatic disease. If suspicious areas are found beyond the uterus and adnexa, samples are sent to pathology for frozen-section evaluation. It is vital in the modern era of endometrial cancer treatment to have good frozen-section availability to assist in the algorithm of current surgical management. Therapy decisions are frequently made at the time of operation when the histologic grade of the tumor and extent of disease can be rapidly and accurately assessed.

After abdominal exploration, all patients undergo extrafascial hysterectomy and bilateral salpingo-oophorectomy. The adnexa and cervix are always removed because they are frequent sites of occult metastatic disease (7% and 8%, respectively). The uterine cavity is examined intraoperatively for the location and size of the tumor as well as depth of invasion. Frozen-section histology is often obtained at this juncture to evaluate for grade and histologic cell type.

Many small endometrial adenocarcinomas with associated atypical endometrial hyperplasia are well differentiated and confined to the inner half of the endometrial cavity. The risk of lymph node metastasis in this group of patients is less than 5% [31]. Most of these patients have an excellent prognosis, and increased morbidity incurred by further surgical staging is not indicated. The remainder of the endometrial cancer patients are considered at higher risk for metastatic disease and deserve thorough surgical staging, including obturator, external iliac, common iliac, para-aortic, and paracaval lymph node sampling (Figure 26-9). As many as 25% of patients with deep myometrial invasion, large tumors filling the uterine cavity, cervical or adnexal involvement, grade 3 lesions, deeply invasive grade 2 lesions, or papillary, serous, or clear-cell histology have lymph node metastasis. Two of these factors can increase the risk of nodal metastasis to as high as 50%. Other high-risk features of endometrial cancers include nondiploid DNA content, overexpression of the *Her-2/Neu* gene, *p53* mutations, lymph-vascular space involvement, and lack of progesterone and estrogen receptors. For all high-risk patients medically fit to undergo surgery, pelvic and para-aortic lymph node sampling, liberal biopsy sampling of suspicious areas, and omental sampling complete surgical staging.

There has been great discord as to whether surgical staging should be performed in all patients, regardless of disease grade. Proponents for surgical staging have reported that lymphadenectomy, in endometrial cancer patients, is not only diagnostic but also therapeutic and correlated with improved survival [32]. However, opponents to surgical staging, except for grade 3 or above, have reported no improved survival rates in those surgically staged with lymph node dissection versus those patients treated empirically following their surgery with adjuvant radiotherapy [33]. After review of all the data, a committee opinion prepared by ACOG advises that most patients with endometrial

High-risk Features of Endometrial Cancer

Poor Prognostic Features

Poorly differentiated (grade 3) disease

Less than 50% myometrial invasion

Papillary serous histology

Clear-cell histology

Cervical involvement

Lymph-vascular space involvement

Adnexal involvement

Tumor > 2 cm in diameter

Negative estrogen progesterone receptors

Lymph node or distant metastatic disease

Nondiploid tumors

Her-2/Neu and *p53* gene mutations

Figure 26-9. High-risk features of endometrial cancer.

cancer undergo complete lymph node evaluation unless young or perimenopausal with grade 1 endometrioid adenocarcinomas associated with atypical hyperplasia and women at increased risk of mortality secondary to comorbidities.

Primary Radiation Therapy

Patients with early endometrial cancer as determined by clinical staging who are not surgical candidates may be treated with moderate success using radiation therapy alone. External-beam radiotherapy and internal radiotherapy (brachytherapy) must be given to achieve maximal tumor control. External radiotherapy is delivered to the entire pelvis, covering the uterus, adnexa, and pelvic lymph nodes, to a dose of 4500 to 5000 cGy. Brachytherapy involves the delivery of radiation directly to the endometrial cavity. The patient is taken to the operating room and given light general or regional anesthesia. Radiation holding devices (Heyman capsules or a Fletcher-Suit tandem and ovoids) are placed directly into the uterine cavity; when the patient returns to her hospital room, the capsules are loaded with cesium or radium for a 48- to 72-hour period.

Directed therapy is difficult with radiation therapy and in 10% to 15% of cases, uterine cancer is not eradicated [27]. Inoperable patients with clinical stage 1 or 2 disease treated with radiotherapy alone have a 5-year survival rate of 60% to 85% compared to 98% 5-year survival rate in stage 1 operable patients. Although the survival rate is higher in those healthier patients who are treated with surgery, these medically complex patients treated with radiation alone would likely have significant operative morbidity and therefore may well have a better overall survival with radiation therapy. Radiation therapy is not without its own significant potential side effects. Patients can develop bowel obstructions or bowel and bladder fistulas even 10 years after treatment. Therefore, due to the lower survival rates and radiation-associated morbidities, each woman should be evaluated carefully before she is denied the benefits of surgery.

Rarely, patients with early endometrial cancer are candidates for neither surgery nor radiation therapy or wish to maintain their fertility. Some gynecologic oncologists have reported moderate success using high-dose progesterone therapy alone. However, continued histologic monitoring is imperative, since recurrence may occur in up to 50% of patients.

Adjuvant Radiation Treatment

Survival rates of patients diagnosed with endometrial cancer and surgically staged are presented in Figure 26-10. As can be seen, most patients with early disease can expect to be cured of their cancer with surgery alone, and adjuvant treatment is not advised. For patients with disease that is more than stage I and grade 1, efforts have been made to find additional therapies that could improve overall survival. Given the reasonable results seen in patients treated with radiation alone, radiotherapy has traditionally been the adjuvant treatment of choice in patients with more advanced stage disease.

Patients with high-risk features as determined by surgical staging and histologic review with no evidence of systemic disease have been given adjuvant external-beam pelvic radiotherapy and brachytherapy to the vaginal cuff. It is clear that radiation given to this group of patients reduces significantly the risk of locally recurrent disease. What remains less clear is the benefit to overall survival. Two prospective randomized trials, the Postoperative Radiation Therapy in Endometrial Cancer (PORTEC) trial and the Gynecologic Oncology Group (GOG #99) trial, could find no survival advantage with adjuvant radiation in patients with stage IB, IC, IIA, or IIB disease [34,35]. Retrospective studies in clinically staged patients have reported conflicting results in high-risk patients, with some studies suggesting a significant survival advantage with adjuvant radiotherapy.

Patients found to have malignant peritoneal cytology with disease otherwise confined to the uterus (stage IIIc) are commonly treated with whole abdominal irradiation to 3000 cGy or intraperitoneal radioactive phosphorus (phosphorus 32). No randomized study has been published to confirm a survival advantage in stage IIIa patients treated with these adjuvant modalities.

Patients who have endometrial cancer and nodal metastases have traditionally been treated with external-beam radiotherapy to the involved lymph node groups. A comparison of treatment and no treatment has not been undertaken in this group of stage IIIc patients; however, most gynecologic oncologists would recommend adjuvant radiation therapy. As is the case with most patients treated with adjuvant radiation, local control is excellent, but disease usually recurs outside the radiation field. A combination of surgery and radiation can be individualized to treat locally advanced disease. Rarely, patients are treated with radiotherapy before surgery. Patients with distant disease at diagnosis can achieve good local control with surgery and abdominal irradiation but must rely on systemic therapy to treat the remaining metastatic disease.

In deciding whether or not to administer radiation therapy, other poor prognostic factors should be considered, including the patient's age, advanced grade, and presence of more than 50% myometrial invasion. If these factors are present,

Endometrial Cancer Rates: Survival

Five-year Survival Rates in Surgically Staged Patients, %

Surgical Stage	Grade 1	Grade 2	Grade 3
IA	96	91	83
IB	95	89	82
IC	90	85	73
IIA	90	81	60
IIB	77	79	55
IIIA	72	—	59
IIIC	59	42	42
IV	35	28	18

Figure 26-10. Endometrial cancer survival rates.

radiation therapy has not been shown to offer a long-term survival advantage [35–37].

Adjuvant Chemotherapy and Hormone Therapy

Adjuvant chemotherapy for advanced endometrial cancer can be delivered after radiation therapy and surgery, especially in the setting of recurrence, in the form of cytotoxic agents. Doxorubicin (Adriamycin, Pharmacia & Upjohn, Kalamazoo, MI), cisplatin, and paclitaxel (Taxol, Bristol-Myers Squibb, New York, NY) are the most active cytotoxic chemotherapeutic agents for endometrial cancer. In a Cochrane review of chemotherapy for endometrial cancer, it was clear that cisplatin, carboplatin, doxorubicin, and taxanes were effective against advanced, metastatic, or recurrent cancer [38]. However, it was unclear which patients would benefit from this regimen, and the authors also pointed out the uncertainty of whether this regimen improved quality of life. Furthermore, the associated side effects were significant and included thrombocytopenia and neurologic toxicity. A recently published randomized trial revealed the superiority of the combination of doxorubicin, cisplatin, and paclitaxel for advanced and recurrent endometrial cancer [39]. Furthermore, GOG protocol 122 recently supported the use of doxorubicin plus cisplatin with paclitaxel over the use of whole abdominal radiation therapy for advanced endometrial cancer [40]. The GOG has examined combination treatment with radiation and chemotherapy in patients with advanced endometrial cancer. Although final results are pending, it would appear that the combination of chemotherapy and radiation in advanced endometrial cancer is superior to either treatment alone. GOG 209 is currently examining whether the addition of doxorubicin, cisplatin, and paclitaxel is superior to paclitaxel and carboplatin regarding survival in advanced and recurrent endometrial cancer.

Hormonal therapy in the form of medroxyprogesterone acetate (MPA), megestrol acetate, and tamoxifen has been evaluated in phase II trials and found to have some activity, particularly in patients with positive estrogen and progesterone receptors. It appears that low-dose MPA had a lower risk of death and marginally improved response compared with high-dose MPA [41].

Follow-up and Treatment of Recurrent Disease

With modern multimodal therapeutic management of endometrial cancer, more than 80% of patients are cured. Of those patients who fail first-line therapy, more than three fourths have recurrent disease within 2 years. The median time to recurrence being detected was 14 months for recurrence in the vagina and 19 months for recurrence distally [27]. Therefore, patients should be encouraged to follow-up at any sign of weight loss, pain, or vaginal bleeding, which may signify recurrence. Close surveillance of these patients is required, including a complete physical examination with rectovaginal examination, Papanicolaou smear, and chest radiograph (in selected high-risk patients) three or four times per year for the first 3 years. Although no increase in survival is seen in symptomatic versus asymptomatic occurrences between visits, there may be a psychological advantage for the patient who is periodically reassured she does not have recurrent disease [42].

The location of recurrent disease depends on the initial treatment as well as the cancer histology. In general, patients who were treated with radiation are less likely to have pelvic and vaginal recurrences and more likely to develop lung, abdomen, liver, brain, and distant lymph node disease. Patients with early grade 1 cancers tend not to be treated with radiation and develop recurrences after a longer interval at the vaginal apex. More than half of the cases of recurrent central pelvic disease with grade 1 histology can be salvaged with radiation therapy and surgical excision.

Therapies for recurrent disease include surgery, chemotherapy, hormonal therapy, and radiation therapy. Treatment of recurrent disease must be individualized and take into account cancer histology, recurrence sites, previous therapy, and patient performance status. Progesterone agents are generally considered first-line treatment for distant metastatic disease, and some patients can have a complete and sustained response. Overall, about 10% of patients live more than 3 years after treatment of recurrent disease.

Hormone Replacement After Treatment of Endometrial Cancer

Hormone replacement in the form of estrogen is a matter of significant controversy for patients diagnosed with endometrial cancer. The benefits of estrogen are well documented and include osteoporosis prevention, decrease in the incidence of colon cancer, and symptomatic relief of hot flashes. Endometrial cancer is frequently thought to be caused by overstimulation of the endometrium by estrogen. The concern, then, is whether replacement estrogen can stimulate residual cancer cells to grow.

There is no evidence that estrogen replacement therapy after treatment of endometrial cancer increases the risk of recurrence [43]. GOG #137A randomized prospective trial was designed to compare estrogen to placebo in women with stage I or II endometrial cancer. However, it was closed prematurely after the results of the World Health Organization were published. Due to this premature closure, it was unable to repudiate or support the use of estrogen. Nevertheless, they did note that the rate of recurrence in the low-risk population was 2.1% [44]. In the ACOG committee opinion on HRT in women treated for endometrial cancer they state: "At this time, the decision to use HRT in these women should be individualized on the basis of potential benefit and risk to the patient" [45].

If patients with endometrial cancer are offered estrogen replacement therapy, informed consent should be obtained. Patients treated for more advanced cancer may wish to wait

2 years before initiating estrogen replacement. In the meantime, symptomatic relief may be achieved with MPA, 10 mg/d, Depo-Provera, 150 mg intramuscularly every 3 months, Bellergal (belladonna extract, phenobarbital, and ergotamine tartrate), or clonidine. Patients may report symptomatic relief with various herbal agents, many of which contain estrogen-like compounds that are as a group called phytoestrogens. Their safety has not been established.

Uterine Sarcomas

Uterine sarcomas constitute 2% to 6% of all uterine cancers and are categorized as mixed mullerian tumors (MMT), leiomyosarcomas (LMS), and endometrial stromal sarcomas (ESS). Most uterine sarcomas are either MMT or LMS. Patients usually present in the postmenopausal years with symptoms of vaginal bleeding, increasing pelvic pressure, or an enlarging pelvic mass. Occasionally, younger patients are diagnosed with a leiomyosarcoma at the time of hysterectomy for presumed benign disease. Diagnosis may be difficult in these patients because endometrial biopsy and even dilation and curettage are commonly nondiagnostic. Uterine sarcomas are clinically and surgically staged similar to endometrial cancers.

Histologically, uterine sarcomas may be composed of a single cell type (pure sarcomas) or more than one cell type (mixed sarcomas). Mixed cell types can have elements normally found only in the uterus (homologous), whereas others have cell types typically not found in the uterus (heterologous). Leiomyosarcoma and endometrial stromal sarcoma are the most common pure uterine sarcomas. MMT uterine malignancies are mixed sarcomas often with heterologous malignant sarcomatous elements like rhabdomyosarcoma and chondrosarcoma. The malignant potential of leiomyosarcomas is directly related to the number of mitotic figures and anaplasia seen histologically. More than 10 mitotic figures per 10 high-power fields denotes a poor prognosis, even for stage I disease. One reason for the poor prognosis seen in sarcomas is that they tend to have a much higher propensity for hematogenous spread earlier in the disease process. Metastatic disease is commonly encountered in lung, liver, and bone, contributing to the generally poor prognosis for all uterine sarcomas.

Treatment of uterine sarcomas begins with abdominal hysterectomy and bilateral salpingo-oophorectomy. Endometrial cancers and uterine sarcomas are staged similarly with surgery. Half of patients in whom malignancy is confined to the uterus die of recurrent disease, as do most patients who have extrauterine disease. Radiation therapy has been effective in controlling local recurrences but does not affect survival. Several trials have evaluated chemotherapy in the treatment of uterine sarcomas. Ifosfamide, platinum, and doxorubicin appear to have the most activity in uterine sarcomas; however, the responses are generally short-lived. Studies evaluating paclitaxel, topotecan, multiagent chemotherapy, and chemotherapy plus radiation therapy for the treatment of uterine sarcomas showed minimal improvement.

Preservation of Fertility

Although endometrial cancer is predominantly a cancer of postmenopausal women, 8% to 14% of endometrial malignancies will occur at less than 45 years of age [46,47]. Risk factors as outlined previously include prolonged use of unconjugated estrogens, excess estrogen production as in polycystic ovarian syndrome, obesity, and an elevated body mass index. Many young women will present with abnormal vaginal bleeding, and it is important to maintain suspicion for endometrial cancer to prevent a delay in diagnosis, especially in women with known risk factors. Conservative management is an option for the highly motivated woman after thorough evaluation and detailed counseling has been done. Definitive treatment requires a hysterectomy.

For women with precancerous lesions or hyperplasia, hysteroscopy and dilation and curettage are recommended to avoid missing any foci of endometrial cancer. These lesions have a favorable prognosis and may regress with progesterone treatment. Megestrol 10 mg two to four times per day, daily for 3 to 12 months, may be used, with regression rates of 94% [47]. The patient should be encouraged to become pregnant as soon as possible and on completion of her child-bearing, the patient should then be encouraged to have her hysterectomy.

Women with invasive disease pose a problem. For the woman that desires to maintain her fertility, again, a progestational agent may be used and only for grade I endometrioid adenocarcinomas after careful evaluation has been performed. This includes a pelvic examination, Papanicolaou smear, dilation and curettage, abdominal-pelvic CT, pelvic MRI, CA 125, and pelvic exploration with laparoscopy. Close follow-up with ultrasound, hysteroscopy, and endometrial curettage every 3 to 6 months should ensue. Conception may be attempted after documented regression of malignancy.

The patient must be counseled carefully and in great detail with all risks explained and with the understanding of the potential serious consequences that may ensue following a delay in treatment. The patient should be made aware of the possibility of understaging, failure of progestin therapy, progression of the malignancy, initial response to progestin followed by recurrence or metastases, and the presence of synchronous ovarian tumors [46]. The patient also should be counseled on fertility options, including the use of ovarian stimulation, with the intent of completing child-bearing as rapidly as possible. Ovarian stimulation has not been reported to increase the risk of endometrial cancer [46]. Finally, the patient should be informed of the need for postpartum treatment and on completion of child-bearing, definitive treatment with a hysterectomy.

Unlike endometrial adenocarcinomas, uterine sarcomas are more aggressive. There have been reports of "conservative" management with a myomectomy, and only one recurrence was seen that resulted in the patient's death [47]. Nevertheless, if this option is to be employed, the patient should have her hysterectomy on completion of child-bearing.

Recently, assessment of patients who are most likely to respond to progestational agents has revealed an association with 17 β-hydroxysteroid dehydrogenase type 2 and progesterone receptors [48]. Elucidation and expansion on these findings may allow us to select those patients most likely to respond to hormonal treatment without the risk of delaying for several months and potential progression of the malignancy.

References

1. Ahmedin JD, Siegel R, Ward E, et al.: Cancer Statistics, 2007. CA Cancer J Clin 2007, 57:43–66.

2. Grady D, Gebretsadik T, Kerlikowske K, et al.: Hormone replacement therapy and endometrial cancer risk: a meta-analysis. Obstet Gynecol 1995, 85:304–313.

3. Meirow D, Schenker JG: The link between female infertility and cancer: epidemiology and possible aetiologies. Hum Reprod Update 1996, 2:63–75.

4. Giudice LC: Endometrium in PCOS: Implantation and predisposition to endocrine CA. Best Pract Res Clin Endocrinol Metab 2006, 20:235–244.

5. Madison T, Schottenfeld D, James SA, et al.: Endometrial cancer: socioeconomic status and racial/ethnic differences in stage at diagnosis, treatment, and survival. Am J Public Health 2004, 94:2104–2111.

6. Persson I, Adami HO, Bergkvist L, et al.: Risk of endometrial cancer after treatment with oestrogens alone or in conjunction with progestogens: results of a prospective study. BMJ 1989, 298:147–151.

7. Tamoxifen and Uterine Cancer. ACOG Compendium 2006, 336(ACOG Committee Opinion).

8. Delmas PD, Bjarnason NH, Mitlak BH, et al.: Effects of raloxifene on bone mineral density, serum cholesterol concentrations, and uterine endometrium in postmenopausal women. N Engl J Med 1997, 337:1641–1647.

9. Vogel VG CJ, Wickerham DL, Cronin WM, et al.: National Surgical Adjuvant Breast and Bowel Project (NSABP). Effects of tamoxifen vs raloxifene on the risk of developing invasive breast cancer and other disease outcomes: the NSABP Study of Tamoxifen and Raloxifene (STAR) P–2 trial. JAMA 2006, 295:2727–2741.

10. Lindor NM, Petersen GM, Hadley DW, et al.: Recommendations for the care of individuals with an inherited predisposition to Lynch syndrome: a systematic review. JAMA 2006, 296:1507–1517.

11. Hampel H, Frankel W, Panescu J, et al.: Screening for Lynch syndrome (hereditary nonpolyposis colorectal cancer) among endometrial cancer patients. Cancer Res 2006, 66:7810–7817.

12. Averette HE, Steren A, Nguyen HN: Screening in gynecologic cancers. Cancer 1993, 72:1043–1049.

13. Grimes DA, Economy KE: Primary prevention of gynecologic cancers. Am J Obstet Gynecol 1995, 172:227–235.

14. Chambers JT, Chambers SK: Endometrial sampling: When? Where? Why? With what? Clin Obstetr Gynecol 1992, 35:28–39.

15. Varner RE, Sparks JM, Cameron CD, et al.: Transvaginal sonography of the endometrium in postmenopausal women. Obstet Gynecol 1991, 78:195–199.

16. Barwick TD, Rockall AG, Barton DP, et al.: Imaging of endometrial adenocarcinoma. Clin Radiol 2006, 61:545–555.

17. Messiou C, Spencer JA, Swift SE: MR staging of endometrial carcinoma. Clin Radiol 2006, 61:822–832.

18. Rockall AG SS, Harisinghani MG, Babar SA, et al.: Diagnostic performance of nanoparticle-enhanced magnetic resonance imaging in the diagnosis of lymph node metastases in patients with endometrial and cervical cancer. J Clin Oncol 2005, 23:2813–2821.

19. Kurman RJ, Kaminski PF, Norris HJ: The behavior of endometrial hyperplasia: a long–term study of "untreated" hyperplasia in 170 patients. Cancer 1985, 56:403–412.

20. Baak JP, Mutter GL: EIN and WHO94. J Clin Pathol 2005, 58:1–6.

21. Mutter GL: Endometrial intraepithelial neoplasia (EIN): will it bring order to chaos? Gynecol Oncol 2000, 76:287–290.

22. Gassel AM, Backe J, Krebs S, et al.: Endometrial carcinoma: immunohistochemically detected proliferation index is a prognosticator of long–term outcome. J Clin Pathol 1998, 51:25–29.

23. Hecht JL, Mutter GL: Molecular and pathologic aspects of endometrial carcinogenesis. J Clin Oncol 2006, 24:4783–4791.

24. Pappa KI, Anagnou NP: Emerging issues of the expression profiling technologies for the study of gynecologic cancer. Am J Obstet Gynecol 2005, 193:908–918.

25. Sherwin R, Catalano R, Sharkey A: Large–scale gene expression studies of the endometrium: what have we learnt? Reproduction 2006, 132:1–10.

26. Cowles TA, Magrina JF, Masterson BJ, Capen CV: Comparison of clinical and surgical staging in patients with endometrial carcinoma. Obstet Gynecol 1985, 66:413–416.

27. Management of Endometrial Cancer. ACOG Compendium 2005, 65:1–13.

28. Chi DS, Abu–Rustum NR, Sonoda Y, et al.: Ten-year experience with laparoscopy on a gynecologic oncology service: analysis of risk factors for complications and conversion to laparotomy. Am J Obstet Gynecol 2004, 191:1138–1145.

29. Barakat RR, Lev G, Hummer AJ, et al.: Twelve-year experience in the management of endometrial cancer: A change in surgical and postoperative radiation approaches. Gynecol Oncol 2007, 105:150–156.

30. Schlaerth AC, Abu-Rustum NR: Role of minimally invasive surgery in gynecologic cancers. Oncologist 2006, 11:895–901.

31. Creasman WT, Morrow CP, Bundy BN, et al.: Surgical pathologic spread patterns of endometrial cancer. A Gynecologic Oncology Group Study. Cancer 1987, 60(Suppl):2035–2041.

32. Kilgore LC, Partridge EE, Alvarez RD, et al.: Adenocarcinoma of the endometrium: survival comparisons of patients with and without pelvic node sampling. Gynecol Oncol 1995, 56:29–33.

33. Aalders JG, Thomas G: Endometrial cancer: revisiting the importance of pelvic and para aortic lymph nodes. Gynecol Oncol 2007, 104:222–231.

34. Creutzberg CL, van Putten WL, Koper PC, et al.: Surgery and postoperative radiotherapy versus surgery alone for patients with stage-1 endometrial carcinoma: multicentre randomised trial. PORTEC Study Group. Post-operative Radiation Therapy in Endometrial Carcinoma. Lancet 2000, 355:1404–1411.

35. Alektiar KM: When and how should adjuvant radiation be used in early endometrial cancer? Semin Radiat Oncol 2006, 16:158–163.

36. Jolly S, Vargas CE, Kumar T, et al.: The impact of age on long-term outcome in patients with endometrial cancer treated with postoperative radiation. Gynecol Oncol 2006, 103:87–93.

37. Macdonald OK, Sause WT, Lee RJ, *et al.*: Adjuvant radiotherapy and survival outcomes in early-stage endometrial cancer: a multi-institutional analysis of 608 women. *Gynecol Oncol* 2006, 103:661–666.

38. Humber C, Tierney J, Symonds P, *et al.*: Chemotherapy for advanced, recurrent or metastatic endometrial carcinoma. *Cochrane Database Syst Rev* 2005, 4:CD003915.

39. Fleming GF, Brunetto VL, Cella D, *et al.:* Phase III trial of doxorubicin plus cisplatin with or without paclitaxel plus filgrastim in advanced endometrial carcinoma: a Gynecologic Oncology Group study. *J Clin Oncol* 2004, 22:2159–2166.

40. Randall M, Filiaci V, Muss H, *et al.*: Randomized phase III trial of whole-abdominal irradiation versus doxorubicin and cisplatin chemotherapy in advanced endometrial carcinoma: a Gynecologic Oncology Group study. *J Clin Oncol* 2006, 24: 36–44.

41. Carey MS, Gawlik C, Fung-Kee-Fung M, *et al.*: Systematic review of systemic therapy for advanced or recurrent endometrial cancer. *Gynecol Oncol* 2006, 101:158–167.

42. Amant F, Moerman P, Neven P, *et al.*: Endometrial cancer. *Lancet* 2005, 366:491–505.

43. Creasman WT, Henderson D, Hinshaw W, *et al.*: Estrogen replacement therapy in the patient treated for endometrial cancer. *Obstet Gynecol* 1986, 67:326–330.

44. Barakat RR, Bundy BN, Spirtos NM, *et al.*: Randomized double-blind trial of estrogen replacement therapy versus placebo in stage I or II endometrial cancer: a Gynecologic Oncology Group Study. *J Clin Oncol* 2006, 24:587–592.

45. ACOG committee opinion. Hormone replacement therapy in women treated for endometrial cancer. Number 234, May 2000 (replaces number 126, August 1993). *Int J Gynaecol Obstet* 2001;73:283–284.

46. Rackow BW, Arici A: Endometrial cancer and fertility. *Curr Opin Obstet Gynecol* 2006, 18:245–252.

47. Maltaris T, Boehm D, Dittrich R, *et al.*: Reproduction beyond cancer: a message of hope for young women. *Gynecol Oncol* 2006, 103:1109–1121.

48. Farthing A: Conserving fertility in the management of gynaecological cancers. *BJOG* 2006, 113:129–134.

27 | Ovarian Cancer

Todd D. Tillmanns

- Ovarian cancer is the fifth most common cause of cancer related mortality in women in the United States.
- Overall it is the second most common cause of gynecologic malignancy, but the number one cause of gynecologic cancer–related death [1].
- One in 70 women will develop ovarian cancer, and one in 100 will die of ovarian cancer in the United States.
- Ovarian cancer is most often derived from epithelial origins in 90% of the cases, although it also may arise from sex cord stromal, germ cell, mixed cell, or metastatic processes.
- The most common metastatic sites are from the breast, gastrointestinal tract, and gynecologic organs (uterus and cervix) with occasional lymphoma metastases.
- Ovarian cancers generally spread by way of direct exfoliation from the ovary into the abdominal cavity with peritoneal implantation; however, lymphatic and hematogenous spread is also noted.

Staging

Ovarian cancer is a surgically staged disease. It is mandatory that patients receive an opportunity to have a surgical procedure directed to cytoreduce their cancer before induction of chemotherapy when possible. The staging information is primarily obtained at the time of exploratory laparotomy (Figure 27-1). Survival rates by stage with 5-year follow-up for patients diagnosed from 1995 to 1998 are from the American College of Surgeons national cancer database (Figure 27-2).

Histology

Ovarian cancer is derived from three major histologic types. The first type is epithelial, which constitutes 90% of all ovarian cancers [2]. The epithelial group can be further subdivided in decreasing order into serous, mucinous, endometrioid, clear cell, transitional cell, squamous, mixed epithelial, and undifferentiated tumors. The second large histologic type is malignant germ cell tumors of the ovary. They arise from the primordial cells in the ovary, account for 3% to 5% of all ovarian cancer, and are most often diagnosed in young women 16 to 20 years of age. The germ cell group can be further subdivided in decreasing order of prevalence into dysgerminomas, teratomas, yolk sac tumor (endodermal sinus tumor), embryonal carcinoma, polyembryomas, choriocarcinomas, mixed germ cell tumors, and tumors composed of germ cells and sex cord stromal tumors [3]. The third histologic type of ovarian cancer is sex cord stromal tumors, which make up approximately 7% of all ovarian neoplasms [4]. These tumors account for almost 90% of all hormonally functioning neoplasms [5]. The sex cord stromal tumors can be further subdivided into granulose stromal cell, Sertoli stromal cell, gynandroblastomas, sex cord tumor with annular tubules, and unclassified [6].

Epidemiology

The incidence of ovarian cancer increases with age, peaking in the eighth decade of life. The median age of diagnosis is 59 years of age, and less than 15% of ovarian cancer cases occur in women less than 50 years of age. The etiology of ovarian cancer remains unclear. Various causes have been implicated including incessant ovulation, endometriosis transforming to malignancy, and a multitude of tumor suppressor genes and oncogenes involved in the pathogenesis [7–10].

The biologic etiology of ovarian cancer remains undefined; however, environmental, endogenous, and hereditary risk factors have been identified. The most notable hereditary disorders associated with ovarian cancer are mutations of the tumor suppressor genes *BRCA-1* and *BRCA-2*. Other genes involved in ovarian cancer include *p53*, *c-myc*, *erbB2*, and *H-ras* [11,12]. Patients with first- and second-degree relatives with ovarian cancer have an increased risk of developing ovarian cancer. The presence of two first-degree relatives or vertically transmitted ovarian cancer within a family indicates hereditary ovarian

International Federation of Gynecology and Obstetrics Staging for Ovarian Cancer

Stage	Description
Stage I	Malignancy limited to the ovaries
IA	Limited to one ovary; no ascites with malignant cells, capsule in tact, no implants on surface of ovary
IB	Limited to both ovaries; no ascites with malignant cells, capsule intact, no implants on surface of ovary
IC	Stage IA or IB with tumor implants on surface of either or both ovaries, rupture of ovarian capsule or ascites with malignant cells, or washing with malignant cells
Stage II	Malignancy involving one or both ovaries with extension to the pelvis
IIA	Metastatic extension to the uterus or fallopian tubes
IIB	Metastatic extension to the other tissue within the pelvis
IIC	Stage IIA or IIB with tumor implants on surface of either or both ovaries, rupture of ovarian capsule or ascites with malignant cells, or washings with malignant cells
Stage III	Malignancy involving one or both ovaries with peritoneal implants outside of the pelvis and/or positive retroperitoneal or inguinal lymph nodes. Superficial histologically proven implants on any of the abdominal organs or tissues outside of the pelvis indicate stage III disease
IIIA	Malignancy within the pelvis with negative nodes but with microscopic superficial histologically proven implants on any of the abdominal organs or peritoneal tissues
IIIB	Malignancy within the pelvis with negative nodes but with superficial implants < 2 cm in diameter on any of the abdominal organs or peritoneal tissues
IIIC	Malignancy within the pelvis with implants > 2 cm in diameter on any of the abdominal organs or peritoneal tissues and/or positive retroperitoneal or inguinal lymph nodes
Stage IV	Malignancy involving one or both ovaries with distant metastatic disease. If pleural effusion is present, then positive cytology must be confirmed. Parenchymal liver disease indicates stage IV disease and warrants histologic confirmation

Figure 27-1. International Federation of Gynecologists and Obstetricians staging for ovarian cancer.

Five-year Survival Rates After Cancer Diagnosis: 1995–1998*

Stage	Relative 5-year Survival Rate, %
IA	92.7
IB	85.4
IC	84.7
IIA	78.6
IIB	72.4
IIC	64.4
IIIA	50.8
IIIB	42.4
IIIC	31.5
IV	17.5

*The 5-year survival rate refers to the percentage of patients who live at least 5 years after their cancer is diagnosed.

Figure 27-2. Five-year survival rates after cancer diagnosis. The numbers are based on patients diagnosed from 1995 to 1998. (*Data from* American College of Surgeons National Cancer Database.)

cancer; this increases the lifetime risk of developing ovarian cancer to approximately 50% [13]. *BRCA-1* and *BRCA-2* genes seem to have a similar function, increasing transcription rates for other genes responding to DNA injury. These *BRCA-1* and *BRCA-2* tumor suppressor genes use the undamaged DNA strand as a template to fix the damaged strand. If these tumor suppressor genes are mutated, then loss of the DNA repair mechanism may occur. Currently the connection between *BRCA-1* and *BRCA-2* mutations leading to malignancy requires the concomitant loss of function in the *P53/21* pathway [14]. Eleven percent of all ovarian cancer patients will be found to have a mutation of *BRCA-1* or *BRCA-2*. Typically the diagnosis of ovarian cancer is made 10 years earlier than in sporadic cases of ovarian cancer, and almost all are papillary serous type for women with *BRCA-1* or *BRCA-2* mutations [14]. Furthermore, women that are of Ashkenazi Jewish descent, previously diagnosed with medullary, high grade, estrogen receptor (ER) negative breast cancer are at significantly increased risk for *BRCA* mutation. Women that demonstrate hereditary ovarian cancer syndrome will have *BRCA-1* mutations 75% of the time, *BRCA-2* mutations in 15% to 20%, and 10% will have mismatch repair genes (*MLH1* or *MSH2*) [15].

Risk reduction modalities for women identified with *BRCA-1* or *BRCA-2* mutation include counseling for the signs and symptoms of ovarian cancer as well as a regimen of oral contraception until pregnancy is desired. In women who do not desire pregnancy, tubal ligation or more definitive bilateral salpingo-oophorectomy with or without hysterectomy is recommended. The risk reduction with bilateral salpingo-oophorectomy is 96% for epithelial ovarian cancer, 50% for breast cancer and combined risk reduction of 80% [15]. Despite this risk reduction, there remains a 4.3% residual risk for developing primary peritoneal cancer in patients with a *BRCA-1* or *BRCA-2* mutation [16].

Theories behind reducing the risk for ovarian cancer mainly focus on decreasing undefined events that lead to transformation by way of accumulation of genetic alteration in the surface epithelium of the ovary. There are several strategies that can be employed or behaviors that can be modified to reduce the development of ovarian cancer (Figure 27-3) [17–26].

Diagnostic Methods

The signs and symptoms of ovarian cancer are often described as insidious. Yet there are defined symptoms that typically herald the development of ovarian cancer as defined by a survey that Goff *et al.* [27] discovered in a group of ovarian cancer patients after the diagnosis had been confirmed. Like Goff, Olson *et al.* [28] found that certain defined symptoms were more common in patients with ovarian cancer when matched with an age-appropriate case-control group (Figure 27-4).

Some of the most common findings on examination are pelvic mass, abdominal distension, or an abdominal mass. The majority of palpable masses detected in a routine examination will not be malignant in postmenopausal women.

The differential diagnosis for ovarian cancer includes malignant and benign alternatives. A commonly used tumor marker, CA-125, is often helpful to distinguish malignant from benign pelvic masses. A serum CA-125 level that is elevated (> 35 U/mL) in combination with a pelvic mass in a postmenopausal

Strategies to Reduce the Risk of Ovarian Cancer

Factor Influencing Risk	RR or OR	Conclusions
Exercise [1]	RR = 0.73 (0.56–0.94)	No clear benefit to exercise
Diet (low fat decreases risk [2])	RR = 0.51	No clear benefit
Parity (nulliparity increases risk; multiparity decreases risk [6–8])	RR = 2.5; OR = 0.4 if ≥ 5 births	Each pregnancy confers a risk reduction of 20%; also true for BRCA-1/2
Breast feeding [10]	OR = 0.6	Most effective in first 6 months
Fertility treatment [9,10]	OR = 2.8; RR = 11	Likely a modest risk of ovarian cancer; one study cited OR of 27 in nulliparous women
HRT	N/A	No compelling evidence; small increased risk if more than 10 years of use [3]
Tubal ligation	OR = 0.6	This benefit extends to BRCA-1 mutation patients [4]
Prophylactic oophorectomy	N/A	Obvious, reduces breast and celomic epithelial cancer
Oral contraception	RR = 0.6 [5]; RR = 0.2 for > 10 years of use	Even for a few months reduces risk by 40% for women ages 20 through 54; reduces number of lifetime ovulations; reduces gonadotropin levels; suppresses androgens, contains progestins; may decrease toxins reaching ovaries from vagina by altering mucous at the cervix
Progesterone	RR = 0.4 for < 3 years of use; RR = 0.2 for > 3 years of use	May be a reason why pregnancy is protective—progesterone levels are very high

Figure 27-3. Strategies to reduce the risk of ovarian cancer. HRT—hormone replacement therapy; N/A—not applicable; OR—odds ratio; RR—relative risk.

woman should elicit consideration for consulting a gynecologic oncologist. Eighty percent to 85% of patients with epithelial ovarian cancers will have elevated serum levels of CA-125. The serous histologic subset has the highest incidence of elevated CA-125 (> 85 %). Mucinous have the lowest incidence of elevated CA-125 levels. In postmenopausal women with an elevated CA-125 (> 65) and an asymptomatic mass, sensitivity is 97%, and specificity is 78% [29]. Preoperative CA-125 levels are extremely useful when elevated to follow postoperative response to therapeutic interventions. Although CA-125 is a very useful marker in postmenopausal women for an ovarian malignancy, it can also be elevated with other forms of malignancy and in benign conditions (Figure 27-5) [30].

No reliable procedures are currently available for the early detection of ovarian cancer. The American Academy of Family Physicians, the American College of Obstetrics and Gynecology, the Canadian Task Force on Periodic Health Examination, and the US Preventative Task Force all state there is no convincing evidence to support routine screening with tumor markers or ultrasound for ovarian cancer at this time [31]. The American College of Obstetrics and Gynecology recommends referral to a gynecologic oncologist in premenopausal women with a pelvic mass who also has one of the following: CA-125 greater than 200 U/mL, ascites,

evidence of abdominal or distant metastatic disease, or family history of one or more first-degree relatives with breast cancer [32]. Routine pelvic examinations on at least a yearly basis are recommended for the general population. The diagnostic evaluation of a patient with a suspected ovarian malignancy begins with a thorough physical examination looking for evidence of extra-abdominal metastasis in the lymph nodes or pleural effusions. Laboratory evaluation includes hematology, complete metabolic panel, as well as serum markers (CA-125 for epithelial tumors; alpha-fetoprotein), β-human chorionic gonadotropin, and lactate dehydrogenase for germ cell tumors. Radiologic evaluation may include ultrasound or CT scan of the abdomen, pelvis, and chest, a chest radiograph to detect pulmonary disease, and a barium enema or colonoscopy if constrictive pelvic disease is suspected. Routine screening with CA-125 or other tumor markers is discouraged. Women with significant hereditary risks for ovarian cancer may benefit from an intensive monitoring program that employs the Risk of Ovarian Cancer Algorithm curve in combination with the necessary ultrasound and CA-125 monitoring. This modality is currently under analysis in the Gynecologic Oncology Group protocol 199 closed for accrual in late 2006.

Rosenthal and Jacobs [33] defined that a screening test for the general population regarding ovarian cancer should have

Comparison of Symptoms in Patients with Ovarian Cancer with Age-matched Control Subjects

Symptoms	Patients with Ovarian Cancer, %	Control Subjects, %
Bloating, fullness, abdominal pressure	71	9
Abdominal or back pain	52	15
Lack of energy	43	16
Frequent urination	33	12
Constipation	21	7
Anorexia	20	3
Diarrhea	16	6
Nausea	13	9

Figure 27-4. Comparison of symptoms in patients with ovarian cancer with age-matched control subjects.

Elevation of CA-125 in Benign and Malignant Conditions Not Associated with Ovarian Cancer

Elevated CA-125 Categories Not Associated with Ovarian Cancer	Conditions
Gynecologic	Endometriosis, leiomyomas, ovarian cysts, menstruation, pelvic inflammatory disease, pregnancy (first trimester)
Gastrointestinal and hepatic disease	Pancreatitis, colitis, hepatitis, cirrhosis, diverticulitis
Malignancy	Bladder, breast, uterine, lung, liver, non-Hodgkin's lymphoma, ovary, pancreas, colon (metastatic)
Miscellaneous	Pericarditis, polyarteritis nodosa, renal disease, Sjögren's syndrome, systemic lupus erythematosus, tuberculosis

Figure 27-5. Elevation of CA-125 in benign and malignant conditions not associated with ovarian cancer.

99.6% specificity to achieve a positive predictive value of 10% (*ie*, 10 operations for each case of ovarian cancer identified). In a separate study by Zurawski *et al.* [34], they defined from serum samples obtained more than 60 months before surgery that 14 of 59 ovarian cancer patients had elevated CA-125 values. The Risk of Ovarian Cancer Algorithm uses an individuals sequential CA-125 values from which a slope and intercept can be determined; the higher the slope or intercept, the higher the risk of ovarian cancer. The Risk of Ovarian Cancer Algorithm achieves a sensitivity of 83%, specificity of 99.7%, and a positive predictive value of 16% in predicting the risk of cancer in the year after the patient's last screen [35]. The utility of panels of markers such as CA-125, CA-72-4, CA-15-3, and LSA combined to improve the positive predictive power has great promise. The usefulness of preoperative CT scans cannot be underestimated to assist the surgeon in preoperative therapeutic planning. Furthermore, CT imaging and ultrasound can assist in confirming the suspicion of ovarian cancer (Figure 27-6) [36–39].

Treatment

SURGERY

Ovarian cancer is surgically staged with an emphasis on optimal debulking. It is essential that the initial surgical procedure is undertaken by a surgeon comfortable and capable of performing the typical staging requirements that include hysterectomy, bilateral salpingo-oophorectomy, pelvic and para-aortic lymph node dissection, abdominopelvic washings, complete omentectomy, and peritoneal biopsies (anterior

Prospective Ultrasound Studies with Scoring Systems to Predict Malignancy					
Study	Sensitivity, %	Specificity, %	Positive Predictive Value, %	Negative Predictive Value, %	Accuracy, %
Sassone *et al.* [36]	65	88	74	83	80
De Priest *et al.* [37]	100	81	74	100	88
Ferrazzi *et al.* [38]	84	83	72	91	83
Alcazar *et al.* [39]	100	95	91	100	97

Figure 27-6. Prospective ultrasound studies with scoring systems to predict malignancy.

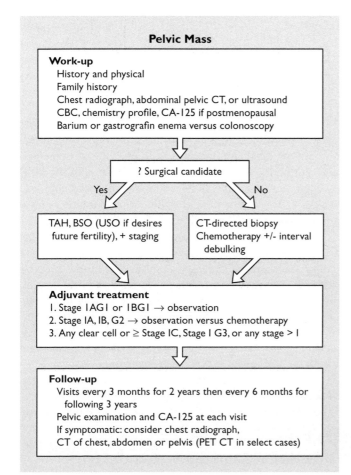

Figure 27-7. Pelvic mass management. BSO— bilateral salpingo-oophorectomy; CBC—complete blood count; PET—positron emission tomography; TAH— total abdominal hysterectomy; USO—unilateral salpingo-oophorectomy.

and posterior cul-de-sac, bilateral pelvic sidewalls, bilateral paracolic gutters, and diaphragm). Further treatment options with chemotherapy are often guided by the initial surgery (Figure 27-7). Furthermore, it is essential that the surgeon have the capability to perform necessary procedures to leave no residual tumor or less than 1-cm (optimal debulking) implants. More than 70% of patients that undergo primary surgery for ovarian cancer are capable of optimal tumor debulking when operated upon by a gynecologic oncologist, which greatly improves their survival. The size of the largest remaining lesion, and not the number of lesions, seems to correlate best with survival [40]. Patients with optimal cytoreduction have a 22-month median survival advantage compared with those with suboptimal cytoreductive efforts: 17 months versus 39 months (optimal vs suboptimal) [41].

Occasionally, initial surgery is met with an inability to significantly debulk the ovarian cancer or it is deemed not amenable to debulking based on patient performance status. In this scenario, some authors have advocated neoadjuvant chemotherapy that is generally followed by an attempt at interval debulking any remaining tumor after three to four cycles of chemotherapy. Neoadjuvant chemotherapy has been shown to decrease blood loss and hospital stay in some small case control series [42,43].

Special interest in fertility-preserving surgery remains for women of reproductive age when diagnosed with an ovarian malignancy or a low malignant potential tumor of the ovary. Generally women in this scenario can be offered preservation of the uninvolved ovary and retention of the uterus, with an otherwise complete staging procedure as defined. Despite the fertility-sparing type of surgery, surgeons should maintain aggressive debulking methods and adhere to standard staging protocols, which will maintain the exceptional survival rates in young women [44]. Standard chemotherapy with platinum-based regimens after surgery will usually allow preservation of fertility [45].

There are various adjuvant chemotherapeutic options for treatment of ovarian malignancy. These treatment options are primarily based on the histologic type of malignancy. More recently, a renewed interest in intraperitoneal chemotherapy has developed for treating patients with advanced-staged epithelial malignancies. After adjuvant chemotherapy has been completed, some authors advocate consolidation therapy.

Chemotherapy

EPITHELIAL OVARIAN CANCER
Treatment for epithelial ovarian cancer has evolved significantly over the past 40 years. Melphalan was the first agent that demonstrated efficacy in the treatment of ovarian cancer in the late 1960s. Cisplatin was subsequently introduced in the 1970s and dramatically improved survival rates. The Gynecologic Oncology Group published the first large randomized study establishing that the addition of cisplatin to multidrug therapy for ovarian cancer improved response [46]. With the addition of paclitaxel to cisplatin, the gold-standard chemotherapy regimen was established [47]. The Gynecologic Oncology Group protocol 158 next established that carboplatin could replace cisplatin with an improvement in toxicity profile and no loss in efficacy [48]. Most recently, Gynecologic Oncology Group protocol 182 sought to determine the best adjuvant therapy for advanced stage ovarian cancer by comparing five separate arms and eight cycles in each regimen: paclitaxel plus carboplatin for eight cycles versus paclitaxel plus carboplatin plus gemcitabine for eight cycles versus an alternating regimen of paclitaxel plus carboplatin for four cycles; with paclitaxel plus carboplatin plus Doxil (Ortho Biotech Products, LP, Raritan, NJ) for four cycles versus topotecan plus carboplatin for four cycles; then paclitaxel plus carboplatin for four cycles versus gemcitabine plus carboplatin for four cycles; then paclitaxel plus carboplatin for four cycles. The end result of Gynecologic Oncology Group protocol 182 indicated no improvement of progression-free survival or overall survival for any of the five different regimens [49]. Treatment recommendations for early-stage disease are different from advanced stage. Low risk—stage IA, IB; grade 1 or 2—do not necessarily require chemotherapy. High risk—all IC, II, clear cell histology, and all grade 3 regardless of IA or IB—may benefit from Taxol (Bristol-Myers Squibb, New York, NY)/carboplatin as their recurrence risk is 20% to 50% [50].

Recently intraperitoneal chemotherapy has gained significant momentum for adjuvant treatment of advanced-stage ovarian cancer. This is based on the data compiled by the Gynecologic Oncology Group and corresponding authors regarding three separate phase 3 trials (Figure 27-8) [51–53]. Based on these trials, adoption of this type of chemotherapy is expanding and in some parts of the country has become standard of care in patients that are eligible. In these patients, it seems to increase overall survival by 25% and progression-free survival by 20%. Patients with poor kidney function, adhesions, or left-sided colon resection are not ideal candidates for intraperitoneal chemotherapy. Furthermore, difficulties administering this modality of chemotherapy have been addressed by Markman and Walker [54] in their critical evaluation of intraperitoneal administration difficulties.

Patients that achieve a complete clinical response after adjuvant chemotherapy may be eligible for consolidation therapy. This form of therapy was shown to improve progression-free survival to 28 months compared with the control arm of the study of 21 months [55]. To achieve this difference the consolidation arm patients received 9 more months of chemotherapy than the control group. The consolidation group of patients received paclitaxel at 175 mg/m^2 every 4 weeks for 12 months. It has never been determined whether patients that receive consolidation therapy actually have an improved overall survival or whether consolidation therapy is beneficial overall [56]. Currently the Gynecologic Oncology Group is investigating the utilization of consolidation treatment with Xyotax (Cell Therapeutics, Inc., Seattle, WA) or paclitaxel versus observation in Gynecologic Oncology Group protocol 212.

Recurrent ovarian cancer is typically the result of chemo-resistant tumor cell clones that evade initial chemotherapy. These cells may remain clinically undetectable for months to years. Treatment for recurrent ovarian cancer is divided into platinum-sensitive and platinum-resistant disease. Platinum-resistant patients are defined as patients that have recurrent disease within 6 months after completion of adjuvant chemotherapy using a platinum agent or progression during initial treatment [57]. Platinum-resistant patients have a very poor prognosis and generally worse response rates to single and combination therapy retreatment when compared with platinum-sensitive patients. Platinum-sensitive patients have much better overall survival rates and typically respond to retreatment with platinum-based therapy, which is not true for platinum-resistant patients. Chemotherapeutic agents that have been utilized for treatment of recurrent disease include numerous agents (Figure 27-9).

In the past several years, metronomic chemotherapy is gaining renewed interest. These regimens involve very low-dose chemotherapy given on a daily basis. The current theories indicate that dosages of this fashion may reduce toxicity while providing antiangiogenic and cytotoxic therapy. Recent success has been shown with cyclophosphamide alone and in combination with newer biologic agents [58].

Phase III Randomized Intraperitoneal Adjuvant Chemotherapy Versus Intravenous Adjuvant Chemotherapy for Ovarian Cancer

Study	Treatment Regimen	Patients, n	Residual Disease	OS, mo	PFS, mo	Toxicity
Alberts et al. 1996 [51]	CDDP 100 mg/m² IV q 3 wk	279	≤ 2 cm	41		IV: increased neurotoxicity and hearing loss; IP: increased abdominal pain
	CDDP 100 mg/m² IP q 3 wk	267		49 (P = 0.02)		
Markman et al. 2001 [52]	CDDP 75 mg/m² IV + paclitaxel 135 mg/m² IV	227	≤ 1 cm	52	22	IP: increased neutropenia, thrombocytopenia, gastrointestinal toxicity, metabolic toxicity
	CDDP 7100 mg/m² IP + paclitaxel 135 mg/m² IV	235		63 (P = 0.05)	28 (P = 0.01)	
Armstrong et al. 2006 [53]	D1: IV paclitaxel 135 mg; D2: IV CDDP 75 mg	210	≤ 1 cm	49.7	18.3	IP: increased myelosuppression, emesis, abdominal pain, neuropathy
	D1: IV paclitaxel 135 mg; D2: IV CDDP 100 mg; D8: IP paclitaxel 60 mg	210		65.6 (P = 0.03)	24 (P = 0.05)	No difference in quality of life at 12 months

Figure 27-8. Phase III randomized intraperitoneal (IP) adjuvant chemotherapy versus intravenous (IV) adjuvant chemotherapy for ovarian cancer. CDDP—cisplatin; OS—overall survival; PFS—progression-free survival.

Treatment Options for Recurrent Ovarian Cancer*

US FDA–approved Second-line Treatment Options	Non–US FDA–approved Second-line Treatment Options
Altretamine	Alkylating agents
Carboplatin	Docetaxel
Cisplatin	Oral etoposide
Gemcitabine	Tamoxifen
Pegylated liposomal doxorubicin	Vinorelebine
Paclitaxel	
Topotecan	

Platinum-based combination therapy can be considered.

Figure 27-9. Treatment options for recurrent ovarian cancer. US FDA—US Food and Drug Administration.

GERM CELL TUMORS

Germ cell tumors make up 20% of all ovarian neoplasms but only 5% of the ovarian malignancies. Serum tumor markers can be very useful to follow response to therapy and for evaluation of germ cell malignancies: alpha-fetoprotein, human chorionic gonadotropin, and lactic acid dehydrogenase (Figure 27-10). Treatment for germ cell tumors is fertility sparing if possible. Adjuvant treatment may consist of radiation or chemotherapy, although chemotherapy is the favored adjuvant treatment. Optimal staging with appropriate platinum-based chemotherapy yields survival rates near 90% for most germ cell tumors.

Bleomycin, etoposide, and cisplatin is currently the favored regimen for treatment of germ cell tumors [59]. The only patients that do not require adjuvant chemotherapy after surgery for germ cell tumors are those that have stage IA G1 dysgerminomas. Three cycles of bleomycin, etoposide, and cisplatin should suffice in patients that have optimally debulked disease after initial surgery. Any patients with significant residual disease should receive four cycles of bleomycin, etoposide, and cisplatin. The development of acute leukemia as a complication of treatment is disturbing and mandates careful long-term follow-up but is unusual and does not alter the risk-to-benefit ratio of treatment.

SEX CORD STROMAL TUMORS

Sex cord stromal tumors tend to present at younger ages with a peak occurrence in the fifth and sixth decade of life. Treatment generally involves typical surgical staging, although fertility preservation is acceptable in appropriate patients. These tumors may characteristically secrete various hormones at elevated levels resulting in precocious puberty, abnormal menstruation, or endometrial cancer, whereas androgen-secreting tumors may cause hirsutism or virilization, with balding, voice deepening, and clitoromegaly. Endometrial sampling should be considered specifically for granulose cell tumors as they have a tendency to secrete estrogen and may cause endometrial hyperplasia or concomitant endometrial cancers. Sex cord stromal tumors generally behave in an indolent manner with characteristic slow growth and late recurrences. Eighty percent of patients will present with stage I or II disease and 11% as stage III, with only 9% stage IV [60]. The overall 5- and 10-year survival rates are 95% and 84% for patients with stage I to II disease compared with 59% and 57% for those with stage III to

IV disease [60]. Stage of disease and age seem to be the most important prognostic indicators of survival [60]. Adjuvant treatment typically involves platinum-based regimens: bleomycin, etoposide, and cisplatin; etoposide and cisplatin; or paclitaxel and carboplatin [61]. Granulose cell tumors are radiosensitive, and benefits have been demonstrated for patients with advanced-stage or recurrent disease [62,63].

Future Directions

The future holds great hope for patients yet to be diagnosed with ovarian cancer as well as those currently fighting the disease. Great emphasis is currently being placed on identifying markers for the disease, as well as methodologies to identify patients at risk for ovarian cancer. The best policy is to identify the disease in its earliest stage before the malignancy has the opportunity to spread and become biologically more resilient to therapy. Current evaluation for potential future screening markers is ongoing utilizing microarray and proteomic assays. Chemotherapeutic treatment regimens continue to develop for cytotoxic therapy. Newer agents such as immunotherapies (ovarex-CA-125 antibody vaccine), angiogenesis inhibitors (thalidomide, bevacizumab, metronomic topotecan, and cyclophosphamide), and biologic modulators (gefitinib [Iressa; AstraZeneca, Wilmington, DE] and imatinib mesylate [Gleevec; Novartis, Annandale, NJ]) hold great promise for augmenting traditional cytotoxic options of treatment. Lastly, we must emphasize the unprecedented support of cancer advocacy and support groups. It is through the united effort of continued education, research, and service that a new hope remains within reach for our heroic patients and families.

Information for Patients

1. National Cancer Institute booklet *Taking Time: Support for People with Cancer*.
2. National Cancer Institute's Information Specialists at 1-800-4-CANCER and at LiveHelp (http://www.cancer.gov/help) can help you locate programs, services, and publications.
3. For a list of organizations offering support, see the NCI fact sheet "National Organizations That Offer Services to People With Cancer and Their Families."

Tumor Markers in Germ Cell Tumors

Tumor	Marker		
	AFP	hCG	LDH
Dysgerminoma	-	+/-	+
Immature teratoma	+/-	-	+/-
Endodermal sinus tumor	+	-	+/-
Embryoma carcinoma	+	+	+/-
Choriocarcinoma	-	+	-

Figure 27-10. Tumor markers in germ cell tumors. AFP—alpha-fetoprotein; hCG—human chorionic gonadotropin; LDH—lactate dehydrogenase.

References

1. Jemal A, Siegel R, Ward E, *et al.*: Cancer statistics, 2006. *CA Cancer J Clin* 2006, 56:106.

2. Scully RE: Recent progress in ovarian cancer. *Hum Pathol* 1970, 1:73.

3. Talerman A: Germ cell tumors of the ovary. In *Blaustein's Pathology of the Female Genital Tract*, edn 5. Edited by Kurman RJ. New York: Springer-Verlag; 2002:967–1034.

4. Koonings PP, Campbell K, Mishell DR Jr, *et al.*: Relative frequency of primary ovarian neoplasms: a 10-year review. *Obstet Gynecol* 1989, 74:921–926.

5. Tavassoli FA: Ovarian tumors with functioning manifestations. *Endocrinol Pathol* 1994, 5:137.

6. Young RH, Scully RE: Sex cord–stromal, steroid cell, and other ovarian tumors with endocrine, paraendocrine, and paraneoplastic manifestations. In *Blaustein's Pathology of the Female Genital Tract*, edn 5. Edited by Kurman RJ. New York: Springer-Verlag; 2002:905–966.

7. Fathala MF: Incessant ovulation: a factor in ovarian neoplasia? *Lancet* 1971, ii:163.

8. Fathala MF: Factors in the causation and incidence of ovarian cancer. *Obstet Gynecol Surv* 1972, 27:751–768.

9. Stern RC, Dash R, Bentley RC, *et al.*: Malignancy in endometriosis: frequency and comparison of ovarian and extraovarian types. *Int J Gynecol Pathol* 2001, 20:133–139.

10. Cvetkovic D, Connolly DC, Hamilton TC: Molecular biology and molecular genetics of ovarian, fallopian tube, and primary peritoneal cancer. In *Gynecologic Cancer: Controversies in Management*. Edited by Gershenson DM, McGuire WP, Gore M, *et al.* Philadelphia: Elsevier; 2004:385–398.

11. Hartmann LC, Podratz KC, Keeney GL: Prognostic significance of p53 immunostaining in epithelial ovarian cancer. *J Clin Oncol* 1994, 12:64.

12. Perez RP, Godwin AK, Hamilton TC, *et al.*: Ovarian cancer biology. *Semin Oncol* 1991, 18:186.

13. Lynch HT, Fitzcommons ML, Conway TA, *et al.*: Hereditary carcinoma of the ovary and associated cancers: a study of two families. *Gynecol Oncol* 1990, 36:48.

14. Werness BA, Eltabbakh GH: Familial ovarian cancer and early ovarian cancer: biologic, pathologic, and clinical features. *Int J Gynecol Pathol* 2001, 20:48–63.

15. Kauff ND, Satagopan JM, Robson ME, *et al.*: Risk-reducing salpingo-oophorectomy in women with a BRCA1 or BRCA2 mutation. *N Engl J Med* 2002, 346:1609–1615.

16. Finch A, Beiner M, Lubinski J, *et al.*: Salpingo-oophorectomy and the risk of ovarian, fallopian tube, and peritoneal cancers in women with a BRCA1 or BRCA2 mutation. *JAMA* 2006 296:185.

17. Cottreau CM, Ness RB, Kriska A: Physical activity and reduced risk of ovarian cancer. *Obstet Gynecol* 2000, 96:609–614.

18. Bosetti C, Negri E, Franceschi S, *et al.*: Diet and ovarian cancer risk: a case-control study in Italy. *Int J Cancer* 2001, 93:911–915.

19. Rodriguez C, Patel AV, Calle EE, *et al.*: Estrogen replacement therapy and ovarian cancer mortality in a large prospective study of US women. *JAMA* 2001, 285:1460–1465.

20. Narod SA, Sun P, Ghadirian P, *et al.*: Tubal ligation and risk of ovarian cancer in carriers of BRCA1 or BRCA2 mutations: a case-control study. *Lancet* 2001, 357:1467–1470.

21. The reduction in risk of ovarian cancer associated with oral-contraceptive use. The Cancer and Steroid Hormone Study of the Centers for Disease Control and the National Institute of Child Health and Human Development. *N Engl J Med* 1987, 316:650–655.

22. Fathala MF: Incessant ovulation: A factor in ovarian neoplasia? *Lancet* 1971, ii:163.

23. Fathala MF: Factors in the causation and incidence of ovarian cancer. *Obstet Gynecol Surv* 1972, 27:751–768.

24. Mosgaard BJ, Lidegard O, Kjaer SK, *et al.*: Infertility, fertility drugs, and invasive ovarian cancer: a case control study. *Fertil Steril* 1997, 67:1005–1012.

25. Rossing MA, Daling JR, Weiss NS, *et al.*: Ovarian tumors in a cohort of infertile women. *N Engl J Med* 1994, 331:771–776.

26. Whittemore AS, Harris R, Itnyre J: Characteristics relating to ovarian cancer risk: collaborative analysis of 12 U.S. case control studies. II. Invasive epithelial ovarian cancers in white women. Collaborative Ovarian Cancer Group. *Am J Epidemiol* 1992, 136:1184–1203.

27. Goff BA, Mandel L, Muntz HG, Melancon CH: Ovarian carcinoma diagnosis. *Cancer* 2000, 89:2068–2075.

28. Olson SH, Mignone L, Nakraseive C, *et al.*: Symptoms of ovarian cancer. *Obstet Gynecol* 2001, 98:212–217.

29. Cannistra SA: Cancer of the ovary. *N Engl J Med* 2004, 351:2519.

30. Lewis E, Wallace S: Radiologic diagnosis of ovarian cancer. In *Ovarian Malignancies*. Edited by Piver MS. Edinburgh: Churchill Livingstone; 1987:59.

31. US Preventive Services Task Force: *Guidelines from Guide to Clinical Preventive Services*, edn 2. Washington, DC: US Preventive Services Task Force; 1996.

32. Creasman WT: Committee Opinion # 280, December 2002. The role of the generalist obstetrician-gynecologist in the early detection of ovarian cancer. In *2007 Compendium of Selected Publications*. Edited by American College of Obstetrics and Gynecology. Washington, DC: American College of Obstetricians and Gynecologists; 2007:203–205.

33. Rosenthal A, Jacobs I: Ovarian cancer screening. *Semin Oncol* 1998, 25:315.

34. Zurawski VR, Orjaseter H, Andersen A, Jellum E: Elevated serum CA 125 levels prior to diagnosis of ovarian neoplasia: relevance for early detection of ovarian cancer. *J Cancer* 1988, 42:677–680.

35. Skates SJ, Fu FJ, Yu YH, *et al.*: Toward an optimal algorithm for ovarian cancer screening with longitudinal tumor markers. *Cancer* 1995, 76:2004–2010.

36. Sassone AM, Timor-Trisch IE, Artner A, *et al.*: Transvaginal sonographic characterization of ovarian disease: evaluation of a new scoring system to predict ovarian malignancy. *Obstet Gynecol* 1991, 78:70–76.

37. De Priest PD, Shenson D, Fried A, *et al.*: A morphology index based on sonographic findings in ovarian cancer. *Gynecol Oncol* 1993, 51:7–11.

38. Ferrazzi E, Zanetta G, Dordoni D, *et al.*: Transvaginal ultrasonographic characterization of ovarian masses: comparison of five scoring systems in a multicenter study. *Ultrasound Obstet Gynecol* 1997, 10:192–197.

39. Alcazar JL, Merce LT, Laparte C, et al.: A new scoring system to differentiate benign from malignant adnexal masses. Am J Obstet Gynecol 2003, 188:685–692.

40. Bristow RE, Tomacruz RS, Armstrong DK, et al.: Survival effect of maximal cytoreductive surgery for advanced ovarian carcinoma during the platinum era: a meta-analysis. J Clin Oncol 2002, 20:1248–1259.

41. Ozols RF, Rubin SC, Thomas GM, Robboy SJ: Epithelial ovarian cancer. In Principles and Practices of Gynecologic Oncology, edn 4. Edited by Hoskins WJ, Perez CA, Young RC, et al. Philadelphia: Lippincott Williams and Wilkins; 2005:895–987.

42. Schwartz PE, Rutherford TJ, Chambers JT, et al.: Neoadjuvant chemotherapy for advanced ovarian cancer: long-term survival. Gynecol Oncol 1999, 72:93–99.

43. Atlas II, Childers JM, Surwit EA: Laparoscopic cytoreductive surgery after chemotherapy for advanced ovarian cancer. J Am Assoc Gynecol Laparosc 1996, 3(Suppl):S2.

44. Chan JK, Urban R, Cheung MK, et al.: Ovarian cancer in younger vs. older women: a population-based analysis. Br J Cancer 2006, 95:1314–1320.

45. Brewer M, Gershenson DM, Herzog CE, et al.: Outcome and reproductive function after chemotherapy for ovarian dysgerminoma. J Clin Oncol 1999, 17:2670.

46. Omura G, Blessing JA, Ehrlich CE: A randomized trial of cyclophosphamide and doxorubicin with or without cisplatin in advanced ovarian carcinoma. Cancer 1987, 56:1725.

47. McGuire WP, Hoskins WJ, Brady MF: Cyclophosphamide and cisplatin compared with paclitaxel and cisplatin in patients with stage III and stage IV ovarian cancer. N Engl J Med 1996, 334:1.

48. Ozols RF, Bundy BN, Greer BE, et al.: Phase III trial of carboplatin and paclitaxel compared with cisplatin and paclitaxel in patients with optimally resected stage III ovarian cancer: a Gynecologic Oncology Group study. J Clin Oncol 2003, 21(17):3194–3200.

49. Copeland LJ, Bookman M, Trimble E, Gynecologic Oncology Group Protocol GOG 182-ICON5: Clinical trials of newer regimens for treating ovarian cancer: the rationale for Gynecologic Oncology Group Protocol GOG 182-ICON5. Gynecol Oncol 2003, 90:S1–S7.

50. Gynecologic Oncology Group: Phase III randomized study of carboplatin and paclitaxel with or without low-dose paclitaxel in patients with early stage ovarian epithelial cancer. National Cancer Institute Web site. http://www.cancer.gov/clinicaltrials/GOG-175#Registry-Info_CDR0000066732.

51. Alberts DS, Liu PY, Hannigan EV, et al.: Intraperitoneal cisplatin plus intravenous cyclophosphamide versus intravenous cisplatin plus intravenous cyclophosphamide for stage III ovarian cancer. N Engl J Med 1996, 335:1950–1955.

52. Markman M, Bundy BN, Alberts DS, et al.: Phase III trial of standard-dose intravenous cisplatin plus paclitaxel versus moderately high-dose carboplatin followed by intravenous paclitaxel and intraperitoneal cisplatin in small-volume stage III ovarian carcinoma: an intergroup study of the Gynecologic Oncology Group, Southwestern Oncology Group, and Eastern Cooperative Oncology Group. J Clin Oncol 2001, 19:1001–1007.

53. Armstrong DK, Bundy B, Wenzel L, et al.: Intraperitoneal cisplatin and paclitaxel in ovarian cancer. N Engl J Med 2006, 354:34–43.

54. Markman M, Walker JL: Intraperitoneal chemotherapy of ovarian cancer: a review, with a focus on practical aspects of treatment. J Clin Oncol 2006, 24:988–994.

55. Markman M, Liu PY, Wilczynski S, et al.: Phase III randomized trial of 12 versus 3 months of maintenance paclitaxel in patients with advanced ovarian cancer after complete response to platinum and paclitaxel-based chemotherapy: a Southwest Oncology Group and Gynecologic Oncology Group trial. J Clin Oncol 2003, 21:2460–2465.

56. McMeekin DS, Tillmanns T, Chaudry T, et al.: Timing isn't everything: an analysis of when to start salvage chemotherapy in ovarian cancer. Gynecol Oncol 2004, 95:157–164.

57. Markman M, Rothman R, Hakes T, et al.: Second-line platinum therapy in patients with ovarian cancer previously treated with cisplatin. J Clin Oncol 1991, 9:389–393.

58. Kerbel RS, Kamen BA: The anti-angiogenic basis of metronomic chemotherapy. Nat Rev Cancer 2004, 4:423–436.

59. Williams S, Blessing JA, Liao S, et al.: Adjuvant therapy of ovarian germ cell tumors with cisplatin, etoposide, and bleomycin: a trial of the Gynecologic Oncology Group. J Clin Oncol 1994, 12:701.

60. Zhang M, Cheung MK, Shin JY, et al.: Prognostic factors responsible for survival in sex cord stromal tumors of the ovary: an analysis of 376 women. Gynecol Oncol 2007, 104:396–400.

61. Schumer ST, Cannistra SA: Granulosa cell tumor of the ovary. J Clin Oncol 2003, 21:1180–1189.

62. Wolf JK, Mullen J, Eifel PJ, et al.: Radiation treatment of advanced or recurrent granulosa cell tumor of the ovary. Gynecol Oncol 1999, 73:35–41.

63. Savage P, Constenla D, Fisher C, et al.: Granulosa cell tumours of the ovary: demographics, survival and the management of advanced disease. Clin Oncol 1998, 10:242–245.

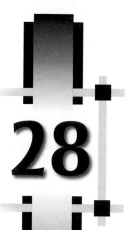

28 | Fallopian Tube Cancer

Brook A. Saunders and Todd D. Tillmanns

- Fallopian tube carcinoma is the rarest gynecologic malignancy.
- It primarily occurs in the 5th and 6th decades of life.
- It is usually asymptomatic; however, most common symptoms are:
  Serosanguinous vaginal bleeding/discharge
  Pelvic pain
  Pelvic mass
  Hydrops tubae profluens
- Fallopian tube cancer is typically diagnosed at the time of surgery for an adnexal mass.
- Staging is performed surgically with total abdominal hysterectomy, bilateral salpingo-ophorectomy, omentectomy, peritoneal biopsies, and peritoneal cytological examination.
- It is treated primarily by surgical tumor debulking and chemotherapy.
- Follow-up every 3 months for 2 years, then every 6 months for 3 years, and annually thereafter.
- Patients followed with routine history and physical examination, CA-125 levels and radiographs, CT as clinically indicated.

Background

Fallopian tube carcinoma is the least common of the gynecologic malignancies [1,2]. Metastatic cancer to the fallopian tubes from the ovaries, endometrium, breast, and gastrointestinal sites occurs with greater frequency than primary fallopian tube cancer. The incidence of fallopian tube carcinoma is approximately 3.6 cases per 1 million women annually [3].

Fallopian tube cancer is typically diagnosed between the ages of 50 and 70 years of age. The direct cause of fallopian cancer is unknown; however, there have been suggestions of an association between tuberculosis salpingitis and prior pelvic inflammatory disease. These associations have not been proven to date. An association between breast cancer (BRCA) genes 1/2 has been identified [4–7]. Patients with BRCA 1/2 were found to develop fallopian tube cancer 120 times more frequently when compared with the general population. Patients with fallopian tube cancer also have primary infertility more frequently with a 40% to 70% increase in nulliparity.

Pathology

Histologically, the most common type of fallopian tube cancer is papillary serous adenocarcinomas [8]. Other histologic types include endometroid, clear cell, adenosquamous, squamous cell, sarcoma, choriocarcinoma, and malignant teratoma. Fallopian tube sarcomas are extremely rare and are usually leiomyosarcomas and carcinosarcomas [9,10].

Fallopian tube cancers typically spread via the tubal ostia to the fimbria into the peritoneal cavity. The intra-abdominal organs are often affected through transcoelomic migration [11,12]. The tumors often spread synchronously to the uterus and ovaries. Lymphatic spread through the rich lymphatic drainage occurs commonly to the pelvic and periaortic lymph nodes. Studies have shown that metastatic disease is present approximately one third of the time [13,14].

Diagnosis

Delay in diagnosis of fallopian tube cancer is common, as the patients often present with vague complaints. The majority of patients are typically diagnosed postoperatively. Women with fallopian tube cancer often present with symptoms resulting in an earlier stage at the time of diagnosis. They usually have common, nondescriptive complaints. The most common and classic symptoms are usually: 1) serosanguinous vaginal discharge, 2) pelvic pain, and 3) a pelvic mass. The classic triad (Latzko's triad) occurs in less than 20% of patients [15]. Hydrops tubae profluens, which is intermittent discharge of clear or blood-tinged fluid, occurs as a result of pressure within the fallopian tube. This discharge followed by shrinkage of an adnexal mass is pathognomonic for fallopian tube cancer. Colicky, abdominal pain as a result of peristalsis of the fallopian tube against the distending tubal mass also is common. The pain from distension of the fallopian tube often causes women with fallopian tube cancer to present to the doctor earlier than those women with ovarian cancer [16].

LABORATORY
Cervical cytology should be performed in all women with a pelvic mass. Women with fallopian tube cancer will have abnormal cervical cytology approximately 10% of the time [17]. CA-125 levels are useful for evaluating response to therapy when elevated preoperatively. Before surgery, the patient should have routine hematologic and metabolic assessments performed.

IMAGING
Patients often have routine pelvic ultrasonography as a result of their symptoms. A solid, cystic, or complex adnexal mass is often seen at the time of the ultrasound examination. The fallopian tube mass is often very difficult to distinguish from an ovarian mass at the time of the ultrasound. The fallopian tube masses are often incorrectly diagnosed as a hydrosalpinx, tubal ovarian abscess, or pelvic inflammatory process. If increased vascularity or ascites is present, the suspicion for fallopian or ovarian cancer should be increased. CT scan or MRI has not been shown to increase the diagnostic accuracy for fallopian tube cancer and the diagnosis should be made definitively by surgery. However, the CT/MRI scans can be beneficial in the evaluation of metastatic disease.

HISTOLOGIC CRITERIA
Histologic criteria to diagnose fallopian tube cancer tissue are required for a definitive diagnosis. The distinction between fallopian and ovarian cancer is often difficult. The criteria established by Hu *et al.* [18] in 1950 continue to be the standard used today to confirm the diagnosis of fallopian tube cancer. These criteria are as follows: 1) the bulk

of the tumor should arise from the endosalpinx with the bulk of the tumor in the tube; 2) the transition from benign to malignant epithelium should show a clear transition within the tube; and 3) there should be no nexus between tubal and ovarian disease.

Staging

The staging of fallopian tube cancer is done surgically. The staging procedure consists of a total hysterectomy, bilateral salpingo-oophorectomy, omentectomy, pelvic and peri-aortic lymph node dissection, peritoneal biopsies, as well as an examination of the peritoneal cytology. In women wishing to retain fertility, a unilateral salpingo-oophorectomy in addition to the additional staging procedures except for the hysterectomy can be an option.

The International Federation of Gynecology and Obstetrics (FIGO) staging system for fallopian tube cancer is similar to that for ovarian cancer and is shown in Figure 28-1. At the time of staging, patients have stage I disease 33 % of the time and stage II disease an additional 33% of the time. Unlike ovarian cancer, only 34% of the patients have stage III/IV disease [19,20].

Treatment

The treatment of fallopian tube cancer consists of the surgical staging procedure done at the time of diagnosis as well as chemotherapeutic options as per ovarian cancer regimens if necessary.

SURGERY
As stated previously, the patient ideally should undergo a total hysterectomy with bilateral salpingo-oophorectomy along with the additional components of a complete staging procedure. Survival rates are increased if the cancer can be completely resected with the patient having less than 1 cm of residual disease at the end the surgery. This is similar to the findings for ovarian cancer.

RADIOTHERAPY
Radiation therapy is not routinely used in the treatment of fallopian tube cancer as the disease is usually spread beyond the pelvis, which would require whole abdominal radiation. There are very few clinical trials evaluating radiotherapy for treatment of fallopian tube cancer.

Prognosis/Follow-Up

The initial stage of fallopian tube cancer is the most important prognostic indicator. Patients with fallopian tube cancer are typically diagnosed at an earlier stage than those with ovarian cancer; therefore, they have a slightly better prognosis. The 5-year survival rates are shown in Figure 28-2. The rates range from 95% to 45% for stage I to IV respectively [21].

CA-125 is used to follow the patients with fallopian tube cancer for treatment success and recurrence. The initial response to chemotherapy with regard to CA-125 levels has a prognostic value. Patients with fallopian tube cancer should be followed every 3 months for the first 2 years. After two years, the follow-up can be decreased to every 6 months for a 3-year period. After 5 years, the follow-up can then be performed at yearly examinations. At each of these examinations, a thorough history and physical examination including a pelvic examination should be performed. If the review of systems or physical examination is positive for any respiratory or abdominal complaints, a recurrence should be suspected, and the clinician should consider evaluating the patient with a chest radiograph or an abdominal/pelvic CT.

FIGO Staging System: Fallopian Tube Carcinoma

Stage 0	Carcinoma in situ (limited to tubal mucosa)
Stage I	Limited to fallopian tubes
Stage IA	Limited to one tube with extension into the submucosa ± muscularis layers; no serosal penetration; negative ascites/peritoneal cytology
Stage IB	Limited to both tubes with extension into the submucosa ± muscularis layers; no serosal penetration; negative ascites/peritoneal cytology
Stage IC	IA or IB tumors but with extension through or onto the tubal serosa or positive peritoneal cytology or malignant ascites
Stage II	Growth involving one or both fallopian tubes with extension to the pelvis
Stage IIA	Extension ± metastasis onto the uterus or ovaries
Stage IIB	Extension to other pelvic tissues
Stage IIC	IA or IB tumors with positive peritoneal cytology or malignant ascites
Stage III	Tumor involving one or both fallopian tubes with peritoneal metastases outside the pelvis ± positive retroperitoneal or inguinal lymph nodes; superficial liver metastases; histologically proven extension outside of the pelvis on the peritoneal surfaces, bowel, or omentum
Stage IIIA	Tumor grossly limited to the true pelvis; negative lymph nodes; histologically proven microscopic disease of the abdominal peritoneal surfaces
Stage IIIB	Tumor involving one or both fallopian tubes with histologically proven abdominal peritoneal implants; none exceeding 2 cm in diameter; negative lymph nodes
Stage IIIC	Tumor involving one or both tubes with histologically proven abdominal peritoneal implants > 2 cm in diameter; positive retroperitoneal or inguinal lymph nodes
Stage IV	Tumor involving one or both tubes with distant metastases; pleural effusion must be positive for malignancy to be stage IV; parenchymal liver metastases are stage IV

Figure 28-1. International Federation of Gynecology and Obstetrics (FIGO) staging system for fallopian tube carcinoma.

Survival Rates for Patients with Fallopian Tube Cancer

Stage	Patients, *n*	5-year Survival Rate, %
I	102	95
II	29	75
III	52	69
IV	151	45

Figure 28-2. Survival rates for patients with fallopian tube cancer.

References

1. Peters WA, III, Anderson WA, Hopkins MP, *et al.*: Prognostic features of carcinoma of the fallopian tube. *Obstet Gynecol* 1988, 71:757–762.

2. Yeung HH, Bannatyne P, Russell P: Adenocarcinoma of the fallopian tubes: a clinicopathological study of eight cases. *Pathology* 1983, 15:279.

3. Rosenblatt KA, Weiss NS, Schwartz SM: Incidence of malignant fallopian tube tumors. *Gynecol Oncol* 1989, 35:236.

4. Brose MS, Rebbeck T, Calzone KA, *et al.*: Cancer risk estimates for *BRCA1* mutation carriers identified in a risk evaluation program. *J Natl Cancer Inst* 2002, 94:1365.

5. Levine DA, Argenta PA, Yee CJ, *et al.*: Fallopian tube and primary peritoneal carcinomas associated with *BRCA* mutations. *J Clin Oncol* 2003, 21:4222.

6. Aziz S, Kuperstein G, Rosen B, *et al.*: A genetic epidemiological study of carcinoma of the fallopian tube. *Gynecol Oncol* 2001, 80:341.

7. Cass I, Holschneider C, Datta N, *et al.*: *BRCA*-mutation-associated fallopian tube carcinoma: a distinct clinical phenotype? *Obstet Gynecol* 2005, 106:1327.

8. Berg JW, Lampe JG: High-risk factors in gynecologic cancer. *Cancer* 1981, 48:429.

9. Abrams J, Kazal HL, Hobbs RE: Primary sarcoma of the fallopian tube. *Am J Obstet Gynecol* 1958, 75:180.

10. Hanjani P, Petersen RO, Bonnell SA: Malignant mixed mullerian tumor of the fallopian tube. *Gynecol Oncol* 1980, 9:381.

11. Hirai Y, Kaku S, Teshima H: Clinical study of primary carcinoma of the fallopian tube: experience with 15 cases. *Gynecol Oncol* 1989, 34:20.

12. Podratz KC, Podczaski ES, Gaffey TA: Primary carcinoma of the fallopian tube. *Am J Obstet Gynecol* 1986, 154:1319.

13. Wolfson AH, Tralins KS, Greven KM, *et al.*: Adenocarcinoma of the fallopian tube: Results of a multi-institutional retrospective analysis of 72 patients. *Int J Radiat Oncol Biol Phys* 1998, 40:71.

14. Tamimi HK, Figge DC: Adenocarcinoma of the uterine tube: Potential for lymph node metastases. *Am J Obstet Gynecol* 1981, 141:132.

15. Sedlis A: Primary carcinoma of the fallopian tube. *Obstet Gynecol* 1961, 16:209.

16. Friedrich M, Villena-Heinsen C, Scweizer J, *et al.*: Primary tubal carcinoma: A retrospective analysis of four cases with a literature review. *Eur J Gynaecol Oncol* 1998, 19:138.

17. Podezaski E, Herbst AL: Cancer of the vagina and fallopian tube. In *Gynecologic Oncology*. Edited by Knapp RC, Berkowitz RS. New York: MacMillan; 1986.

18. Hu CY, Taymor ML, Hertig AT: Primary carcinoma of the fallopian tube. *Am J Obstet Gynecol* 1950, 59:58.

19. Rosenblatt KA, Weiss NS, Schwartz SM: Incidence of malignant fallopian tube tumors. *Gynecol Oncol* 1989, 35:236.

20. Pfeiffer P, Mogensen H, Amtrup F, *et al.*: Primary carcinoma of the fallopian tube. *Acta Oncol* 1989, 28:7.

21. Kosary C, Trimble EL: Treatment and survival for women with fallopian tube carcinoma: a population-based study. *Gynecol Oncol* 2002, 86:190.

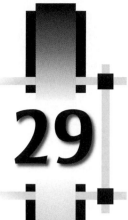

29 Gestational Trophoblastic Disease

David B. Engle and Todd D. Tillmanns

- Gestational trophoblastic disease describes a group of rare tumors including complete and partial moles, invasive moles, choriocarcinoma, and placental site trophoblastic tumors.
- It is paramount to follow β-human chorionic gonadotropin (β-hCG) values after a molar pregnancy, and to determine β-hCG levels in patients with delayed postpartum hemorrhage and in reproductive-age women presenting with disseminated metastatic disease.
- Excellent response to chemotherapy can be expected in almost all cases.
- Reproductive function can be preserved in 99% of cases.
- Patients with malignant gestational trophoblastic disease should be managed by a physician experienced in the disease.

Gestational trophoblastic disease (GTD) describes a group of rare tumors that arise from the fetal placenta. Thus, they are a type of tumor that arises from a pregnancy. Hydatidiform moles (complete and partial), invasive moles, choriocarcinoma, and placental site trophoblastic tumors comprise this group. These tumors range from benign to extremely malignant.

All of these tumors secrete β-human chorionic gonadotropin (β-hCG), which can be used to follow the disease. Additionally, these tumors respond to cytotoxic chemotherapy. Today, many women with malignant GTD may be cured and their fertility preserved.

Epidemiology

Gestational trophoblastic disease is very rare in the United States, with reports varying from one in 1000 to one in 1500 pregnancies. The incidence of choriocarcinoma in the United States is one in 20,000 to 40,000 pregnancies. Approximately 50% of choriocarcinoma occurs after a term pregnancy, 25% after molar pregnancies, and the remainder from other gestational events [1]. Reports from other countries, especially from Southeast Asia, have a higher incidence of GTD. Some of these differences may be related to statistical collection methods. The figures in hospital-based studies are usually higher than population-based studies. Whereas the highest incidences are reported from Asian countries, such as Indonesia, Taiwan, China, and the Philippines, most of these reports are also hospital-based studies. In the United States, there are conflicting reports regarding the incidence of molar pregnancy rates in African-American women compared with white women. However, the risk of choriocarcinoma is approximately two times greater in African-Americans compared with whites [2].

Patient age also has been attributed as a risk factor for GTD. There is an increased risk for complete molar gestations at the beginning and end of a woman's reproductive life. Women over the age of 40 have a higher incidence, as well as women less than 20, although the risk is greater in the group over the age of 40 [3].

Partial moles do not have an age distribution and occur at any time during a woman's reproductive life with similar frequency. Because partial moles can often be mistaken for an early spontaneous miscarriage, their numbers may be under-reported.

The greatest risk factor for molar pregnancy is having a prior molar pregnancy. The risk increases from a 0.1% baseline risk to 1.0 to 2.6% for a subsequent pregnancy. The risk of a third molar pregnancy is approximately 28% [4]. Term pregnancies after molar pregnancies reduce the risk of having further molar pregnancy.

Hydatidiform Moles

Hydatidiform moles come in two varieties based on their histologic findings: complete and partial. The differences between the two types of moles are displayed in Figure 29-1; however, their treatment and follow-up are essentially the same. Complete, or classic, moles have a 46, XX chromosome complement 95% of the time, all of paternal origin. This occurs when either a single sperm enters a hollow egg and replicates or when two separate sperm enter a hollow egg (dispermic fertilization). In the latter, which occurs in approximately 25% of the cases, complete moles can have either a 46, XX or 46, XY chromosome complement.

Complete moles will have a uterus larger than expected for dates 50% of the time, and β-hCG levels are usually greatly increased with values often seen greater than 200,000 mIU/mL [1]. Due to the similarity between β-hCG and thyroid-stimulating hormone (TSH), some patients will actually present with signs and symptoms of hyperthyroidism brought on by the high circulating level of β-hCG. Pathologic evaluation of the molar specimen reveals significant hyperplasia of the cytotrophoblasts and the syncytial trophoblasts. The villi are edematous; however, they do not contain fetal blood cells. The rate of post molar malignant sequelae for a complete mole ranges from 6% to 32% [1].

Partial moles occur through dispermic fertilization of a normal (23, X haploid) egg. Therefore, the resulting chromosome pattern is trisomic with 69, XXX or 69, XXY being the most common. A fetus will often form; however, fetal death will usually occur by the end of the first trimester. Additionally, fetal red blood cells will also form; therefore, an RH-negative mother will require rhogam. In the fetal placenta, only focal hydropic villi are present, and there is less trophoblastic proliferation. Therefore, these patients often present with a normal to slightly "small for gestation age" size uterus. Additionally, β-hCG is not as elevated as with a complete mole. The clinical and ultrasound picture often point toward a missed abortion and, therefore, the preoperative diagnosis of gestational trophoblastic disease is often missed. The rate of malignant transformation is lower for partial moles than complete moles and is less than 5% [1].

Diagnosis

The most common presenting symptom of a molar pregnancy is vaginal bleeding. The vaginal bleeding usually occurs late in the first trimester or during the first half of the second trimester. Sometimes with vaginal bleeding, grape-like clusters of villi will be expressed through the cervical os. Other presenting symptoms can include absent heart tones, greater than expected uterine enlargement, bilateral ovarian cysts, hyperthyroidism, and exceptionally high β-hCG. The diagnosis of a molar pregnancy is typically made during the first trimester [1].

Molar pregnancy is now almost exclusively diagnosed by ultrasound. However, early complete moles or partial moles may be diagnosed as a missed abortion. The ultrasound will often have an absence of fetal parts and a classic "snowstorm" appearance. This appearance is due to the hydroptic villi seen inside the uterus. Once a molar pregnancy has been diagnosed, an appropriate laboratory and radiologic workup is necessary.

Treatment

The initial preoperative work-up should include complete blood count, electrolytes, liver function, renal function, clotting

Features of Partial and Complete Hydatidiform Moles

Feature	Partial Mole	Complete Mole
Karyotype	Most commonly 69,XXX or 69,XXY	Most commonly 46,XX or 46,XY
Pathology		
Fetus	Often present	Absent
Amnion, fetal red blood cells	Usually present	Absent
Villous edema	Variable, focal	Diffuse
Trophoblastic proliferation	Focal, slight to moderate	Diffuse, slight to severe
Clinical presentation		
Diagnosis	Missed abortion	Molar gestation
Uterine size	Small for gestational age	50% larger for gestational age
β-hCG value	Low to normal	High
Theca lutein cysts	Rare	15% to 25%
Medical complications	Rare	< 25%
Postmolar malignant sequelae	< 5%	6% to 32%

Figure 29-1. Types of moles. β-hCG—β-human chorionic gonadotropin. (*Adapted from* Soper *et al.* [11].)

studies, blood type and screen, quantitative β-hCG, and chest radiograph [1]. If the patient is showing signs or symptoms of hyperthyroidism, then evaluation of a TSH level is recommended. Clotting and coagulopathy studies can also be considered. The primary treatment is evacuation of the uterus. This is often done today with suction curettage. In the event a patient desires no further reproductive potential, then a simple hysterectomy can be considered. Hysterectomy will reduce the risk of postmolar malignancy, but it does not eliminate the risk; therefore these patients should receive the same follow-up as patients that do not undergo a hysterectomy. Medical methods used to evacuate the uterus (prostaglandins, anti-progesterones) are not recommended as these methods have been linked to a more likely need for chemotherapy [5].

Complications from the dilation and curettage for a molar pregnancy can be severe. Pitocin should be routinely added to the intravenous fluid as soon as the procedure starts to help decrease blood loss. Additionally, uterine perforation, infection, toxemia, anemia, and pulmonary complications can occur. An overall complication rate of 67% has been reported after evacuation of a molar pregnancy [6]. Respiratory insufficiency has been reported to occur in up to 16% of patients [6]. The risk of respiratory insufficiency is perhaps greater if the evacuation is completed in the second trimester rather than the first trimester. The incidence of pulmonary complications peaks approximately 4 hours after the dilation and curettage is completed. Therefore, these patients should be closely observed postoperatively with continuous pulse oximetry [7]. Pulmonary insufficiency is most often due to massive embolization of fetal cells into the maternal circulation [7].

Follow-Up

A repeat β-hCG should be obtained within 48 hours after dilation and curettage and then every week while elevated. Once the value has returned to negative, β-hCG can be checked every 1 to 2 months for up to 1 year [8••]. It is imperative that the patient be placed on reliable contraception during the follow-up period. A rising β-hCG from a pregnancy can cloud the issue of postmolar malignant sequelae. The Gynecologic Oncology Group performed a randomized trial and confirmed that oral contraceptives do not increase the incidence of postmolar malignancy and are effective at preventing pregnancy [9].

The International Federation of Gynecology and Obstetrics (FIGO) published the β-hCG requirements for the diagnosis of post molar gestational trophoblastic disease (Figure 29-2) [10]. The role of repeat dilation and cutterage for rising or plateau of β-hCG is very controversial and until further studies are done should probably be avoided [1,8••]. "Phantom" β-hCG is a erroneous laboratory value brought on by heterophilic antibodies that crossreact with the hCG test. These values are usually very low β-hCG values, but values up to 700 mIU/mL have been reported. Because these antibodies do not pass into the urine, a negative urine β-hCG can be used to help confirm these antibodies. Dilutional assays done by the laboratory also may be used.

Chemotherapy is indicated when β-hCG values plateau or rise after a molar evacuation, for the histologic diagnosis of choriocarcinoma or invasive mole, or for clinical or radiographic evidence of metastasis [1,8••].

Malignant Gestational Trophoblastic Disease

Malignant GTD includes invasive moles, choriocarcinoma, and placental site trophoblastic tumor. Approximately 10% of molar pregnancies are actually invasive moles. Unlike complete or partial moles, invasive moles actually invade into the myometrium of the uterus and its blood vessels. They contain chorionic villi and trophoblastic proliferation. Invasive moles also have the potential to metastasize to the vagina and lung.

Choriocarcinoma is an epithelial cancer that contains neoplastic trophoblasts but not villi. Choriocarcinomas tend to metastasize early in their course; therefore, chemotherapy is indicated when the diagnosis is made. It is especially important to expedite treatment given that areas of metastasis have a propensity to bleed [11].

The final cause of malignant GTD is a very rare form called placental site trophoblastic disease. Histologically, it is characterized by placental site (intermediate) trophoblasts, which are a separate and distinct form compared to villous trophoblasts. Because the syncytiotrophoblasts are frequently absent, β-hCG levels are usually very low, and therefore not a reliable tumor marker [12]. Observing levels of β-hCG and human placental lactogen may assist the clinician in determining response to therapy. Additionally, these tumors are notoriously unresponsive to chemotherapy.

2000 FIGO Criteria for Diagnosis of Postmolar GTD

1) An hCG level plateau of four values ± 10% recorded over a 3-week duration (days 1, 7, 14, and 21)

2) An hCG level increase of more than 10% of three values recorded over a 2-week duration (days 1, 7, and 14)

3) Persistence of detectable hCG for more than 6 months after molar evacuation

Figure 29-2. International Federation of Gynecology and Obstetrics (FIGO) postmole B-human chorionic gonadotropin (β-hCG) criteria. GTD—gestational trophoblastic disease.

Evaluation of Malignant Gestational Trophoblastic Disease

The evaluation of malignant GTD closely follows the initial work-up for a molar pregnancy. These include laboratory studies for complete blood count, electrolytes, liver and renal function, clotting function, and a type and screen. Lung metastasis will almost always precede disseminated metastasis, therefore a CT scan of the chest is required [13,14]. Additional imaging would include CT of the abdomen and pelvis and a CT or MRI of the head.

Today there are three different staging systems for patients with malignant GTD: the 2000 revised FIGO staging system, World Health Organization Prognostic Index Score, and the Clinical Classification System developed from the National Institutes of Health (NIH) [10,15,16]. The new FIGO staging system includes a modified version of the World Health Organization Prognostic Index Score and has been shown in a retrospective review to correlate better with outcome than the original World Health Organization classification [17]. The FIGO scoring system is currently the one most frequently used [8••].

The FIGO scoring system gives a numerical risk score that is based on points given for eight different prognostic indicators. Points of 0, 1, 2, and 4 are awarded for each of the eight different prognostic indicators, and these points are then summed.

A total score of 0 to 6 is considered low risk, whereas 7 or greater is high risk (Figure 29-3). Under the FIGO system, an anatomic stage (I to IV) is given based on location of the tumor, and a risk score is also calculated (Figure 29-4). Most deaths related to GTD are among women who fall into the high-risk category. For this reason, any high-risk patient should be transferred to a physician with experience in this field.

Treatment of Malignant Gestational Trophoblastic Disease

LOW RISK

Malignant GTD was the first solid tumor cured by chemotherapy. Li et al. [18•], at the NIH, successfully treated and cured a case of choriocarcinoma with methotrexate in 1956. Many other chemotherapy drugs have now been used successfully as single agents or in combination. These include dactinomycin, etoposide, 5-flourouracil, 6-mercaptopurine, and cisplatin [8••].

Nonmetastatic GTD can often be successfully treated with single-agent chemotherapy. A Gynecologic Oncology Group prospective phase 2 trial examined single-agent, once-weekly intramuscular injections of 30 to 50 mg/m^2 of methotrexate and found a 70% to 80% primary remission rate [19]. This schedule

Revised FIGO Scoring System

FIGO Score	0	1	2	4
Age, y	< 39	> 39		
Antecedent pregnancy	Hydatidiform mole	Abortion	Term pregnancy	
Interval from index pregnancy, mo	< 4	> 4	7–12	> 12
Pretreatment human chorionic gonadotropin level, mIU/mL	< 1000	1000–10,000	> 10,000–100,000	> 100,000
Largest tumor size including uterus, cm	3–4	5		
Site of metastases	Lung, vagina	Spleen, kidney	Gastrointestinal tract	Brain, liver
Number of metastases identified	0	1–4	4–8	> 8
Previous failed chemotherapy			Single-drug	Two or more drugs

The total score for a patient is obtained by adding the individual scores for each prognostic factor. Total score 0–6 = low risk; > 7 = high risk.

Figure 29-3. Revised International Federation of Gynecology and Obstetrics (FIGO) scoring system. (*Adapted from* Kohorn [10].)

FIGO Staging for Gestational Trophoblastic Disease

Stage	Characteristics
I	Confined to the uterus
II	Extends outside of the uterus, but limited to genital structures
III	Lung extension
IV	Any other metastatic site

Figure 29-4. International Federation of Gynecology and Obstetrics (FIGO) staging system.

is continued until the patient's β-hCG returns to baseline. If additional doses are given after the β-hCG normalizes, a less than 5% recurrence rate can be expected [20].

For patients wishing to maintain their fertility, hysterectomy is not required. However, if a patient no longer desires fertility, then a hysterectomy will shorten the duration and, therefore, the amount of chemotherapy needed [21]. This operation is often performed between the first and second doses of chemotherapy.

In patients who have a rising or plateau in their β-hCG, a different single-agent chemotherapy should be attempted. If the alternative single agent fails or there is evidence of metastasis, then multiagent chemotherapy is warranted. Hysterectomy can still be considered as long as there is no evidence of spread outside of the uterus [22]. Primary remission rates for nonmetastatic GTD approaches 100% [1].

Metastatic low-risk GTD, like the nonmetastatic variant, also can usually be cured with chemotherapy [1,8••]. Initial treatment usually consists of single-agent methotrexate or dactinomycin [23,24]. Unfortunately, almost 40% of these patients will require additional treatment [24]. Recurrence rates are usually less than 5% [20].

HIGH RISK

High-risk malignant GTD is found in those patients with a FIGO risk score of 7 or greater. These patients are treated aggressively with multiagent chemotherapy. Radiation and surgery also may be required as part of their treatment. Survival has been reported as high as 84% by trophoblastic disease centers [1,10]. Classically, in the United States, triple-agent chemotherapy with methotrexate, dactinomycin, and chlorambucil or cyclophosphamide was the standard [1,8]. Many centers across the country are now using a chemotherapy combination referred to as EMA/CO (etoposide, methotrexate, and dactinomycin alternating with cyclophosphamide and vincristine) [25]. To date, no direct comparison has been made between triple-agent chemotherapy and EMA/CO.

The treatment of brain metastasis is still controversial. Currently, radiation to the head along with multiagent chemotherapy or multiagent chemotherapy and intrathecally administered chemotherapy are being used [26,27]. Additionally, there is no clear consensus for the treatment of liver metastasis. Chemoresistant areas of metastasis may require radiation or surgical removal. These treatments also can be used for areas of hemorrhage [1,8••].

Chemotherapy is continued for at least two to three additional cycles after the β-hCG normalizes. As many as 13% of patients with high-risk disease will recur, even after their β-hCG reaches zero [20].

Follow-up from Malignant Gestational Trophoblastic Disease

Patients should have serial β-hCG drawn every 2 weeks for 3 months, and then every month for 1 year after they complete

their treatment. The risk of later recurrence is around 1% [20]. As with a molar pregnancy, patients should be encouraged to utilize hormonal contraception during this follow-up period. An early transvaginal ultrasound should be performed to confirm a normal intrauterine pregnancy in the event of subsequent pregnancy after a preceding molar pregnancy.

References

Papers of particular interest have been highlighted as follows:
• Of interest
•• Of outstanding interest

1. Diagnosis and treatment of gestational trophoblastic disease. ACOG Practice Bulletin No. 53. *Obstet Gynecol* 2004, 103:1365–1377.

2. Freedman RS, Tortolero-Luna G, Pandey DK, *et al.*: Gestational trophoblastic disease. *Obstet Gynecol Clin North Am* 1996, 23:545.

3. Grimes DA: Epidemiology of gestational trophoblastic disease. *Am J Obstet Gynecol* 1984, 150:309.

4. Bracken MB: Incidence and aetiology of hydatidiform mole: an epidemiological review. *Br J Obstet Gynaecol* 1987, 94:1123.

5. Tidy JA, Gillespie AM, Bright N, *et al.*: Gestational trophoblastic disease: a study of mode of evacuation and subsequent need for treatment with chemotherapy. *Gynecol Oncol* 2000, 78: 309–312.

6. Schlaerth JB, Morrow CP, Month FJ, Ablaing G: Initial management of hydatidiform mole. *Am J Obstet Gynecol* 1998, 158:1299–1306.

7. Miller BE: Gestational trophoblastic disease. In *Obstetrics & Gynecology Principles for Practice*. Edited by Ling FW, Duff P. New York: McGraw-Hill; 2001.

8.•• Soper JT: Gestational trophoblastic disease. *Obstet Gynecol* 2006, 108:176–187.
Excellent article looking at specific treatments for advanced gestational trophoblastic disease.

9. Curry SL, Schlaerth JB, Kohorn EL, *et al.*: Hormonal contraception and trophoblastic sequelae after Hydatidiform mole. *Am J Obstet Gynecol* 1989, 160:805–811.

10. Kohorn EL: The new FIGO 2000 staging and risk factor scoring system for gestational trophoblastic disease: description and clinical assessment. *Int J Gynecol Cancer* 2001, 11:73–77.

11. Soper JT, Lewis JL Jr, Hammond CB: Gestational trophoblastic disease. In *Principles and Practice of Gynecologic Oncology*, 2nd ed. Edited by Hoskins WJ, Perez CA, Young RC. Philadelphia: Lippincott-Raven; 1997:1039–1077.

12. Papadopoulos AL, Foskett M, Seckl MJ, *et al.*: Twenty-five years' clinical experience with placental site trophoblastic tumors. *J Reprod Med* 2002, 47:460–464.

13. Soper JT, Clarke-Pearson DL, Hammond CB: Metastatic gestational trophoblastic disease: prognostic factors in previously untreated patients. *Obstet Gynecol* 1988, 71:338–343.

14. Mutch DG, Soper JT, Baker ME, *et al.*: Role of computed axial tomography of the chest in staging patients with non-metastatic gestational trophoblastic disease. *Obstet Gynecol* 1986, 68:348–352.

15. World Health Organization Scientific Group: Gestational trophoblastic disease. *World Health Organ Tech Rep Ser* 1983, 692:1–80.

16. Soper JT, Evans AC, Conaway MR, *et al.*: Evaluation of prognostic factors and staging in gestational trophoblastic tumor. *Obstet Gynecol* 1994, 84:969–973.

17. Hancock BW, Welch EM, Gillespie AM, Newlands ES: A retrospective comparison of current and proposed staging and scoring systems for persistent gestational trophoblastic disease. *Int J Gynecol Cancer* 2000, 10:318–322.

18.• Li MC, Hertz R, Spencer DB: Effect of methotrexate therapy upon choriocarcinoma and chorioadenoma. *Proc Soc Exp Biol Med* 1956, 93:361.
Seminal article showing effective treatment of a neoplastic condition using chemotherapy.

19. Homesley HD, Blessing JA, Rettenmaier M, *et al.*: Weekly intramuscular methotrexate for nonmetastatic gestational trophoblastic disease. *Obstet Gynecol* 1988, 72:413–418.

20. Mutch DG, Soper JT, Babcock CJ, *et al.*: Recurrent gestational trophoblastic disease: experience of the Southeastern Regional Trophoblastic Disease Center. *Cancer* 1990, 66:978–982.

21. Suzuka K, Matsui H, Iitsuka Y, *et al.*: Adjuvant hysterectomy in low-risk gestational trophoblastic disease. *Obstet Gynecol* 2001, 97:431–434.

22. Hammond CB, Weed JC Jr., Currie JL: The role of operation in the current therapy of gestational trophoblastic disease. *Am J Obstet Gynecol* 1980, 136:844–858.

23. Roberts JP, Lurain M: Treatment of low-risk metastatic gestational trophoblastic tumors with single-agent chemotherapy. *Am J Obstet Gynecol* 1996, 174:1917–1923.

24. Soper JT, Clarke-Pearson DL, Berchuck A, *et al.*: Five-day methotrexate for women with metastatic gestational trophoblastic disease. *Gynecol Oncol* 1994, 54:76–79.

25. Bower M, Newlands ES, Holden L, *et al.*: EMA/CO for high-risk gestational trophoblastic tumors: Results from a cohort of 272 patients. *J Clin Oncol* 1997, 15:2636–2643.

26. Evans AC Jr, Soper JT, Clarke-Pearson DL, *et al.*: Gestational trophoblastic disease metastatic to the central nervous system. *Gynecol Oncol* 1995, 59:226–230.

27. Rustin GJ, Newlands ES, Begent RH, *et al.*: Weekly alternating etoposide, methotrexate, and actinomycin/vincristine and cyclophosphamide chemotherapy for the treatment of CNS metastases of choriocarcinoma. *J Clin Oncol* 1989, 7:900–903.

Stress Urinary Incontinence

30

Renée M. Ward and Deborah L. Myers

- Stress urinary incontinence can greatly impact quality of life. It is associated with significant social and economic burdens as well as higher rates of depression, and in the elderly, institutionalization.
- Evaluation of stress urinary incontinence in women should include an evaluation for other co-existing defects in the pelvic floor.
- Urodynamics can be used to confirm urodynamic stress incontinence and to evaluate for other disorders such as detrusor overactivity. Urodynamics are not essential for the routine evaluation of stress incontinence in an uncomplicated patient, especially before trying conservative treatment modalities.
- Successful treatment can often be achieved with conservative measures such as physical and behavioral therapy. Continence pessaries can also be used effectively.
- For patients desiring surgical treatment, retropubic midurethral slings are safe and effective. This is now the most common surgical treatment for stress incontinence, although other treatments may be preferred in certain populations.

Introduction

Stress urinary incontinence (SUI) is estimated to affect 12.2% of adult women [1]. In the United States, the estimated annual direct cost for female urinary incontinence is $12.43 billion, the majority of which is due to the costs of sanitary protection, laundry, and caregiver labor [2]. Although many women do not discuss incontinence with health care providers because they have only mild symptoms, others are reluctant to broach the subject due to shame and embarrassment [3].

Women with urinary incontinence indicate that it negatively impacts their quality of life [4–6]. Specifically, activities involving unfamiliar locations where the availability of restrooms is unknown can be distressing [7]. Among women with SUI, 77.5% report their symptoms to be bothersome, with 28.8% reporting their symptoms to be moderately to extremely bothersome. As would be expected, the degree of bother is associated with the severity of SUI [8]. The majority of patients seek out protective undergarments as a first step in managing the problem [5]. Women may complain of the odor and of the fear of public accidents. Additionally, urinary incontinence is a major burden for caregivers of women with other disabling conditions. The additional hygienic concerns, laundry, and cost of protective

undergarments often overwhelms family caregivers and leads to institutionalization, poignantly attested to by the fact that 50% of nursing home residents are incontinent of urine [9].

There are multiple types of urinary incontinence, but the main types seen in adult women are stress, urge, and mixed incontinence (Figure 30-1). SUI, as defined by the International

Classification of Urinary Incontinence

Stress incontinence

Urge incontinence

Mixed incontinence

Overflow incontinence

Anatomic abnormalities

  Fistula

  Urethral diverticulum

  Ectopic ureter

Functional incontinence

Figure 30-1. Classification of urinary incontinence.

Continence Society, is the complaint of involuntary leakage on effort or exertion, or on sneezing or coughing [10]. Typically, it is small volume leakage, but can be of large volume if excessive Valsalva activities occur. Urge incontinence is leakage associated with the sensation of urgency and can be the result of involuntary detrusor contractions. Mixed incontinence is a combination of both stress and urge and is treated by addressing the pathophysiology of both components. Therapeutically, it is important to distinguish which type of incontinence is present, as this will guide management. Although history alone is not adequate for diagnosis, complaints suggestive of SUI are relatively specific for its presence [11]. This chapter will focus on SUI.

Epidemiology

The prevalence of SUI depends on the strictness of the criteria used (Figure 30-2). Among women with urinary incontinence, SUI predominates until 59 years of age. At more advanced ages, mixed incontinence is the most prevalent, followed by SUI, and urge incontinence, respectively [12].

Among women with weekly incontinence, only 40% will seek treatment from a physician. In fact, women with moderate to severe incontinence are more likely to use a coping strategy than a medical therapy for their symptoms. Over 60% use protective undergarments or absorbent pads, and 12% avoid activities which aggravate their symptoms [5]. The first step in medically helping women with SUI is for the physician to ask the patient if she has bothersome leakage.

There are multiple risk factors for SUI: advanced age, parity, smoking, and higher body mass index [1,13–15]. Although the cause of a woman's incontinence is often attributed to child bearing, the effects of parity are not straightforward. Most

studies show a decreased risk of SUI after cesarean delivery when compared to a vaginal delivery [1,16], but the benefit of a cesarean delivery appears to wane when patients reach 65 years of age [17]. During pregnancy, there is a higher incidence of SUI due to the added pressure of the gravid uterus resting on the bladder. Postpartum, transient urinary incontinence is very common. This resolves or lessens in the majority of women as normal anatomic relationships resume and the pelvic floor regains strength.

Multiple studies show that depression is more common among women with urinary incontinence [18,19]. Of middle-aged women (50–69 years), those with mild to moderate incontinence are 40% more likely to have depression, whereas those with severe incontinence are 80% more likely to have depression as compared to continent women [19].

Mild physical activities are protective. For instance, the prevalence of SUI is lower among women who regularly do low impact physical activity such as walking [14,20]. This protective benefit persists even when controlling for body mass index.

Nearly 60% of institutionalized women 65 years of age or older have urinary incontinence [21]. In fact, just the presence of urinary incontinence increases the risk of hospitalization and admission to a nursing home, independent of the presence of other diseases [22]. Early identification and treatment of urinary incontinence may allow family caregivers to be able to continue home care. Moreover, nursing home staff spend a considerable amount of time caring for incontinence. Diagnosis and treatment of the incontinence not only helps the patient, but may free care givers for other responsibilities. Although the topic of urinary incontinence is discussed more openly today than in the past, patients are still often reluctant to volunteer their symptomatology.

Diagnostic Methods

In taking the history, the health care provider should ask the woman whether she leaks urine during times of increased activity. Pertinent questions include inquiring about the duration of symptoms, amount of leakage, and whether pads are required for protection. Questions about aggravating factors and precipitating events before leakage episodes can help distinguish stress from urge incontinence. In SUI, women typically complain of leakage with coughing, sneezing, laughing, and running. Urge incontinence tends to be larger volume leakage which often cannot be predicted. Urge incontinence can be triggered by cues such as running water, "pulling into the driveway," or "putting the key in the door." Patients with urge incontinence also tend to have urinary frequency, urgency, and nocturia. It is important to ask about any history of bladder problems, recurrent urinary tract infections, hematuria, or pelvic organ prolapse. One should query about voiding problems, urinary hesitancy, and incomplete bladder emptying. Information about drinking habits is very pertinent. On should ask how much water, soda, caffeine, and artificially sweetened beverages does she consume daily? Caffeine is a bladder irritant and can relax smooth muscle. Although more often considered as

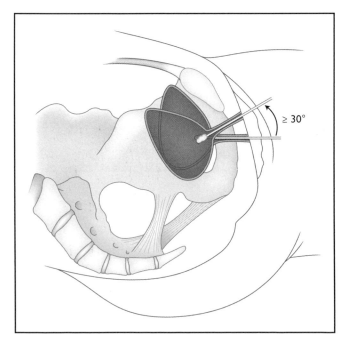

Figure 30-2. Cotton swab test demonstrating urethral hypermobility.

part of the treatment for urge incontinence, limiting its intake can help people with SUI as well.

Objectively assessing the patient begins with evaluating her mobility and body mass index. Patients who are unable to reach the bathroom in a timely manner have functional incontinence, which can coexist with SUI. The physical examination needs to involve an abdominal examination to evaluate for any masses which could be pressing on the bladder, a neurologic evaluation, and a pelvic examination.

The neurologic examination should evaluate mental status, sensory and motor function of the lower extremities, and sacral nerves S2–S4, which control micturition. Sensory function of the sacral nerves can be evaluated by sharp and light touch discrimination over the inner thigh and perineum. One can evaluate for intact anal and bulbocavernosus reflexes; however, these reflexes can be absent, even in neurologically intact women. The anal reflex is tested by gently stroking the perianal skin and watching for contraction of the external anal sphincter. In the bulbocavernosus reflex, gently tapping the labia near the clitoris results in contraction of the bulbocavernosus and ischiocavernosus muscles.

On the pelvic examination, one should look for any vulvar rash secondary to urine, urethral or vaginal masses, and vaginal atrophy. To check for a urethral diverticulum, the urethra should be palpated and milked in order to express urine from the diverticulum; pain may or may not be present. Urethral hypermobility can be detected by placing a cotton-tipped swab into the urethra such that the tip rests at the urethrovesical junction (Figure 30-2). A result of 30 degrees or more with Valsalva indicates hypermobility.

Inspect for any pelvic organ prolapse, especially a cystocele. This can be done with a monovalve speculum placed against the posterior vaginal wall and then observing the degree of anterior vaginal wall descent that occurs with Valsalva. When the anterior vaginal wall descends within 1 cm of the hymen, patients often become symptomatic from the prolapse, and the concurrent treatment of the cystocele and SUI should be considered. Also, check pelvic floor muscle strength by having the patient perform a Kegel squeeze. Place two fingers in the vagina and instruct the patient to squeeze and internally lift the vagina. A proper Kegel squeeze is performed without holding the breath, squeezing the buttocks, or adducting the thighs. The strength of a Kegel squeeze can be qualitatively described as strong, weak, or absent or by a validated grading system such as the Oxford scale of 1 through 5 [10].

Next, one should examine for leakage. This can be done initially with an empty bladder and having the patient cough. Visible leakage confirms a positive empty cough stress test and is indicative of significant SUI (Figure 30-3). A catheter can then be placed to measure the postvoid residual, or alternatively, one can perform a bladder ultrasound. Less than 50 mL is considered normal and greater than 200 mL is abnormal. Values in between need to be interpreted in the context of each individual patient [23].

With the catheter still in place (useful items are a red rubber catheter or a 14-French, long female catheter), filling cystometry can be performed. The end of a 60 mL catheter-tip syringe can be attached to the tubing and the bladder is filled with sterile water. Typically patients are filled to capacity or to approximately 300 mL. Then, with the catheter removed, examine for leakage with a large cough. This cough stress test can be repeated in a standing position if no leakage is seen while in lithotomy. If the patient has significant prolapse, this test should be performed both with and without reduction of the prolapse. Long proctoswabs supporting the vaginal walls, a monovalved speculum or a pessary may be used to reduce the prolapse. If leakage occurs only with reduction of the prolapse, this indicates that occult stress incontinence is present. The patient is unlikely to be bothered by the incontinence unless her prolapse is treated.

Another way to objectively evaluate for incontinence is with a pad test. A preweighed pad is worn for 1 hour while the woman is active. The pad is then weighed, thus quantifying the amount of leakage in 1 hour. Provocative maneuvers, such as coughing, should be performed during the test period. An alternative is to weigh pads that have been collected for a 24-hour period. Typically the used pads are transported or mailed in a resealable bag.

Few laboratory tests are needed in the evaluation of SUI, but a urinalysis and urine culture from a midstream, clean catch, or catheterized specimen are helpful. If other urologic abnormalities are detected, such as microscopic hematuria, this merits its own evaluation. Serum creatinine and blood urea nitrogen should be evaluated in any patient at risk of compromised renal function.

A bladder diary can be very helpful when assessing complaints of incontinence. Times of micturition, the amount voided, incontinence episodes, pad usage, and fluid intake are recorded on a timed log for 48 to 72 hours. The degree of incontinence can be graded as dampness, a wet pad/undergarment, or soaking/complete emptying of the bladder. The patient also records what activity she was doing when leakage occurred. This assists the provider in categorizing leakage as stress or urge related. A specipan to collect and measure the urine enhances the utility of the diary. Often keeping the diary assists the patient in identifying problematic behaviors such as drinking large volumes of fluid.

Additional information about how the bladder functions can be obtained with multichannel urodynamics. This is

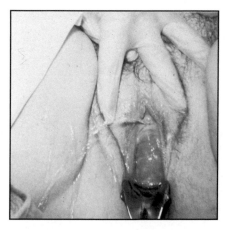

Figure 30-3. Leakage in a woman with stress urinary incontinence.

particularly useful for women contemplating surgical management, with complaints of mixed incontinence, a history of prior anti-incontinence procedures, advanced prolapse, neurologic symptoms, or advanced age. In some patients, cystoscopy to evaluate for bladder lesions or a foreign body due to prior anti-incontinence procedures will be indicated.

Treatment

Surgical and nonsurgical treatments for SUI are listed in Figures 30-4 and 30-5.

BEHAVIORAL/PHYSICAL THERAPY

Stress incontinence does not need to be treated unless it is bothersome to the patient. For those desiring treatment, first-line management is behavioral and physical therapy.

Strengthening the pelvic floor muscles provides enhanced urethral support and is effective at curing, or at least improving, stress urinary incontinence. These changes can be long-standing for two thirds of women if they regularly perform pelvic floor muscle exercises [24].

Pelvic floor muscle training, also known as Kegel exercises, needs to be done on a daily basis. To strengthen both the slow- and fast-twitch muscle fibers of the pubococcygeus muscle, two different types of exercises are needed. The first are slow, long squeezes for up to several seconds. The second are repetitive, fast squeezes. Pelvic floor muscle strength training mimics the generalized strength training of other muscle groups by building up to 10 slow and 10 fast squeezes three to four times a day. Instructing patients to tighten and internally lift can be useful. Additionally, patients should isolate the muscle and should not involve their abdominal, gluteal, or adductor muscles. Patients who mistakenly perform Valsalva when instructed to do Kegel exercises can exacerbate pelvic floor disorders. These patients need to learn how to properly tighten the pubococcygeous muscles. Verbal encouragement from the physician has been helpful and motivating for patients. Motivation can also come from measuring the strength of the Kegel squeeze and documenting this at each visit.

Low-technology ways to teach Kegel exercises can be as simple as having the patient perform a digital examination or use a mirror to confirm that the pelvic floor is contracting. There are multiple devices—vaginal weights, balls, and cones— designed to assist patients with performing Kegel exercises. The exercises can be performed equally well without these devices, but some patients may find them helpful. Ensure that reputable products are used as there are some commercialized products advertised for the pelvic floor that actually work the adductors of the thigh. For patients who are unable to contract the pelvic floor, working with a pelvic floor physical therapist may be needed. Physical therapists use biofeedback and electrical stimulation to help patients learn when they are contracting and relaxing the pelvic floor.

Bladder irritants such as caffeine and artificial sweeteners should be limited. Moreover, education about water intake can be helpful. The recommendation for six to eight glasses of water daily refers to the total water intake needed, including that from food sources [25••]. Generally, if patients are not thirsty, they do not need to force the intake of water.

CONSERVATIVE TREATMENT/PUBOURETHRAL SUPPORT

In SUI, the pubourethral connective tissue is weakened. Normally, during Valsalva, the female urethra is compressed against the pubourethral fascia; thus allowing for continence to be maintained. Strong pubococcygeal muscles help bolster the pubourethral tissues. Devices placed in the vagina can also augment this support.

Some pessaries, such as the continence ring or dish, are made to provide extra support under the urethra. These are particularly useful for patients with a concurrent cystocele. Some women complain of SUI only with specific activities such as running or aerobics. For these women, the placement of a super-sized tampon may provide enough urethral support for them to stay dry during these activities. Another option is a urethral plug, such as FemSoft (Rochester Medical Corporation, Stewartville, MN).

Nonsurgical Treatment of Stress Urinary Incontinence

Behavior modification
  Timed voids
  Limit caffeine intake
Physical therapy
  Pelvic floor muscle training (Kegel exercises)
  Biofeedback
  Pelvic floor electrical stimulation
Mechanical devices
  Absorbent products (pads)
  Continence pessaries
  Urethral plugs
Pharmacologic therapy
  Alpha-adrenergic agonists
  Tricyclic antidepressants

Figure 30-4. Nonsurgical treatment of stress urinary incontinence.

Surgical Treatment of Stress Urinary Incontinence

Minimally invasive slings
  Retropubic approach (TVT)
  Transobturator approach
Burch retropubic urethropexy
Traditional bladder neck sling
Urethral bulking agents

Figure 30-5. Surgical treatment of stress urinary incontinence. TVT—tension-free vaginal tape.

MEDICATIONS

Medical management for urinary incontinence is usually reserved for urge incontinence, as the anticholinergics are very useful for this disorder. There are medical treatments for stress incontinence; however, their success is often limited.

Alpha agonists work by constricting the urethra. Pseudo-ephedrine hydrochloride can be used for this purpose. Side effects include drowsiness, hypertension, and dry mouth. Treatment can start at 30 mg by mouth twice a day. Phenylpropanolamine hydrochloride has been taken off the market.

Imipramine hydrochloride is a tricyclic antidepressant with alpha-agonist and anticholinergic effects. Serious side effects include orthostatic hypotension, syncope, and multiple cardiovascular effects, especially in the elderly. Common side effects include drowsiness, tachycardia, dry mouth, constipation, and blurred vision. Dosing is lower than that used to treat depression, starting at 10 to 25 mg in the evening and increasing to a maximum of 75 mg twice a day.

For years, estrogen was cited as a treatment for SUI. Multiple studies now show that it does not improve [26] and may aggravate [27,28] SUI. Whereas topical estrogen is appropriate in the treatment of atrophic vaginitis, which may coexist with SUI, it should not be used for the treatment of SUI.

SURGERY

For patients who have failed other treatments, surgery may be a very appropriate choice. Historically, over 100 different surgeries have been described for the management of female SUI; however, today only procedures with over 80% effectiveness at 48 months or procedures with very minimal morbidity are typically used. This means that the anterior repair, Kelly plication, and transvaginal needle suspensions should no longer be used in the treatment of SUI [29•]. More recent data suggest that the Marshall-Marchetti-Krantz urethropexy has long-term success rates of 60%; so it has fallen out of favor as well [30,31]. The Burch retropubic urethropexy, traditional pubovaginal slings, and minimally invasive midurethral slings are commonly used modern surgical treatments for SUI. With the introduction of the minimally invasive midurethral slings and their relative ease of use, shorter length-of-stay, and high efficacy, they have become a popular choice. Urethral bulking agents, although they have a low success rate, are still used due to their minimal surgical morbidity.

The Burch retropubic urethropexy is used to treat SUI in the setting of urethral hypermobility. A retropubic dissection is performed, typically through an abdominal incision. Sutures are placed through the periurethral fascia and attached to Cooper's ligament to help stabilize the bladder neck. The Burch urethropexy has been the gold standard for the surgical treatment of SUI; however, randomized controlled trials have shown that minimally invasive retropubic midurethral slings are of equivalent efficacy and have lower rates of blood loss, less analgesic requirements, and fewer postoperative complications [32•,33]. When comparing a laparoscopic Burch to a retropubic midurethral sling, the sling had better subjective and objective success with equivalent complication rates [34]. For patients wishing to avoid the use of permanent mesh or

who plan to have an abdominal surgery, the Burch urethropexy is still a valid option.

Traditional bladder neck slings have become less popular due to the increased dissection needed and the efficacy of the newer, minimally invasive slings; however, traditional slings are still an effective alternative. Cadaveric or autologous fascia can be used as an alternative to mesh in these procedures.

An array of minimally invasive midurethral slings now exist, but the tension-free vaginal tape (TVT; Ethicon, Somerville, NJ) sling was the first that was well-tolerated, with a low risk of erosion and a high rate of efficacy [35]. Long-term data have shown cure rates of 78% to 85% [32•,36]. Designed to create a firm backboard for the urethra to be compressed against during a Valsalva maneuver, these slings are placed loosely so as to minimize postoperative urinary retention. They require minimal dissection and thus can be performed on an outpatient basis under local anesthesia. Moreover, these slings are placed at the midurethra, not the bladder neck, which is a change from traditional sling procedures.

Because of the success of the retropubic midurethral slings, there are now multiple variations to this procedure. These vary in how they are placed, as well as the materials used for the sling. In general, permanent, macroporous, monofilament mesh seems well-tolerated. Meshes with small pores and braided materials have been more prone to erosions and postoperative infections. Complications of midurethral slings include bleeding, infection, erosion, neuropathy, bladder injury, and urinary retention. Cystourethroscopy must be performed at the time of placement to ensure that there is no bladder injury. Most complications can be managed, but there are case reports of patient death due to hemorrhage, bowel injury, and sepsis [37].

In an attempt to minimize the risk of bleeding and bladder injury from retropubic midurethral slings, a transobturator approach was introduced in 2001 [38]. Currently, there is insufficient data to determine if the retropubic or transobturator approach has better objective outcomes, but subjective success rates are similar. There are lower rates of peri-operative hematoma, infection, vascular, and bladder injuries with the transobturator approach [39], but there are higher rates of vaginal erosions and groin pain [40].

Urethral bulking agents are often chosen for women with multiple comorbidities and who are poor surgical candidates. Cross-linked bovine collagen has been used for many years and can be injected transurethrally or periurethrally to bulk up the walls of the urethra. Because collagen is a biologic material, it is eventually degraded, so repeat injections are usually needed. When effective, patients may be dry for 3 to 6 months, with rare cases of longer results. Among women with severe SUI, objective incontinence as assessed by pad weight is improved after collagen injections, but between 50% and 75% will have persistent symptoms [41].

Multiple attempts have been made to create a permanent urethral bulking agent. Carbon-coated beads and calcium hydroxylapatite are two materials currently on the market. A downside of carbon-coated beads is bead migration. The initial data regarding calcium hydroxyapatite are promising, but studies which are independently funded and have long-term follow-up are needed.

New products are continually being developed. As with all new medical technology, products need to be rigorously tested and compared to current treatments before being used on a widespread basis.

Conclusions

Stress urinary incontinence is a common and treatable condition. Conservative treatments, including behavioral and physical therapy, should be the first approach for all patients. Referral to a urogynecologist or female urologist is appropriate when patients have refractory symptoms, desire surgical therapy, and have had prior anti-incontinence surgery, neurologic disease, or associated pelvic organ prolapse.

References

Papers of particular interest have been highlighted as follows:
• Of interest
•• Of outstanding interest

1. Rortveit G, Dalveit AK, Hannested YS, Hunskaar S: Urinary incontinence after vaginal delivery or cesarean section. *N Engl J Med* 2003, 348:900–907.

2. Wilson L, Brown JS, Shin GP, Luc KO, Subak LL: Annual direct cost of urinary incontinence. *Obstet Gynecol* 2001, 98:398–406.

3. Minassian VA, Drutz HP, Al-Badr A: Urinary incontinence as a worldwide problem. *Int J Gynaecol Obstet* 2003, 82:327–338.

4. Subak LL, Brown JS, Kraus SR, et al.: The "costs" of urinary incontinence for women. *Obstet Gynecol* 2006, 107:908–916.

5. Huang AJ, Brown JS, Kanaya AM, et al.: Quality-of-life impact and treatment of urinary incontinence in ethnically diverse older women. *Arch Intern Med* 2006, 166:2000–2006.

6. Dubeau CE, Simon SE, Morris JN: The effect of urinary incontinence on quality of life in older nursing home residents. *J Am Geriatr Soc* 2006, 54:1325–1333.

7. Wyman JF, Harkins SW, Choi SC, et al.: Psychosocial impact of urinary incontinence in women. *Obstet Gynecol* 1987, 70:378–381.

8. Fultz NH, Burgio K, Diokno AC, et al.: Burden of stress urinary incontinence for community-dwelling women. *Am J Obstet Gynecol* 2003, 189:1275–1282.

9. Ouslander JG, Kane RL, Abrass IB: Urinary incontinence in elderly nursing home patients. *JAMA* 1982, 248:1194–1198.

10. Abrams P, Cardozo L, Fall M, et al.: The standardization of terminology of lower urinary tract function: report from the Standardization Subcommittee of the International Continence Society. *Am J Obstet Gynecol* 2002, 187:116–126.

11. Weidner AC, Myers ER, Visco AG, et al.: Which women with stress incontinence require urodynamic evaluation? *Am J Obstet Gynecol* 2001, 184:20–27.

12. Hannestad YS, Rortveit G, Sandvik H, Hunskaar S: A community-based epidemiological survey of female urinary incontinence: the Norwegian EPINCONT study. Epidemiology of Incontinence in the County of Nord-Trondelag. *J Clin Epidemiol* 2000, 53:1150–1157.

13. Brown JS, Grady D, Ouslander JG, et al.: Prevalence of urinary incontinence and associated risk factors in post-menopausal women. Heart & Estrogen/Progestin Replacement Study (HERS) Research Group. *Obstet Gynecol* 1999, 94:66–70.

14. Hannestad YS, Rortveit G, Daltveit AK, Hunskaar S: Are smoking and other lifestyle factors associated with female urinary incontinence? The Norwegian EPINCONT Study. *Br J Obstet Gynecol* 2003, 110:247–254.

15. Bump RC, McClish DK: Cigarette smoking and urinary incontinence in women. *Am J Obstet Gynecol* 1992, 167:1213–1218.

16. Kuh D, Cardozo L, Hardy R: Urinary incontinence in middle aged women: childhood enuresis and other lifetime risk factors in a British prospective cohort. *J Epidemiol Comm Health* 1999, 53:453–458.

17. Rortveit G, Hannestad YS, Daltveit AK, Hunskaar S: Age- and type-dependent effects of parity on urinary incontinence: the Norwegian EPINCONT study. *Obstet Gynecol* 2001, 98:1004–1010.

18. Melville JL, Delaney K, Newton K, Katon W: Incontinence severity and major depression in incontinent women. *Obstet Gynecol* 2005, 106:585–592.

19. Nygaard I, Turvey C, Burns TL, et al.: Urinary incontinence and depression in middle-aged United States women. *Obstet Gynecol* 2003, 101:149–156.

20. Danforth KN, Shah AD, Townsend MK, et al.: Physical activity and urinary incontinence among healthy, older women. *Obstet Gynecol* 2007, 109:721–727.

21. Aggazotti G, Pesce F, Grassi D, et al.: Prevalence of urinary incontinence among institutionalized patients: a cross-sectional epidemiologic study in a midsized city in northern Italy. *Urology* 2000, 56:245–249.

22. Thom DH, Haan MN, Van den Edeen SK: Medically recognized urinary incontinence and risks of hospitalization, nursing home admission and mortality. *Age Aging* 1997, 26:367–374.

23. Urinary Incontinence Guideline Panel: *Urinary Incontinence in Adults. Clinical Practice Guideline No. 2, 1996 Update.* Rockville, MD: U.S. Department of Health and Human Services; 1996. AHCPR Publication No. 96-0682.

24. Hay–Smith EJ, Dumoulin C: Pelvic floor muscle training versus no treatment, or inactive control treatments, for urinary incontinence in women. *Cochrane Database Syst Rev* 2006, CD005654.

25.•• Norton P, Brubaker L: Urinary incontinence in women. *Lancet* 2006, 367:57–67.
This is an excellent, up-to-date review on female urinary incontinence. It includes useful online websites.

26. Waetjen LE, Brown JS, Vittinghoff E, et al.: The effect of ultralow–dose transdermal estradiol on urinary incontinence in postmenopausal women. *Obstet Gynecol* 2005, 106:946–952.

27. Hendrix SL, Cochrane BB, Nygaard IE, et al.: Effects of estrogen with and without progestin on urinary incontinence. *JAMA* 2005, 293:935–948.

28. Steinauer JE, Waetjen LE, Vittinghoff E, et al.: Postmenopausal hormone therapy: does it cause incontinence? *Obstet Gynecol* 2005, 106:940–945.

29.• Leach GE, Dmochowski RR, Appell RA, *et al.*: Female Stress Urinary Incontinence Clinical Guidelines Panel summary report on surgical management of female stress urinary incontinence. The American Urological Association. *J Urol* 1997, 158:875–880.

This report reviewed different surgical techniques for the treatment of stress incontinence and led to a marked decrease in the use of needle suspensions.

30. Hegarty PK, Power PC, O'Brien MF, Bredin HC: Longevity of the Marshall-Marchetti-Krantz procedure. *Ann Chir Gynaecol* 2001, 90:286–289.

31. Demirci F, Yildirium U, Demirci E, *et al.*: Ten-year results of Marshall-Marchetti-Krantz and anterior colporraphy procedures. *Aust N Z J Obstet Gynaecol* 2002, 42:513–514.

32.• Ward KL, Hilton P: A prospective multicenter randomized trial of tension-free vaginal tape and colposuspension for primary urodynamic stress incontinence: two-year follow-up. *Am J Obstet Gynecol* 2004, 190:324–331.

This study showed that the minimally invasive retropubic midurethral slings were as effective as the Burch urethropexy.

33. Ward K, Hilton P: Prospective multicentre randomised trial of tension-free vaginal tape and colposuspension as primary treatment for stress incontinence. *Br Med J* 2002, 325:67.

34. Paraiso MF, Walters MD, Karram MM, Barber MD: Laparoscopic Burch colposuspension versus tension-free vaginal tape: a randomized trial. *Obstet Gynecol* 2004, 104:1249–1258.

35. Ulmsten U, Henriksson L, Johnson P, Varhos G: An ambulatory surgical procedure under local anesthesia for treatment of female urinary incontinence. *Int Urogynecol J Pelvic Floor Dysfunct* 1996, 7:81–85; discussion 85–86.

36. Nilsson CG, Kuuva N, Falconer C, *et al.*: Long-term results of the tension-free vaginal tape (TVT) procedure for surgical treatment of female stress urinary incontinence. *Int Urogynecol J Pelvic Floor Dysfunct* 2001, 12(Suppl 2):S5–S8.

37. Deng DY, Rutman M, Raz S, Rodriguez LV: Presentation and management of major complications of midurethral slings: are complications under-reported? *Neurourol Urodyn* 2007, 26:46–52.

38. Delorme E: Transobturator urethral suspension: mini-invasive procedure in the treatment of stress urinary incontinence in women. *Prog Urol* 2001, 11:1306–1313.

39. Sung VW, Schleinitz MD, Rardin C R, *et al.*: Comparison of retropubic versus transobturator approach to midurethral slings: A systematic review and meta-analysis. *Am J Obstet Gynecol*, 2007, 197:3–11.

40. Latthe PM, Foon R, Toozs-Hobson P: Transobturator and retropubic tape procedures in stress urinary incontinence: a systematic review and meta-analysis of effectiveness and complications. *Br J Obstet Gynecol* 2007, 114:522–531.

41. Groutz A, Blaivis JG, Kesler SS, *et al.*: Outcome results of transurethral collagen injection for female stress incontinence: assessment by urinary incontinence score. *J Urol* 2000, 164:2006–2009.

31 Urinary Tract Infections

Thomas G. Stovall and Erin J. Saunders

- Urinary tract infections affect approximately 25% to 35% of women between the ages of 20 and 40 years.
- Dysuria, urinary frequency, urgency, nocturia, suprapubic pain, hematuria, and incontinence are the most common symptoms.
- *Escherichia coli* is the most common cause of urinary tract infections.
- Asymptomatic bacteriuria should not generally be treated unless the woman is pregnant.
- An uncomplicated urinary tract infection may be diagnosed by symptoms alone and treated with a 3-day course of antibiotics.

Bacteriuria

Traditionally, bacteriuria is defined as 10^5 or greater uropathogens per mL of a voided midstream clean-catch urine culture. However, recent studies have demonstrated that 30% to 50% of women with symptoms of acute cystitis have less than 10^5 bacteria per mL [1,2]. Significant bacteriuria, defined as at least 10^2 bacteria per mL, has a sensitivity of 95% and specificity of 85% for diagnosing acute cystitis in women [1,3]. Women found to have counts less than 10^5 per mL, if left untreated, have more pronounced symptoms and counts higher than 10^5 per mL a few days later [4•]. The Infectious Diseases Society of America consensus definition of cystitis is bacteriuria of at least 10^3 colony-forming units (CFU)/mL and a sensitivity of 80% and specificity of 90% [5].

There may be many reasons why less than 10^5 bacteria per mL are found on a culture: the infection may have been caught at a subsiding stage, it may have been only partially treated, the patient may have just voided, the patient may be taking a diuretic, or the infection may be confined to the urethra. The urinary tract may also be obstructed below the infected area, or the patient may be taking subtherapeutic antibiotics, which would lower the count [1,6••].

Asymptomatic bacteriuria occurs in 3% to 6% of premenopausal women, and is defined as more than 10^5 bacteria per mL of one or more organisms on two clean-catch cultures taken on separate days in the absence of symptoms. Nicolle [7] showed that asymptomatic bacteriuria is overdiagnosed by 10% when only one culture is done.

Asymptomatic Bacteriuria

Asymptomatic bacteriuria is defined as more than 10^5 bacteria per mL of one or more organisms on two clean-catch cultures taken on separate days in the absence of symptoms. The significance and treatment of asymptomatic bacteriuria is dependent on age, comorbidities such as diabetes, renal insufficiency, or the presence of an indwelling catheter, and the history of complicated urinary tract infections (UTIs). In general, unless the woman is pregnant, asymptomatic bacteriuria is not treated.

Asymptomatic bacteriuria is often a dynamic process; that is, it may wax and wane in any particular woman. Whether patients with asymptomatic bacteriuria who have symptomatic episodes should be classified as having symptomatic bacteriuria with asymptomatic episodes, intermittent asymptomatic bacteriuria, or asymptomatic bacteriuria with symptomatic episodes is unclear. Approximately one third of women with asymptomatic bacteriuria eventually have symptomatic episodes.

The prevalence of asymptomatic bacteriuria in full-term infants is less than 10%. During preschool years, asymptomatic bacteriuria occurs in approximately 0.8% of girls, and increases to approximately 5% by age 15. In children, asymptomatic bacteriuria in the absence of reflux or obstruction is benign; however, the presence of reflux can cause focal cortical scars with distortion of the calices. This is a common cause of renal damage during the first 5 years of life. Reflux is not necessarily caused by infection, but infection can increase its severity. Asymptomatic bacteriuria in children may not only be a marker for the presence of underlying reflux or renal damage but also may potentiate existing reflux or renal damage. Young children with asymptomatic bacteriuria should always be investigated for anatomic anomalies of the upper and lower urinary tracts.

The progression in school-aged girls from asymptomatic bacteriuria to renal disease is rare. In one study, girls with asymptomatic bacteriuria and anatomically normal urinary tracts were randomized to treatment and non-treatment groups and were followed for 3 years [8]. Renal growth was normal in both groups. A similar study during the same year confirmed these findings. A trial of 208 girls, aged 5 to 12, randomized to treatment and non-treatment groups and followed over 4 years found no difference between the groups with respect to renal growth, renal function, or frequency of symptomatic infections; thus, the authors could not establish that antimicrobial therapy served any benefit [9].

In approximately 30% of adult, non-pregnant women with asymptomatic bacteriuria, the disease progresses to clinical UTI by 1 year. This does not lead to renal damage in otherwise healthy women, but merely to discomfort and the inconvenience of a bladder infection and should not be treated unless the patient develops symptoms. Population studies have shown that most women with screening asymptomatic bacteriuria previously had symptomatic infection.

Asymptomatic bacteriuria occurs approximately three times more frequently in diabetic women. The cause is most likely related to impaired leukocyte function, recurrent vaginitis, and diabetic microangiopathy. Traditionally, the teaching has been that the bacteriuria is associated with glucose control. However, more recent studies have shown that the prevalence of asymptomatic bacteriuria is not significantly influenced by the duration of diabetes or the quality of its control. In addition, the prevalence of asymptomatic bacteriuria in long-term follow-up studies has not been correlated with the progression or development of diabetic nephropathy [10]. The consequences of untreated asymptomatic bacteriuria in this population are not known.

Risk Factors That Suggest A Complicated Urinary Tract Infection

Indwelling urinary catheter

Functional or anatomic abnormality of the urinary tract

Childhood urinary tract infection

Recent antibiotic use

Symptoms lasting longer than 7 days

Diabetes or other neuropathy

Immunosuppression

Pregnancy

Recent pelvic surgery

Pseudomonas, *Proteus*, or *Klebsiella* species infection

Figure 31-1. Risk factors that suggest a complicated urinary tract infection. (*Adapted from* Johnson and Stamm [11].)

Chronic illness may also contribute to asymptomatic bacteriuria. The most likely contributing factor is a neurologic disease, such as diabetic autonomic neuropathy, Parkinson's disease, Alzheimer's disease, and cerebrovascular disease. These conditions typically cause incomplete voiding, leading to increased residual volume and reflux. The greater the neurologic impairment, the higher the prevalence of bacteriuria.

Acute Cystitis

Acute cystitis, more commonly known as a UTI, is an infection of the mucosal lining of the bladder. Acute cystitis is further classified as uncomplicated and complicated. This distinction is important for diagnosis, treatment, and follow-up. A UTI is uncomplicated if there are no underlying structural or neurologic lesions; it is complicated if obstruction, stones, or neurologic lesions are present or if there is residual inflammation from repeated bacterial invasion (Figure 31-1).

Urethritis is associated with pyuria, rarely hematuria, and bacterial counts of less than 10^2 organisms per milliliter [1]. The most common organisms associated with urethritis are *Neisseria gonorrhoeae*, *Chlamydia trachomatis*, and herpes simplex virus [11]. The patient usually reports the gradual onset of symptoms. Urine cultures typically show negative results [6••]. Vaginitis can be detected by noting that the vaginal discharge has an odor, and there is vulvovaginal itching if yeast is present. Vaginitis is rarely associated with pyuria and hematuria. Urine cultures obtained from patients with vaginitis are usually negative; if positive, the colony counts are less than 10^2 organisms per mL of urine. Patients with, or suspected of having, vaginitis should be evaluated as follows: vaginal pH, whiff test performed on the vaginal discharge, and microscopic examination of the vaginal discharge.

Acute bacterial pyelonephritis is characterized by fever, flank pain, tenderness, increased white blood cell count, leukocyte casts, and bacteriuria. However, upper tract disease may be entirely asymptomatic. Uncomplicated pyelonephritis is associated with bacteremia in 12% of patients [12]. Histologically, acute pyelonephritis is marked by an acute neutrophilic exudate within the tubules and the renal substance. The cortical surface may be dotted with little abscesses. After the acute phase, healing occurs. The inflammatory foci are eventually replaced by scars that can be seen on the cortical surface as fibrous depressions. Chronic or recurrent pyelonephritis appears to be the result of bacterial infection, superimposed on obstructive urinary abnormalities, or vesicoureteral reflux. The latter, in particular, plays a critical role in the spread of infection to the kidney. On intravenous pyelogram, pyelonephritis shows dilation and blunting of the calices.

Incidence and Epidemiology

Urinary tract infections affect approximately 25% to 35% of women between the ages of 20 and 40 years [13], and 50% to 60% of women report having a UTI at some time during their life [14]. UTIs account for more than six million office visits in the United States per year, with an annual health cost exceeding $1 billion. Twenty percent of women who have a UTI have more than three recurrences a year, and approximately 250,000 present initially as acute pyelonephritis. Approximately 15% to 50% of patients with symptoms of acute cystitis are also found to have involvement of the upper urinary tract [1]. Of patients who experience their first episode of acute cystitis, 27% have a recurrence within 6 months [15]. In another study of women aged 17 to 82 years, 44% had a recurrence within 1 year [16••]. Recurrent infection places the patient at risk for pyelonephritis; the ratio of cystitis to pyelonephritis in this setting has been found to be 18:1 to 28:1 [15,16••]. For adult women, having three or more UTIs in 1 year is classified as recurrent or chronic. Evaluation of the bladder and upper urinary tract is necessary to exclude urinary retention, obstruction, and bladder or kidney lesions. As mentioned previously, the presence of an underlying neurologic or structural abnormality is classified as a complicated UTI and alters treatment.

Particular subsets within the group of normal women who may have increased UTIs are those who use a diaphragm and spermicide for birth control. Women using this combination have increased vaginal *Escherichia coli* colonization, and it is thought this is because they decrease the vaginal hydrogen peroxide-producing lactobacilli. This results in increased adherence of *E. coli* to epithelial cells [17–19]. The current hypothesis is that the spermicide jelly or foam introduced into the vagina when used in conjunction with a diaphragm or condom may alter the vaginal pH and flora.

In a study published by Hooton *et al.* [18], the prevalence of *E. coli* bacteriuria increased dramatically in foam, condom, and diaphragm spermicide users after intercourse and persisted 24 hours later. Of note, concentration of *Lactobacillus* species in the vagina did not change after intercourse in this study. None of the patients developed a symptomatic UTI. No relation was seen between early post-intercourse voiding (less than 1 hour) and the prevalence of *E. coli* bacteriuria at the follow-up visits in the latter two groups. Acquisition of bacteriuria and vaginal colonization with *E. coli* was not associated with a history of previous UTIs, duration of intercourse, duration of wearing a diaphragm, or number of ejaculations.

Pathophysiology

Escherichia coli, the most common cause of UTI, originates from the fecal flora. Contamination can result in the colonization of the periurethral area. UTIs are the result of ascension of bacteria into the urethra and bladder. Hematogenous seeding of the kidney occurs under some circumstances, such as in association with septicemia or endocarditis. Experimentally, when *E. coli* are introduced into the bloodstream, only small numbers (approximately one in 10,000) of bacteria are trapped by the kidney, and these are destroyed by antibacterial mechanisms within the kidney without causing injury. If the kidney is injured in some way, however, such as by ligation of a ureter, blood-borne organisms localize in the obstructed

kidney, multiply, and produce a unilateral acute pyelonephritis without affecting the opposite unaffected kidney.

E. coli accounts for approximately 80% to 85% of acute cystitis in sexually active women [20]. Uropathogenic *E. coli* belong to a relatively small group of bacterial clones that have accumulated multiple virulent properties that enhance their ability to colonize and infect the urinary tract. These properties include adhesions, hemolysin, or aerobactin. Adhesions include type I pilae, P-fimbria, or X-adhesions, which are composed of proteins with the ability to attach to host cell receptors [21–23]. This facilitates their colonization of vaginal, periurethral, and bladder epithelial cells. Specific proteins can attach to these adhesions and, therefore, prevent their attachment to the bladder. These kinds of blocking proteins include urinary oligosaccharides, immunoglobulin G and A, and glycosaminoglycans.

Staphylococcus saprophyticus is a coagulase-negative staphylococcus, once considered a skin contaminant. It is now known to be the second most common cause of community-acquired UTI in women of reproductive age. In fact, it is more aggressive than *E. coli* because almost half of patients present with upper tract involvement, and infection with this organism is more likely to be recurrent, relapsing, and persistent [24,25].

Urea-splitting bacteria include *Proteus*, *Klebsiella*, coagulase-negative *Staphylococcus*, and *Pseudomonas* species. Urea-splitting bacteria have the enzyme urease, which breaks down urea into ammonia and carbon dioxide. The ammonia causes the urine to become alkaline, which causes precipitation of magnesium, ammonium, and phosphate salts and forms struvite stones. Some authorities recommend treating asymptomatic bacteriuria caused by these organisms in all cases.

Chlamydial infections account for more than 30% of nonbacterial UTIs. They are associated with pyuria and are best diagnosed with urethral culture or nucleic acid detection tests. They are also commonly associated with coexisting cervical infection.

Differential Diagnosis

Sexually active women who develop symptoms of a UTI, namely dysuria, may have one of the following infections: acute urethritis, acute cystitis, or vaginitis. Women with vaginal trichomoniasis may also have involvement of the urethra and complain of dysuria [3].

Dysuria, urinary urgency, frequency, nocturia, suprapubic discomfort, hematuria, and incontinence are the most common symptoms associated with bacteriuria (Figure 31-2) [6••]. Between 40% and 60% of patients with acute cystitis have microscopic hematuria. Microscopic hematuria is uncommon in other dysuric syndromes, such as interstitial cystitis, chronic pelvic pain, vulvitis, or vaginitis.

Diagnostic Studies

Routine culture of urine obtained from patients with symptoms of a UTI is not recommended. Patients can be treated based on symptoms alone or screened with a rapid dipstick test for the nitrite and leukocyte esterase tests. Nitrites are derived from the dietary nitrates that are concentrated in the urine. Nitrate-reducing bacteria, such as *E. coli*, *Klebsiella*, and *Proteus*, reduce the nitrates into nitrites. Nitrites then react with an amino acid on a dipstick pad. The leukocyte esterase dipstick test detects white blood cells. Leukocyte esterase is found in the primary neutrophil granules and reacts with a clear acetate stain in the pad. A false-negative nitrite test can result if the uropathogen is a non-nitrate-reducing organism, such as *S. saprophyticus*, or if the urine is too dilute.

When a rapid screening test, urine analysis, or urine culture is used to determine if bacteriuria is present, appropriate collection of the urine specimens is essential. If the patient has a copious vaginal discharge, a tampon can be inserted into the vagina before collecting the urine specimen. The introitus should also be cleansed by wiping from front to back, and the labia should be kept apart while collecting the urine specimen.

When to evaluate a patient for structural or neurologic cause of her UTIs depends on her age, associated symptoms such as hematuria, pelvic examination, and surgical history (Figure 31-3). Studies evaluating the routine use of excretory urography, cystography, and cystoscopy in the diagnosis and management of women with UTIs have found little to no benefit [26–28].

A woman who develops a UTI along with feelings of urinary retention or other neurologic complaints should have a postvoid residual measured. This is an easy and inexpensive test to check for retention secondary to neuropathy or obstruction. A woman rarely has obstruction unless she has undergone surgery or has 'kinking' of her urethra from pelvic organ prolapse. In addition, if a woman develops recurrent UTIs after surgery near her bladder, a cystoscopy should be performed to exclude the presence of a stitch in her bladder acting as a nidus for infection. Other indications for evaluation of the lower and upper urinary tract include the presence of bacteria suspicious for contributing to stones, such as *Proteus*, *Pseudomonas*, or *Klebsiella* or persistent hematuria.

Children under the age of 5 diagnosed with a first UTI, males of any age with a first UTI, and children with recurrent UTIs should be evaluated with a renal ultrasound or intravenous pyelogram and voiding cystourethrogram as recommended by the American Academy of Pediatrics. Ultrasound is less invasive and can detect obstruction, ureteral duplication, and decreased medullary or cortical echogenicity. An intravenous pyelogram evaluates for function as well as anatomic abnormalities. The voiding cystourethrogram determines ureteral reflux. CT scan is the diagnostic procedure of choice in patients suspected of having a renal abscess.

Treatment

The principles of treatment are based on decades of treating UTIs and research. Women with acute cystitis, including those who experience frequent recurrences and are not pregnant, rarely undergo progression to upper tract infection [29]. A recent placebo-controlled study of acute cystitis revealed that 26% of women in the placebo group experienced spontaneous resolution of their bacteriuria by 2 weeks [30]. Although prolonged outcomes were not reported in this study, long-term adverse outcomes on renal function do not appear to be associated with untreated acute cystitis [31]. Antibiotic therapy, however, is still recommended for those with acute cystitis. A short-course 3-day antimicrobial therapy is effective in treating acute uncomplicated cystitis. Short-course, single-dose therapy, compared with 3- and 7-day regimens, was originally thought to be equally effective. The advantages of short-course, single-dose therapy are better compliance, economy, and reduced risk of adverse reactions. Recent studies have shown, however, that single-dose regimens are not as effective as 7- and 14-day regimens [9,32–35].

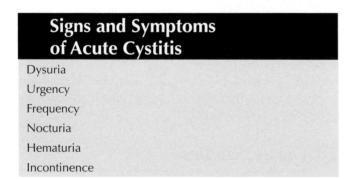

Signs and Symptoms of Acute Cystitis

Dysuria

Urgency

Frequency

Nocturia

Hematuria

Incontinence

Figure 31-2. Signs and symptoms of acute cystitis.

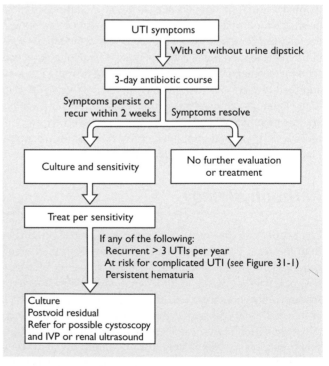

UTI symptoms

With or without urine dipstick

3-day antibiotic course

Symptoms persist or recur within 2 weeks | Symptoms resolve

Culture and sensitivity | No further evaluation or treatment

Treat per sensitivity

If any of the following:
Recurrent > 3 UTIs per year
At risk for complicated UTI (see Figure 31-1)
Persistent hematuria

Culture
Postvoid residual
Refer for possible cystoscopy and IVP or renal ultrasound

Figure 31-3. Algorithm for the treatment of symptomatic bacteriuria in adult women. IVP—intravenous pyelogram; UTI—urinary tract infection.

Further analyses of single-dose regimens have uncovered several factors that are associated with failures. These include a recent history of a UTI, use of diaphragm and spermicide, and colony counts of more than 10^5 CFU/mL [9].

Several studies demonstrated that 3-day regimens were more effective than single-dose regimens in general. This did not appear to be the case when a single 5.63-g oral dose of fosfomycin tromethamine was used. A single 5.63-g oral dose of fosfomycin tromethamine appears to be as effective as a 3-day course of trimethoprim-sulfamethoxazole [36]. Three-day regimens with trimethoprim-sulfamethoxazole were found to be more effective than β-lactams [32,34]. In addition, several studies have not only supported the effectiveness of 3-day regimens of trimethoprim-sulfamethoxazole, but have also shown similar cure rates when compared to prolonged therapy. A meta-analysis of close to 10,000 patients proved that 3-day regimens are similar to prolonged therapy in providing symptomatic cures [37].

A variety of antibiotics have been effective for the treatment of acute cystitis (Figure 31-4). These antibiotics are all suitable for use but are not all of equal efficacy when used in 3-day regimens. Trimethoprim-sulfamethoxazole administered for 3 days should be considered as the first-line agent for uncomplicated cystitis. In patients who fail to respond to a 3-day regimen, the urine should be cultured, and antimicrobial susceptibility testing should be performed. If treatment is to be empiric, the patient should be administered an agent different from the initial agent. Patients whose symptoms resolve after treatment but recur within 2 weeks should also have their urine cultured. If a bacterium grows, antimicrobial sensitivity testing should be performed. It appears that β-lactam penicillins and the cephalosporins are not as effective as the agents listed in Figure 31-4. Nitrofurantoin has not been shown to be as effective as trimethoprim-sulfamethoxazole when used as a single dose or 3-day regimen. Nitrofurantoin is not active against *Proteus mirabilis* and some *Enterobacter* and *Klebsiella* species but is active against gram-positive bacteria.

RECURRENT OR CHRONIC CYSTITIS

Recurrent or chronic cystitis, characterized by three or more UTIs within 1 year, can be managed with a 3-day course of antibiotics or by prophylactic therapy. Women with recurrent cystitis have an 85% reliability rate for identifying infection recurrence based on symptoms alone, and self-treatment is associated with a 90% cure rate [38]. Routine cultures before therapy are not necessary unless the patient fails to respond to treatment. Prophylactic therapy is efficacious in the management of women with recurrent symptomatic cystitis, decreasing recurrences by 95% [39]. Prophylaxis is recommended if more than two symptomatic episodes occur within a 6-month period or more than three episodes occur in a year. The most widely used regimens are nitrofurantoin, 100 mg/d, and trimethoprim-sulfamethoxazole, 40 to 200 mg/d, for 6 to 12 months. For patients who identify intercourse as a precipitating event, a single-dose postcoital prophylaxis is effective [40].

PYELONEPHRITIS

Patients with pyelonephritis should be treated for 10 to 14 days. All patients diagnosed as having pyelonephritis should have pre-treatment and post-treatment urine cultures. Patients who develop pyelonephritis typically have a history of having had cystitis. For mild acute uncomplicated pyelonephritis, outpatient oral antibiotic therapy is appropriate. The recommended treatment of choice is a fluoroquinolone, such as ciprofloxacin or levofloxacin [41].

For patients with complicated pyelonephritis or with pyelonephritis associated with catheterization, hospitalization, pregnancy, or surgery, hospitalization is required for parental antibiotics, pain management, and intravenous hydration.

PREGNANCY

Bacteriuria in pregnancy can have severe complications. The overall prevalence of bacteria in pregnancy ranges from 4% to 7% [42,43]. The incidence of asymptomatic bacteriuria in pregnancy is between 2% and 7%. If left untreated, approximately 25% of patients with asymptomatic bacteriuria would develop pyelonephritis during the pregnancy or in the postpartum period [44,45]. Therefore, all women with bacteriuria during pregnancy should be treated, regardless of their symptoms.

Although the relation between symptomatic bacteriuria and preterm labor is well-established, the role of asymptomatic bacteriuria in preterm labor has not been elucidated.

Antimicrobial Therapy for Uncomplicated Urinary Tract Infection

Oral 1-day regimen

Fosfomycin tromethamine as powder mixed in water—5.63 g

Oral 3-day regimens

Trimethoprim-sulfamethoxazole as tablet q 12 h

Trimethoprim 100 mg q 12 h

Ciprofloxacin 250 mg q 12 h

Levofloxacin 250 mg q day

Ofloxacin 200 mg q 12 h

Norfloxacin 400 mg q 12 h

Lomefloxacin 400 mg q day

Enoxacin 400 mg q 12 h

Sparfloxacin 400 mg on day 1, then 200 mg q day

Cefixime 400 mg q day

Cefpodoxime proxetil 100 mg q 12 h

Oral 7-day regimens

Nitrofurantoin macrocrystals 100 mg q 12 h

Nitrofurantoin macrocrystals 50–100 mg qid

Figure 31-4. Antimicrobial therapy for uncomplicated urinary tract infection. qid—four times daily.

Many factors contribute to the development of pyelonephritis in pregnancy, including decreased ureteral and vesicle muscle tone, mechanical obstruction of the ureters at the pelvic brim, increased bicarbonate secretion causing the urine to become alkaline, glycosuria, and a decreased immune response. Pyelonephritis is known to cause preterm labor in pregnancy. This is thought to be because the endotoxin may stimulate the prostaglandin pathway to cause myometrial contractility. In addition, the combination of endotoxin and the infectious response can cause destruction of the uterine and placental vasculature. It should be stated that current literature supports inpatient treatment of pyelonephritis during pregnancy [46].

Commonly used antibiotics have some specific problems in pregnancy. Nitrofurantoin (Macrodantin; Proctor and Gamble Pharmaceuticals, Cincinnati, OH) can cause hemolysis if a fetus has glucose phosphate deficiency. Sulfas and other drugs with very high protein binding, such as ceftriaxone, compete with bilirubin for albumin and therefore should not be used in the third trimester because of the risk of kernicterus after delivery. Trimethoprim-sulfamethoxazole (Bactrim; Mutual Pharmaceutical Company, Philadelphia, PA; Septra; Monarch Pharmaceuticals, Inc., Bristol, TN) can cause folate antagonism in the fetus, and is only recommended after the first trimester. Quinolones cause cartilage problems in animals. Current recommendations for the treatment of UTIs during pregnancy include amoxicillin, nitrofurantoin, and trimethoprim-sulfamethoxazole after the first trimester.

SYMPTOMATIC AND ASYMPTOMATIC BACTERIURIA IN ELDERLY WOMEN

Asymptomatic bacteriuria occurs in 1% to 2% of young women; in women older than 60 years, the prevalence is between 4% and 43% [47,48]. Elderly women living in institutions are more likely to have bacteriuria than those living at home (prevalence, 20% to 53%) [49]. In the absence of structural abnormalities, bacteriuria does not lead to renal damage. Studies conflict on whether the eradication of bacteriuria in the elderly improves survival rates.

Symptomatic postmenopausal women have particularly high reinfection rates with treatment. One symptom of UTI that is fairly unique to elderly women is incontinence. Laboratory studies done in Sweden showed that the *E. coli* 06 endotoxin could inhibit α-adrenergic receptor contractions induced by phenylephrine and norepinephrine in the bladder neck. This is a potential explanation for the incontinence that is sometimes seen in UTIs in elderly women. In addition, elderly women may be more predisposed to UTIs because of atrophic vaginitis from lack of estrogen. Estrogen causes accumulation of glycogen in vaginal epithelial cells. This stimulates the growth of lactobacilli and thereby the production of lactic acid. This in turn makes the vaginal secretions acidic, which suppresses the vaginal growth of urinary pathogens. *Lactobacillus* is also considered a blocker because it can adhere to the uroepithelial cells and inhibit attachment of *E. coli* and *Klebsiella* and *Pseudomonas* species. This is one reason that postmenopausal women without estrogen replacement may have more UTIs.

Privette *et al.* [50] studied 12 postmenopausal women with frequent UTIs. In the 2 years before estrogen therapy was begun, there were 89 infections in 258 patient-months. After the patients began taking Premarin (Wyeth Pharmaceuticals, Inc., Philadelphia, PA) 0.625 mg orally or Premarin 2 to 4 g intravaginally twice a week, there were only four infections in 288 patient-months.

CATHETER-ASSOCIATED INFECTION

Use of urinary catheters is common in hospitalized patients. It is estimated that 15% to 25% of patients will have a catheter placed in the bladder through the urethra. The mean duration of catheterization is 2 days [51,52]. Among this group of patients, there is a 3% to 10% incidence of bacteriuria per day [51–53].

Cross-contamination among catheterized patients was the main mode of spread in several nosocomial outbreaks of UTI caused by *Serratia* and *Proteus* species. Nosocomial UTIs are important because approximately 1% of patients develop bacteremia, and approximately 10% of these patients die. Cross-contamination occurs when the same collecting jug is used to empty leg bags from multiple patients. The less the drainage system is interrupted, the lower the chance of nosocomial UTI.

All patients with symptomatic catheter-associated UTIs should receive systemic antimicrobial therapy. This eradicates UTIs in approximately 80% of patients who acquire catheter-associated bacteriuria and maintains sterile urine during the catheterization in about 65%. Schaeffer and Chmiel [54] examined whether the urine should be cultured before the catheter is discontinued. Because the incidence of bacteriuria is approximately 5% to 7% per day, approximately 15% to 25% of patients develop bacteriuria within 3 to 4 days after beginning catheterization. These authors therefore recommend that, if the catheter is left in place for more than 3 days, a culture and sensitivity should be done 1 day before the catheter is removed. If there are more than 1000 CFU/mL, they recommend that the catheter not be removed until the sensitivity is back and the patient has begun drug therapy. They do not recommend empiric treatment because so many nosocomial UTIs are caused by resistant bacteria. However, even if urine is sterile at the time of discontinuing the catheter, recently catheterized patients have an increased susceptibility to bacteriuria. Most patients with indwelling Foley catheters develop symptomatic catheter-associated UTI on the first day that bacteremia appears [55].

In patients with long-term indwelling Foley catheters, the administration of antibiotics for the treatment of asymptomatic bacteriuria does not reduce the prevalence of febrile episodes but does result in an increase in the acquisition of resistant bacteria [56]. Likewise, antimicrobial irrigation of the bladder is not recommended because it does not prevent or delay infection. Studies suggest that it may result in infections with more resistant organisms [57].

Summary

Urinary tract infections in women usually originate from bacteria ascending from the periurethral microflora. Asymptomatic bacteriuria, except in pregnant patients, does not need to be treated. *E. coli* is the most common bacterium to cause UTI and can usually be treated with oral antibiotics. Patients who are hospitalized with an indwelling Foley catheter or have undergone instrumentation tend to be infected with a bacterium other than *E. coli*.

Patients with uncomplicated cystitis can be treated effectively with an oral antibiotic (*see* Figure 31-4) for 3 days. Patients who fail empiric therapy or have a recurrence within 2 weeks of treatment should undergo culture and sensitivity tests before retreatment. Referral for further evaluation, including postvoid residual, cystoscopy, and renal ultrasound or intravenous pyelogram, should be considered for patients with recurrent UTIs and those at risk for complicated UTIs.

References

Papers of particular interest have been highlighted as follows:
- • Of interest
- •• Of outstanding interest

1. Johnson JR, Stamm WE: Urinary tract infections in women: diagnosis and treatment. *Ann Intern Med* 1989, 111:906–917.

2. Kunin CM, White LV, Hua TH: A reassessment of the importance of "low-count" bacteriuria in young women with acute urinary symptoms. *Ann Intern Med* 1993, 119:454–460.

3. Stamm WE, Counts GW, Running KR, *et al.*: Diagnosis of coliform infection in acutely dysuric women. *N Engl J Med* 1982, 307:463–468.

4.• Arav-Bozer H, Leibovici RL, Danon YL: Urinary tract infections with low and high colony counts in young women: spontaneous remission and single-dose vs. multiple-day treatment. *Arch Intern Med* 1994, 154:300–305.

An example of a well-designed study looking at antibiotic success by dose and colony counts, as well as natural course of colony counts if left untreated. This prospective randomized study evaluates spontaneous resolution of a culture-proven UTI versus a one-time or 7-day course of norfloxacin. Results of treatment were analyzed based on initial colony counts. Spontaneous resolution was rare at 7%. Single-dose treatment was 84% successful at 1 week vs 98% for a 7-day course. The efficacy of single-dose treatment in patients with low urinary colony counts (10^2 to 10^4) was similar to those with high counts and less than that achieved by 7 days of treatment.

5. Rubin VH, Shapiro ED, Ardiole VT, *et al.*: Evaluation of new anti-infective drugs for the treatment of urinary tract infection. *Clin Infect Dis* 1992, 15:S216–S221.

6.•• Stamm WE, Hooton TM: Management of urinary tract infections in adults. *N Engl J Med* 1993, 329:1328–1334.

An excellent review article with 60 references summarizing the diagnosis and treatment of acute and recurrent UTIs, along with management of catheter-associated UTIs.

7. Nicolle LE: Asymptomatic bacteriuria in the elderly. *Infect Dis Clin North Am* 1997, 11:647–662.

8. Lindberg U, Claesson I, Hanson LA, *et al.*: Asymptomatic bacteriuria in school girls. VIII. Clinical course during a 3-year follow up. *J Paediatr Scand* 1978, 92:194–199.

9. Sequelae of covert bacteriuria in schoolgirls: a four-year follow-up study. *Lancet* 1978, i:889–893.

10. Sobel J: Pathogenesis of urinary tract infections. *Infect Dis Clin North Am* 1997, 11:531–549.

11. Johnson JR, Stamm WE: Diagnosis and treatment of acute urinary tract infections. *Infect Dis Clin North Am* 1987, 1:773–791.

12. Johnson JR, Lyons MG, Pearce W, *et al.*: Therapy for women hospitalized with acute pyelonephritis: a randomized trial of ampicillin versus trimethoprim-sulfamethoxazole for 14 days. *J Infect Dis* 1991, 163:325–330.

13. Kunin CM: Urinary tract infections in females. *Clin Infect Dis* 1984, 18:1–14.

14. Foxman B: Epidemiology of urinary tract infections: incidence, morbidity, and economic costs. *Am J Med* 2002,113(Suppl 1A):5S–13S.

15. Ikaheimo R, Siitonen A, Heistzanen T, *et al.*: Recurrence of urinary tract infection in a primary care setting: analysis of a one-year follow up of 179 women. *Clin Infect Dis* 1996, 22:91–99.

16.•• Stamm WE, McKevitt M, Roberts PL, *et al.*: Natural history of recurrent urinary tract infections in women. *Rev Infect Dis* 1991, 13:77–84.

The authors followed 51 infection-prone women for a median of 9 years. The women had on average 2.6 UTIs per year when not on prophylaxis and an 18:1 ratio of cystitis to pyelonephritis episodes. Prophylaxis was highly effective in preventing acute UTIs.

17. Hooton TM, Fennel CL, Clark AM, *et al.*: Nonoxynon-9 differential antibacterial activity and enhancement of bacterial adherence to vaginal epithelial cells. *J Infect Dis* 1991, 164:1216–1219.

18. Hooton TM, Hillier S, Johnson C, *et al.*: *Escherichia coli* bacteriuria and contraceptive method. *JAMA* 1991, 265:64–69.

19. Hooton TM, Roberts PL, Stamm WE: Effects of recent sexual activity and use of a diaphragm on the vaginal microflora. *Clin Infect Dis* 1994, 19:274–278.

20. Hooton TM, Besser R, Foxman B, *et al.*: Acute uncomplicated cystitis in an era of increasing antibiotic resistance: a proposed approach to empirical therapy. *Clin Infect Dis* 2004, 39:75–80.

21. DeMan P, Jodal U, Lincoln K, *et al.*: Bacterial attachment and inflammation in the urinary tract. *J Infect Dis* 1988, 158:29–35.

22. Linder H, Engberg I, Hoschützby H, *et al.*: Adhesion dependent activation of mucosal IL-6 production. *Infect Immunol* 1991, 59:4357–4362.

23. Duguid J, Smith I, Dempster G, *et al.*: Non-flagellin filamentous appendages (fimbriae) and hemagglutinating activity in *Bacterium coli*. *J Pathol Bacteriol* 1955, 7:335–348.

24. Fowler JE: *Staphylococcus saprophyticus* as the cause of infected urinary calculus. *Ann Intern Med* 1985, 102:342–344.

25. Hovelius B, March PA: *Staphylococcus saprophyticus* as a common cause of urinary tract infections. *Rev Infect Dis* 1984, 6:328–337.

26. Fowler JE, Pulaski ET: Excretory urography, cystography, and cystoscopy in the evaluation of women with urinary tract infections. *N Engl J Med* 1981, 304:462–465.

27. Fair WR, McClennan BL, Jost RG: Are excretory urograms necessary in evaluating women with urinary tract infections? *J Urol* 1979, 121:313–315.

28. Engel G, Schaeffer AJ, Grayhack JT, *et al.*: The role of excretory urography and cystoscopy in the evaluation and management of women with recurrent urinary tract infection. *J Urol* 1980, 123:190–191.

29. Nicolle LE: The optimal management of lower urinary tract infections. *Infection* 1990, 19(Suppl 2):S50–S52.

30. Asbach HW: Single dose oral administration of cefixime 400 mg in the treatment of acute uncomplicated cystitis and gonorrhoeae. *Drugs* 1991, 42:10–13.

31. Fihn SD, Johnson C, Roberts PL, *et al.*: Trimethoprim-sulfamethoxazole for acute dysuria in women: a single dose or 10-day course. *Ann Intern Med* 1988, 108:350–357.

32. Andriole VT: Use of quinolones in treatment of prostatitis and lower urinary tract infections. *Eur J Clin Microbiol Infect Dis* 1991, 10:342–350.

33. Masterton RG, Bochsler JA: High-dosage co-amoxiclav in a single dose versus 7 days of cotrimoxazole as treatment of uncomplicated lower urinary tract infection in women. *J Antimicrob Chemother* 1995, 35:129–137.

34. Norrby SR: Short-term treatment of uncomplicated lower urinary tract infections in women. *Rev Infect Dis* 1990, 12:458–467.

35. Philbrick JT, Bracikowski JP: Single-dose antibiotic treatment for uncomplicated urinary tract infections: less for less? *Arch Intern Med* 1985, 145:1672–1678.

36. Crocchiolo P: Single-dose fosfomycin trometamol versus multiple-dose cotrimoxazole in the treatment of lower urinary tract infections in general practice. Multicenter Group of General Practitioners. *Chemotherapy* 1990, 36:37–40.

37. Katchman EA, Milo G, Paul M, *et al.*: Three-day vs longer duration of antibiotic treatment for cystitis in women: systematic review and meta-analysis. *Am J Med* 2005, 118:1196–1207.

38. Wong ES, McKevitt M, Running K, *et al.*: Management of recurrent urinary tract infections with patient-administered single-dose therapy. *Ann Intern Med* 1985, 102:302.

39. Nicolle LE, Ronald AR: Recurrent urinary tract infection in adult women: diagnosis and treatment. *Infect Dis Clin North Am* 1987, 1:793.

40. Vosti KL: Recurrent urinary tract infections: prevention by prophylactic antibiotics after sexual intercourse. *JAMA* 1975, 231:934.

41. Warren JW, Abrutyn E, Hebel JR, *et al.*: Guidelines for antimicrobial treatment of uncomplicated acute bacterial cystitis and acute pyelonephritis in women. Infectious Diseases Society of America (IDSA). *Clin Infect Dis* 1999, 29:745–758.

42. Norden CW, Kass EH: Bacteriuria of pregnancy: a critical appraisal. *Ann Rev Med* 1968, 19:431–470.

43. Stenqvist K, Dahlen-Nilsson I, Lindin-Jansen G, *et al.*: Bacteriuria in pregnancy. *Am J Epidemiol* 1989, 129:372–379.

44. Harris RE: The significance of eradication of bacteriuria during pregnancy: an introspective study. *Obstet Gynecol* 1979, 53:71–73.

44. Harris RE, Gilstrap LC, Pretty A: Single-dose antimicrobial therapy for asymptomatic bacteriuria during pregnancy. *Obstet Gynecol* 1982, 59:546–549.

46. American College of Obstetricians and Gynecologists: *Antimicrobial Therapy for Obstetric Patients*. Washington, DC: American College of Obstetricians and Gynecologists; 1998.

47. Brocklehurst JC, Dillane JB, Griffiths L, *et al.*: The prevalence and symptomatology of urinary infections in an aged population. *Gerontol Clin* 1968, 10:345–347.

48. Kunin CM, McCormack RC: An epidemiologic study of bacteriuria and blood pressure among nuns and working women. *N Engl J Med* 1968, 278:635–642.

49. Nicolle LE: Urinary tract infections in long-term care facilities. *Infect Control Hosp Epidemiol* 1993, 14:220–225.

50. Privette M, Cade R, Peterson J, *et al.*: Prevention of recurrent urinary tract infections among nursing home patients. *Nephron* 1988, 50:24–27.

51. Haley RW, Hooten TM, Culver DH, *et al.*: Nosocomial infections in US hospitals, 1975-1976: estimated frequency by selected characteristics of patients. *Am J Med* 1981, 70:947–959.

52. Hartstein AI, Gacher SB, Ward TT, *et al.*: Nosocomial urinary tract infection: a prospective evaluation of 108 catheterized patients. *Infect Control* 1981, 2:380–386.

53. Kunin CM, McCormack RC: Prevention of catheter-induced urinary tract infections by sterile closed drainage. *N Engl J Med* 1966, 274:1155–1161.

54. Schaeffer AJ, Chmiel J: Urethral meatal colonization in the pathogenesis of catheter-associated bacteriuria. *J Urol* 1983, 130:1096–1099.

55. Garibaldi RA, Mooney BR, Epstein BJ, *et al.*: An evaluation of daily bacteriologic monitoring to identify preventable episodes of catheter-associated urinary tract infection. *Infect Control* 1982, 3:466–470.

56. Warren JW, Anthony WB, Hoopes JM, *et al.*: Cephalexin for susceptible bacteriuria in afebrile, long-term catheterized patients. *JAMA* 1982, 248:454–458.

57. Warren JW, Platt R, Thomas RJ, *et al.*: Antibiotic irrigation and catheter-associated urinary-tract infections. *N Engl J Med* 1978 299:570–573.

32 | Overactive Bladder

Thao Nguyen and AnnaMarie Connolly

- The prevalence of overactive bladder increases with age. With an increasing number of citizens 65 years of age and older in the United States, primary care physicians can expect to see an increasing number of patients with overactive bladder.
- The initial evaluation of women with overactive bladder symptoms should rule out pathologic etiologies.
- A cystometrogram is a simple and inexpensive test that can be used to confirm a diagnosis of detrusor overactivity.
- Pharmacologic and behavior therapy (diet/behavior changes, bladder retraining, pelvic floor muscle exercise, with or without biofeedback) are first-line treatment options for patients with overactive bladder.
- Uncertain diagnosis, prior incontinence surgery, prior pelvic radiation or radical pelvic surgery, elevated postvoid residual, pelvic organ prolapse, failed initial therapy, hematuria without infection, planned pelvic surgery, and comorbid conditions are reasons for referring incontinent patients to a specialist.

Introduction

Overactive bladder (OAB) is a syndrome of lower urinary problems which may present as urinary frequency, urgency, nocturia, with or without urge urinary incontinence. The term *overactive bladder* often implies detrusor overactivity as the underlying etiology, but it may also be caused by other forms of urethra-vesicle dysfunction. According to the International Continence Society of Standardization of Terminology report, the term *overactive bladder* "can be used if there is no proven infection or other obvious pathology." As the population of the United States ages, primary care physicians can expect to see an increasing number of patients with OAB. Therefore, a working knowledge of this disorder is an important element of the general health maintenance care of the aging female population.

This chapter focuses on the evaluation and management of OAB in women, paying particular attention to the etiology of detrusor overactivity. We aim to assist primary care physicians in differentiating detrusor overactivity from other common causes of lower urinary symptoms, to provide a guideline of possible treatment options without the need for referral, and to identify clinical situations in which referral to incontinence specialists is prudent.

Basic Terminology

According to the International Continence Society terminology, detrusor overactivity is the observation of involuntary detrusor contraction on urodynamic studies [1]. It was previously known as "detrusor instability." When detrusor overactivity is the result of a neurogenic condition, it is called neurogenic detrusor overactivity.

A patient with OAB often experiences urinary frequency. This is usually defined as having more than eight voids per day. Urinary urgency is the strong desire to void that is difficult to defer. When urinary incontinence occurs immediately after or in association with urgency, it is termed *urge urinary incontinence*. Nocturia is the symptom of waking up at night to void. Nocturia becomes clinically significant when it occurs more than once per night.

Epidemiology

The prevalence of OAB in women varies from 10% to 50%, depending on the definitions used and the population studied [2–4]. Using the International Continence Society terminology, a telephone survey of more than 5000 noninstitutionalized American adults revealed a prevalence of OAB, with or without urge incontinence in the United States, of 17% [5]. The incidence of urge incontinence increases with age, with a marked increase after 44 years of age.

A similar national survey estimated that the total financial cost of OAB in 2000 was $12 billion [6]. The physical and psychologic burden of OAB on individuals suffering from the disorder is also significant. OAB is associated with lower quality-of-life scores, higher depression scores, and poorer sleep quality [5].

Pathophysiology

NORMAL NEUROPHYSIOLOGIC BLADDER PATHWAYS

Urine is stored in and emptied from the bladder in an orderly process known as the micturition cycle (Figure 32-1). The reciprocal relationship between the bladder and urethra is controlled by an on-off switching process. The sympathetic nervous system promotes bladder relaxation and internal urethral sphincter contraction for urine storage, whereas the parasympathetic nervous system controls bladder contractions and the passage of urine. Abnormalities along any part of this path-

way lead to bladder dysfunction, which may result in urgency, frequency, nocturia, and urinary incontinence.

As urine fills the bladder, sensory information is transmitted to cerebral cortex through visceral afferents. In order to allow urine storage in the bladder, sympathetic efferent nerve fibers from T11-L2 spinal cord segments travel with the hypogastric nerve to presynaptically inhibit the parasympathetic nerve supply to prevent bladder contraction. These sympathetic efferents synapse with a small number of β-receptors in the bladder wall to directly mediate relaxation of the bladder. Sympathetic fibers also synapse with α-receptors to tonically contract the internal urethral sphincter during bladder filling to prevent urine outflow. To urinate, parasympathetic nerve fibers from S2–S4 synapse on smooth muscle cholinergic receptors in the bladder wall to produce contraction. The somatic efferent nerve fibers from the pudendal nucleus of S2-S4 supply the external periurethral sphincter. The external sphincter is under voluntary control and normally contracts in response to coughing, Valsalva maneuver, or active voluntary prevention of urine outflow.

Three areas of the central nervous system (*ie*, the sacral micturition center, the pontine micturition center, and the cerebral cortex) control bladder function. The sacral micturition center at the S2-S4 levels is responsible for bladder contraction. The

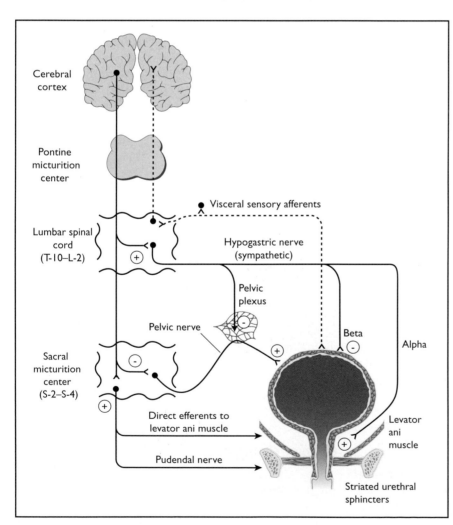

Figure 32-1. The neurophysiologic pathways responsible for urine storage. As the bladder fills, sensory information is transmitted to the cerebral cortex through visceral afferents, which travel through the pelvic plexus with the hypogastric nerve to enter the spinal cord at T-10 to T-12. Urine is stored in the bladder through cortical and spinal inhibition of the bladder's parasympathetic nerve supply and through excitation of the bladder's sympathetic nerve supply and somatic efferents to the intrinsic and extrinsic urethral sphincters. The sympathetic nervous system promotes urine storage by a presynaptic inhibition of the bladder's parasympathetic nerve supply and an increase in urethral resistance mediated by a smooth muscle contraction (β-adrenergic receptor). A limited number of β-adrenergic receptors, which directly inhibit the detrusor when excited, are located in the bladder wall.

pontine micturition center may play a role in coordinating relaxation of the external urethral sphincter at the time of bladder contraction while the cerebral cortex helps to inhibit the activity of the sacral micturition center.

NEUROGENIC PATHOPHYSIOLOGY

Lesions of the peripheral nerves or the sacral micturition center may cause detrusor areflexia and tonic contraction of the urethral sphincter. This can lead to bladder overdistension and overflow incontinence. Lesions between the sacral and pontine micturition centers lead to uninhibited bladder contractions with uncoordinated sphincter activity, a problem known as *detrusor sphincter dyssynergia*. However, in acute settings immediately after spinal injuries, spinal shock often causes areflexic detrusor. With recovery and reorganization of synaptic connections in the spinal cord, women often develop uninhibited bladder contractions with urgency, frequency, and urge incontinence through the spinal micturition reflex [7•]. Lesions above the pontine micturition center lead to lack of inhibition from the cerebral cortex and result in uninhibited bladder contractions, but voluntary relaxation of the urethral sphincter remains intact. Suprapontine lesions may include cerebrovascular accident, intracranial tumors, head injury, Parkinson disease, or multiple sclerosis [8].

Myogenic Pathophysiology

Alteration in detrusor smooth muscle is a postulated cause of OAB [9]. Detrusor muscle from patients with detrusor overactivity patients was found to have abnormal mechanical activity, including increased spontaneous fused titanic contractions [10], supersensitivity to agonists [11], and increased sensitivity of direct electrical stimulation [9]. A histologic study by Elbadawi *et al.* [12] showed a distinctive disjunction structural pattern on bladder biopsies obtained from patients with voiding dysfunction on urodynamic studies. Further light microscopic studies on detrusor smooth muscle also demonstrated changes in innervation, cell-cell junction, and cell structure [9]. Further investigation is warranted to validate these findings in patients with OAB and develop strategies to counteract these abnormalities.

Obstruction

Urge incontinence resulting from outlet obstruction is a well-known entity. This is seen more often in spinal cord injury patients or those with prostate hypertrophy. One hypothesis is that outlet obstruction leads to overdistension of the bladder, causing cholinergic denervation, and subsequently, supersensitivity of cholinergic receptors in the detrusor muscle [11,13]. In the presence of acetylcholine, the obstructed bladder is stimulated to contract to a greater degree than would be expected in an unobstructed case.

In women, severe pelvic organ prolapse can cause bladder outlet obstruction from urethral kinking, and this can lead to OAB symptoms. Similarly, bladder outlet obstruction as a complication of bladder neck suspension for the treatment of stress urinary

incontinence can cause postoperative OAB symptoms. However, de novo detrusor overactivity may arise in the absence of bladder outlet obstruction after an anti-incontinence procedure [14,15].

Psychogenic

Evidence for psychogenic causes of detrusor overactivity is supported by the fact that treatments such as behavioral modification are often effective [16–18]. A single incontinent episode may alter bladder habits in a patient with normal bladder function. Increased stress caused by fear of losing bladder control and increased awareness of bladder sensation and fullness lead to more frequent voiding. This may result in lower bladder capacity and worsening of frequency and urgency [19].

Evaluation

The diagnosis of OAB is made when potential pathologic etiologies have been excluded. Often the diagnosis of OAB can be made based on medical history, physical examination, and simple studies without the need for referral. One of the most common causes of urinary frequency, urgency, nocturia, and urinary incontinence is lower urinary tract infection. Inflammation from infection can irritate the detrusor muscle and may provoke urinary symptoms. Bladder lesions or foreign bodies can trigger detrusor contractions. Overly sedated patients or patients with restricted mobility may develop overflow urinary incontinence as a result of inability to reach the bathroom. Figure 32-2 summarizes common causes of urinary incontinence.

History

It is important to obtain a complete medical and surgical history to identify factors that can affect the urinary system. Figure 32-3 summarizes differential diagnoses for OAB symptoms. In addition to a complete history with a special focus on urogenital and neurologic systems, the history should help physicians to characterize the patient's urinary symptoms and the effects

Common Reversible Causes of Urinary Incontinence

Urinary tract infection

Urogenital atrophy

Medications

Delirium or diminished mental status

Stroke

Immobility

Pelvic organ prolapse

Fecal impaction

Figure 32-2. Common reversible causes of urinary incontinence.

Differential Diagnoses for Overactive Bladder Symptoms

Urethral factors
  Urethral instability
  Urethral syndrome
  Urethral diverticulum
  Urethritis
  Urinary tract fistula
Bladder factors
  Bladder calculi
  Bladder tumor
  Intravesical suture from continence surgery
  Interstitial cystitis
  Urinary tract infection
Gynecologic factors
  Atrophy (menopause)
  Pregnancy
  External compression (pelvic, tumor, fibroids)
Medical factors
  Endocrine disorders
    Diabetes mellitus
    Diabetes insipidus
  Neurologic disorders
    Cerebrovascular accident
    Intracranial tumor
    Head injury
    Parkinsonism
    Spinal cord injury or tumor
    Multiple sclerosis
    Myelomeningocele
  Medications
  Congestive heart failure
  Chronic venous insufficiency
  Pelvic irradiation
Surgical factors
  Prior continence surgery
  Prior prolapse surgery
  Radical pelvic surgery
Behavioral factors
  Habitual voiding
  Excessive caffeine intake
  Excessive fluid intake

Figure 32-3. Differential diagnoses for overactive bladder symptoms.

these symptoms have on the patient's daily life. Examples of focused questions include:

Do you experience leaking of urine? (Yes/No). If yes, how long has it been a problem for you?

Do you lose urine associated with activities such as heavy lifting, sneezing, coughing, or laughing?

Do you lose urine associated with an uncontrollable urge to urinate?

How many times do you leak urine per day?

Do you usually experience frequent urination?

Do you experience urinary dribbling after voiding?

How often do you void during the daytime?

How many times do you wake up at night to void?

Do you have difficulty emptying your bladder or have a strong desire to empty your bladder after immediately doing so?

How many pads do you use per day for urine leakage?

Do you wet the bed while sleeping?

Do you have pain or burning with urination?

Do you have blood in your urine?

How many urinary tract infections have you had in the last two years?

Have you ever had kidney infections?

Have you ever had kidney stones?

To what degree do you limit your daily activities because of urine leakage?

The patient's medications should be reviewed in an attempt to identify pharmacologic agents that may contribute to symptoms of OAB (Figure 32-4). The list of medications that affect the lower urinary tract is exhaustive. It is unrealistic to expect that the patients can be taken off all of these medications without adversely affecting general medical health. However, primary care physicians can be guided by some basic tenets in an attempt to minimize the effects of these drugs. Women with hypertension should be asked about incontinence before starting diuretics. Patients with nocturia or nocturnal enuresis could take their diuretics in the

Medications That May Affect Overactive Bladder Symptoms

Medication	Mechanism of Effect
Diuretics	Increased urine output
Sedatives/narcotics	Sedation or altered mental status
Anticholinergics	Decrease in bladder contractility
Antipsychotics	Sedation; impaired motility
Alpha-adrenergics	Increased urethral sphincter construction
Calcium channel blockers	Decrease in bladder contractility

Figure 32-4. Medications that may affect overactive bladder symptoms.

morning. Alternatively, these medications can be given at dinnertime to prevent the supine diuresis seen in elderly patients that can exacerbate symptoms. Because they cause urethral smooth muscle relaxation, α-adrenergic receptor antagonists such as prazosin (Minipress; Pfizer, Inc., New York, NY) and terazosin (Hytrin; Abbott Laboratories, Abbott Park, IL) should be avoided if possible. Anticholinergic medications are contraindicated in patients with urinary retention.

Physical Examination

The major components of the physical examination for a woman with OAB symptoms include a neurologic examination and an abdominal/pelvic examination. The woman's mental status, gait, and gross movement should be noted to rule out obvious causes such as cerebrovascular accidents, Parkinsonism, dementia, or sedation. Abdomen or pelvic masses can cause external bladder compression and hence exacerbate urinary symptoms. A pelvic examination identifies vulva or vaginal lesion, evidence of vaginal atrophy from hypoestrogenic status, pelvic muscle strength, and the extent of pelvic organ prolapse that may cause urethral obstruction. Urogenital abnormalities such as urethral diverticula or fistula may or may not be detectable on physical exam. The bulbocavernosus reflex, innervated by S1 through S3, and the anal reflex, innervated by S4 and S5, can be used to indirectly assess for spinal cord integrity. A postvoid residual (PVR) volume can be checked using sterile catheterization technique after the woman empties her bladder. A PVR of 100 mL or more is considered abnormal if the voided volume is greater than 200 mL. High PVR may suggest urethral obstruction or inadequate detrusor contraction. The catheterized urine can be sent for urine analysis and microscopic evaluation, as well as urine culture in all women with symptoms of OAB. Urinary cytology should be sent in women with hematuria.

Voiding Diary

The objective data gained from reviewing a patient's voiding diary is invaluable as it can assist the physician in differentiating between types of incontinence. The diary is a record of the woman's fluid intake, voiding habits, and circumstances of incontinence episodes (Figure 32-5). Usually, a three-day diary is needed. Women with OAB tend to have greater frequency of urination with lower mean voided volumes (total voided volume divided by frequency) compared with asymptomatic women [20]. Circumstances around the time of incontinence episodes (such as coughing, laughing, or urinary urgency) can help differentiate symptoms of stress from urge incontinence.

A focused medical history and physical examination, urine analysis and culture, and a completed voiding diary offer the health care provider great insight into possible etiologies of OAB symptoms. Treatable etiologies can be appropriately addressed. Physicians should recognize the limitations of patient history in diagnosing urinary incontinence. Compared with findings on urodynamic testing, symptoms of urge incontinence have a positive and negative predictive value of 56% and 73%, respectively [21]. Because the predictive value is so poor, further testing may be warranted if the risks to an improperly diagnosed patient are high. Thus, medical decision

Voiding diary					
Time	Amount voided	Activity	Leak volume	Urge present	Amount/type of intake
					water 4 oz
					coffee 12 oz
10:30				yes	
11:22	7 oz				water 12 oz
11:30		cough	1	no	
11:58		cough	1	no	
12:55		cough	2	no	
1:25		cough			pop 16 oz
1:40					
1:40	8 oz	cough	3		
3:05					
↓	6 oz				
8:00					
↓	26 oz			yes	
7:18					

A

Figure 32-5. A, Example of a voiding diary from a patient with genuine stress incontinence. Note the large functional bladder capacity and the infrequent voids. Patient notes urine leakage with cough.

Continued on the next page

making should be based on a risk and benefit assessment of available treatment options. Treatment options with a low side-effect profile may be instituted without further testing.

Cystometrogram

The cystometrogram is a simple and inexpensive method to evaluate the capacity and function of the bladder (Figure 32-6A). A cystometrogram can help the primary care physician to confirm a diagnosis of detrusor overactivity before instituting therapy. It should be considered in patients who have failed empiric therapy based on history and physical findings alone.

A simple cystometrogram measures bladder pressure in response to bladder filling. "Eyeball" cystometry is an example of an incremental simple cystometrogram using 1000 mL of sterile saline, a Toomey syringe, and a red rubber catheter. As saline is poured into the syringe, one can measure the volume when the patient has the first sensation, first desire to void, strong desire to void, and uncontrollable desire to void (capacity). Usually, the first urge occurs at 150 to 200 mL, and capacity occurs at 400 to 500 mL. During the filling phase, a normal bladder expands to accommodate the volume, and intravesical pressure remains low. A rise in the water column in response to filling is suggestive of an elevated bladder pressure caused by detrusor overactivity. A single channel cystometry can be assembled in a similar fashion using a 1000 mL intravenous saline bag connected through intravenous tubing to a filling catheter, with a pressure catheter placed in the bladder to measure intravesical pressure (Figure 32-6B and C). Phasic pressure elevation may represent detrusor overactivity. A diagnosis of urge incontinence secondary to detrusor overactivity can be made when leakage is associated with these phasic bladder pressure elevations (Figure 32-7A). A continuous but slow rise in pressure may be suggestive of low bladder compliance (Figure 32-7B). A major limitation of single channel cystometry is that of artifacts caused by increases in intra-abdominal pressure during bladder filling. These artifacts

24 hr period		**Voiding diary**			
Time	Amount voided	Activity	Leak volume	Urge present	Amount/type of intake
9:00 p.m.	1 cup	toilet		yes	water 10 oz
9:55	50 mL	toilet		yes	water 8 oz
1:15 a.m.	2 cups	toilet		yes	water 8 oz
5:00	2 cups	toilet		yes	water 8 oz
5:13	—	standing	drops	cough/no	—
5:14	40 mL	toilet			water 8 oz
5:16	—	—	—	—	? 8 oz
6:10	6 oz	toilet		yes	water 8 oz
6:30	4 oz	toilet		yes	water 8 oz
7:00	75 mL	toilet	drops	yes	
7:31	50 mL	toilet		yes	
7:40	—	sitting in bathtub	drops	yes	
7:50	25 mL	toilet			
7:55	—	blowing nose-standing	drops		
8:25	—		—	—	orange juice 6 oz
8:55	—				skim milk 8 oz
9:00	50 mL	toilet		yes	water 9 oz
9:45	200 mL	toilet		yes	
10:05		sitting-cough	drops		
10:10	75 mL	toilet		yes	? 10 oz
11:00	90 mL	toilet		yes	
11:05					
11:15					warm water 8 oz
11:30	50 mL	toilet			cranberry juice 4 oz
Noon	75 mL	toilet		yes	
12:30	100 mL	toilet		yes	
1:35					water 8 oz
2:40	200 mL	toilet		yes	
3:00	50 mL	toilet		yes	
3:25	50 mL	toilet		yes	
3:26		blowing nose-standing	drops		
4:10	50 mL	toilet		yes	water 8 oz
6:30	50 mL	toilet			
8:00	50 mL	toilet			

B

Figure 32-5. *(Continued)* **B**, Example of a voiding diary from a patient with bladder overactivity. Note the small, frequent voids. The cause of this patient's bladder overactivity appears to be excessive fluid intake, which may warrant evaluation for diabetes mellitus or insipidus. The voiding diary also may be used as a form of biofeedback for this patient. Once she is able to decrease her fluid intake, she can be instructed to fill out subsequent diaries and find that her voiding frequency and incontinent episodes decrease.

can be reduced by complex cystometry, which requires special instrumentation and specialty training and will not be discussed in this chapter.

The positive and negative predictive values of simple cystometry are 74% and 81%, respectively [22]. Therefore, simple cystometry may be used to exclude detrusor insta-bility in 80% of incontinent patients. The negative predictive value can be improved by repeating the test, having the woman change positions (sit to stand) during testing, or by performing provocative maneuvers such as heel-bouncing, washing hands, coughing, or running water during bladder filling.

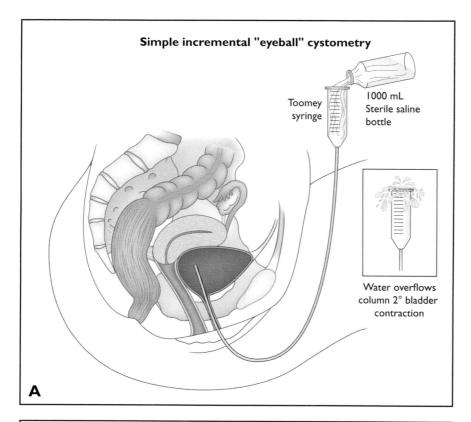

Simple incremental "eyeball" cystometry

Toomey syringe

1000 mL Sterile saline bottle

Water overflows column 2° bladder contraction

A

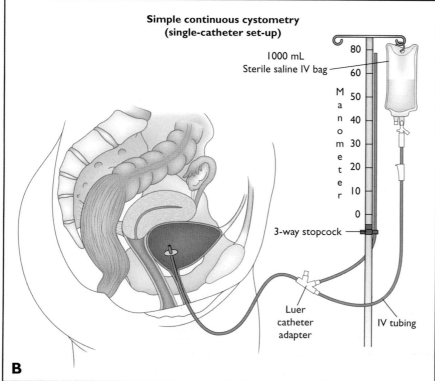

Simple continuous cystometry (single-catheter set-up)

1000 mL Sterile saline IV bag

Manometer
80
60
50
40
30
20
10
0

3-way stopcock

Luer catheter adapter

IV tubing

B

Figure 32-6. Examples of simple and complex cystometrograms. **A,** During eyeball cystometry, 50 to 60 mL of saline is infused through a red rubber catheter while the water column is monitored. A rise in the water column during bladder filling may be suggestive of detrusor overactivity.

Continued on the next page

Stress (Bonney) Test

After the bladder has been filled to capacity, the catheter is removed, and the patient is asked to perform a standing cough stress test. The combination of a negative cystometrogram (no detrusor overactivity) and a positive stress test (leakage with cough) has a specificity of 100%, a positive predictive value of 100%, and a negative predictive value of 76% for the diagnosis of genuine stress incontinence [23].

Management

Figure 32-8 presents an algorithm for the evaluation and treatment of patients with symptoms of OAB. The first step in managing these women is to treat identifiable causes as summarized in Figure 32-3. Women should be made aware of all treatment options, including pharmacologic and nonpharmacologic therapies for OAB.

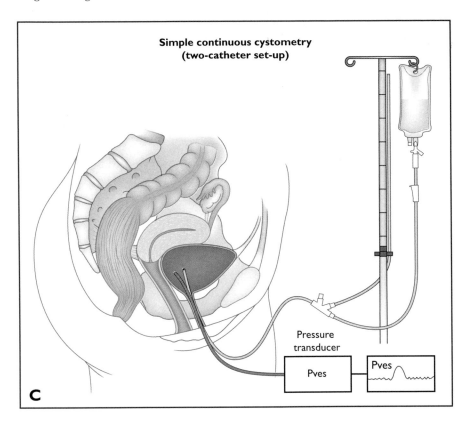

Figure 32-6. *(Continued)* **B** and **C**, Continuous cystometry can be performed using a one- or two-catheter set-up, with pressure fluctuations measured by a transducer or manometer placed and zero-calibrated at the level of the patient's bladder. Pves—vesicular pressure.

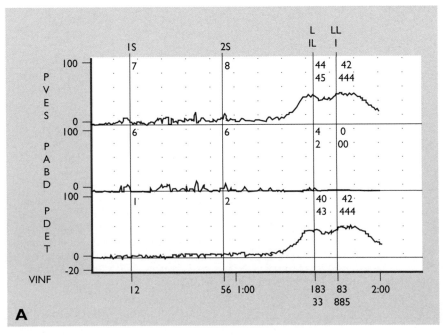

Figure 32-7. A, A complex cystometrogram demonstrating a phasic bladder pressure elevation typical of detrusor instability and hyper-reflexia. The patient leaked urine as a result of this uninhibitable detrusor contraction.

Continued on the next page

Diet and Habit

Overactive bladder has been shown to be associated with carbonated drinks and tobacco use [24]. This association also holds true for high caffeine intake and detrusor overactivity [25]. Decreased fluid and caffeine intake improves urinary symptoms, incontinence episodes, and quality of life in patients with detrusor overactivity [26]. Patients with urgency, frequency, or urge incontinence should restrict their fluid intake to six to eight 8-ounce glasses of fluid per day. Patients with nocturia or nocturnal enuresis should be counseled not to drink any fluid or alcohol after dinner.

Bladder Retraining

Bladder retraining is one of the most common behavioral therapies available for the treatment of detrusor overactivity. Bladder training has a proven success rate of up to 80% [17,27]. Complete resolution of OAB symptoms can be expected in 15% of women, with 50% of women showing a 50% to 75% reduction in symptoms. Bladder retraining (or bladder retraining drills) is a form of behavioral modification whereby the patient is asked to pursue scheduled voiding with conscious suppression of the urinary urge between voids. The woman's 24-hour voiding diary is reviewed to determine the shortest time interval between voids. The woman is then advised to void at the prescribed time. When she feels an urge between the timed voids, the woman is instructed to sit down, purposely distract herself by counting or focusing on other tasks, and to perform ten quick pelvic floor muscle contractions (Kegel exercises.) The voiding interval can be increased by 30 minutes each week if the patient is able to comply with the previous week's schedule and symptoms improve. The goal is to void every 3 to 4 hours without incontinent episodes.

Pelvic Muscle Rehabilitation

Pelvic muscle therapy (Kegel exercises) is an effective treatment for motor and sensory urgency. It helps to increase urethral resistance and to inhibit involuntary detrusor contractions, and hence reduces the number of incontinent episodes. Unfortunately, only half of women are capable of performing a pelvic floor contraction after brief verbal instruction. One fourth of women instead perform Valsalva maneuvers or strain in an attempt to perform a contraction; this may increase their risk of an incontinent episode [28]. Physicians can help the patient to identify appropriate pelvic floor muscles during pelvic examination by manually locating pubococcygeus muscles at 3 and 9 o'clock just behind the hymen. The patient is then asked to contract these muscles around the examiner's finger without using abdominal muscles concurrently.

Biofeedback (verbal, auditory, or visual) is appropriate for patients who have weak pelvic floor musculature but can identify the correct muscles to contract. It is also appropriate for patients who have good pelvic floor strength but use accessory muscles to assist in the exercise. Biofeedback has been shown to augment the efficacy of pelvic muscle therapy by 20% [29]. With this type of therapy, patients are given verbal, auditory, or visual cues about how well or poorly they are performing the required task. These cues enable women to make the necessary adjustments. Computer programs are available for the biofeedback specialist to assess and treat pelvic floor disorders through a combination of pressure probes and electromyogram patches. Typically, women are begun on a series of quick "flick-like" pelvic floor contractions. Once they are successful at completing this task, they can be advanced to a series of contract and hold exercises. Women are encouraged to continue this therapy at home with or without the use of home biofeedback units.

Electrical stimulation may be an effective treatment option for patients with weak pelvic floor muscles who are not able to identify the correct muscles to contract. Electrical stimulation can be used concurrently with biofeedback. The cure rate of electrical stimulation for patients with detrusor overactivity is approximately 50% [29,30].

Pharmacologic Therapy

Figure 32-9 lists medications considered as first-line therapy for the treatment of OAB, along with their dosage, side effects, side effect incidence, and special considerations.

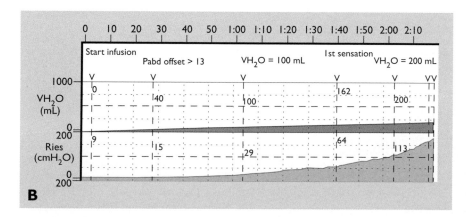

Figure 32-7. *(Continued)* **B**, A simple cystometrogram demonstrating the slow, steady bladder pressure elevation typical of low bladder compliance. This patient had a history of pelvic irradiation for cervical cancer. Pabd—abdominal pressure; Pdet—detrusor pressure; Pves—vesicular pressure.

ANTICHOLINERGICS

Current US Food and Drug Administration–approved anticholinergic medications for OAB include oxybutynin, tolterodine, trospium, solifenacin, and darifenacin. They also are the most commonly used medications for urinary incontinence. The medication choices depend on efficacy, cost, side effects, and patient comorbidities. Anticholinergic side effects, such as dry mouth, blurred vision, constipation, tachycardia, nausea and vomiting, and drowsiness are common. Adverse effect rates generally increase with higher medication dosage. One study showed that up to 80% of women placed on anticholinergic medications discontinued therapy within 6 months [31]. Thus, primary care physicians should develop strategies to improve compliance with these medications. One option is to begin at a low dosage and titrate until the desired effect is achieved. Another option is to select an anticholinergic medication with a lower adverse effect profile regarding the particular symptoms that bother the woman. Adding a low dose of anticholinergic

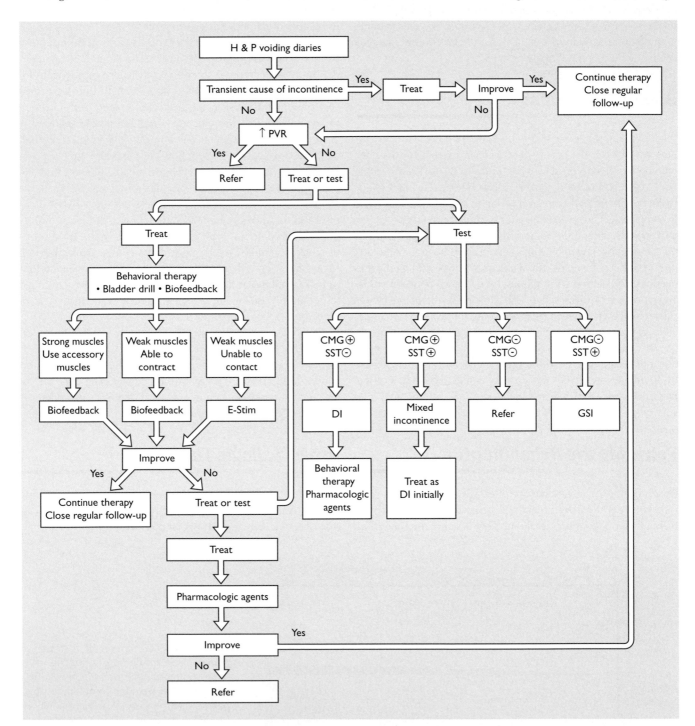

Figure 32-8. Algorithm for the evaluation and management of patients with detrusor overactivity. CMG—cystometrogram; DI—detrusor incontinence; GSI—genuine stress incontinence; E-Stim—transvaginal electrical stimulation; H & P—history and physical examination; PVR—postvoid residual; SST—standing stress test.

medications to behavioral therapy has been shown to improve efficacy in some patients [32,33].

Oxybutynin and tolterodine are the most frequently used medications for urinary incontinence. Oxybutynin can be taken orally or transdermally. The oral extended-release (ER) formulation can be taken daily, whereas the immediate-release (IR) formulation can be taken three to four times per day. Whereas the IR and ER formulations provide similar reductions in urge incontinence and total incontinence episodes, the incidence for dry mouth is lower in the ER oxybutynin [34]. The transdermal formulation bypasses the hepatic and gastrointestinal metabolism, leading to less N-desethyloxybutynin, which is thought to be responsible for anticholinergic side effects. Transdermal oxybutynin (Oxytrol; Watson Laboratories, Corona, CA) has been shown to be efficacious with improved adverse effect profile in patients with OAB; the dry mouth incidence was as low as 3% to 7% [35–37].

Tolterodine provides similar clinical efficacy compared to oxybutynin [38,39•]. Dry mouth is less common in tolterodine compared to oxybutynin [38,39•,40]. Compared with placebo, tolterodine had a 20% reduction in the number of micturitions per 24 hours and a 40% to 60% reduction in the mean daily incontinence episodes [41]. However, tolterodine should be used cautiously in the elderly due to association with memory

Medications for the Treatment of Overactive Bladder

Medication	Mechanism	Dosage	Elimination Route	Common Side Effects	Special Considerations
Oxybutynin	Anticholinergic	IR tablet: 5 mg po bid/tid; IR syrup: 5 mg/5 mL syrup po bid/tid; ER tablet: 5–15 mg po qd; transdermal: 3.9 mg/d patch, 1 patch twice per week	Hepatic	Dry mouth (7%–90%), constipation (50%), blurred vision (50%), heartburn (60%), application-side erythema and pruritus in transdermal formulary (5%–15%)	Start dosage at 2.5 mg po bid/tid in elderly patients; use with caution in patients with hepatic impairment
Tolterodine	Anticholinergic	IR tablet: 2 mg po bid; ER capsule: 4 mg po qd (take 1 hour before meals on empty stomach)	Hepatic	Dry mouth (25%–50%), headache (5%–10%), constipation (5%)	Dosage 1 mg po bid in patients with significantly impaired hepatic function
Trospium	Anticholinergic	Tablet: 20 mg po bid	Renal	Dry mouth (20%), constipation (10%), blurred vision (5%)	Dosage 20 mg po qd in patients with renal impairment (CrCl < 30)
Solifenacin	Anticholinergic	Tablet: 5–10 mg po qd	Hepatic and renal	Dry mouth (8%–15%), constipation (3%–10%), blurred vision (3%–6%)	Decreased dosage in patients with moderately impaired hepatic or severely impaired renal function, should not be used in patients with severely impaired hepatic function
Darifenacin	Anticholinergic	ER tablet: 7.5–15 mg po qd	Hepatic	Dry mouth (20%–30%), constipation (20%–25%)	Should not be used in patients with severe hepatic impairment; decreased dosage in patients with moderately impaired hepatic function
Imipramine	Alpha-adrenergic agonist; anticholinergic	Tablet: 10–25 mg po qd to qid	Hepatic	Urinary retention, blurred vision, dry mouth, constipation, tachycardia, orthostatic hypotension, cardiovascular changes	Use with caution in patients with hepatic impairment; use with caution in elderly patients

Figure 32-9. Medications for the treatment of overactive bladder. bid—twice daily; CrCl—creatinine clearance; ER—extended release; IR—immediate release; po—by mouth; qd—every day; tid—three times daily.

impairment and hallucination [42] and in patients on warfarin due to an association with unexpected international normalized ratio elevation [43,44].

Trospium, solifenacin, and darifenacin were approved by the US Food and Drug Administration for detrusor overactivity in 2004. They have been proven to be effective in patients with OAB over placebo [11,45–47,48•]. In head-to-head studies comparing these new agents with older drugs (*ie*, oxybutynin and tolterodine), they have been shown to have similar efficacy with better tolerance [49–53]. Dry mouth occurs in 20% of patients taking trospium [54•]. This side effect occurs in 14% with solifenacin 5 mg and in 21% with solifenacin 10 mg, compared with 19% tolterodine 2 mg twice daily [52]. Trospium is water soluble with reduced blood-brain barrier penetrance [55]. Therefore, in theory it should have minimal central nervous system adverse effects (such as cognitive impairment, drowsiness) compared to other anticholinergics. However, this has not been shown by head-to-head studies [49,53]. Trospium should be taken with an empty stomach, and the dose should be reduced by half in patients with renal impairment. Solifenacin and darifenacin are selective M3 muscarinic receptor antagonists, which potentially impose fewer side effects on the gastrointestinal tract such as dry mouth and constipation [51,56].

ALPHA-ADRENERGIC AGONIST

Imipramine has alpha-agonist and anticholinergic effects. It should be reserved for children and for adults suffering from nocturnal enuresis. It should not be given to elderly who are sensitive to the anticholinergic side affects.

Other Therapies: Sacral Nerve Root Stimulation

Sacral nerve root stimulation is an effective therapy for patients with OAB who have failed behavioral and pharmacologic interventions. It also may be beneficial in patients with OAB complicated by elevated PVRs. Electrodes are surgically inserted into the sacral foramina and connected to an external (test device) or implantable (permanent device) electrical stimulator. Patients are fitted with a test device and asked to complete a series of objective testing used to quantitate the frequency and severity of their disorder. Patients with a 50% improvement in symptoms are fitted with the permanent device. Improvement was seen in more than 66% of patients with refractory urinary incontinence [57].

Surgery

Patients with an OAB who fail pharmacologic and behavioral therapy should be referred to an incontinence specialist. The primary care physician should be aware of the therapeutic options available on referral. Bladder augmentation (enterocystoplasty) with a detubularized bowel segment and autoaugmentation (detrusor myomectomy) are last resorts for treatment for patients with intractable disease or low bladder compliance.

When to Refer

Most incontinent women can be evaluated and managed by primary care physicians without referral. Some women are best managed by specialists who use multichannel urodynamic testing to determine the physiologic changes in bladder function responsible for urinary symptoms. Referrals for multichannel urodynamic testing should be reserved for women with an uncertain diagnosis after a basic evaluation, history of prior continence surgery, history of previous pelvic radiation or radical pelvic surgery, elevated postvoid residual, pelvic organ prolapse, failed initial therapeutic interventions, hematuria without infection, or comorbid conditions (*eg*, diabetes, multiple sclerosis, spinal cord disease).

References

Papers of particular interest have been highlighted as follows:
- • Of interest
- •• Of outstanding interest

1.   Abrams P, Cardozo L, Fall M, *et al.*: The standardisation of terminology of lower urinary tract function: report from the Standardisation Subcommittee of the International Continence Society. *Neurourol Urodyn* 2002, 21:167–178.

2.   Irwin DE, Milsom I, Hunskaar S, *et al.*: Population-based survey of urinary incontinence, overactive bladder, and other lower urinary tract symptoms in five countries: results of the EPIC study. *Eur Urol* 2006, 50:1306–1314.

3.   Temml C, Heidler S, Ponholzer A, Madersbacher S: Prevalence of the overactive bladder syndrome by applying the International Continence Society definition. *Eur Urol* 2005, 48:622–627.

4.   Wein AJ, Rovner ES: Definition and epidemiology of overactive bladder. *Urology* 2002, 60:7–12.

5.   Stewart WF, Van Rooyen JB, Cundiff GW, *et al.*: Prevalence and burden of overactive bladder in the United States. *World J Urol* 2003, 20:327–336.

6.   Hu TW, Wagner TH, Bentkover JD, *et al.*: Costs of urinary incontinence and overactive bladder in the United States: a comparative study. *Urology* 2004, 63:461–465.

7.•   Andersson KE: Mechanisms of Disease: central nervous system involvement in overactive bladder syndrome. *Nat Clin Pract Urol* 2004, 1:103–108.

This is a good review of the neurophysiology of the lower urinary tract.

8.   de Groat WC: A neurologic basis for the overactive bladder. *Urology* 1997, 50:36–52.

9.   Brading AF: A myogenic basis for the overactive bladder. *Urology* 1997, 50:57–67.

10.   Mills IW, Greenland JE, McMurray G, *et al.*: Studies of the pathophysiology of idiopathic detrusor instability: the physiological properties of the detrusor smooth muscle and its pattern of innervation. *J Urol* 2000, 163:646–651.

11.   Yokoyama O, Nagano K, Kawaguchi K, Hisazumi H: The response of the detrusor muscle to acetylcholine in patients with infravesical obstruction. *Urol Res* 1991, 19:117–121.

12.   Elbadawi A, Yalla SV, Resnick NM: Structural basis of geriatric voiding dysfunction. III. Detrusor overactivity. *J Urol* 1993, 150:1668–1680.

13. Harrison SC, Hunnam GR, Farman P, *et al.:* Bladder instability and denervation in patients with bladder outflow obstruction. *Br J Urol* 1987, 60:519–522.

14. Sevestre S, Ciofu C, Deval B, *et al.:* Results of the tension–free vaginal tape technique in the elderly. *Eur Urol* 2003, 44:128–131.

15. Vierhout ME, Mulder AF: De novo detrusor instability after Burch colposuspension. *Acta Obstet Gynecol Scand* 1992, 71:414–416.

16. Burgio KL, Robinson JC, Engel BT: The role of biofeedback in Kegel exercise training for stress urinary incontinence. *Am J Obstet Gynecol* 1986, 154:58–64.

17. Fantl JA, Wyman JF, McClish DK, *et al.:* Efficacy of bladder training in older women with urinary incontinence. *JAMA* 1991, 265:609–613.

18. Burgio KL: Influence of behavior modification on overactive bladder. *Urology* 2002, 60:72–76.

19. Hunt J: Psychological approaches to the management of sensory urgency and idiopathic detrusor instability. *Br J Urol* 1996, 77:339–341.

20. Fitzgerald MP, Ayuste D, Brubaker L: How do urinary diaries of women with an overactive bladder differ from those of asymptomatic controls? *BJU Int* 2005, 96:365–367.

21. Jensen JK, Nielsen FR Jr, Ostergard DR: The role of patient history in the diagnosis of urinary incontinence. *Obstet Gynecol* 1994, 83:904–910.

22. Sand PK, Brubaker LT, Novak T: Simple standing incremental cystometry as a screening method for detrusor instability. *Obstet Gynecol* 1991, 77:453–457.

23. Swift SE, Ostergard DR: Evaluation of current urodynamic testing methods in the diagnosis of genuine stress incontinence. *Obstet Gynecol* 1995, 86:85–91.

24. Dallosso HM, McGrother CW, Matthews RJ, Donaldson MM: The association of diet and other lifestyle factors with overactive bladder and stress incontinence: a longitudinal study in women. *BJU Int* 2003, 92:69–77.

25. Arya LA, Myers DL, Jackson ND: Dietary caffeine intake and the risk for detrusor instability: a case-control study. *Obstet Gynecol* 2000, 96:85–89.

26. Swithinbank L, Hashim H, Abrams P: The effect of fluid intake on urinary symptoms in women. *J Urol* 2005, 174:187–189.

27. Frewen WK: A reassessment of bladder training in detrusor dysfunction in the female. *Br J Urol* 1982, 54:372–373.

28. Bump RC, Hurt WG, Fantl JA, Wyman JF: Assessment of Kegel pelvic muscle exercise performance after brief verbal instruction. *Am J Obstet Gynecol* 1991, 165:322–327.

29. Wang AC, Wang YY, Chen MC: Single-blind, randomized trial of pelvic floor muscle training, biofeedback-assisted pelvic floor muscle training, and electrical stimulation in the management of overactive bladder. *Urology* 2004, 63:61–66.

30. Brubaker L, Benson JT, Bent A, *et al.:* Transvaginal electrical stimulation for female urinary incontinence. *Am J Obstet Gynecol* 1997, 177:536–540.

31. Kellcher CJ, Cardozo LD, Khullar V, Salvatore S: A medium-term analysis of the subjective efficacy of treatment for women with detrusor instability and low bladder compliance. *Br J Obstet Gynaecol* 1997, 104:988–993.

32. Song C, Park JT, Heo KO, *et al.:* Effects of bladder training and/or tolterodine in female patients with overactive bladder syndrome: a prospective, randomized study. *J Korean Med Sci* 2006;21:1060–1063.

33. Alhasso AA, McKinlay J, Patrick K, Stewart L: Anticholinergic drugs versus non-drug active therapies for overactive bladder syndrome in adults. *Cochrane Database Syst Rev* 2006:CD003193.

34. Anderson RU, Mobley D, Blank B, *et al.:* Once daily controlled versus immediate release oxybutynin chloride for urge urinary incontinence. OROS Oxybutynin Study Group. *J Urol* 1999, 161:1809–1812.

35. Dmochowski RR, Nitti V, Staskin D, *et al.:* Transdermal oxybutynin in the treatment of adults with overactive bladder: combined results of two randomized clinical trials. *World J Urol* 2005, 23:263–270.

36. Cartwright R, Cardozo L: Transdermal oxybutynin: sticking to the facts. *Eur Urol* 2007, 51:907-914.

37. Sand P, Zinner N, Newman D, *et al.:* Oxybutynin transdermal system improves the quality of life in adults with overactive bladder: a multicentre, community–based, randomized study. *BJU Int* 2006, 99:836-844.

38. Diokno AC, Appell RA, Sand PK, *et al.:* Prospective, randomized, double-blind study of the efficacy and tolerability of the extended–release formulations of oxybutynin and tolterodine for overactive bladder: results of the OPERA trial. *Mayo Clin Proc* 2003, 78:687–695.

39.• Drutz HP, Appell RA, Gleason D, *et al.:* Clinical efficacy and safety of tolterodine compared to oxybutynin and placebo in patients with overactive bladder. *Int Urogynecol J Pelvic Floor Dysfunct* 1999, 10:283–289.

This is a good study comparing tolterodine to oxybutynin and placebo.

40. Armstrong RB, Luber KM, Peters KM: Comparison of dry mouth in women treated with extended-release formulations of oxybutynin or tolterodine for overactive bladder. *Int Urol Nephrol* 2005, 37:247–252.

41. Appell RA: Clinical efficacy and safety of tolterodine in the treatment of overactive bladder: a pooled analysis. *Urology* 1997, 50:90–96.

42. Tsao JW, Heilman KM: Transient memory impairment and hallucinations associated with tolterodine use. *N Engl J Med* 2003, 349:2274–2275.

43. Colucci VJ, Rivey MP: Tolterodine–warfarin drug interaction. *Ann Pharmacother* 1999, 33:1173–1176.

44. Taylor JR: Probable interaction between tolterodine and warfarin. *Pharmacotherapy* 2006, 26:719–721.

45. Cardozo L, Chapple CR, Toozs–Hobson P, *et al.:* Efficacy of trospium chloride in patients with detrusor instability: a placebo–controlled, randomized, double–blind, multi-centre clinical trial. *BJU Int* 2000, 85:659–664.

46.• Cardozo L, Lisec M, Millard R, *et al.:* Randomized, double-blind placebo controlled trial of the once daily antimuscarinic agent solifenacin succinate in patients with overactive bladder. *J Urol* 2004,172:1919–1924.

This is a good study on solifenacin.

47. Frohlich G, Bulitta M, Strosser W: Trospium chloride in patients with detrusor overactivity: meta-analysis of placebo-controlled, randomized, double-blind, multi-center clinical trials on the efficacy and safety of 20 mg trospium chloride twice daily. *Int J Clin Pharmacol Ther* 2002, 40:295–303.

48.• Haab F, Corcos J, Siami P, *et al.:* Long–term treatment with darifenacin for overactive bladder: results of a 2–year, open–label extension study. *BJU Int* 2006, 98:1025–1032.

This is a good study on side effects and efficacy of darifenacin.

49. Halaska M, Ralph G, Wiedemann A, *et al.*: Controlled, double–blind, multicentre clinical trial to investigate long–term tolerability and efficacy of trospium chloride in patients with detrusor instability. World *J Urol* 2003, 20:392–399.

50. Zinner N, Tuttle J, Marks L: Efficacy and tolerability of darifenacin, a muscarinic M3 selective receptor antagonist (M3 SRA), compared with oxybutynin in the treatment of patients with overactive bladder. *World J Urol* 2005, 23:248–252.

51. Chapple CR, Martinez–Garcia R, Selvaggi L, *et al.*: A comparison of the efficacy and tolerability of solifenacin succinate and extended release tolterodine at treating overactive bladder syndrome: results of the STAR trial. *Eur Urol* 2005, 48:464–470.

52. Chapple CR, Rechberger T, Al–Shukri S, *et al.*: Randomized, double-blind placebo- and tolterodine-controlled trial of the once-daily antimuscarinic agent solifenacin in patients with symptomatic overactive bladder. *BJU Int* 2004, 93:303–310.

53. Madersbacher H, Stohrer M, Richter R, *et al.*: Trospium chloride versus oxybutynin: a randomized, double-blind, multicentre trial in the treatment of detrusor hyper-reflexia. *Br J Urol* 1995, 75:452–456.

54.• Zinner N, Gittelman M, Harris R, *et al.*: Trospium chloride improves overactive bladder symptoms: a multicenter phase III trial. *J Urol* 2004, 171:2311–2315.

This is a good study on effectiveness of trospium.

55. Todorova A, Vonderheid–Guth B, Dimpfel W: Effects of tolterodine, trospium chloride, and oxybutynin on the central nervous system. *J Clin Pharmacol* 2001, 41:636–644.

56. Zinner N, Susset J, Gittelman M, *et al.*: Efficacy, tolerability and safety of darifenacin, an M(3) selective receptor antagonist: an investigation of warning time in patients with OAB. *Int J Clin Pract* 2006, 60:119–126.

57. Shaker HS, Hassouna M: Sacral nerve root neuromodulation: an effective treatment for refractory urge incontinence. *J Urol* 1998, 159:1516–1519.

33 | Pelvic Organ Prolapse

Robert L. Summitt, Jr.

- Pelvic organ prolapse is a common problem, but only a small portion of affected women seek medical care.
- A general understanding of pelvic anatomy and the supporting structures of the pelvis is essential to management decisions regarding pelvic floor dysfunction.
- Use of the Pelvic Organ Prolapse Quantification vaginal profile at the time of vaginal examination to describe prolapse is encouraged to standardize the examination of all women who have or will develop symptomatic pelvic organ prolapse.
- Surgical and nonsurgical treatment options are available for all women with varying extent of symptomatic pelvic organ prolapse.
- Regardless of the extent of prolapse, a symptomatic patient should be referred to a gynecologist skilled in all techniques of reconstructive pelvic surgery.

Historical Perspective

Gynecologists have studied and managed pelvic relaxation for centuries, but there are many unanswered questions regarding etiology, treatment, and therapeutic outcomes. Pelvic relaxation—now more appropriately referred to as pelvic organ prolapse—is a common condition and has been affecting women for centuries. Early treatments included chemicals and emollients to induce contraction of the vaginal musculature and resolve the prolapse, scare tactics with a hot iron to induce retraction of the prolapse, and even hanging upside down by a suspension apparatus to restore the prolapse [1]. Later, less barbaric nonsurgical treatments arose including various devices used as pessaries to hold the prolapsed vagina in place [1].

The first surgical procedures to correct pelvic organ prolapse were developed at the end of the 19th century and were directed toward suspension or obliteration of the vagina. Current surgical treatments are still directed in this manner and include various vaginal and abdominal approaches to restore normal anatomy and suspend the prolapsed vagina. Vaginal obliterative procedures, including resection of the vagina with closure of the genital hiatus, are less commonly used.

Introduction

Epidemiologic data regarding the incidence of pelvic organ prolapse are limited. It has been estimated that half of parous women have some amount of pelvic floor dysfunction, probably secondary to childbirth, which results in pelvic organ prolapse. About 10% to 20% of women seek medical care for their symptoms [2]. The lifetime risk of undergoing a single operation for pelvic organ prolapse by 80 years of age has been reported to be 11.1%, and the National Center for Health Statistics reports that almost 400,000 operations are performed annually for pelvic organ prolapse [3,4].

The severity and symptoms of pelvic organ prolapse vary and are manifest when the pelvic contents, including reproductive organs, bladder, rectum, and small intestines, herniate through defects in the pelvic floor. These herniations can result in genital tract and urinary tract dysfunction as well as significant bowel dysfunction. More severe degrees of pelvic organ prolapse can distort body image, impair sexual function, and negatively impact professional and recreational activities.

Many opinions exist as to the etiology of pelvic organ prolapse. (Figure 33-1). Most authorities agree that vaginal delivery is the primary and most important event leading to subsequent problems with pelvic organ prolapse or urinary incontinence.

Obstetric trauma may cause direct damage to muscles and indirect damage through denervation of the pelvic floor [5–7]. Other conditions that promote chronic increases in intra-abdominal pressure, such as obesity, ascites, and chronic respiratory conditions with cough, can be precipitating factors of pelvic organ prolapse [3]. Finally, smoking, underlying connective tissue disease, and neuropathies have also been implicated as risk factors for the development and promotion of pelvic organ prolapse [3,8,9]. Aging has its effect on pelvic organ prolapse, and some authorities recognize prolapse as a progressive process with a known acceleration after menopause. The cumulative incidence of operative intervention for pelvic organ prolapse increases dramatically after 50 years of age, with more than half of these operations being performed in those women [3].

The average age of menopause is 50 years, and most women spend one third of their life after menopause. Currently, 15% of the population is 65 years of age or older, and this percentage is expected to increase to more than 20% after the year 2000. Furthermore, life expectancy for women is now 83 years, and women who are healthy at age 60 can expect to live into their ninth decade.

Pelvic Anatomy

An understanding of the anatomy of the pelvis and its muscular components is essential to understanding how the pelvic organs, including the vagina, bladder, rectum, and small intes-

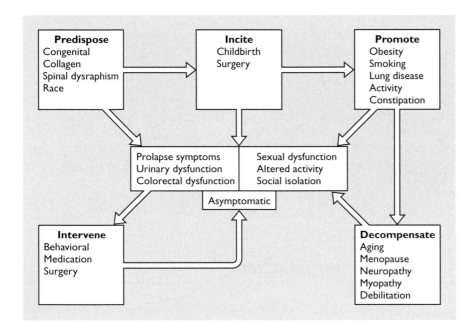

Figure 33-1. Pelvic organ prolapse paradigm. (*Adapted from* Theofrastus [24].)

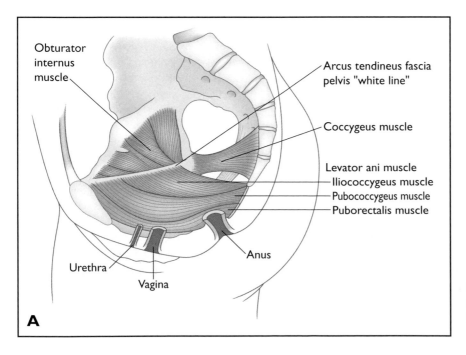

Figure 33-2. A and **B**, Pelvic floor anatomy. (*Adapted from* Shingleton and Hurt [25].)

Continued on the next page

tines, are held in their respective anatomic positions. Only then can one fully comprehend how a compromise in the pelvic support system can lead to pelvic organ prolapse.

Figure 33-2 provides an anatomic representation of the bony pelvis and its muscular components. The reproductive organs, bladder, and rectum are supported by and rest on the pelvic diaphragm, which is formed by the puborectalis, pubococcygeus, and iliococcygeus muscles that compose the levator ani and the coccygeus muscle. The condensation of tissue at the junction of the levator ani and obturator internus muscle is called the arcus tendineus fascia pelvis (ATFP). The lateral vagina attaches here and forms an important landmark in reconstructive pelvic surgery.

A three-level support system was described in detail by DeLancey [10•] in 1992, who dissected 74 fresh and fixed female cadavers. This system represents an easy and reason-able means to understand pelvic floor support. The bladder, uterus, vagina, and rectum are all supported by connective tissue, and this tissue forms identifiable structures that support each pelvic organ. Levels of support are described below and depicted in Figures 33-3 and 33-4.

Level I support corresponds to the primary support for the uterus, which is the cardinal and uterosacral ligament complex. These "ligaments" are not made up of the same type of ligamentous tissues that compose ligaments in other parts of the body, such as the knee, but instead are composed mostly of blood vessels, nerves, and connective tissue, from which they derive strength [11,12]. Broad attachments arise from the pelvic walls originating near the greater sciatic foramen and lateral sacrum and insert along the lateral margin of the vagina, enveloping its anterior and posterior surfaces.

Level II support is a direct attachment of the vagina to the pelvic wall that is in closer proximity at this level. No "ligaments" are found here. Instead, the lateral attachments are created by the encapsulating endopelvic "fascia" of the vagina, which is not the same type of fascia as in other parts of the body, such as the anterior abdominal wall fascia, but instead is mostly smooth muscle, attaching directly to the pelvic wall at the ATFP. This attachment supports the midportion of the vagina and extends from the more proximal 2 to 3 cm of the vagina to 2 to 3 cm above the hymenal ring.

Level III extends from the area 2 to 3 cm proximal to the hymenal ring to the genital hiatus. Here, the vagina is fused directly with the surrounding structures: laterally to the medial border of the levator ani muscles, posteriorly to the perineal body, and anteriorly with the urethra, which is normally adherent to the pubic bone by the pubourethral ligament. Because the vagina directly adheres to these structures, damage to any of them may cause subsequent vaginal defects. Weakening of the urethral attachments may cause urethral mobility and therefore an anterior vaginal wall defect and possibly urinary incontinence. Likewise, compromises in the functional integrity of the levator ani muscles from direct insult or denervation may lead to a more open introitus, predisposing the pelvic organs to prolapse.

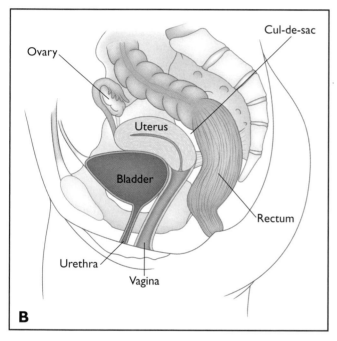

Figure 33-2. (Continued).

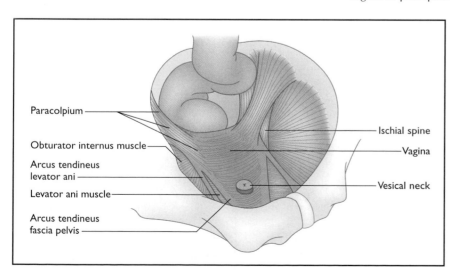

Figure 33-3. Depiction of levels of support. (*Adapted from* DeLancey [10•].)

Although presented here as separate entities, these levels are intertwined in the support and function of the pelvic floor. Each level is intimately connected to the other, with no clear separation, and each depends on the others for additional strength. Specific weakness at any one level can cause specific defects, but often more than one level of support is compromised.

Diagnostic Studies

HISTORY
A constellation of symptoms can plague the woman with pelvic organ prolapse, with worse degrees of prolapse usually causing more severe symptoms. Anterior vaginal wall defects, that is, defects involving the bladder or urethra (cystocele or urethrocele), can present with complaints similar to those associated with a urinary tract infection, including frequency or dysuria, difficulty initiating a stream, incomplete bladder emptying, or urinary incontinence. Defecatory dysfunction, such as fecal incontinence, soiling, or incomplete evacuation, may be the primary symptomatology associated with a posterior defect (rectocele). Prolapse of the apex, that is, uterus and vaginal vault (procidentia), can cause sexual dysfunction, pelvic pressure or fullness, lower back pain, and sometimes bleeding from abrasions and erosions of the prolapsed cervix or vaginal epithelium.

PHYSICAL EXAMINATION
Differences in describing clinical findings at physical examination have been an impediment to comparing preoperative and postoperative outcomes for pelvic surgeons. Epidemiologic data are scarce and have been difficult to apply in different populations because of various untested and unproven mea-

surement techniques. Brubaker and Norton [13] reported that in 103 articles about pelvic organ prolapse, 16 different systems for description had been used, no two of which were similar enough to be used in comparison with the others. In 47 articles, no grading system was defined, and consistent grading systems were used in only 10% of the articles.

In an attempt to address these problems, in 1996 the International Continence Society, American Urogynecologic Society, and Society of Gynecologic Surgeons adopted standardized terminology for pelvic organ prolapse [14••]. This system, called the Pelvic Organ Prolapse Quantification (POP-Q) examination system, was designed to replace more imprecise descriptions of vaginal defects, such as cystocele, rectocele, and enterocele, and also to replace more subjective descriptions, such as mild, moderate, or severe, with more precise measurements. The POP-Q system is a modification of the Baden and Walker [15] halfway grading system that was in itself a major advance from previous systems. Baden and Walker [15] used a precise site-specific description of defects, but there remained potential for variation among examiners. The POP-Q system identifies specific points along the midline of the vagina in a sagittal plane on both the anterior and posterior vaginal walls as well as points denoting apical support. The genital hiatus, perineal body, and total vaginal length are also measured (Figure 33-5). All points except total vaginal length are measured with maximal straining to examine the prolapse and vaginal defects at their maximum extent.

The POP-Q examination can be represented by a list of the measured points, a three-by-three grid (Figure 33-6), or a grid and line diagram (Figure 33-7). Six vaginal points outline the profile of the vagina, with the hymenal ring used as the reference point for all measurements. Points cephalad to the hymen are represented as negative numbers, whereas those caudal to

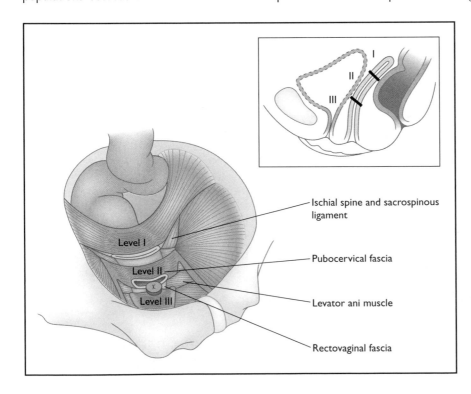

Ischial spine and sacrospinous ligament

Pubocervical fascia

Levator ani muscle

Rectovaginal fascia

Level I

Level II

Level III

Figure 33-4. Depiction of levels of support. (*Adapted from* DeLancey [10•].)

the hymen are positive. The six vaginal points that represent the pelvic examination profile are as follows:

Aa: The position of the most distal anterior vaginal wall. It begins at the urethral meatus and extends 3 cm into the vagina, representing the approximate location of the urethrovesical crease. Because it is only 3 cm long, by definition, it can only have values ranging from -3 (no prolapse) to +3 (maximally prolapsed). It would have a value of 0 if it descended to the hymen (reference point).

Ba: The most distal (*ie*, most dependent) part of the anterior vaginal wall from the vaginal cuff (posthysterectomy) or anterior fornix to point Aa. It is -3 with no prolapse (equal to point Aa) and would have a positive value equal to the position of the vaginal cuff with vaginal vault eversion after a hysterectomy (the most dependent portion of the anterior vaginal wall would now be at the vaginal cuff). It would have a value of 0 (zero) if the most dependent point descended to the hymen.

C: The most distal (*ie*, most dependent) edge of the cervix or vaginal cuff after hysterectomy.

D: The position of the posterior fornix in a woman with a cervix. This describes the attachment of the cardinal and uterosacral ligaments to the posterior cervix and uterus. It distinguishes between an apical support failure of the cardinal–uterosacral complex (point D positive) and cervical elongation (point C positive but point D negative). This point is obviously omitted after hysterectomy.

Ap: The position of the most distal posterior vaginal wall. It begins at the posterior hymen and extends 3 cm cephalad into the vagina. It can only have values ranging from -3 (no prolapse) to +3 (maximally prolapsed). Extension to the hymen (reference point) would be given a value of 0.

Bp: The most distal (*ie*, most dependent) position of any part of the posterior vaginal wall from the vaginal cuff (post hysterectomy) or posterior vaginal fornix to point Ap. By definition, it is -3 in the absence of prolapse and equal to the position of the vaginal cuff in a woman with total posthysterectomy vaginal vault eversion. It

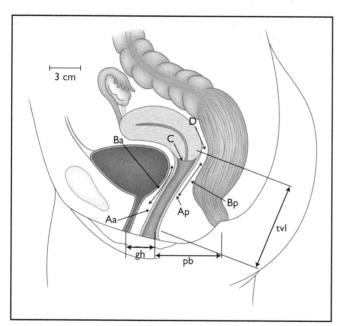

Figure 33-5. Sites of measurement for vaginal defects (*Adapted from* Bump *et al.* [14••].)

Anterior wall **Aa**	Anterior wall **Ba**	Cervix or cuff **C**
Genital hiatus **gh**	Perineal body **pb**	Total vaginal length **tvl**
Posterior wall **Ap**	Posterior wall **Bp**	Posterior fornix **D**

Figure 33-6. Three-by-three grid for pelvic organ prolapse. (*Adapted from* Bump *et al.* [14••].)

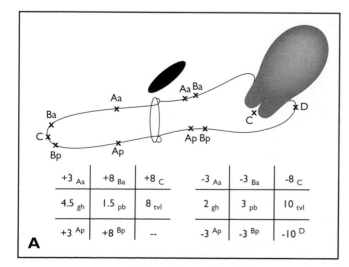

+3 Aa	+8 Ba	+8 C		-3 Aa	-3 Ba	-8 C
4.5 gh	1.5 pb	8 tvl		2 gh	3 pb	10 tvl
+3 Ap	+8 Bp	--		-3 Ap	-3 Bp	-10 D

A

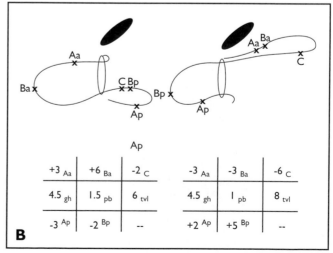

+3 Aa	+6 Ba	-2 C		-3 Aa	-3 Ba	-6 C
4.5 gh	1.5 pb	6 tvl		4.5 gh	1 pb	8 tvl
-3 Ap	-2 Bp	--		+2 Ap	+5 Bp	--

B

Figure 33-7. A and **B**, Grid and line diagram for pelvic organ prolapse. (*Adapted from* Bump *et al.* [14••].)

would have a value of 0 (zero) if the most dependent point extended to the hymen, -1 if it is 1 cm above the hymen, +2 if it is 2 cm beyond the hymen, and so forth.

The three other points of measurement are genital hiatus (gh), perineal body (pb), and total vaginal length (tvl). All except the total vaginal length are measured with maximal straining, and their measurements are obtained as follows: genital hiatus (gh): The distance from the middle of the external urethral meatus to the posterior hymen; perineal body (pb): The length from the posterior hymen to the midanal opening; total vaginal length (tvl): the greatest vaginal depth when point C (anterior fornix or vaginal cuff) or D (posterior fornix) is reduced to its full normal position.

Anterior Vaginal Wall

The anterior vaginal wall is best visualized by using a speculum that has been taken apart. Using the bottom portion of the speculum, pressure is applied to the posterior vagina to optimize visualization anteriorly (Figure 33-8). This allows for full evaluation and description of the anterior vaginal wall points Aa and Ba. Characterization of the defect as being urethrocele, cystocele, or cystourethrocele is discouraged unless ancillary techniques have been used to characterize the defect further because these terms may imply an unrealistic certainty about the structure underneath the vaginal bulge. Anterior defects can be caused by separation of the endopelvic fascia from the ATFP laterally (paravaginal defect); loss of the vaginal attachment to the vaginal cuff or cervix, possibly with intervening small bowel contents (enterocele); or tears within the anterior endopelvic fascia (pubocervical fascia) with bulging of the bladder through this defect (cystocele). Each of these defects presents as bulging of the anterior vaginal wall and should be characterized quantitatively using the POP-Q system. The examiner may state that the defect appears to be a cystocele or enterocele, but this should not preface representation of the anterior defect in the POP-Q grid.

Uterus and Vaginal Apex

The cervix or apex of the vagina is easily visualized with a speculum. Gently separating the bills of the speculum permits adequate visualization for examination of the cervix or vaginal cuff. Straining or having the patient bear down maximally permits assessment of the amount of cervical or vaginal cuff (point C) or posterior fornix (point D) descent toward the hymen using the POP-Q system. Complete eversion of the vagina and uterus is often referred to as uterovaginal prolapse or complete uterine procidentia and implies complete failure of apical supports (Figure 33-9). Likewise, posthysterectomy cuff eversion is commonly referred to as vaginal vault prolapse.

Posterior Vaginal Wall

Examination of the posterior vaginal wall is similar to that of the anterior vaginal wall. The bottom portion of the speculum is used to retract the anterior wall upward to visualize the posterior vagina (Figure 33-10). Bearing down, or straining, is performed by the patient to maximize visualization of any defect that is present. Again, the defined points along the posterior wall are represented in the POP-Q profile. Further characterization by the examiner can be made, which should include performance of a digital rectal examination to determine if the defect involves only the rectum (rectocele), or if there is an enterocele component. Qualification as an enterocele may also be determined by seeing peristaltic movement of small bowel within the defect; this should be described by the examiner after the posterior defect has been appropriately expressed within the POP-Q grid.

Ancillary Tests

Only rarely do defects of pelvic support require ancillary evaluation, and this falls beyond the scope of the initial workup by the primary care physician. Interpretation is sometimes difficult, and the necessity of these tests is best determined by those more familiar with reconstructive pelvic surgery. Indeed,

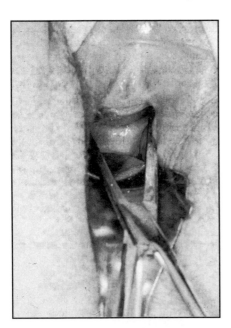

Figure 33-8. Anterior wall defect.

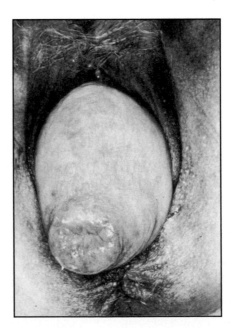

Figure 33-9. Complete uterovaginal eversion (procidentia).

it is beneficial at times to distinguish the underlying prolapsing structure more definitely so that better determination can be made of the appropriate surgical alternative. MRI [16] and fluoroscopic techniques [17] (eg, evacuation proctography) can help demonstrate occult enteroceles, further evaluate rectoceles or sigmoidoceles, and better demonstrate other anatomic alterations in the position of the bladder and rectum, especially in patients with previous reconstructive surgery.

In cases of total prolapse or large anterior vaginal wall defects, complex urodynamic testing can play an important role and should be considered. Large defects can cause kinking of the urethra and mask underlying genitourinary dysfunction such as urinary incontinence. One study [18] revealed that 59% of patients with pelvic organ prolapse had abnormal urodynamic findings with pessary reduction of their prolapse. Of these, 35% had genuine stress incontinence, 35% had detrusor instability, and 30% had mixed urinary incontinence. Consideration for formal testing should be given to the elderly, those with prior reconstructive or incontinence surgery, patients with lower urinary tract symptomatology that is not straightforward, and those with prolapse beyond the hymen.

Management

NONSURGICAL TREATMENT

Nonsurgical therapies for prolapse have existed for thousands of years. Vaginal pessaries are perhaps the most common alternative to surgery and have proved to be effective in alleviation of pelvic organ prolapse symptoms, especially for those with comorbid conditions that may preclude safe surgical intervention. Pessaries come in a variety of shapes and sizes, and each has a specific role in the treatment of various types of prolapse. They are now composed of siliconized rubber, making

them very pliable, and thus more resistant to formation of erosions of the vagina. The Gellhorn pessary is pacifier-shaped and is useful in cases of total prolapse. Other types of pessaries include doughnuts, cubes, and rings, with multiple variations of each. Ring pessaries may be more useful for sexually active women because they allow for coitus without the need for removal. However, ring pessaries are also the most easily removable, and therefore are associated with fewer complications. Pessaries should be fitted by an experienced physician and should adequately reduce the defect with no significant pressure on the vagina or discomfort to the patient. Postmenopausal patients should be on estrogen therapy to help prevent abrasions and erosions, and all patients should be checked within 1 week after fitting for evidence of such. Each patient should be taught proper care for her pessary and should be comfortable with removal, cleaning, and replacement. For those unable to remove the pessary, regular follow-up visits every 2 to 3 months should be maintained.

Other nonsurgical options include estrogen replacement for postmenopausal patients with irritative urogenital symptoms, such as urinary frequency or incontinence [19]. The trophic effects of estrogen on the vaginal epithelium may also be beneficial if future surgery is planned. Alterations in lifestyle, such as alleviation of constipation, cessation of smoking, weight loss for obese patients, or activity modifications to decrease stress and strain, may improve symptoms significantly without need for further interventions.

SURGICAL TREATMENT

Patients with symptoms that do not respond to nonsurgical therapies may opt for surgical intervention. Numerous surgical options are available to women with symptomatic pelvic relaxation. Surgical correction, approached vaginally or abdominally, is directed toward correction of the specific defect in the anterior, posterior, or apical compartment and

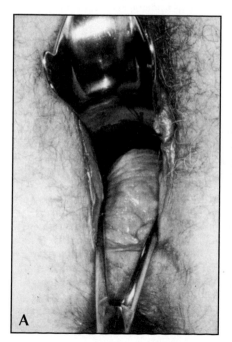 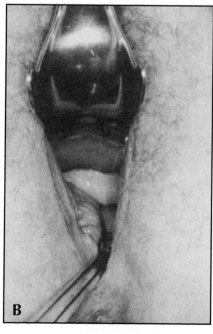

Figure 33-10. A and **B**, Posterior vaginal wall defect.

should only be considered if the patient is complaining of associated symptoms.

Anterior Defects

Vaginal reconstruction of the anterior vaginal wall has been the mainstay of anterior compartment defects. Defects within the anterior wall can be midline, paravaginal, or combined. The more common midline defects, referred to as cystoceles, are caused by midline separation or attenuation of the anterior endopelvic fascia (pubovisceral fascia). Kelly in 1912 advocated midline plication of this fascia under the hypermobile urethra and bladder for correction of the midline defect, and this operation is still commonly performed today. Paravaginal defects, as described earlier, form when the lateral edge of the endopelvic fascia becomes detached from the ATFP, or "white line." These defects cause the lateral vaginal wall to sag or drop, also resulting in a cystocele. Vaginal and abdominal operations exist for correction of paravaginal defects, and these defects can be adequately identified and repaired at the time of operation by reattaching the laterally detached anterior endopelvic fascia along the ATFP from the ischial spine to the pubic bone.

Posterior Defects

There is some disagreement among pelvic surgeons regarding the best way to correct posterior vaginal defects surgically. In the past, correction of posterior defects included plication of the levator ani muscles across the midline between the vagina and rectum, and many still practice this technique. Recent investigators have challenged this tenet based on the fundamental anatomic fact that the levator ani muscles do not normally separate the vagina and rectum, and their plication could potentially lead to dyspareunia or altered defecatory function. Alternatively, they recommend identification and repair of specific defects within the posterior endopelvic fascia in a more anatomic fashion [20]. Repair of the perineal body is performed if there is disruption of these muscles or detachment from the distal end of the posterior endopelvic fascia. Whatever the choice of operative approach, overcorrecting should be avoided to prevent possible future coital dysfunction.

Apical Defects

Perhaps no defect provokes more thought and apprehension from the reconstructive pelvic surgeon than that of surgical correction of uterine or vaginal vault prolapse. This trepidation is in part related to the potential for failure and the subsequent negative impact this can have on an otherwise healthy woman. Repair may be accomplished through the vaginal or abdominal route. Vaginal procedures include the prespinous suspension [21], which reattaches the apex of the vagina unilaterally or bilaterally to the fascia overlying the iliococcygeus muscle, and sacrospinous ligament suspensions [22•], whereby the vaginal apex is attached, usually unilaterally, to the sacrospinous ligament deep within the pelvis. Both procedures have reported good long-term success rates [21,22•]. Abdominal sacral colpopexy is performed through an abdominal incision and uses a synthetic mesh, usually Mersilene (Ethicon, Inc., Somerville, NJ) or polypropylene, as a prosthesis to suspend the vagina to the presacral ligamentous tissue near the sacral promontory. This procedure restores anatomy and avoids vaginal incisions that could lead to subsequent scarring and dyspa-reunia or could further compromise vaginal depth, especially in women with previous pelvic surgery and an already fore-shortened vagina. Success rates of greater than 90% have been reported [23•]. Obliterative procedures are good options for women who are no longer sexually active. Complete or partial removal of the vagina (colpectomy) with closure of the genital hiatus (colpocleisis) results in less morbidity, and at times can even be performed under local anesthesia if necessary. These procedures are effective, require less operative time, and usually allow for easier recovery than reconstructive procedures.

Conclusions

Pelvic organ prolapse commonly occurs in many reproductive and post-reproductive age women. The associated symptoms may be devastating personally, socially, and even sexually, and a woman's embarrassment over this may preclude her from seeking help. Thus, it is the duty of all physicians to inquire about such problems and be reassuring to these patients. This is especially true for primary care physicians since the bulk of these women will likely present with other primary medical complaints and problems. It is important that the physician have an understanding of the basic pathophysiology and available therapeutic options so that women with symptomatic pelvic organ prolapse can receive appropriate counseling and referral as needed.

References

Papers of particular interest have been highlighted as follows:
* Of interest
•• Of outstanding interest

1. Emge LA, Durfee RB: Pelvic organ prolapse: four thousand years of treatment. *Clin Obstet Gynecol* 1966, 9:997–1032.

2. Olsen AL, Smith VJ, Bergstrom JO, *et al.*: Epidemiology of surgically managed pelvic organ prolapse and urinary incontinence. *Obstet Gynecol* 1997, 89:501–506.

3. Beck RP: Pelvic relaxational prolapse. In *Principles and Practice of Clinical Gynecology*. Edited by Kase NG, Weingold AB. New York: John Wiley & Sons, 1983:677–685.

4. *National Center for Health Statistics Figures for 1987*. Atlanta, GA: National Center for Health Statistics at the Centers for Disease Control and Prevention; 1987.

5. Koelbl H, Strassegger H, Riss PA, *et al.*: Morphologic and functional aspects of floor muscles in patients with pelvic relaxation and genuine stress incontinence. *Obstet Gynecol* 1989, 74:789.

6. Snooks SJ, Barnes PRH, Swash M: Damage to the innervation of the voluntary anal and periurethral sphincter musculature in incontinence: an electrophysiologic study. *J Neurol Neurosurg Psychiatry* 1984, 47:1269.

7. Sharf B, Zilberman, Sharf M, *et al.*: Electromyogram of pelvic floor muscles in genital prolapse. *Int J Gynaecol Obstet* 1976, 14:2–4.

8. Dewhurst J, Toplis PJ, Shepherd JH: Ivalon sponge hysteropexy for genital prolapse in patients with bladder extrophy. *Br J Obstet Gynaecol* 1980, 87:67–69.

9. Stanton SL: Gynecologic complications of epispadias and bladder exstrophy. *Am J Obstet Gynecol* 1974, 119:749–754.

10.• DeLancey JOL: Anatomic aspects of vaginal eversion after hysterectomy. *Am J Obstet Gynecol* 1992, 166:1717.
Levels of vaginal support from surrounding pelvic structures are graphically demonstrated as well as common vaginal defects manifested by injury to these levels of support.

11. Campbell RM: The anatomy and histology of the sacrouterine ligaments. *Am J Obstet Gynecol* 1950, 59:1–12.

12. Range RL, Woodburne RT: The gross and microscopic anatomy of the transverse cervical ligament. *Am J Obstet Gynecol* 1964, 90:460–467.

13. Brubaker L, Norton P: Current clinical nomenclature for description of pelvic support defects. *Int J Urogynecol* 1993, 4:399.

14.•• Bump RC, Matiasson A, Bo K, *et al.*: The standardization of terminology of female pelvic organ prolapse and pelvic floor dysfunction. *Am J Obstet Gynecol* 1996, 175:10–17.
This article presents the standardized terminology and method of measurement for the clinical description of pelvic organ prolapse.

15. Baden WF, Walker TA: Genesis of the vaginal profile: a correlated classification of vaginal relaxation. *Clin Obstet Gynecol* 1972, 15:1048.

16. Goodrich MA, Webb MJ, King BF, *et al.*: Magnetic resonance imaging of pelvic floor relaxation: dynamic analysis and evaluation of patients before and after surgical repair. *Obstet Gynecol* 1993, 82:883.

17. Brubaker L, Retzky S, Smith C, *et al.*: Pelvic floor evaluation with dynamic fluoroscopy. *Obstet Gynecol* 1993, 82:863.

18. Rozenzweig BA, Pushkin S, Blumenfeld D, *et al.*: Prevalence of abnormal urodynamic test results in continent women with severe genitourinary prolapse. *Obstet Gynecol* 1992, 79:539.

19. Fantl JA, Cardozo L, McClish DK, and the Hormones and Urogenital Therapy Committee: Estrogen therapy in the management of urinary incontinence in postmenopausal women: a meta-analysis. First report of the Hormones and Urogenital Therapy Committee. *Obstet Gynecol* 1994, 83:12.

20. Richardson AC: The rectovaginal septum revisited: its relationship to rectocele and its importance in rectocele repair. *Clin Obstet Gynecol* 1993, 36:976.

21. Meeks GR, Washburne JF, McGehee RP, *et al.*: Repair of vaginal prolapse by suspension of the vagina to iliococcygeus (prespinous) fascia. *Am J Obstet Gynecol* 1994, 171:1444–1452.

22.• Morley GW, DeLancey JOL: Sacrospinous ligament fixation for eversion of the vagina. *Am J Obstet Gynecol* 1988, 158:872.
This article reports the effectiveness of sacrospinous ligament fixation for pelvic organ prolapse.

23.• Addison WA, Timmons MC: Abdominal approach to vaginal eversion. *Clin Obstet Gynecol* 1993, 36:976.
The effectiveness of an abdominal approach to vaginal vault eversion is proven in this study.

24. Theofrastus JP: Pelvic organ prolapse: relationship to pelvic floor dysfunction. *Postgraduate Obstet Gynecol* 1994, 14:3.

25. Shingleton HM, Hurt WG: *Postreproductive Gynecology*. New York: Churchill Livingstone, 1990:414.

26. Shull BL: Clinical evaluation of women with pelvic support defects. *Clin Obstet Gynecol* 1993, 36:945.

34 | Menopause

Frank W. Ling

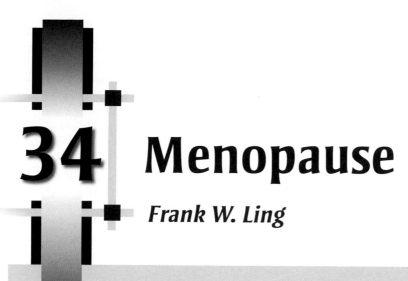

- Menopause is associated with a significant reduction in estrogen after cessation of ovarian function.
- Adverse long-term health effects accompany menopause and women should be treated for symptoms and prevention of diseases common to women.
- Estrogen replacement remains a therapeutic option, but should be used at the lowest dose for the shortest length of time possible based on the needs of the individual patient.

In 1990 there were approximately 36 million women in the United States over age 50. With the median age of menopause in the United States at 50 and the life expectancy for women 83 years, more women live a third of their lives in an estrogen-deficient state. As this population grows, addressing healthier living after menopause becomes a greater priority.

With an ever-increasing number of women seeking health care during the menopause, it is important to provide these women with complete information about hormone replacement therapy (HRT) and its alternatives. Risks and benefits for each patient should be reviewed. Helping the patient understand both pharmacologic interventions and life style changes will greatly improve her knowledge of the therapies chosen.

Definitions

Menopause is cessation of menstruation, but this event is only one point in the continuum of declining ovarian function. It signals the time in a woman's life when reproductive function is lost. The process of transition is termed the climacteric or perimenopause. Prominent during the climacteric are the symptoms of menopause. Premature menopause, also called premature ovarian failure, is the cessation of menses before age 40.

The age of menopause is genetically determined and is not related to the number of prior ovulations (ie, pregnancy, lactation, use of hormonal contraceptives, or anovulatory cycles). The age of menopause is also unrelated to race, socioeconomic status, level of education, height, weight, age of menarche, or age at last pregnancy. Menopause occurs earlier in women who smoke cigarettes, live at high altitudes, and those with poor nutritional status.

Menopausal Changes

Symptoms of irregular menses, hot flashes, night sweats, and mood swings often begin sometime after age 40. When a patient complains of these symptoms and she is over 40, she is likely experiencing symptoms of estrogen fluctuation and possibly estrogen deficiency. Until a patient is known to be estrogen deficient, the approach to treatment should be directed at relieving her complaints.

Vasomotor, mood and changes
Hot flashes and night sweats
Increased perspiration
Sleep disturbance
Anxiety and a feeling of tension
Depression and irritability
Skin changes
Reproductive tract
Vaginal dryness
Dyspareunia
Urinary frequency
Recurrent urinary tract infection
Loss of libido and sexual dysfunction
Health risks
Bone loss progressing to osteopenia and osteoporosis
Cardiovascular disease

Changes in Menstrual Bleeding Patterns

Complaints of increasing length between periods with infrequent very short cycles are common. Finally, menses completely stop. This is the usual change in the bleeding pattern as the climacteric progresses. However, many women will experience more frequent, heavier or prolonged bleeding prior to the onset of oligomenorrhea. This is due to the decrease in length of the follicular phase of an ovulatory cycle.

The diagnosis of the last menstrual period is made only retrospectively and requires 6 to 12 months of amenorrhea to confirm. Once elevated gonadotropin levels confirm the menopause, subsequent bleeding must be viewed as "postmenopausal bleeding" and evaluated to rule out endometrial pathology.

Hot Flashes and Night Sweats

A hot flash may be described as a sudden perception of intense upper body warmth which usually begins in the chest region and rises to the neck and face, followed commonly by intense sweating in the upper body. They can be accompanied by lightheadedness and a rapid heart beat. Hot flashes are often preceded by prodromal symptoms such as increasing head pressure. They are particularly disturbing at night and cause night sweats, insomnia, and fatigue the next day. Hot flash frequency varies from every 20 minutes to once or twice per month. The duration can be as short as seconds or as long as an hour. Over 80% of menopausal women continue to experience hot flashes after 1 year and 25% after 5 years.

TThe mechanisms responsible for the hot flash are not well understood. Although skin temperature rises with the flash, the core body temperature actually falls. The vasomotor hot flash is experienced by nearly 75% of menopausal women.

Mood Changes and Memory

The relationship between anxiety, irritability, nervousness, headaches, fatigue, joint and muscle pain, dizziness, depression, and estrogen deficiency is unknown. Certain symptoms may be due to vasomotor symptoms at night causing sleep disorders and subsequent mood alteration. This may explain why some of these symptoms may improve with estrogen therapy or other effective nonhormonal treatment. There is some evidence of improvement of memory with HRT, leading to increased interest among patients who wish to improve their cognitive function.

Early reports suggested that Alzheimer's disease and dementia may occur less frequently in women on HRT. In contrast, older patients started on HRT had a slightly increased risk of dementia. This area of investigation, like so many others related to HRT, remains controversial.

Vaginal Atrophy

Estrogens and progestins influence normal vaginal moisture. Estrogens increase blood flow to the vagina and produce the sensation of vaginal moisture. The absence of estrogen results in thinning of the vaginal mucosa, decreased rugae and vascularity, shortening of the vaginal canal and changes in the normal bacterial flora. Pelvic examination may reveal a pale sometimes friable epithelium. The vaginal pH increases above 4.5, whereas premenopausally it is less than 3.4. Altered vaginal pH allows recolonization of the vagina with enteric bacteria and may result in pruritus and discharge. Inflammation of the vaginal mucosa due to progressive estrogen loss, known as atrophic vaginitis, can cause the mucosa to have a "strawberry" appearance.

These atrophic changes are responsible for the common complaints of dysuria (secondary to a thinned urethral mucosa), urinary frequency and urgency (caused by atrophic trigonitis), vaginal dryness, and dyspareunia. Urinary frequency can occur day and night. It is commonly accompanied by urinary urgency. Stress urinary incontinence (worsened by diminished sphincter tone) and urge incontinence due to atrophic trigonitis, which are common in this age group, can be worsened by estrogen deficiency.

Skin Changes

There is no question that estrogen influences the epidermis and dermis. Collagen synthesis and maturation are estrogen sensitive. Estrogen may preserve collagen content and thickness. Loss of endogenous estrogen may result in new skin wrinkles and dry skin.

Loss of Libido

There are many determinants of libido, with endocrinologic, environmental, sociocultural beliefs, and emotional factors all impacting a woman's sexual function.

Simultaneous with the decline of estrogens in the menopause, there is also a 50% to 75% drop in the production of all four androgens: dehydroepiandrosterone sulfate, dehydroepiandrosterone, androstenedione, and testosterone. This decrease of androgens has been implicated in loss of sexual drive as women approach menopause.

Sexual interest is decreased and there is a diminution of orgasmic and coital frequency. Diminished sexual sensation and dyspareunia compound the dysfunction. Many times the cause of sexual dysfunction is multifactorial and therapy requires counseling, education, and medication.

Cardiovascular Disease

Among women over age 50, heart disease and stroke are responsible for more than 50% of deaths each year. Coronary heart disease in women occurs 10 to 12 years later in life than men. Because their rates approach those of men in the older ages, and there are more old women than men, about half of all coronary deaths occur in women. Almost all these deaths occur in postmenopausal women.

Heart palpitations are the most common cardiovascular complaint in the menopausal transition. Their cause is unknown, but they often improve with estrogen replacement. The first symptom of coronary heart disease may be chest pain or angina. Chest pain caused by reduced blood flow in the coronary arteries typically occurs behind the sternum and may travel to the left arm or up the neck, or be a squeezing, pressing sensation that does not change with breathing. It is usually caused and made worse by exercise and eased by rest. Pain usually lasts two to five minutes. Reduced blood flow to the heart can cause symptoms other than chest pain such as shortness of breath and indigestion.

Although the incidence of cardiovascular disease does increase with advancing age, there is some evidence to suggest that the process is affected by the loss of estrogen. There is an increase in total cholesterol, low-density lipoprotein cholesterol and lipoprotein(a), whereas high-density lipoprotein cholesterol is reduced. Postmenopausal women also gain weight with a shift from peripheral to central. Hemostatic factors are also altered after menopause.

Smoking cessation and other lifestyle changes, such as the reduction of dietary fat intake and regular aerobic exercise, should be recommended in all women, regardless of risk status.

OSTEOPENIA AND OSTEOPOROSIS

Osteopenia is low bone mass and osteoporosis is a reduction in bone mass per unit volume of bone tissue and is characterized by microarchitectural deterioration of bone. This leads to increased bone fragility and fracture risk. The two most significant determinants for its development are the peak bone mass (achieved by middle to late adolescence) and the rate of bone loss after menopause.

Back or hip pain in a menopausal woman should alert the clinician to possible osteopenia or osteoporosis. Loss of height can be documented with regular office visits. Spontaneous vertebral fractures can result from everyday activities such as lifting, walking, or rising from a reclining position. Pain can be acute or chronic and can present as sharp or a dull ache.

Bone remodeling predominates after linear growth ends and helps to keep bone dynamic and elastic. After peak bone mass is achieved, remodeling ensures that the amount of bone resorbed by osteoclasts is equal to the amount formed by osteoblasts. During this time, bone mineral density (BMD) remains relatively constant. Bone remodeling is affected by various factors including parathyroid hormone, growth hormone, 1,25 dihydroxyvitamin D, and estrogen deficiency.

Pathologic processes increase resorption or decrease formation. The decline in bone mass begins sometime after age 35 and accelerates with estrogen deficiency. After age 40, bone resorption exceeds formation by 0.5% to 5% for trabecular bone and 1.5% of cortical bone each year after menopause. The greatest loss in bone mass occurs in the first 2 to 3 years postmenopause, so early assessment and initiation of therapy is important. A combination of low BMD and a single traumatic event can result in an osteoporotic fracture of the hip, spine, or wrist. Untreated bone loss may also result in the osteoporotic syndrome of pain and disability.

There may be other causes for bone loss during menopause. Endocrine disorders such as hyperthyroidism, primary hyperparathyroidism, hypercortisolism, and gastrointestinal disorders, such as biliary cirrhosis and malabsorption syndromes, may result in bone loss. Screening should be performed when bone loss is suspected to assess osteoporosis risk.

Osteoporosis remains a significant cause of morbidity and mortality in menopausal women. More than one million fractures are reported each year in menopausal women and nearly 15% of women with hip fractures die within 3 months.

Factors contributing to development of osteoporosis (Figure 34-1) include age, calcium metabolism, and estrogen. Fracture risk is difficult to assess and depends upon bone mass and rate of bone loss at the time of menopause. Women who decline therapy for prevention of osteoporosis in the menopause can expect to shrink approximately 2.5 inches. Calcium supplementation alone does not prevent loss of bone mineral content.

Diagnostic Approaches and Risk Assessment

LABORATORY TESTS FOR ESTROGEN DEFICIENCY

The first step is to determine if the patient is estrogen deficient and in need of replacement therapy. This can be done by measuring the primary premenopausal estrogen, 17β estradiol (E_2) and serum follicle stimulating hormone (FSH). After the cessation of menses, circulating serum E_2 levels fall to less than 30 pg/mL (most of which is derived from the peripheral conversion of estrone) and estrone levels fall to less than 70 pg/mL (most of which is derived from the peripheral conversion of androstenedione). The androgen-estrogen ratio increases because of a marked decline in estrogen and complaints of mild hirsutism are common. In the time just prior to menopause, which can range from 2 to 10 years, estradiol levels can fluctuate widely, giving rise to the symptoms of perimenopause.

In response to the decreasing ability of the ovary to produce estradiol and inhibin, FSH levels rise, then fluctuate during the perimenopausal period until menopause is established, when levels remain elevated greater than 40 mIU/mL. Menopause is thus characterized by declining E_2 levels and subsequent rise in FSH. FSH and estrogen levels are readily available and, besides symptoms, provide the best evidence that a patient is estrogen deficient.

The maturation index of the vaginal smear is a measure of the ratio of superficial cells and intermediate cells over parabasal cells. Before serum estrogen testing was easily available, it was used as an indicator of relative estrogen deficiency. With estrogen depletion, there is diminution of the superficial cells and prevalence of the parabasal cells, or a shift to the left. This cellular distribution is reversed by the addition of estrogen. The clinical reliability of this test is limited by the experience of the clinician. FSH levels are more useful in most clinical settings.

EVALUATION OF BONE DENSITY

Bone mineral density is the most accurate measure of bone mass and the strongest predictor of osteoporotic fracture. The two most common methods for measurement of BMD are dual-energy radiograph absorptiometry (DXA) and quantitative CT (QCT). DXA has become the usual screening technique because it has a better precision than QCT as well as shorter scanning time and lower radiation dose. Measurement of BMD generally should only be performed when the result will affect patient management, that is, to confirm or exclude the presence of osteoporosis or allow decisions about treatment. It is recommended that women over 50 years of age, or menopausal women, or those at significant risk for osteoporosis have routine DXA scans every 2 years.

Using DXA, BMD is usually measured at two or three sites (the lumbar spine, hip, and forearm) whereas by QCT, BMD is usually measured only in the spine. BMD measured by DXA is not a true density but rather an apparent density (g/cm^2) corrected for length and width. The risk of fracture primarily relates to how a subject's value compares to a young normal population and consequently BMD is usually expressed as a T score or the number of standard deviations from the mean of young normal values. Thus a T score of -2 is a 2 SD below the young normal mean. The T score cut off points for diagnostic categories as proposed by the World Health Organization are shown in Figure 34-2.

Using these cutoffs, the term *severe osteoporosis* is used when a patient has a low BMD as well as having already sustained an atraumatic fracture. This latter category is analogous to the older term, *established osteoporosis*, which should be avoided, since it implies osteoporosis is only present after a fracture occurs, whereas a markedly reduced BMD is an indication for treatment to prevent future fractures.

Treatment of Specific Problems

HOT FLASHES AND NIGHT SWEATS

Estrogen replacement therapy (ERT) is approximately 95% successful in the treatment of hot flashes. Conjugated estrogen, 0.625 mg daily or its equivalent (*eg*, estradiol 1 mg), generally controls hot flash episodes, but higher doses may be neces-

Common Risk Factors for Osteoporosis

Genetic

Family history of osteoporosis

White, Asian

Hypogonadism

Early menopause

Drugs

Corticosteroids

Anticonvulsants

Nutritional

Low dietary calcium intake

Malabsorption

Lifestyle

Smoking

Low body weight

Immobility/sedentary lifestyle

High risk of falls

History of previous fractures after age 50

Other

Figure 34-1. Common risk factors for osteoporosis.

sary. Estrogen replacement appears to also increase rapid-eye-movement sleep, thus improving sleep. Medroxyprogesterone acetate (MPA), 10 mg daily, can also be effective and is a reasonable alternative therapy in women for whom estrogen therapy is contraindicated. Megestrol acetate 10–40 mg/d, has also been shown to be effective in the treatment of hot flashes. There are no long-term data on the effect of these drugs on bone mass. They should not be used as substitutes for proven methods unless other methods are contraindicated. Abnormal bleeding can occur in 25% to 50% of women, so this treatment is primarily of benefit in women who have previously had a hysterectomy. If HRT is to be used, combinations of estrogen and progestin are recommended for women with a uterus.

Other agents have been used with varying success. Bellergal-S, a mixture of ergotamine tartrate, levorotatory alkaloids of belladonna, and phenobarbital, given twice daily, has been used in the treatment of hot flashes. The patient should be warned about the drug's sedative effects, as well as its addictive potential.

Clonidine is an α-adrenergic agonist commonly used as an antihypertensive agent and has been shown effective in reducing the frequency and severity of hot flashes. Initiation of therapy begins with 0.1 mg/d patch to be worn for 1 week. The dose can be increased as needed but blood pressure must be monitored when increasing the dosage. Side effects are mild and tend to decrease with continued therapy. Common complaints include dizziness, drowsiness, localized skin irritation, and dry mouth. The use of propanolol to treat hot flashes has been associated with conflicting outcomes. Neither clonidine nor propanolol is approved by the US Food and Drug Administration. Serotonergic antidepressants have also been used effectively to treat vasomotor symptoms. Similarly, gabapentin has been useful in selected patients.

VAGINAL ATROPHY

Symptomatic vaginal atrophy is usually relieved with estrogen therapy. In the event estrogen is not an option, over-the-counter preparations are available to increase vaginal moisture but none reverses vaginal atrophy. Such agents include Astroglide, Lubrin, Replens, K-Y Jelly, Gyne-Moistrin, and Moist Again.

OTHER CHANGES

Psychologic symptoms of the menopause have been one of the most contentious issues in menopause research. These symptoms include, but are not limited to, inability to concentrate,

T Score Results

Result	T Score
Normal	Values greater than 1 SD below the young adult mean
Low bone density or osteopenia	Values between 1 to 2.5 SD below the young adult mean
Osteoporosis	Values > 2.5 SD from the mean of young normal values

Figure 34-2. T score results.

mood lability, irritability, anxiety, insomnia, mood depression, memory loss, lack of energy, aggressiveness, nervousness, and headache. Accompanying these symptoms can be complaints of myalgia, joint aches, lack of libido, and palpitations. These symptoms are often ill defined and nonspecific. Although the relationship between the biologic and psychosocial nature of these complaints is not well understood, they are none-the-less real and need attention.

Estrogen therapy is often accompanied by decreases in insomnia, anxiety, irritability and improvement of memory. In decreasing hot flushes during sleep, the quality of sleep is improved, preventing chronic sleep insomnia. Thus estrogen improves many psychologic symptoms in addition to relieving hot flushes. Nonhormonal management of these symptoms is similarly used on an individualized basis.

OSTEOPOROSIS

If estrogen replacement therapy is to be used, it should start as soon as possible after natural menopause or oophorectomy, because estrogen slows the rate of bone loss, although estrogen replacement will not restore bone mass to pretreatment levels. Conjugated estrogen (0.625 mg), ethinyl estradiol (20 µg), and micronized estradiol (1 mg) have proven efficacy in the prevention of osteoporosis. Bone loss can also be slowed when lower doses of estrogen (0.3 mg conjugated estrogen) and higher doses of calcium (1.5 g/d) are used. Transdermal administration of 17β-estradiol has been equally effective in arresting bone loss.

Other antiresorptive agents such as calcitonin and bisphosphonates (etidronate, alendronate, and risedronate) have similar effects on bone density and appear to protect against fractures. Calcitonin prevents osteoporosis from causing more bone breakdown. Bisphosphonates are bound to mineralized bone surface and inhibit osteoclast activity, thus the term *antiresorptive agent* is applied to these drugs. Weekly and even monthly dosing of these medications helps to minimize the effect of gastrointestinal irritation that plagues women who take the medication in daily doses.

Raloxifene has gained popularity as an alternative for the management of patients with findings of bone thinning. Although it is associated with significant vascular symptoms, it does not have adverse effects on the endometrium.

Possible Adverse Effects of Estrogen

CARDIOVASCULAR DISEASE

Despite observational and epidemiologic studies that suggested a cardioprotective effect, randomized trials have not confirmed those data. The Heart and Estrogen/Progestin Replacement Study (HERS) trial did not show any benefit of combined estrogen and progestin if started after a myocardial infarct or angioplasty. The Women's Health Initiative (WHI) did not demonstrate any advantage of combined estrogen/progestin treatment over placebo in prevention of cardiovascular disease, and, in fact, showed a slight increased risk of nonfatal myocardial infarction and nonfatal ischemic

stroke in the first year of treatment. These data originally caused great alarm among clinicians and the public alike, but, with time, and further analysis of the results, a more balanced view of the studies has come forth, that is, this is only a single dataset among many, and the great consternation caused by the initial release of the data needs to be tempered until more data are available. A current hypothesis is that early initiation of estrogen after the menopause may prove cardioprotective whereas a later start may prove less beneficial.

VENOUS THROMBOEMBOLISM

With advancing age, the risk of venous thromboembolism increases. The HERS and WHI studies showed an increased risk with estrogen alone or in combination with a progestin. In the HERS trial, the attributable risk was 2.3 per 1000 woman-years. The increased risk appears to be in the first year of therapy, possibly owing to the unmasking in some women of inherited thrombophilias.

ENDOMETRIAL HYPERPLASIA AND CANCER

Estrogen is a known cellular mitogen in the endometrium, and endometrial hyperplasia and cancer have been associated with unopposed estrogen use. This effect is dose- and duration-dependent, with an increase of 1.8-fold and 12.7-fold with conjugated estrogen dosages of 0.625 mg and 1.25 mg, respectively. Furthermore, when unopposed estrogen was given for 5 to 10 years or longer, the relative risk for endometrial cancer rose from 4.1 to 11.6. However, the development of endometrial cancer while using unopposed estrogen is associated with a better prognosis. Women diagnosed with stage I, grade 1 adenocarcinoma demonstrated a 96.7% 5-year survival rate. The PEPI Trial confirmed the need for the addition of a progestin to estrogen therapy for women with a uterus.

The addition of progestin to estrogen therapy has been shown to decrease the occurrence of endometrial hyperplasia and cancer. This effect also appears to be dose and duration dependent. The addition of norethindrone for 7 and 10 days each month decreased the incidence of endometrial hyperplasia from 32% in the estrogen alone group to 4% and 2%, respectively. It appears that therapy for greater than 12 days each cycle is required to reduce the rate of endometrial hyperplasia to zero. This makes intuitive sense, because in ovulating women progesterone secretion affects the endometrium for 13 to 14 days. The most efficacious dose of progestin for endometrial stabilization with minimal metabolic impact on lipoprotein profiles remains to be determined.

BREAST CANCER

Epidemiologic research over the past 20 years has attempted to determine if there is an association between postmenopausal estrogen use and breast cancer. The determination of this relationship is difficult because of the confounding variables of estrogen type, dose, and duration of exposure. However, there is the suggestion of an increased risk if estrogen use is greater than 20 years. The type of estrogen may be of importance. One

European study reported a significant increase in the breast cancer rate among women using ethinyl estradiol for longer than 9 years. Using meta-analytic techniques, data from separate investigations can be analyzed to generalize conclusions. One report using meta-analysis to review 556 articles found no significant increase in the risk of breast cancer with conjugated estrogen use. Another report that used this technique to analyze specific types of estrogen reported a 30% increase in the risk of breast cancer among women taking estradiol.

A large observational study in the United Kingdom reported an increase in breast cancer risk in estrogen users and combined hormone users. This study was widely criticized, however, on methodologic grounds.

In the large WHI trial, patients received placebo or estrogen alone (if the subject did not have a uterus) or combined estrogen/progestin. For those patients receiving combination therapy who had never taken hormones, there was no increase in the breast cancer risk. For those who had taken hormones in the past, there was a slight increase in the breast cancer risk during the first 5 years of treatment. In those taking estrogen only, there was a lower rate of reported breast cancer, but it failed to reach statistical significance. The data do not support the notion that estrogen therapy increases the risk of breast cancer in women with benign breast disease. Similarly, the use of estrogen does not increase breast cancer risk in patients with a family history of the malignancy.

In summary, the case for a causal effect of estrogen and breast cancer remains to be clarified. Currently, the practitioner and patient can be reassured that hormone therapy for troublesome symptoms related to the loss of estrogen is relatively safe during the early menopausal years. These findings should be discussed with each patient before estrogen therapy is instituted.

Absolute Contraindications to Hormone Replacement Therapy

Suspected or previously diagnosed estrogen-dependent neoplasia (breast or advanced-stage uterine cancer)

Active thrombosis or embolic disease

Undiagnosed uterine bleeding

Active liver disease or severely impaired hepatic function

Figure 34-3. Absolute contraindications to hormone replacement therapy.

Estrogen Use in Preexisting Conditions

Chronic liver dysfunction (may use smaller and less frequent doses of estrogen)

Preexisting symptomatic uterine leiomyomas or active endometriosis

Acute intermittent porphyria (estrogens precipitate attacks)

Figure 34-4. Estrogen use in preexisting conditions.

Estrogen Replacement Therapy

Because exogenous estrogen therapy in estrogen-deficient women lessens and possibly prevents undesirable potentially life-threatening sequelae, therapy should be seriously considered for selected menopausal women. Therapy should be at the lowest dosage possible that will maximize relief from symptoms and prevent other problems.

CONTRAINDICATIONS
The medical history is used to determine if absolute contraindications are present (Figure 34-3). Relative contraindications are listed in Figure 34-4. Progestin-only therapy may be beneficial in patients who cannot undergo estrogen therapy. There is no reason to deny use of HRT in women with controlled hypertension, diabetes mellitus, or biliary stones.

AVAILABLE ESTROGEN PREPARATIONS
Estrogen preparations commonly used for menopausal ERT or HRT are natural estrogens (found in a plant or animal), whereas estrogens used in oral contraceptive preparations are synthetic (Figure 34-5). Synthetic estrogens differ from natural estrogens in their increased target tissue potency.

The rationale for any medical therapy is to prescribe the lowest possible dose to achieve the desired clinical effect. Studies have shown that 5 µg of ethinyl estradiol is comparable in biologic potency to 0.625 mg of conjugated equine estrogens. Low-dose oral contraceptives for hormone replacement provide four to seven times the amount of estrogen in traditional HRT.

Unopposed estrogen therapy is an option as long as proper precautions are taken. Therapy is often reserved for the patient who suffers intolerable adverse side effects from progestin component. If estrogen-alone therapy is ultimately desired in a woman with a uterus refusing progestin, discussion regarding the increased risk of endometrial hyperplasia and cancer should be undertaken. Pretreatment and annual endometrial biopsies are warranted. If abnormal endometrial histology is identified, then estrogen therapy should be stopped, and the patient appropriately treated with observation or high-dose progestin therapy.

Conjugated equine estrogens (Premarin, PMB) (Figure 34-6 to 34-8) are derived from pregnant mares' urine, which

Natural and Synthetic Estrogens

Natural Estrogens	Synthetic Estrogens
Estrones	17β-ethinyl estrogens
Conjugated equine	Mestranol
Estrogens	Diethylstilbestrol
Estropipate	
Estradiols	
Micronized estradiol	
Estradiol valerate	

Figure 34-5. Natural and synthetic estrogens.

contains estrone, equilin, and a mixture of other estrogen metabolites. Equilin is a potent estrogen, and because it is stored in fat, is also long lasting. Conjugated equine estrogen starting dose is 0.625 mg. When applied vaginally or transdermally, estrogens bypass the liver and act directly on the target tissue. After prolonged treatment with conjugated equine estrogens, serum equilin levels can remain elevated for 13 weeks or more post-treatment because of storage and slow release from adipose tissue.

Estradiol (Estrace, Estraderm, and Climara) is a synthetically produced natural 17β-estradiol. Estrace is the micronized form of estradiol. The recommended starting dose is 1 mg. Estraderm is a transdermal patch applied twice weekly (Figure 34-7). The recommended starting dose is 0.05 mg, and the patch is applied to the skin of the lower trunk and changed once every 3.5 days. Serum levels remain constant for 84 hours, then fall rapidly. Although Climara contains the same estrogen as Estraderm, the patch is manufactured differently and it is applied once weekly. Topical creams and gels are new products which can be used in similar fashion.

Estropipate (Ogen, Ortho Est) is a naturally produced estrogen prepared from purified crystalline estrone. The recommended starting dose for estropipate is 0.625 (0.75 mg estropipate). Esterified estrogens (Estratab, Menest) are plant estrogens.

Available Oral Estrogens

Generic Name	Trade Name	Usual Dose	Manufacturer
Conjugated equine estrogens	Premarin	0.625–1.25 mg	Wyeth-Ayerst
17β-estradiol	Estrace	1–2 mg	Bristol-Myers Squibb
Estropipate	Ogen, Ortho-Est	0.625–1.25 mg	Upjohn
Esterified estrogens	Estratab, Menest	0.3, 0.625, 1.25, 2.5 mg	Solvey/SmithKline Beecham
Estrogen/progestin combinations	Prempro, Premphase	0.625 mg Premarin, 2.5 mg MPA	Wyeth-Ayerst
Estinyl estradiol	Estinyl	0.02, 0.05, or 0.5 mg	Schering-Plough
Estrone	Estrone (no longer available)	2 mg (no longer available)	Legere
Estradiol cypionate	Cypionate	5 mg (no longer available)	Legere
Quinestrol	Estrovis	100 µg/wk	Warner Lambert Parke-Davis

Figure 34-6. Available oral estrogens. MPA—medroxyprogesterone acetate.

Transdermal Estrogen Replacement Therapy

Generic Name	Trade Name	Estrogen	Usual Dose	Site	Manufacturer
17β-estradiol	Estraderm	0.05, 0.1 mg/d	0.05–0.1 mg every 3.5 d	Skin	Ciba
17β-estradiol	Climara	0.05, 0.1 mg/d	0.05–0.1 mg once weekly	Skin	Berlex
Conjugated equine estrogens	Premarin vaginal cream	0.625 mg	1–4 g daily	Vagina	Wyeth-Ayerst
Estropipate	Ogen vaginal cream	1.5 mg	1–4 g daily	Vagina	Upjohn
17β-estradiol	Estrace vaginal cream	1 mg	3 g weekly	Vagina	Bristol-Myers Squibb
Dienestrol	Ortho Dienestrol cream	0.1 mg	3–18 g weekly	Vagina	Ortho

Figure 34-7. Transdermal estrogen replacement therapy.

Injectable Estrogens

Generic Name	Trade Name	Usual Dose	Manufacturer
Conjugated equine estrogens	Premarin injection	25 mg/mL	Wyeth-Ayerst
Estradiol cypionate	Estro V injection	0.5 mg/mL	Legere
Polyestradiol phosphate	Estradurin (no longer available)	40 mg/mL IM q 2–4 wks	Wyeth-Ayerst

Figure 34-8. Injectable estrogens.

Esterified estrogens and methyltestosterone (Estratest, Estratest HS shown in Figure 34-9) are the only available estrogen/androgen combination capsules.

Vaginal creams are also available. Estrogen is readily absorbed through the vaginal epithelium, but circulating levels of estrogen are only one fourth the levels of an equivalent oral dose. Disadvantages include messy application and variable absorption patterns resulting in widely different bioavailability.

ESTROGEN SIDE EFFECTS

Known side effects of estrogen include nausea, breast tenderness, and edema. These usually decrease in intensity and resolve with continued therapy.

REGIMENS

Before initiating therapy, a thorough discussion should include the indications for therapy, dosing schedule, possible side effects and alternative therapy, and the possible change in recommendations as new information becomes available. The information should be presented as an issue of prophylaxis and/or therapy. The concern about increased risk for breast cancer, and other conditions, however, must also be presented during informed consent. The informed patient is more likely to remain compliant with the recommended therapy.

Patients who have previously undergone hysterectomy for benign tumors can be placed on estrogen therapy alone. The addition of progestin in these patients is not necessary. Common oral therapeutic regimens include conjugated equine estrogens, 0.625 to 1.25 mg, or estradiol, 1 mg, all days. Transdermal application of estrogen 0.05 or 0.1 mg maintains a relatively constant circulatory drug level. It has added advantages of lower overall dose of estradiol with precise control, reduced frequency of dosing, and convenient administration and termination. Transdermal delivery systems avoid first-pass metabolism in the liver, thereby leaving more available to target tissues.

For patients with an intact uterus, progestin is added to the regimen for endometrial protection against atypical changes. A routine pretreatment endometrial biopsy is not necessary. Estrogen/progestin regimens can be sequential or continuous. The success of the therapy depends largely on the history of the patient. If the patient is bleeding monthly on a regular or semi-regular schedule, sequential therapy offers a window for withdrawal bleeding and lessens the chance of intermittent abnormal uterine bleeding. Cyclic bleeding will continue as long as therapy does. Combined continuous therapy, although having the initial disadvantage of up to a year of irregular bleeding, offers the patient eventual relief from monthly bleeding episodes. If she has been amenorrheic for 6 months or more, then combined continuous therapy offers her the benefits of replacement without the added worry of monthly withdrawal bleeding, and is the only logical choice.

Sequential Combined Therapy

Sequential therapy is defined by a hormone-free period when withdrawal bleeding is allowed to occur. Estrogen therapy can be administered continuously with the addition of a progestin for 10, 12, 14, or 25 days of the patient's cycle. Continuous daily estrogen therapy provides for patient convenience and avoids annoying cyclic postmenopausal symptoms. There is no evidence that continuous combined estrogen therapy is associated with an increase in endometrial hyperplasia when compared with a cyclic combined regimen.

Common regimens include conjugated equine estrogens, 0.625 to 1.25 mg, or estradiol, 1 mg, each day with 10 to 14 days of MPA 5 to 10 mg or 25 days of MPA 2.5 mg. Menses usually ensue within 5 to 6 days after progestin withdrawal.

Medroxyprogesterone acetate 10 mg/d is a commonly used progestin that can be associated with the side effects of depression, fluid retention, and bloating in nearly 25% of women. Reducing the dosage to 5 mg/d often eliminates these complaints. Micronized progesterone for menopausal treatment was used successfully in the Postmenopausal Estrogen/Progestin Intervention trial in a cyclic fashion with minimal side effects. Effects on HDL cholesterol were better in the natural progesterone group than in the synthetic progesterone groups. Alternative progestin therapies may also be substituted to ameliorate these untoward effects (Figure 34-10). Norethindrone, 0.7 mg, is endometrial protective when added to estrogen therapy and is less commonly associated with the side effects that are found with MPA. Megestrol acetate 10 mg/d also appears to have less unwanted side effects, although there is no evidence on benefits or risks.

Continuous Combined Therapy

Continuous combined therapy administers estrogen and progestin on a continuous daily basis. The major benefit of this therapy is possible avoidance of cyclic bleeding and therefore better compliance as well as a lower progestin dose. Daily progestin causes endometrial atrophy and protection from atypical changes. Because the progestin is administered at a lower total dose (MPA 75 mg continuous versus 100 to 140 mg sequential dosing), its adverse effects on lipoproteins and side effects such as breast tenderness, bloating, headache, and emotional lability are minimized.

Oral Estrogen/Testosterone Preparations

Generic Name	Trade Name	Usual Dose	Manufacturer
Conjugated equine estrogens and methyltestosterone	Premarin and Testosterone	0.625 mg/5 mg	Wyeth-Ayerst
		1.25 mg/10 mg	
Esterified estrogen and methyltestosterone	Estratest, Estratest H.S.	0.625 mg/5 mg	Solvay
		1.25 mg/10 mg	

Figure 34-9. Oral estrogen/testosterone preparations.

Minimal spotting may occur during the first 6 months of therapy; however, 33% of patients will not experience bleeding at all, and 80% of patients who bleed will stop within the first year. Continuous dosing may decrease the incidence of additional problems associated with premenstrual symptoms and uterine fibroids. Varying doses of progestin (MPA 2.5 to 5 mg. or norethindrone 0.35 to 1.45 mg) have been examined using the continuous combined regimen. For example, in one study, 2 mg of micronized estradiol and 1 mg of norethindrone continuously for 12 months yielded persistent decrease in LDL over the study period.

Early evidence suggests that combined continuous therapy may have similar protective effect on bone as combined sequential therapy. A combination of conjugated equine estrogens 0.625 mg with MPA 2.5 mg for combined continuous therapy is now available. In addition, a 0.625/5 mg version has recently been introduced. The potential advantages of continuous, daily administration of estrogen and progestin are summarized in Figure 34-11.

Alternatives to Estrogen Therapy

SELECTIVE ESTROGEN RECEPTOR MODULATORS

Selective estrogen receptor modulators are synthetic estrogen lookalikes. They act as agonist or antagonist to specific tissues and therefore promise an exciting future for the prevention and treatment of many menopausal disorders. Many are just beginning early clinical trials primarily for the treatment of osteoporosis. Some are being studied as alternatives to traditional HRT, because they are more acceptable than estrogens because of their antiestrogenic effects on the breast.

Most have beneficial effects on bone mass and lipids and are appealing as a bleed-free form of HRT (because they do not stimulate the endometrium). Raloxifene is US Food and Drug Administration approved for the prevention of osteoporosis.

Raloxifene is only half as effective in bone as estrogen and has a side effect profile of increased hot flashes, leg cramps and venous thromboembolism risk. These factors remain stumbling blocks for its mainstream use. A beneficial effect may be a reduction in breast cancer risk.

Idoxifene is an iodinated descendant of tamoxifen, which has estrogen agonist and antagonist activity. It is in nononcologic clinical trials and because of its long half-life, may have less undesirable vasomotor side effects than other drugs in this class. It appears to have antagonist effects on the breast and endometrium, as well as agonist effects on the bone and heart. Other agonist/antagonist agents with similar profiles include raloxifene, droloxifene, and toremifene. Toremifene has a profile similar to tamoxifen and because of increased vasomotor flushing is probably not an alternative for treatment of menopausal symptoms.

PHYTOESTROGENS

Phytoestrogens are weak estrogens of plant origin. The precursors of the biologically active compounds originate in soybean products (mainly isoflavonoids), and whole grain cereals, seeds, and nuts (mainly ligands). These plant glycosides are converted by intestinal bacteria to weak estrogen-like compounds.

Epidemiologic investigations have suggested that they are natural anticancer compounds because the highest concentrations of these compounds are found in the diet of countries with low cancer rates. They have antiestrogenic effects in much the same way as selective estrogen receptor modulators, competitively binding to the estrogen receptor and displacing more potent endogenous estrogens (estrone). This hypothesis is corroborated by the low rates of breast cancer in Hispanic women despite their increased adiposity, a breast cancer risk factor.

High dietary intake of these plant estrogens not only appears to reduce risk for breast cancer, but has also been linked to fewer menopausal symptoms. In a small study of 58

Progesterone and Progestins

Generic Name	Trade Name	Usual Dose	Manufacturer
Medroxyprogesterone acetate	Provera, Cycrin	2.5, 5, or 10 mg	Upjohn, ESI, Lederle
Norethindrone acetate	Aygestin	5 mg	ESI, Lederle
Norethindrone tablets	Micronor	0.35 mg	Ortho
Micronized progesterone	Prometrium	100 mg hs continuous	Solvay
		200 mg hs continuous days 12–25	

Figure 34-10. Progesterone and progestins.

Potential Advantages of Continuous Dosing

Amenorrhea

Endometrial atrophy (protection from atypical changes and pregnancy)

Uterine atrophy (asymptomatic fibroids)

Less adverse effect on blood lipoproteins

Convenience and, therefore, better compliance

Figure 34-11. Potential advantages of continuous dosing.

postmenopausal women, soy (daidzein) and wheat (entero-lactone) reduced hot flashes 40% and 25%, respectively; however, it is unclear if these estrogens may be potent enough to stimulate the growth of estrogen dependent tumors.

Suggested Bibliography

Albrecht BH, Schiff I, Tulchinsky D, et al.: Objective evidence that placebo and oral medroxyprogesterone acetate therapy diminish menopausal vasomotor flashes. Am J Obstet Gynecol 1981, 139:631–635.

Alcoff JM, Campbell D, Tribble D, et al.: Double blind placebo controlled cross-over trial of propanolol as treatment for menopausal vasomotor symptoms. Clin Ther 1981, 3:356–364.

Barrett-Connor E, Brown WV, Turner J, et al.: Heart disease risk factors and hormone use in postmenopausal women. JAMA 1979, 241:2167.

Brincat M, Moniz CF, Studd JW, et al.: Long-term effects of the menopause and sex hormones on skin thickness. Br J Obstet Gynecol 1985, 92:256–259.

Bush TL, Barrett-Connor E, Crowan L, et al.: Cardiovascular mortality and noncontraceptive use of estrogen in women: Results from the Lipid Research Clinics Program Follow-up Study. Circulation 1987, 74:1102–1107.

Castelli WP: Cardiovascular disease in women. Am J Obstet Gynecol 1988, 158:1553–1560.

Chetkowski RJ, Meldrum DR, Steingold KA, et al.: Biologic effects of transdermal estradiol. N Engl J Med 1986, 314:1615–1620.

Christensen C: What should be done at the time of menopause? Am J Med 1995, 98:2A–56S–59S.

Colditz GA, Hankinson SE, Hunter DJ, et al.: The use of estrogens and progestins and the risk of breast cancer in postmenopausal women. N Engl J Med 1995, 332:1589–1593.

Coope J, Williams S, Parreson JS: A study of the effectiveness of propanolol in the menopausal hot flash. Fr J Obstet Gynecol 1978, 85:472–475.

Crailo MD, Pike MC: Estimation of the distribution of age at natural menopause from prevalence data. Am J Epidemiol 1983, 117:356.

Dewhurst J: Postmenopausal bleeding from benign causes. Clin Obstet Gynecol 1983, 26:769.

Ettinger B, Genant HK, Cann CE: Postmenopausal bone loss is prevented by treatment with low-dosage estrogen with calcium. Ann Intern Med 1987, 106:40–45.

Hunt K, Vessey M, McPherson K, Coleman M: Long-term surveillance of mortality and cancer incidence in women receiving hormone replacement therapy. Br J Obstet Gynaecol 1987, 94:620–635.

Kaplan NM: Hypertension induced by pregnancy, oral contraceptives and postmenopausal replacement therapy. Cardiol Clin 1988, 6:475–482.

Lindsay RL, Heart DM: The minimum effective dose of oestrogen for prevention of postmenopausal bone loss. Obstet Gynecol 1984, 63:759–763.

Lobo RA, Pickar JH, Wild RA, et al.: Metabolic impact of adding medroxyprogesterone acetate to conjugated estrogen therapy in postmenopausal women. Obstet Gynecol 1994, 8:987–995.

Magos AL, Brincat M, Studd JWW, et al.: Amenorrhea and endometrial atrophy with continuous oral estrogen and progesterone therapy in postmenopausal women. Obstet Gynecol 1985, 65:496–499.

Mashchack CA, Lobo RA, Dozono-Takano R, et al.: Comparison of pharmacodynamic properties to various estrogen formulations. Am J Obstet Gynecol 1982, 144:511.

Murkies AL, Lombard C, Strauss BJ, et al.: Dietary flour supplementation decreases post-menopausal hot flushes: effect of soy and wheat. Maturitas 1995, 21:189–195.

Quigley MET, Martin PL, Burnier AM, Brooks P: Estrogen therapy arrests bone loss in elderly women. Am J Obstet Gynecol 1987, 156:1516–1523.

Rebar RW, Thomas MA, Gass M, Liu J: Problems of hormone therapy: evaluations, follow-up, complications. In Menopause. Edited by Korenman SG. Boston: Serona Symposia; 1989.

Riis B, Thomsen K, Christiansen C: Does calcium supplementation prevent postmenopausal bone loss? A double-blind controlled clinical study. N Engl J Med 1987, 316:173–177.

Schiff I, Regestein Q, Tulchinsky D, et al.: Effects of estrogens on sleep and the psychologic state of hypogonadal women. JAMA 1979, 242:2405–2407.

Schiff I, Tulchinsky D, Cramer D, Ryan K: Oral medroxyprogesterone in the treatment of postmenopausal symptoms. JAMA 1979, 242:2405–2407.

Sherwin BB: Affective changes with estrogen and androgen replacement therapy in surgically menopausal women. J Affect Dis 1988, 14:177–187.

Siseles NO, Halperin H, Benencia HJ, et al.: A comparative study of two hormone replacement therapy regimens on safety and efficacy variables. Maturitas 2995, 21:201–210.

Stampfer MJ, Colditz GA: Estrogen replacement and coronary heart disease: a quantitative assessment of the epidemiologic evidence. Prev Med 1991, 20:47–63.

Stanford JL, Weiss NS, Voigt LF, et al.: Combined estrogen and progestin hormone replacement therapy in relation to risk of breast cancer in middle-aged women. JAMA 1995, 274:137–142.

Tataryn IV, Lomax P, Bajorek JG, et al.: Postmenopausal hot flashes: a disorder of thermoregulation. Maturitas 1980, 2:101–107.

The Writing Group for the PEPI Trial: Effects of estrogen or estrogen/progestin regimens on heart disease risk factor in postmenopausal women. JAMA 1995, 273:199–208.

The Writing Group for the PEPI Trial: Effects of hormone replacement therapy on endometrial histology in postmenopausal women. JAMA 1996, 275:370–375.

Walsh BW, Schiff I, Rosner B, et al.: Effects of postmenopausal estrogen replacement on the concentrations and metabolism of plasma lipoproteins. N Engl J Med 1991, 325:1196–1204.

Weinstein L, Bewtra C, Gallagher CJ: Evaluation of continuous combined low dose regimen of estrogen-progestin for treatment of the menopause patient. Am J Obstet Gynecol 1990, 162:1534–1542.

Whitehead MI, King RB, McQueen J, et al.: Endometrial histology and biochemistry in the climacteric woman during estrogen and estrogen/progesterone therapy. J R Soc Med 1979, 72:322–327.

Williams SR, Frenchek B, Speroff T, Speroff L: A study of combined continuous ethinyl estradiol and norethindrone acetate for postmenopausal hormone replacement. Am J Obstet Gynecol 1990, 162:438–497.

Ziel HK, Finkle WD: Increased risk of endometrial carcinoma among users of conjugated estrogen. N Engl J Med 1975, 293:1167–1170.

35 | The Pelvic Mass

Thomas G. Stovall and C. Bryce Bowling

- Ovarian tumors account for 1% of childhood tumors; the most common is the benign cystic teratoma.
- In adolescent and premenopausal women pregnancy must be considered in the differential diagnosis of pelvic masses.
- Ectopic pregnancy is a potentially life-threatening condition that should be considered whenever a patient presents with a positive pregnancy test, an adnexal mass, pain, and vaginal bleeding.
- Cystadenomas are the most common neoplasm in the reproductive years.
- Tubo-ovarian abscess is one of the most common causes of pelvic masses in reproductive-aged women.
- Epithelial ovarian cancer now affects 2 in 70 women in their lifetime.
- Uterine sarcoma may present in the postmenopausal woman as a rapidly enlarging mass in the pelvis.
- CA-125 should not be used as a random screening test for ovarian cancer.
- In management of pelvic mass, ultrasound is probably the most helpful imaging study and relatively easy to obtain.
- Serial ultrasound follow-up without surgical intervention may play a role in management of patients with postmenopausal ovarian cysts that are smaller than 5 cm.

Pelvic masses may arise from a gynecologic or nongynecologic origin. The adnexal region is composed of the ovary, fallopian tube, broad ligament, and associated blood and nerve supply. The ovary is a common source of cystic findings from childhood to menopause. Masses can also arise from the uterus and its round ligament and uterosacral ligament attachments. Nongynecologic sources of masses in the abdomen and pelvis must also be considered. Those masses can arise from the bladder, colon, intestine, or kidney.

This chapter discusses the evaluation of pelvic masses in broad terms across the spectrum of age groups. Dividing the patients into age groups based on reproductive function should help guide the primary care physician's approach to the diagnosis and evaluation of the pelvic mass.

Childhood

INCIDENCE AND EPIDEMIOLOGY

The presence of a pelvic mass is occasionally detected on abdominopelvic examination of the newborn or may have been noted in utero on fetal ultrasound. Commonly, these masses, related to maternal estrogen stimulation, are simple follicular cysts and occur in approximately 2% to 5% of prepubertal females [1]. These cysts generally regress after the first few months of life. Ovarian tumors are the most common genital neoplasm that occurs during childhood; fortunately, they are rare. Ovarian tumors account for 1% of childhood tumors; of the benign neoplastic tumors, the most common is the benign cystic teratoma. The percentage of benign vs malignant neoplasms in childhood is unclear. Breen and Maxson [2] noted that the majority of childhood neoplasms are benign—only 35% of ovarian tumors in children are malignant. Gallup and Talledo [3•] reported that the frequency of malignant ovarian tumors in children and young adolescents changes with age (Figure 35-1), and recently Van Winter *et al.* [4•] reported on a similar incidence. However, Norris and Jensen [5] noted that of the primary ovarian neoplasms found under the age of 15, approximately 80% are malignant.

DIFFERENTIAL DIAGNOSIS

In children, abdominopelvic masses usually are non-gynecologic in origin and often are related to Wilms tumor or neuroblastomas. The finding of an adnexal mass in a child is rare and usually represents a dysgerminoma or teratoma [6]. The differential diagnosis of a pelvic mass in children is given in Figure 35-2.

HISTORY AND PHYSICAL EXAMINATION

In newborns, the follicular cyst is found on abdominopelvic examination, which is then generally followed by abdominal ultrasound. The ultrasound usually reveals a simple ovarian follicular cyst. These cysts typically resolve once hormonal stimulation from the mother is removed, generally in the first few months of life. Observation is an appropriate method of treatment, and parents should be cautioned about symptoms of ovarian torsion.

In children, the symptoms of ovarian neoplasm may be nonspecific and include nausea, vomiting, abdominal pain, urinary complaints, or abdominal fullness. If the ovarian neoplasm is of germ cell origin, it may produce estrogen or testosterone, resulting in precocious puberty or masculinization. The child may also present with acute abdominal pain related to torsion or infarction of the mass. The most common preoperative diagnosis resulting in referral identified in a recent study by Van Winter *et al.* [4•] was acute appendicitis. Intermittent abdominal pain may represent intermittent torsion of the adnexal mass or even a normal ovary. In children, the

evaluation of a pelvic mass must include abdominal palpation with a rectoabdominal examination. A mass high in the pelvis may represent a pelvic kidney or other anomaly. In the child with an acute abdomen or severe abdominal pain, immediate referral is appropriate. In patients in whom the mass is felt to be stable, a pelvic ultrasound may be obtained, and timely referral to the appropriate specialist should be considered. Serum tumor markers need not be obtained by the primary care provider in children because they generally do not affect preoperative management. An algorithm for the work-up of pelvic masses found in newborns and children is provided in Figure 35-3.

Adolescents

INCIDENCE AND EPIDEMIOLOGY

With the onset of menarche, the finding of a pelvic mass is more commonly encountered. Most adnexal masses in this age group are functional cysts related to physiologic function of the ovary. Ovarian cysts are the fourth most common gynecologic cause of admission to the hospital. Approximately 65% of young women operated on for an ovarian enlargement had a postoperative diagnosis of functional ovarian cyst [7••]. The functional ovary also allows the adolescent to become fertile, which can result in pregnancy. Pregnancy in the intrauterine or extrauterine location is a major cause for a pelvic mass in this age group.

Neoplasm, whether benign or malignant, is always a possibility and must be excluded. The most common neoplasm found in this age group is the benign cystic teratoma, which is commonly referred to as a dermoid cyst. These tumors tend to be slow growing, and usually are asymptomatic.

Relative Frequency of Malignant Ovarian Tumors in Children and Young Adolescents

Tumor Type	Frequency By Age, %		
	0–5 y	7–9 y	10–14 y
Germ cell	45	62	72
Epithelial	5	5	30
Gonadal stromal (sex cord)	48	30	8
Miscellaneous	7	3	7

Figure 35-1. Relative frequency of malignant ovarian tumors in children and young adolescents. (*Adapted from* Gallup and Talledo [3•].)

Differential Diagnosis of a Pelvic Mass in Newborns and Children

Newborns
  Functional ovarian cysts
Children
  Ovarian
   Teratoma
   Dysgerminoma
  Wilms tumor
  Neuroblastoma
  Lymphoma
  Burkitt's tumor
  Gastrointestinal
  Musculoskeletal

Figure 35-2. Differential diagnosis of a pelvic mass in newborns and children.

They generally range in size between 5 cm and 10 cm and are bilateral in 15% to 25% of cases [7••].

DIFFERENTIAL DIAGNOSIS

Compared with premenarchal patients, the differential diagnosis in adolescent girls becomes much more complex for many reasons, including the onset of menses, the functioning ovary, and the possibility of pregnancy (Figure 35-4). During this period, abnormalities of müllerian development may first become apparent. Obstruction of the reproductive outflow tract may result in the accumulation of menstrual blood in the vagina (hematocolpos) or in the uterus (hematometra), which will then result in a palpable mass.

The ovary begins to produce physiologic ovarian cysts during this time frame and may become a source of a symptomatic pelvic mass. Although rare, benign and malignant neoplasms of the ovary must be considered, and pregnancy must be considered in the differential diagnosis. Because a large number of adolescents are becoming sexually active at younger ages, for some in this age group pelvic infection and

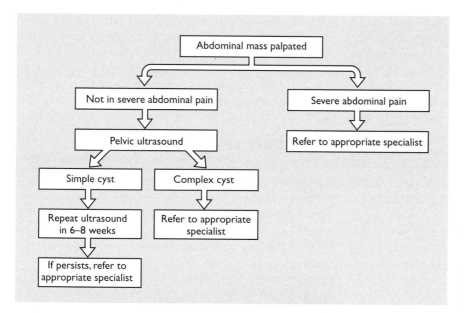

Figure 35-3. Algorithm for the evaluation and treatment of pelvic mass in newborns and children.

Differential Diagnosis of a Pelvic Mass in Adolescent Girls

Obstructive genital lesion

  Imperforate hymen

  Blinded uterine horn

Ovarian

  Functional

  Germ cell tumor

  Other ovarian neoplasm

Tubal

  Paratubal cyst

  Ectopic gestation

  Tubo-ovarian abscess

  Pyosalpinx

Uterine

  Cornual ectopic gestation

  Leiomyoma

  Pregnancy, including molar gestation

Gastrointestinal

  Appendiceal abscess

Figure 35-4. Differential diagnosis of a pelvic mass in adolescent girls.

salpingitis may progress to pyosalpinx or tubo-ovarian abscess presenting as an adnexal mass. When evaluating an adolescent with an infectious etiology, appendiceal abscess must also be considered in the differential diagnosis.

HISTORY AND PHYSICAL EXAMINATION

A complete menstrual history should be obtained within a complete history and physical examination. This includes the date of the last menstrual period, the length of menses, and the age of onset of menses. A patient who presents with a mass at about midcycle could have a functional ovarian cyst; if she is in the latter half of her menstrual cycle, she could have a hemorrhagic corpus luteum cyst. A patient who presents with secondary amenorrhea may be pregnant, and this should be excluded with a pregnancy test. The presence of dysmenorrhea should also be questioned. Congenital obstruction of the reproductive outflow tract often presents with absent menstrual cycles but cyclic lower abdominal pain. On physical examination, the primary care provider identifies a blue mass in the vagina or hematocolpos secondary to an imperforate hymen. A blind uterine horn can present with cyclic menstrual bleeding, but the evaluation reveals severe cyclic pain and a pelvic mass. After hemodynamic stability is ensured, these adolescents should be referred in a timely manner to a gynecologist.

A functional ovarian cyst is a common cause of pelvic mass in adolescents and is frequently treated by the primary care provider. If the patient is not in acute distress and an adnexal mass is palpated that is less than 5 cm, the patient can be re-examined in 4 to 6 weeks. Patients with adnexal masses greater than 5 cm that do not appear to be resolving should have a pelvic ultrasound performed and be referred to a gynecologist. Patients in severe pain and those with a cyst greater than 8 cm to 10 cm should be referred to a gynecologist. Functional cysts may be followed and managed with symptomatic relief of pain with nonsteroidal anti-inflammatory drugs. Oral contraceptives are helpful in suppressing future ovulatory cysts; however, this treatment in adolescents is usually accompanied by additional counseling with the parent or guardian.

Although most adnexal masses in this age group are benign, it is important to make the diagnosis early to improve prognosis for malignant lesions. Any patient with complex or solid components of the cyst found on ultrasound should be referred in a timely fashion to a gynecologist. Patients with masculinization should be referred because of increased risk of Sertoli-Leydig cell tumors. Teratomas arise from germ cells and can therefore have a number of structures within them, such as hair, teeth, sebaceous material, and neural elements. A flat plate of the abdomen can be helpful in identifying calcified structures in the adnexa. Dysgerminomas and malignant teratomas are much less common but can also occur.

Other possible causes of pelvic masses in adolescents include pregnancy and infection. Intrauterine pregnancy, ectopic pregnancy, and gestational trophoblastic disease can all present as a pelvic mass. It is important to obtain a complete history of sexual activity. This may present a challenge because adolescents often deny sexual activity as a result of family pressure, embarrassment, or fear. So, as always, in the adolescent with a pelvic mass, a pregnancy test should be ordered. Ectopic pregnancy is a potentially life-threatening condition that should be considered whenever a patient presents with a positive pregnancy test, an adnexal mass, pain, and vaginal bleeding. Prompt referral to a gynecologist is indicated because early therapy may avoid surgery.

In patients who present with signs of infection and a pelvic mass, the differential diagnosis must include pyosalpinx, tubo-ovarian abscess, and appendiceal abscess. A complete blood count should be obtained, and examination of the cervix for frank pus and cultures for sexually transmitted diseases should be part of the initial examination. In general, these patients should be hospitalized and started on intravenous antibiotics in the hope of preserving fertility. If there is a question of appendicitis versus pelvic inflammatory disease, then general surgery in conjunction with gynecology can be consulted.

Reproductive-Aged Women

INCIDENCE AND EPIDEMIOLOGY

In the reproductive years, in addition to the causes already presented, consideration should be given to the possibility of leiomyomas or fibroids, endometriomas, and malignancies, the latter of which have an increasing incidence in older women. Leiomyomas can be seen in the uterus, ovary, cervix, pelvic ligaments, or other pelvic organs. They are common and often asymptomatic. In the United States, myomas are found in at least 10% of white women and 30% to 40% of black women older than 35 years of age [7••]. These numbers increase to around 70% of white women and greater than 80% of black women by age 50 [8].

Adnexal masses in reproductive women are most often ovarian in origin. Cystadenomas are the most common neoplasm in the reproductive years, followed by benign teratomas. Endometriosis is most commonly found in this age group, and classically is seen in white, nulliparous women between the ages of 35 and 45 years. In severe cases, endometriosis can form cysts on the ovaries, which can become large and be easily mistaken for malignancy. These endometriomas, or "chocolate cysts," can present as an adnexal mass.

Ovarian cancer is unusual before the age of 40 years; however, the diagnosis must always be entertained in the patient presenting with an adnexal mass. The lifetime risk for a woman in the United States of developing ovarian carcinoma is approximately one in 70, although epithelial ovarian cancer is currently affecting two in every 70 women in the United States, which increases to 4% to 6% if there is a family history of the disease (one first-degree relative) [7••]. Unfortunately, more than two thirds of women are diagnosed with advanced disease. Approximately 75% of patients with early-stage (stage I or II) disease can be cured, whereas the 5-year survival rate for patients with more advanced disease is only 5% to 15% [9,10••]. The most common ovarian malignancy is cystadenocarcinoma.

DIFFERENTIAL DIAGNOSIS

The differential diagnosis for the reproductive years is similar to that of adolescence. Pregnancy should always be considered. Functional cysts are the most common adnexal mass in this age group. Conditions involving the fallopian tube, such as pyosalpinx, hydrosalpinx, and tubo-ovarian abscess, must be considered. In this age group, the pelvic mass may also be related to the uterus (Figure 35-5).

HISTORY AND PHYSICAL EXAMINATION

Pregnancy, normal and abnormal, should be considered in this age group. The evaluation and treatment of intrauterine pregnancy, ectopic pregnancy, or functional ovarian cysts is the same in reproductive-aged women and adolescents (Figure 35-6).

A pregnancy test is obtained; if positive with no evidence of ectopic pregnancy, appropriate obstetric care can be provided. If the patient has pain, or vaginal bleeding, or the ultrasound suggests an ectopic pregnancy, referral to a gynecologist should be made. Risk factors for the development of ectopic pregnancy include a history of pelvic infection (ruptured appendix, pelvic inflammatory disease), previous ectopic pregnancy, tubal or abdominal surgery, and assisted reproductive technology. If a patient has had a tubal ligation and has a positive pregnancy test, she has a 50% chance of

Differential Diagnosis of a Pelvic Mass in Women of Reproductive Age

Ovarian
  Functional
  Neoplastic
  Endometrioma
Uterine
  Leiomyoma
  Cornual ectopic
  Pregnancy, including molar gestation
Tubal
  Paratubal cyst
  Ectopic gestation
  Tubo-ovarian abscess
    Pyosalpinx
    Hydrosalpinx

Figure 35-5. Differential diagnosis of a pelvic mass in women of reproductive age.

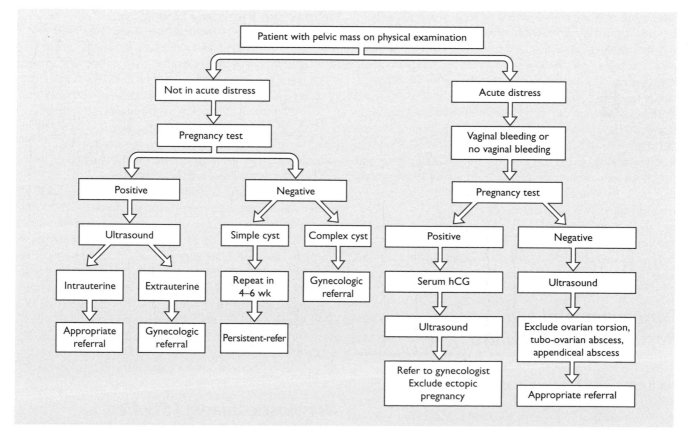

Figure 35-6. Algorithm for the evaluation and treatment of intrauterine pregnancy, ectopic pregnancy, or functional ovarian cysts in adolescents and reproductive-aged women. hCG—human chorionic gonadotropin.

having an ectopic; referral to a gynecologist to rule out ectopic pregnancy should be the top priority.

Functional ovarian cysts (discussed previously) are managed the same in the reproductive years as in adolescence. A history of pelvic infection or salpingitis can pose a problem in women of reproductive age. In patients who had prior salpingitis, occlusion of the tube can result in hydrosalpinx, pyosalpinx, or tubo-ovarian abscess, all of which may present as a pelvic mass. Tubo-ovarian abscess, an acute infection, may present as pelvic masses in reproductive-aged women and is the most common intra-abdominal abscess in premenopausal women [11]. Tubo-ovarian abscess often presents as severe abdominal pain and fever. The pain is often so severe that it may be difficult to perform a thorough abdominal and pelvic examination. Patients with ovarian torsion present in similar fashion but without fever. Because of the inability to perform a thorough pelvic examination, the use of ultrasound can be invaluable. It can often delineate the complex tubo-ovarian abscess or show lack of Doppler flow and therefore help distinguish an ovarian torsion.

As in adolescents, the most common neoplastic ovarian mass is the benign cystic teratoma [11]. Ovarian malignancy is rare but must be considered. Endometriosis commonly is seen in the reproductive years, and these patients have a history of pelvic pain that often worsens with menses. On pelvic examination, the primary care provider may palpate nodularity at the uterosacral ligament beneath the uterus. An adnexal mass may be palpated, and ultrasound may reveal a complex ovarian cyst suspicious for endometrioma. Referral for gynecologic surgery should be considered so that the definitive diagnosis can be made with laparoscopy.

The evaluation of the uterus in reproductive-aged woman is essential in any physical examination. Leiomyomas or fibroids can be seen in the uterus, ovaries, cervix, and broad ligaments. A pedunculated fibroid can grow in the broad ligaments and other locations outside the uterus and may be indistinguishable from an adnexal mass. The fibroid uterus can grow to a significant size in the absence of abnormal uterine bleeding. The patient may complain only of symptoms related to increasing uterine size, which can include pelvic pain, pressure, increasing abdominal girth, early satiety, and bladder and bowel problems.

Perimenopausal and Postmenopausal Women

INCIDENCE AND EPIDEMIOLOGY
As patient age increases, so does the concern for malignancy. In perimenopausal and postmenopausal women, the presence of a pelvic mass carries an increased risk of neoplasm. Unfortunately, over the past few decades the overall survival rate for patients with ovarian cancer has essentially remained the same, a dismal 35%. Epithelial ovarian cancer now affects 1 in 70 women in their lifetime [7••]. Two thirds of these cases are diagnosed in advanced stages. Benign conditions, such as leio-

myomas and endometriosis, are also seen but less frequently require surgical therapy. By menopause, the incidence of leiomyoma increases to 30% in white women and 50% in black women [7••]. Usually, these tumors shrink after menopause. In older age groups, masses from other organs must be considered. Colon cancer and breast cancer are seen more commonly in elderly patients and can be the primary source of a metastatic pelvic mass.

DIFFERENTIAL DIAGNOSIS
Concern is heightened when a pelvic mass is palpated in a postmenopausal woman. The differential diagnosis of pelvic masses in perimenopausal and postmenopausal patients includes those disorders listed previously for reproductive-aged women as well as gastrointestinal tract disorders, such as diverticula and colon cancer, and primary tumors from the genitourinary, musculoskeletal, and lymphatic tracts, which are more common in the older age group. Uterine leiomyomas and endometriosis, more commonly found in reproductive-aged women, can also be considered. The malignant uterine tumors, such as adenocarcinoma, sarcoma, and mixed mesodermal tumors, are more commonly present in the postmenopausal age group. Uterine sarcoma may present as a rapidly enlarging mass in the pelvis in this age group.

HISTORY AND PHYSICAL EXAMINATION
The postmenopausal patient with a pelvic mass requires a thorough history with particular attention to other organ systems. Specific questions should be asked concerning urinary symptoms, change in bowel habits, and fluctuations in weight. Weakness, constipation, and abdominal bloating should alert the clinician to possible colon involvement. A history of any previous gynecologic surgery or tumors needs to be obtained. Operative reports and pathology records can be helpful. The date of the last gynecologic examination is helpful in determining if the pelvic mass is growing rapidly.

Because breast cancer can be metastatic to the ovary, all women should have a thorough breast examination. The vulva, vagina, and cervix should be inspected closely, and any visible abnormality should undergo biopsy. A Papanicolaou smear should be obtained if not screened recently. Postmenopausal bleeding or menstrual irregularities should be evaluated with endometrial biopsy. A negative endometrial biopsy associated with an enlarged uterus or pelvic mass should be referred to a gynecologist for evaluation. The physical examination should always include a rectovaginal examination, with testing for occult blood. A mass felt high in the pelvis, especially on the left side, may represent a diverticular abscess or colon cancer.

Diagnostic Imaging Studies

Several different imaging modalities are available that can help in management of the pelvic mass. Ultrasonography, CT, and MRI can all help delineate the mass and define soft tissue shapes in the pelvis. Ultrasound is probably the most helpful imaging study and is relatively easy to obtain. The female pelvis can be viewed transabdominally or transvaginally. The transvaginal view can provide more detail regarding pelvic structures.

On ultrasound, functional cysts typically appear as thin-walled, unilocular structures without evidence of internal echoes. In general, the more solid and irregular the internal and external features of a mass, the more likely it is malignant. Bilateral adnexal masses are more worrisome. The presence of papillations, thick septations, or irregular surface heightens the concern for malignancy. In addition to transvaginal ultrasound, color-flow Doppler is a useful tool that helps characterize the pelvic mass. Tumors are generally rich in neovascularization, and there is diminished resistance to blood flow across these vessels. In the future, color-flow Doppler may help in delineating the benign from the malignant ovarian tumor [12••].

Tumor Markers

Various tumor markers can be ordered when a pelvic mass is encountered. Typically, they are not helpful in the initial evaluation and are best left to the consultant physician. The most touted test is CA-125, which is used as a tumor marker in managing patients with epithelial ovarian cancer. However, it should not be used as a screening test. This test lacks specificity as CA-125 counts can often be elevated in endometriosis, adenomyosis, leiomyomas, pregnancy, diverticulitis, cirrhosis, and pelvic infections. In the premenopausal patient, this test is not particularly useful. In the postmenopausal patient with adnexal pathology, an elevated CA-125 would certainly increase the suspicion of malignancy [13].

Some germ cell tumors produce human chorionic gonadotropin, lactate dehydrogenase, or α-fetoprotein, but most early stage ovarian neoplasms are not associated with reliable tumor markers [7••]. Carcinoembryonic antigen, which was originally used as a marker for colon cancer, can be elevated in some ovarian cancers and is used as a marker for mucinous cancers of the ovary [14••]. CA 19-9 is elevated in pancreatic cancers but has also been found to be elevated in mucinous ovarian tumors in European studies [14••]. All these markers may be more helpful in following postoperatively the patient who has a known cancer diagnosis than in identifying preoperatively a patient with cancer. None are recommended for wide-scale screening.

Treatments and Controversies

It is important for the primary care provider to be knowledgeable in the various treatments that are available in caring for the patient with a pelvic mass. Not only will it help prepare the patient for her encounter with the referral physician but it also may alleviate fears that might potentially delay patient follow-up and treatment. With increased access to information via the Internet, patients may become more knowledgeable about the various treatments available than at any previous time.

Many treatment options are available for patients with a pelvic mass associated with a fibroid uterus. Hysterectomy has received much attention in recent times and has been wrongfully deemed an unnecessary procedure. In women who have completed their childbearing years and who have symptomatic fibroids, hysterectomy is a viable option. The patient should be aware of alternative therapies when malignancy is not a issue, including administration of gonadotropin-releasing hormone agonists, endometrial ablation, myomectomy, and uterine artery embolization [15•].

During the reproductive years, the most common cause of a pelvic mass is a functional ovarian cyst. If the cyst is smaller than 5 cm, freely movable, smooth-surfaced, and mildly tender, it is safe to observe these patients through the next menstrual cycle. Indications for surgery are shown in Figure 35-7.

The classic approach to the management of adnexal masses has been laparotomy, but in recent years, operative laparoscopy has emerged as an alternative procedure. In patients younger than 40 years with a preoperative ultrasound suggestive of a benign ovarian cyst, laparoscopy is a reasonable therapy [16•]. Some authorities have recommended aspiration of ovarian cysts and cytologic examination of cyst fluid as an alternative to surgical removal. The accuracy of cytology from ovarian cyst aspirates in excluding malignancy is still arguable. There is always the possibility of carcinogenesis with benign appearing cystic ovarian tumors [17]. The puncture of a benign-appearing cyst can always lead to tumor cell spill, resulting in extensively disseminated ovarian carcinoma [18•], thus altering the stage and subsequent treatment of the cancer.

The controversy remains concerning how to treat the postmenopausal woman with a palpable ovary and a benign-appearing cyst on ultrasound. The classic teaching is that a palpable ovary in a postmenopausal woman is considered cancerous until proved otherwise, but advances in ultrasound and its more widespread use have shown that up to 17% of these postmenopausal patients have a cystic adnexal mass [12••]. Commonly, serial ultrasound follow-up without surgical intervention may play a role in the clinical management of patients with postmenopausal ovarian cysts that are smaller than 5 cm, unilocular, unilateral, and without any excrescences, septations, or ascites [12••]. All postmenopausal patients with a palpable ovary should be referred to a gynecologist for further evaluation with ultrasonography.

Adnexal Mass: Indications for Surgery

Ovarian cystic structure larger than 5 cm that has been followed 6 to 8 weeks without regression

Any solid ovarian lesion

Any ovarian lesion with papillary vegetation on the cyst wall

Any adnexal mass greater than 10 cm in diameter

Ascites

Palpable adnexal mass in a premenarchal or postmenopausal patient

Suspected torsion or rupture

Figure 35-7. Adnexal mass: indications for surgery. (*Adapted from* Disaia and Creasman [7••].)

In conclusion, a primary care physician confronted with a pelvic mass should consider different diagnoses, prognoses, and concerns for patients of different ages. The lack of truly effective screening tools for ovarian malignancy makes an aggressive approach to diagnosis and early referral for ovarian masses extremely important. Likewise, the persistent severe hemorrhage rate and occasional death from ectopic pregnancy makes constant concern for this diagnosis an essential part of the evaluation of every woman in her reproductive years. In a managed care environment, the key to effective management of any pelvic mass in the female patient is prompt recognition, diagnosis, and appropriate referral at the primary care level.

References

Papers of particular interest have been highlighted as follows:
•   Of interest
•• Of outstanding interest

1.   Russell DJ: The female pelvic mass: diagnosis and management. *Med Clin North Am* 1995, 79:1481–1493.

2.   Breen JL, Maxson WS: Ovarian tumors in children and adolescents. *Clin Obstet Gynaecol* 1977, 20:607.

3.•   Gallup DG, Talledo OE: Benign and malignant tumors. *Clin Obstet Gynaecol* 1987, 30:662–669.
This article gives an excellent overview of benign and malignant tumors in female children and young adolescents.

4.•   Van Winter JT, Simmons PS, Podratz KC: Surgically treated adnexal masses in infancy, childhood, and adolescence. *Am J Obstet Gynecol* 1994, 170:1780.
A retrospective study advocating conservative management of adnexal masses in infants, children, and young adolescents.

5.   Norris, HJ, Jensen RD: Relative frequency of ovarian neoplasms in children and adolescents. *Cancer* 1972, 30:713.

6.   Asadourian LA, Taylor HB: Dysgerminoma: an analysis of 105 cases. *Obstet Gynecol* 1969, 33:370–379.

7.•• Disaia PJ, Creasman WT: Management of endometrial adenocarcinoma stage I with surgical staging followed by tailored adjuvant radiation therapy. *Clin Obstet Gynaecol* 1986, 13:751–765.
Key text on clinical gynecologic oncology.

8.   Day-Baird D, Dunson DB, Hill MC, *et al.*: High cumulative incidence of uterine leiomyoma in black and white women: ultrasound evidence. *Am J Obstet Gynecol* 2003, 188:100–107.

9.   National Institutes of Health Consensus Conference: Ovarian cancer: screening, treatment, and follow-up. *JAMA* 1995, 273:491–497.

10.• Wiesenfeld HC, Sweet RL: Progress in the management of tuboovarian abscess. *Clin Obstet Gynecol* 1993, 36:433–444.
An excellent discussion of current therapy for tubo-ovarian abscess.

11.   Peterson WF: Benign cystic teratoma of the ovary: a clinico-statistical study of 1007 cases with a review of the literature. *Am J Obstet Gynecol* 1955, 70:568.

12.•• Goldstein S: Conservative management of small postmenopausal cystic masses. *Clin Obstet Gynecol* 1993, 36:399.
A landmark article for conservative management of small postmenopausal cystic mass.

13.   ACOG Committee Opinion No. 185. September 1997.

14.•• Swartz P: The role of tumor markers in the preoperative diagnosis of ovarian cysts. *Clin Obstet Gynecol* 1993, 36:390.
Excellent discussion on use of tumor markers in the management and diagnosis of adnexal masses.

15.• Bradley E, Reidy J: Transcatheter uterine artery embolization to treat large uterine fibroids. *Br J Obstet Gynaecol* 1998, 105:235–240.
European results in treatment of pelvic mass with uterine artery embolization, which may become another accepted form of therapy in the future.

16.• Marana R: Operative laparoscopy for ovarian cysts. *J Reprod Med* 1996, 41:436.
Advocates operative laparoscopy in selected patients for treatment of ovarian cysts.

17.   Gerber B: Simple ovarian cysts in premenopausal patients. *Int J Gynecol Obstet* 1997, 57:49.

18.• Trimbos JB, Hacker NF: The case against aspirating ovarian cysts. *Cancer* 1993, 72:828–831.
Offers an argument for not aspirating ovarian cysts.

36 Uterine Leiomyomas

Thomas G. Stovall, MD

- Uterine leiomyoma is a common tumor of unknown etiology that may be symptomatic or asymptomatic.
- Asymptomatic leiomyomas of less than 12 weeks' gestational size require no treatment other than annual examination.
- The most common symptom of leiomyoma is heavy menstrual bleeding.
- Symptomatic leiomyomas can be treated medically, radiologically, or surgically.
- Medical management of leiomyomas may include nonsteroidal anti-inflammatory drugs, combination estrogen and progestin therapy, antiestrogen agents, progestins, tranexamic acid, antiprogesterone agents, or gonadotropin-releasing hormone agonists.
- Surgical management of leiomyomas may include myomectomy or hysterectomy by several techniques.
- Radiographic treatment alternatives include bilateral uterine artery embolization and MRI-guided focused ultrasound.
- After myomectomy, a significant number of patients develop recurrent symptoms and require reoperation.

Leiomyomata uteri (more commonly called uterine leiomyomas, leiomyomas, myomas, or fibroids) are pseudoencapsulated, smooth-muscle tumors arising from proliferation of a single smooth muscle cell of the uterine stroma or blood vessels. They are more commonly multiple than solitary and vary in size from microscopic to the size of a term pregnancy (Figure 36-1). Leiomyomas are artificially classified by uterine location as submucous, intramural, or subserosal (Figure 36-2) but may occur within the folds of the broad ligament, in the cervix, or attached to other organs in the pelvis (parasitic). They may be broad-based or attached to the uterus by a vascular pedicle.

pause or other estrogen-deprivation states are associated with a regression in size of leiomyomas. During pregnancy, approximately one third of uterine leiomyomas increase in size [2]. Estrogen and progesterone receptors have been studied in uterine leiomyomas, but whether they are increased, decreased, or unchanged has not been proved [3,4]. Investigators have suggested that peptide growth factors and their receptors may regulate leiomyoma growth [2].

Symptomatic uterine leiomyomas account for approximately one third of all hysterectomies performed in the United States and for more than 1 billion health care dollars spent per year [5•].

Incidence and Epidemiology

The cause is unknown, but cytogenetic studies show that approximately 40% of uterine leiomyomas have chromosomal rearrangements. They are the most common tumor of the female reproductive tract, are present in 20% or more of women older than 35 years, and are more common in African-American than in white women [1].

Uterine leiomyomas are thought to be estrogen dependent, seldom arising before pubarche or after menopause. Meno-

Symptoms

Most uterine leiomyomas are asymptomatic. Symptoms associated with leiomyomas may include abnormal uterine bleeding, pelvic pressure, urinary frequency, voiding difficulty, constipation, infertility, pregnancy wastage, preterm delivery, and pain (Figure 36-3) [5•,6••]. When symptoms are present, they are related to the location, size, or degenerative changes of the tumor. The location of leiomyomas is the most important factor responsible for clinical symptoms.

The symptom most commonly associated with uterine leiomyomas is menorrhagia, defined clinically as menstrual bleeding resulting in anemia, lasting more than 8 days per cycle, or heavy enough to interfere with the woman's normal daily activity. Submucosal leiomyomas are the most symptomatic and are commonly associated with abnormal uterine bleeding. The pathophysiology of leiomyoma-associated menorrhagia is unknown but may be related to leiomyomas altering endometrial microvasculature so that they prevent normal endometrial hemostasis. Intramural leiomyomas may also cause abnormal bleeding by expanding the uterine wall and interfering with contraction of the uterine muscle. Patients with uterine leiomyomas are not predisposed to anovulation or midcycle bleeding. The presence of leiomyomas or other intrauterine pathology should be suspected when patients continue to have problems with bleeding while receiving hormonal therapy [7].

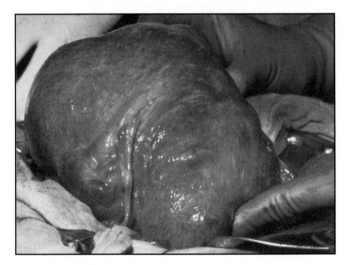

Figure 36-1. This large uterus (compare it to the surgeon's hands) contains several leiomyomas.

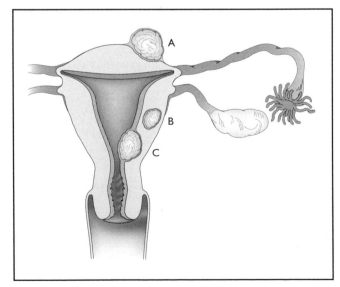

Figure 36-2. Locations of leiomyomas. Submucosal (A); intramural (B); and subserosal (C).

Leiomyomas cause pelvic pressure by impinging on adjacent organs. They should cause no more pressure-related symptoms than a comparable-sized pregnant uterus. Urinary frequency, urgency, or incontinence may be experienced. Leiomyomas that involve the anterior aspect of the uterus can exert pressure on the bladder, causing an increase in the frequency of urination. Leiomyomas can also cause ureteral obstruction and lead to hydronephrosis.

Urinary tract symptoms should be evaluated to determine other causes of symptoms before surgical management of the leiomyomas is performed. Myomectomy or hysterectomy should not be expected to cure urinary incontinence [6••,8•]. Urethral obstruction and hydronephrosis are reported, but complete ureteral obstruction secondary to leiomyomas has not [6••,9]. Posteriorly located large uterine leiomyomas may cause rectal pressure or difficulty passing stool, but this is rare.

Infertility, recurrent pregnancy loss, and preterm delivery are often attributed to uterine leiomyomas, but this is based solely on anecdotal and observational evidence [6••,7]. Term delivery rates of 40% are reported in women undergoing myomectomy for infertility or recurrent pregnancy loss [8•]. This is similar to the delivery rate in untreated patients] with infertility or habitual abortion not associated with leiomyomas. Treating leiomyomas as a cause of infertility or fetal wastage should be done only after other causes of infertility, male and female, are excluded. Although leiomyomas rarely are the cause of a couple's inability to conceive, those involving the intrauterine cavity can interfere with embryo implantation or placentation and can be a factor in recurrent pregnancy loss. Leiomyomas involving the uterotubal junction or the broad ligament can distort the fallopian tube and interfere with conception. They also can distort the position of the cervix, thereby interfering with the opportunity for the cervical os to be bathed in seminal fluid during coitus.

Uterine leiomyomas cause pain when they become infarcted. Infarction is caused by a loss of blood supply, secondary to internal (called carneous or red) degeneration or to torsion of a pedunculated myoma. The pain is most commonly localized to the area of the myoma, and the specific area of degeneration is tender on physical examination. Leiomyoma degeneration

Common Symptoms of Uterine Leiomyomas

Abnormal uterine bleeding—most commonly menorrhagia

Pelvic pressure

Voiding difficulty

Constipation

Infertility

Pregnancy wastage

Preterm delivery

Pain

Partial urethral obstruction

Figure 36-3. Common symptoms of uterine leiomyomas.

as a cause of pain is uncommon and self-limited, most often managed with observation and analgesics. Other causes of pain should be excluded before the diagnosis of a degenerating leiomyoma is made. Symptom resolution takes from a few days to 2 weeks.

Degeneration is more common during pregnancy and should be considered as a cause of localized abdominal or pelvic pain in the gravida. When myomectomy is required during pregnancy, a favorable maternal and fetal outcome should be expected [10•].

Pain may occur after administration of gonadotropin-releasing hormone (GnRH) analogs as a result of degeneration of the leiomyoma. Pressure exerted from leiomyomas on the nerves exiting the lumbar or sacral spine can be a source of lower back or leg pain.

Ulceration and secondary infection of a prolapsing cervical leiomyoma is occasionally seen. Ascites has been reported as a consequence of torsion of a pedunculated subserosal or parasitic leiomyoma. The latter is the result of attachment and vascularization of a pedunculated tumor, which eventually becomes detached from the uterus. Polycythemia is associated with leiomyomas and is believed to be secondary to the autonomous production of erythropoietin by this tumor [3].

Diagnosis

PALPATION
Leiomyomas are diagnosed most commonly during pelvic examination of a symptom-free woman when the examiner palpates an enlarged, irregular, firm pelvic mass contiguous with the uterus. Leiomyomas may also be inside the uterus and not detected by palpation or nonpalpable because of small size.

IMAGING
Pelvic ultrasonography, hysterosonography, or hysterography may help confirm the diagnosis of leiomyomas (Figure 36-4).

Routine ultrasonographic imaging provides adnexal evaluation, assessment of dimensions, number, and locations of tumors, but most information indicates ultrasonographic imaging has little clinical benefit to the patient because it does not improve long-term therapeutic outcomes [11]. Ultrasonography helps most when physical examination is difficult or the adnexa cannot be palpated during physical examination, such as in the obese patient or the patient who, for whatever reason, cannot cooperate with examination.

Magnetic resonance imaging is an effective imaging tool. CT scanning, abdominal flat plate, barium enema, and intravenous pyelogram are seldom as helpful as ultrasonography or MRI.

Hysterosonography is a technique performed by infusing saline into the uterine cavity immediately preceding or during transvaginal ultrasonography. It is especially helpful in identifying submucous leiomyomas and in differentiating them from intrauterine polyps, adhesions, or anomalies (Figure 36-5).

No imaging study is completely reliable in diagnosing leiomyomas. When an unequivocal diagnosis is required, laparoscopy or hysteroscopy may be needed to identify uterine leiomyomas.

LABORATORY STUDIES
Laboratory studies are nondiagnostic for leiomyomas. In cases of abnormal uterine bleeding, Papanicolaou smear, hematocrit level, coagulation studies, and endometrial biopsy should be performed based on patient age, history, and physical examination. Urinalysis should be performed when a bladder tumor is included in the differential diagnosis. The measurement of serum tumor markers, such as CA-125, human chorionic gonadotropin, carcinoembryonic antigen, and lactate dehydrogenase level are generally of no benefit.

Serum CA-125 levels are often slightly elevated in patients with leiomyomas. These slightly elevated values may cause clinicians to act on these false-positive results, resulting in surgical extirpation for fear of missing the diagnosis of ovarian or intrauterine cancer.

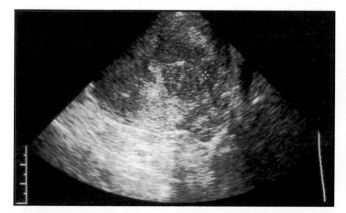

Figure 36-4. Ultrasound photography demonstrating several rounded densities (leiomyomas) of slightly different echogenicity than the normal uterine wall. They have been marked by the radiologist for easier identification and measurement.

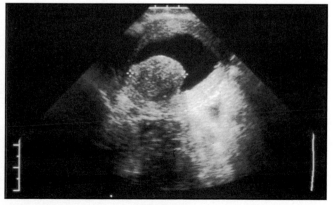

Figure 36-5. A hysterosonogram is an ultrasound examination of the uterus with fluid infused into the cavity. Here, a broad-based submucous leiomyoma is seen that would not be well identified using standard ultrasonography.

Differential Diagnosis

The differential diagnosis of palpable leiomyomas includes common disorders, such as adenomyosis, ovarian tumors, tubo-ovarian abscess, or bicornuate uterus, and less common disorders, such as uterine sarcoma, pelvic kidney, bladder tumors, colonic diverticula, or colon cancer. The differential diagnosis of intramural or subserosal leiomyomas includes intrauterine polyps, adhesions, septa, endometrial hyperplasia, and malignancy.

Leiomyosarcoma, although rare, is the most common malignancy found in uterine leiomyomas. Leiomyomas are not a pre-existing condition of sarcoma, and women with leiomyomas are not at increased risk for developing leiomyosarcomas. Leiomyosarcomas are usually associated with intermenstrual bleeding and may be associated with rapid uterine enlargement.

The diagnosis of leiomyosarcoma is based on histologic criteria, including an increased mitotic figure count and cellular atypia within the tumor. When a leiomyosarcoma is found within a leiomyoma at the time of hysterectomy or in the postsurgical pathology report, no further treatment is indicated. This is because staging and adjuvant therapy have been of no greater benefit than simple hysterectomy for the treatment of this condition [12•].

Treatment

Because most women with leiomyomas do not have symptoms, they require nothing more than physical examination and continued observation. The patient diagnosed with leiomyomas may be examined again in 3 to 6 months as a precautionary measure. If the tumor size is stable and less than the size of a comparable 12-week gestation, the patient with no symptoms may be examined yearly as follow-up.

When the patient is symptomatic, treatment is indicated. Treatment of menorrhagia is the same whether or not the patient has leiomyomas. Nonsteroidal anti-inflammatory agents, combination estrogen and progestin agents, danazol, progestins, tranexamic acid, depomedroxyprogesterone acetate, antiprogesterone (RU-486), and GnRH agonists have all been used in the medical management of menorrhagia (Figure 36-6) [13,14•].

Nonsteroidal anti-inflammatory drugs inhibit prostaglandin synthesis and reduce menstrual blood loss by 30% to 50%. Androgenic agents such as danazol, progestins (medroxyprogesterone acetate, depomedroxyprogesterone acetate, norethindrone), and the antiprogesterone RU-486 are used to create an atrophic endometrial lining. Combination hormonal agents (oral contraceptives and postmenopausal estrogen therapy) are used to stabilize the endometrium, creating a lining that does not slough irregularly. GnRH agonists are used to induce a menopause-like hormonal state. None of these medical agents cause the leiomyomas to regress permanently. Exogenous hormones were once thought to increase the growth rate of leiomyomas, but this is no longer believed [6••].

Gonadotropin-releasing hormone agonists are the most effective medication to control uterine bleeding. When administered continuously, a median reduction in uterine volume of 30% to 50% is obtained after 12 weeks of therapy. Most of the uterine size reduction results from reduced uterine blood flow and cell size, not a reduced cell number or a cytotoxic effect. With cessation of therapy, rapid regrowth of tumors is seen [13]. Extended administration of GnRH agonists with the addition of low-dose cyclic or continuous estrogen and progestin ("add-back" therapy) is being used therapeutically by many practitioners but must be regarded as investigational, and it is certainly expensive.

Gonadotropin-releasing hormone agonists are recommended only for treating a submucous tumor to facilitate hysteroscopic resection, when awaiting the onset of menopause in a perimenopausal woman, or to decrease size and symptoms before surgery. There are insufficient data to support the use of GnRH agonists for the primary treatment of uterine leiomyomas [6••].

Summary of Treatments for Uterine Leiomyomas

Medical

  Observation

  Nonsteroidal anti-inflammatory agents

  Combination estrogen and progestin agents (oral contraceptive pills, sequential or combined hormone replacement therapy)

  Danazol (anti-estrogen agent)

  Progestins (medroxyprogesterone acetate, depomedroxyprogesterone acetate, norethindrone)

  Tranexamic acid (fibrinolytic agent)

  Antiprogesterone agents (RU-486)

  Gonadotropin-releasing hormone agonists

Surgical

  Uterine artery embolization

  Myomectomy

   Hysteroscopic

   Laparoscopic

   Laparotomy

  Hysterectomy

   Vaginal

   Laparoscopic

    Subtotal (leaves uterine cervix in place)

    Total

   Transabdominal

    Subtotal (leaves uterine cervix in place)

    Total

Figure 36-6. Summary of treatments of uterine leiomyomas.

Bilateral embolization of the uterine arteries is an interventional radiographic procedure that may be used to treat leiomyomas. In a series of 12 patients, an average 60% reduction in uterine size and 80% improvement in symptoms were reported. The major deterrent to this procedure is the immediate postoperative pain, severe enough in some cases to require hospitalization and administration of parenteral narcotics [15]. In a more recent study, Spies *et al.* [16] reported a series of 200 consecutive patients treated with uterine artery embolization and followed for 5 years. At 5 years, 73% had continued symptoms control. Twenty-five patients (13.7%) had undergone hysterectomy, eight (4.4%) had undergone myomectomy, and 1.6% had undergone a second embolization procedure. Overall, 25% of patients had a failure of symptom control or recurrence over the course of 5 years. Patients undergoing this procedure have significant reduction of symptom and overall improved life-quality [17].

Magnetic resonance–guided focused ultrasound is a new innovative treatment for selected patients with uterine leiomyoma. Focused ultrasound is a thermal ablation method that uses sound waves created in tissue as a source of thermal injury. Using MRI technology to focus the point of injury, the fibroid can be ablated. The US Food and Drug Administration approved this procedure in October 2004. This treatment method has an excellent safety profile with treatment results similar to that for myomectomy [18].

A woman with symptomatic leiomyomas wishing to preserve fertility may choose to undergo myomectomy. Myomec-

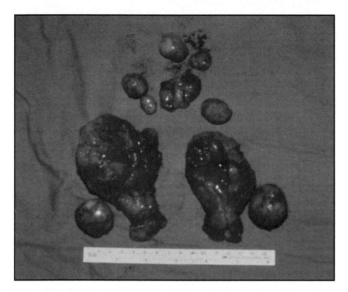

Figure 36-7. Photograph of a postsurgical specimen showing the positions of multiple leiomyomas as they existed before being shelled out to facilitate removal of the uterus during vaginal hysterectomy.

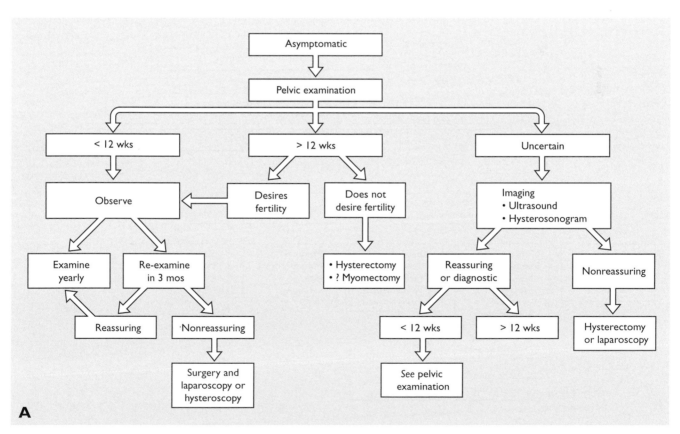

Figure 36-8. Algorithms for the evaluation of leiomyomas. **A,** Asymptomatic. **B,** Symptomatic. GnRH—gonadotropin-releasing hormone; NSAIDs—nonsteroidal anti-inflammatory drugs.

Continued on the next page

tomy successfully treats menorrhagia in about 80% of patients, but 15% again develop symptoms, and 10% require reoperation [8•]. It is therefore essential to inform patients choosing to undergoing myomectomy that there is a significant risk of recurrence of leiomyomas after surgery. Recent ultrasound studies show leiomyoma recurrence rates of 25% for women with three or fewer leiomyomas resected and 90% for women with four or more leiomyomas resected [19].

In a series of patients reported in 1981, approximately one fifth of women undergoing myomectomy required blood transfusion [8•]. With the more cautious current use of blood products and the expanded role of operative hysteroscopy for the treatment of submucous leiomyomas and laparoscopic treatment of subserosal leiomyomas, transfusion rates and operative morbidity for myomectomy may be decreasing. This, however, is speculative on the author's part and not proved.

In the United States, approximately 175,000 hysterectomies are performed yearly for leiomyomas [20]. Hysterectomy is the only absolute cure for leiomyomas and their symptoms. Current indications for hysterectomy to treat leiomyomas include tumors palpable through the abdomen that are of concern to the patient, excessive uterine bleeding, or pelvic discomfort.

Before hysterectomy, the practitioner should confirm the absence of cervical and endometrial malignancy, eliminate other causes of abnormal bleeding, assess surgical risks, and assess the patient's medical and psychological risks. Contraindications to hysterectomy include a desire by the patient to remain fertile or asymptomatic leiomyomas of less than 12 weeks gestational size [6••].

The type of hysterectomy performed depends on the operator's experience, familiarity with current surgical techniques, and patient circumstances. Figure 36-7 shows a uterus removed transvaginally with concomitant myomectomy to accomplish the procedure. For some gynecologic surgeons, this would be a routine operation; others would think it is contraindicated. Similarly, laparoscopic techniques can be used to facilitate hysterectomy, but only in the hands of a skilled laparoscopic surgeon.

Summary

In deciding how to evaluate and treat uterine leiomyomas, many factors need to be considered. The caregiver must determine whether the patient has symptoms, the size and location of existing leiomyomas, the patient's desire for fertility, and the goals of therapy as determined by the patient and caregiver (Figure 36-8). Leiomyomas represent the most common reproductive tract tumor in women; therefore, evaluation and treatment of this condition should be familiar to all who provide health care to women.

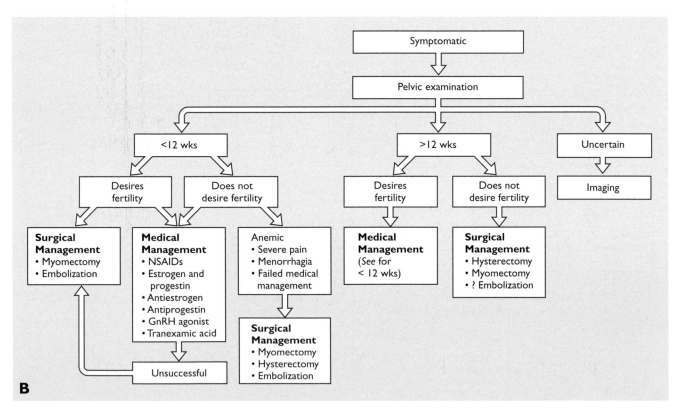

Figure 37-8. *(Continued)*

References

Papers of particular interest have been highlighted as follows:
- *Of interest*
- •• *Of outstanding interest*

1. Brosens I, Hohannisson E, Dal Cin P, *et al.*: Analysis of the karyotype and deoxyribonucleic acid content of uterine myomas in premenopausal, menopausal, and gonadotropin-releasing hormone agonist treated females. *Fertil Steril* 1996, 66:376–379.

2. Aharoni A, Reiter A, Golan D, *et al.*: Patterns of growth of uterine leiomyomas during pregnancy: a prospective longitudinal study. *Br J Obstet Gynaecol* 1988, 95:510–523.

3. Lumsden MR, West CP, Hawkins RA, *et al.*: The binding of steroids to myometrium and leiomyomata (fibroids) in women treated with the gonadotropin-releasing hormone agonist Zoladex (ICI 118630). *J Endocrinol* 1989, 121:389–396.

4. Pollow K, Geilfuss J, Boquoi E, *et al.*: Estrogen and progesterone binding proteins in normal human myometrium and leiomyoma tissue. *J Clin Chem Clin Biochem* 1978, 16:503–511.

5.• Wilcox LS, Koonin LM, Pokras R, *et al.*: Hysterectomy in the United States, 1988–1990. *Obstet Gynecol* 1994, 83:549–555.

This article provides demographic and epidemiologic information about hysterectomy, the most commonly done major surgical procedure in the United States.

6.•• American College of Obstetricians and Gynecologists: *Uterine Leiomyomata. Educational Bulletin No. 192.* Washington, DC: American College of Obstetricians and Gynecologists; May 1994.

This technical bulletin for gynecologists offers perhaps the best single overview about uterine leiomyomas—etiology, clinical behavior, and treatment options.

7. Vollenhoven BJ, Lawrence AS, Healy DL: Uterine fibroids: a clinical review. *Br J Obstet Gynaecol* 1990, 97:285–298.

8.• Buttram VC Jr, Reiter RC: Uterine leiomyomata: etiology, symptomatology, and management. *Fertil Steril* 1981, 6:433–445.

Though an older reference, this is probably the most commonly cited article in the gynecologic literature about uterine leiomyomas.

9. Weinberger MW, Julian TM: Voiding dysfunction and incontinence caused by uterine retroversion. *J Reprod Med* 1995, 40:387–390.

10.• Burton CA, Grimes DA, March CM: Surgical management of leiomyomata during pregnancy. *Obstet Gynecol* 1989, 74:707–709.

This article dispels many of the commonly-held myths about the behavior of uterine leiomyomas during pregnancy.

11. Andolf E, Jorgensen C, Astedt B: Ultrasound examination for the detection of ovarian carcinoma in risk groups. *Obstet Gynecol* 1990, 75:106–109.

12.• Reiter RC, Wagner PL, Gambone JC: Routine hysterectomy for large asymptomatic uterine leiomyomata: a reappraisal. *Obstet Gynecol* 1994, 79:481–484.

This paper discusses whether the commonly-held belief-that large, asymptomatic uterine leiomyomas must be removed-is based in fact or clinical superstition.

13. Murphy AA, Morales AL, Kettel LM, *et al.*: Regression of uterine leiomyomata to the antiprogesterone RU 486: dose response effect. *Fertil Steril* 1995, 64:187–190.

14.• Friedman AJ, Hoffman DI, Comite F, *et al.*: Treatment of leiomyomata uteri with leuprolide acetate depot: a double-blind, placebo-controlled, multi-center study. *Obstet Gynecol* 1991, 77:720–725.

This is one of the earliest and the best controlled studies examining what GnRH agonists will and will not do in the treatment and evaluation of uterine leiomyomas.

15. Skolnick AA: Interventional radiological treatments tested. *JAMA* 1997, 277:1424–1425.

16. Spies JB, Czeyda-Pommersheim F, Magee ST, *et al.*: Long-term outcome of uterine artery embolization of leiomyomata. *Obstet Gynecol* 2005, 106:933–939.

17. Smith WJ, Upton E, Shuster EJ, *et al.*: Patient satisfaction and disease specific quality of life after uterine artery embolization. *AJOG* 2004, 190:1697–1706.

18. Stewart EA, Rabinovici J, Tempany YI, *et al.*: Clinical outcomes of focused ultrasound surgery for the treatment of uterine fibroids. *Fertil Steril* 2006, 85:22–29.

19. Friedman AJ, Daly M, Juneau-Norcross M, *et al.*: Recurrence of myomas following myomectomy in women treated with a gonadotropin-releasing hormone agonist. *Fertil Steril* 1992, 58:205–208.

20. Easterday CL, Grimes DA, Riggs JA: Hysterectomy in the United States. *Obstet Gynecol* 1983, 62:203–212.

37 | Chronic Pelvic Pain

Frank W. Ling and C. Paul Perry

- To be considered chronic, pelvic pain must be present for at least 6 months.
- Psychologic and physical components are present in chronic pelvic pain.
- A multidisciplinary approach to chronic pelvic pain is necessary to achieve the best therapeutic response.
- All components of tissue injury and nerve stimulation must be identified and treated.
- The goals of therapy are to reduce the level of pain and to return the patient to normal functional levels.
- The complete elimination of pain may be impossible.

Women with chronic pelvic pain (CPP) represent a challenge to even the most experienced practitioner. They have often seen multiple physicians, endured many diagnostic procedures, and undergone several surgical procedures. Some have been told that their pain is "all in their head." These patients lose confidence in medical professionals and may be skeptical of any new therapy. Despite the difficult nature of treating CPP, these patients deserve the practitioner's best efforts.

Unlike acute pain, CPP is usually multifactorial. The transition from acute to chronic may take months to years. The pain must be present for at least 6 months to meet the definition of CPP. The initiating visceral nerve pain often results in somatic and musculoskeletal involvement. This complex can cause incomplete diagnosis and delays in treatment. All visceral and somatic components must be accurately diagnosed and treated for best results. The longer chronic pain is inadequately relieved, the less likely is complete resolution to occur. Certain principles of CPP management are foundational. A detailed history is required that includes location of pain, intensity, and aggravating and ameliorating factors (Figure 37-1). The physical examination must include a careful search for trigger points and muscle spasm (Figure 37-2). A Q-tip test can be used to exclude vulvar vestibulitis. Single-digit vaginal examination is required before a bimanual examination to isolate vaginal, urethral, bladder, uterocervical, and parametrial tenderness.

Because pain can be out of proportion to tissue injury, diagnostic studies are less productive in the management of CPP (Figure 37-3). Ultrasound examinations can clarify mass effects, but cannot identify adhesions or endometriosis. Likewise, CT and MRI have limited value. Pain mapping under conscious sedation can be helpful in patients who can tolerate it.

A multidisciplinary approach to pain management renders the best results. Numerous disciplines—for example, gynecology, urology, physical therapy, gastroenterology, and psychiatry—may be needed. One physician should take responsibility for coordinating the referrals to other team members. Ideally, this team leader also manages prescription medications. If controlled substances are used, a drug contract may prove useful. This requires the patient to present to the physician's office on a regular basis to receive written prescriptions. The contract should include provisions for: 1) dismissal if prescriptions are procured elsewhere, 2) stipulation that no telephoned prescriptions will be issued, and 3) stipulation that there will be no reissuing of lost prescriptions.

It is the purpose of this chapter to look at the most common causes of CPP and to describe a thorough approach. There is a popular misconception that a patient with CPP has a psychologic illness or a physical illness. This mind body separation model should be abandoned. Because of the prolonged suffering associated with CPP, there will always be a psychologic component to this disease. Practitioners should avoid the "all in your head" prejudice.

Neuroanatomy of Chronic Pelvic Pain

Pain perception occurs at the cerebral cortex. Two areas of the brain are involved in interpreting nociceptive signals: the

History of the Patient who has Chronic Pelvic Pain

1. When did the pain begin?
2. How has it changed?
3. Where is it located?

   Did it start in one location and move to another?

   Does it radiate to another region?
4. Is the pain associated with menses?

   When does it begin in relation to menstrual flow?
5. Does it occur with intercourse?

   Is there painful penetration, deep thrust, or both?
6. Does it occur with physical activity?
7. Is there associated nausea, diarrhea, or constipation?
8. What medications have been prescribed?

   What has worked and what has not?
9. What surgical therapy has been tried?
10. What do you think is causing the pain?
11. How does your family respond to the pain?
12. How has the pain altered your lifestyle?

Figure 37-1. History of the patient who has chronic pelvic pain.

Physical Examination of the Patient who has Chronic Pelvic Pain

1. Perform general examination of the respiratory, cardiovascular, and integumentary systems
2. Perform examination of the musculoskeletal system

   Check for tender points: occipital, posterior nuchal, trapezius, subscapular, paraspinous, iliolumbar, gluteal, forearm, medial knee muscles

   Check for abdominal wall trigger points
3. Perform q-tip mapping of the vestibule
4. Examine the pelvic floor muscles

   Check for tenderness on each side with single-digit palpation: pubococcygeus, piriformis, obturator muscles
5. Examine bladder and urethra

   Perform single-digit palpation of the urethra, trigone, and each ureteral insertion into the bladder
6. Exert single-digit pressure on the cervix
7. Perform bimanual palpation of the uterine fundus and adnexa
8. Perform rectovaginal examination of the cul de sac and uterosacral ligaments

Figure 37-2. Physical examination of the patient who has chronic pelvic pain.

somatosensory cortex determines the location and quality of the pain, and the limbic system modulates the emotional response to the pain. This is the neurophysiologic basis for the mind–body response to CPP.

Two types of nerves in the female pelvis are capable of initiating and sustaining CPP: somatic and autonomic. Both are usually implicated. Somatic involvement can be primary or secondary. Some peripheral nerves can be trapped in scar tissue, and neuroma formation can occur; this is primary somatic nociception or neuralgia. If the somatic nerve is reflexly stimulated as a response to visceral nerve stimulation, as in vaginismus, it is secondary [1••]. The somatic nerves of the pelvis include the iliohypogastric (T12-L1), ilioinguinal (L1-2), genitofemoral (L1-2), and pudendal (S2-4). Each nerve can be discriminated by its specific dermatome (Figure 37-4).

The autonomic nervous system of the pelvis is mostly efferent or motor (Figure 37-5). However, afferent fibers that travel with the motor fibers respond to noxious stimuli. The sympathetic portion of the autonomic nervous system is supplied by the hypogastric or presacral nerve (T10-L2). Additional sympathetic innervation is supplied by the paravertebral chain. The parasympathetic pelvic nerves also carry afferent nociceptors through the nervi erigentes (S2-4).

Visceral pain is more diffuse and less well localized than somatic pain. There are many fewer visceral nociceptors than somatic nociceptors. Light touch and temperature receptors are absent in the nonsomatic nerves. Stretch and chemoreceptors predominate in the autonomic sensory nerves. True visceral pain is usually accompanied by autonomic reflexes, such as nausea, tachycardia, and diaphoresis. As a result of a phenomenon called projection and convergence, visceral pain is often perceived in a dermatome remote from the actual origin of nociception (Figure 37-6). Convergence occurs as somatic and visceral nerves synapse on the same dorsal horn neuron of the spinal cord. These dorsal horn transmission cells relay the impulse to the cortex. When stimulated, there is no discrimination of the origin of the noxious stimulus. The perception is the same for a visceral structure or a somatic structure at the same

Diagnostic Studies Used in Patients who have Chronic Pelvic Pain

Study	Diagnostic Value
Kidney, ureter, and bladder radiographs	Poor
Abdominal ultrasound	Poor
Pelvic ultrasound	Fair
CT	Good
MRI	Good
Laparoscopy	Very good
Pain mapping	Very good

Figure 37-3. Diagnostic studies used in patients who have chronic pelvic pain.

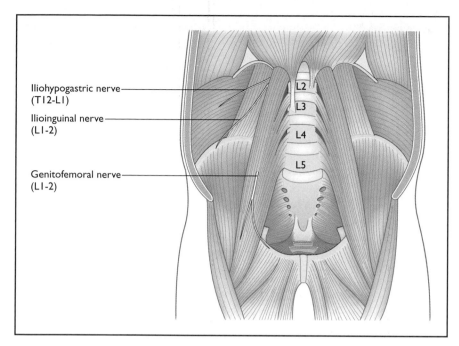

Iliohypogastric nerve (T12-L1)

Ilioinguinal nerve (L1-2)

Genitofemoral nerve (L1-2)

L2
L3
L4
L5

Figure 37-4. Most common peripheral nerves involved in chronic pelvic pain and their respective dermatomes. (*Adapted from* Rogers [1●●].)

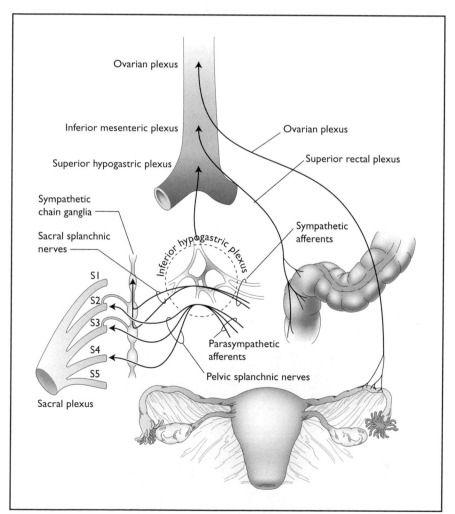

Ovarian plexus

Inferior mesenteric plexus

Superior hypogastric plexus

Ovarian plexus

Superior rectal plexus

Sympathetic chain ganglia

Sacral splanchnic nerves

Inferior hypogastric plexus

Sympathetic afferents

S1
S2
S3
S4
S5

Parasympathetic afferents

Pelvic splanchnic nerves

Sacral plexus

Figure 37-5. The autonomic nervous system of the pelvis. (*Adapted from* Rogers [1●●].)

dermatome level. Therefore, the visceral pain may be perceived to come from an area other than the site of tissue injury. This is termed *referred pain* or *projection* [2].

Patients with CPP should be referred if the primary care physician is uncertain about available treatment options or if efficient pain management cannot be offered. Rarely does any one clinician maintain the skills required to address all aspects of these complicated cases.

Endometriosis

Endometriosis is the most common cause of CPP, estimated to affect 10% to 15% of premenopausal women. Painful periods are usually a result of intense uterine contractions mediated by prostaglandins; this is called primary dysmenorrhea. Secondary dysmenorrhea is painful menstruation from other causes, such as endometriosis. Cramping that starts before the menstrual flow begins is predysmenorrhea. The origin of this pain is intraperitoneal release of chemicals that stimulate nociceptors. Prostanoids, interleukins, and lymphokines are implicated [3]. This pain can be present in young patients and is often ignored by clinicians. If the usual measures of antiprostaglandins or oral contraceptives fail to relieve predysmenorrhea, endometriosis should be considered. Even the very young adolescent should be considered at high risk for developing CPP if predysmenorrhea is uncontrolled. Prevention of the CPP syndrome depends on early diagnosis (possibly including laparoscopy) and treatment.

In the older menstruating patient, other symptoms may be present. In addition to predysmenorrhea, dyspareunia and dyschezia become common complaints. Deep-thrust dyspareunia results from cul de sac lesions of endometriosis. Penetration dyspareunia may be a result of reflex vaginismus or vestibulitis. Older lesions can infiltrate pelvic tissues and elicit tenderness by neural distortion and pressure [4]. Dyschezia is produced by rectal involvement (Figure 37-7).

Treatment of endometriosis can be medical or surgical. Operative laparoscopy can be performed if endometriosis is suspected. This can be diagnostic and therapeutic. Conservative surgery has goals of decreasing pain and preserving fertility. Excision of endometriosis is more effective than laser vaporization or electrodesiccation. Many lesions are much deeper than they appear [4].

Medical therapy may be used to reduce the pain. Gonadotropin-releasing hormone (GnRH) agonist is the most effective agent. As a result of bone loss by production of menopausal estrogen levels, the use of GnRH agonist is currently limited to a 6-month course of therapy. Symptoms usually return to pretreatment levels within 18 months of stopping therapy. The patient with infertility may benefit from medical therapy as a stopgap until conception is desired.

Adhesions

Not all adhesions are painful, but some can cause significant CPP. Adhesion formation is a surface event that is formed in the first 5 days after injury, most commonly infection or surgery. The two pivotal events of adhesion formation are apposition of damaged tissue surfaces and fibrinolysis. Strategies of adhesion prevention are aimed at one of these two points.

Sixty-seven percent of all patients undergoing laparotomy develop adhesions. Parietal peritoneum has somatic innervation, which may be stimulated by traction. In addition, the adhesions themselves have demonstrated afferent innervation by the sympathetic and parasympathetic nervous system [5]. Pain location has correlated with the presence of adhesions found at laparoscopy. Adhesions most likely to be symptomatic are those under tension or restricting organ mobility [6]. Patients with adhesion pain often complain of pain with sudden movements. Pelvic pain may be experienced with intercourse or certain physical activities. The most difficult diagnostic dilemma is differentiating adhesion pain from musculoskeletal pain. Surgery should be avoided if possible because of the high recurrence rate.

Laparoscopic examination is the gold standard to establish the diagnosis. Pain mapping may be helpful to discriminate between asymptomatic and noxious adhesions. Laparoscopic

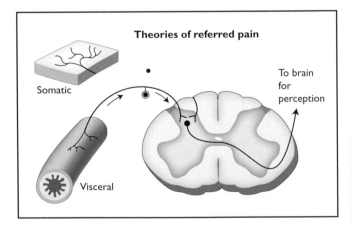

Theories of referred pain

Somatic

Visceral

To brain for perception

Figure 37-6. Convergence–projection phenomenon. Visceral and somatic nociceptors converge on the same dorsal horn transmission neuron. The brain is unable to discriminate the signal from the spinal cord as having a visceral or somatic origin. (*Adapted from* Fields [2].)

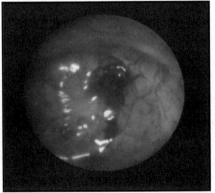

Figure 37-7. A rectovaginal nodule, which is commonly responsible for dyschezia.

lysis of adhesions produces fewer de novo adhesions than laparotomy and effectively relieves most painful adhesions. After adhesiolysis, strategies to prevent recurrence should be employed. Barrier and pharmaceutical measures are now available. To date, no adjuvant has proved uniformly effective.

Pelvic Inflammatory Disease

Pelvic inflammatory disease (PID) can be viewed as a spectrum of diseases beginning with cervical disease and progressing to endometritis, with eventual involvement of the parametria. *Neisseria gonorrhoeae* infection is usually acute and requires immediate attention. *Chlamydia trachomatis* can be particularly devastating because of its relatively indolent clinical presentation (Figure 37-8). After initial tissue injury, other organisms may be responsible for recurrent infections and produce further damage. Tubo-ovarian complexes can develop that induce more scarring and pain.

Unlike acute pelvic pain caused by the inflammatory stimulation of pelvic nociceptors, CPP is usually caused by mechanical pressure and distortion.

Adhesion formation is consistently found in chronic PID. This is independent of any organisms. The severity of adhesion formation is more severe when chronic inflammation is present or when multiple bouts are experienced. Pain may also result from distention of a hydrosalpinx. Prevention of CPP from PID depends on early diagnosis and proper treatment of acute episodes. This diagnosis should be considered in any woman complaining of lower abdominal pain, excessive vaginal discharge, menorrhagia, metrorrhagia, fever, or chills. Cervical, rectal, and urethral cultures for these sexually transmitted diseases should be taken. Single-dose therapy can be administered while awaiting culture results. Ceftriaxone, 125 mg intramuscularly for *N. gonorrhoeae*, and azithromycin, 1 g orally for *C. trachomatis*, have been shown to be effective [7].

Treatment of CPP from PID ranges from conservative laparoscopic lysis of adhesions to complete hysterectomy. If fertility is salvageable, lysis of adhesions with tuboplasty can be an option in some patients with less severe tubal damage. When the fallopian tubes are unsalvageable, bilateral salpingectomy with preservation of at least one ovary permits in vitro conception if the patient wishes to keep this option open. When fertility is not a consideration, hysterectomy is the treatment of choice for chronic pain caused by extensive damage to the tubes and ovaries.

Adenomyosis

Dysmenorrhea and menorrhagia are the cardinal signs of adenomyosis. The ingrowth of endometrium into the uterine musculature produces this condition. Pain is always associated with the menses. Dysmenorrhea developing after one or more pregnancies is often from adenomyosis. The painful cramping may initially occur with the onset of flow, but when CPP is present, it begins one to several days before flow. Periods become increasingly heavy, and clotting is common. The cause is uncertain but is probably related to gestation and placentation. There are no known preventive measures for adenomyosis.

Diagnosis of this condition is usually by exclusion. The uterus is tender and mildly enlarged. Imaging techniques are unreliable. Rarely, ultrasound can pick up severe adenomyosis in the form of a nodular myometrial tumor (adenomyoma). MRI has been somewhat successful but is rarely used because of the expense. The preoperative diagnosis is confirmed in only about half of patients undergoing surgery [7]. Prehysterectomy diagnosis of adenomyosis can be made pathologically if transcervical resection of the endometrium is performed to control menorrhagia.

Conservative treatment with antiprostaglandins and oral contraceptives may reduce symptoms. If fertility is desired, GnRH agonist therapy may be temporizing. Resolution of CPP often requires hysterectomy. Adenomyosis commonly occurs along with endometriosis. The preservation of ovarian function is usually indicated unless endometriosis is extensive.

Vulvodynia

It is estimated that at least 200,000 women in the United States suffer from chronic vulvar pain [8]. Vulvodynia is defined as chronic vulvar discomfort, especially that characterized by the patient's complaint of burning, stinging, irritation, or rawness [9]. There are four categories of this symptom complex: periorificial dermatitis, vestibulitis, dysesthetic vulvodynia, and vulvar neuroma formation. This is one of the most common conditions seen by the primary care physician and one of the most commonly misdiagnosed.

PERIORIFICIAL DERMATITIS
Periorificial dermatitis can be from cyclic vulvovaginitis, steroid-induced dermatitis, or lichen sclerosis. Cyclic vulvitis is characterized by recurrent itching and burning, which is often premenstrual. The vulva appears erythematous, and edema may be present. Fissures may occur with intercourse. Perspiration, semen, and vaginal discharge aggravate the symptoms. Wet

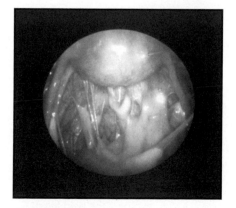

Figure 37-8. Extensive adhesions produced by an asymptomatic chlamydial infection.

preps or cultures of the vaginal discharge often yield *Candida* species. Long-term treatment with ketoconazole, 150 mg once per week for 4 weeks, followed by dosing every other week for 8 weeks, is usually effective.

Steroid-induced dermatitis occurs after prolonged use of topical potent steroids. The symptoms are described as irritation that is temporarily relieved by reapplication of the steroid medication. Rebound discomfort occurs each time that the medication is discontinued. The tissues appear erythematous with telangiectasis. Treatment consists of slowly tapering the topical steroid and prophylactically using long-term ketoconazole to prevent candidiasis while this vulnerable tissue is healing.

Lichen sclerosis produces depigmentation, atrophy, and contraction around the introitus. The patient may complain of tearing and bleeding with intercourse. Usually, burning and dyspareunia bring the patient to the primary care physician, but this condition can be completely asymptomatic in the early stages. It should be verified by a vulvar biopsy. Clobetasol 0.05% applied twice a day offers good relief.

VESTIBULITIS

The cause of vulvar vestibulitis is unknown and may be multifactorial. Factors thought to contribute to this condition include infections, irritants, psychologic stress, and neuropathic changes. Neuropathic changes are commonly thought to be responsible for the allodynia found in the patient's minor vestibular glands. Recurrent candidal infection is often proposed, but no such link has been found. Similarly, bacterial infections and viral infections have been sought but not found consistently. Herpes simplex and human papilloma viruses have also been eliminated as primary agents in the development of vestibulitis.

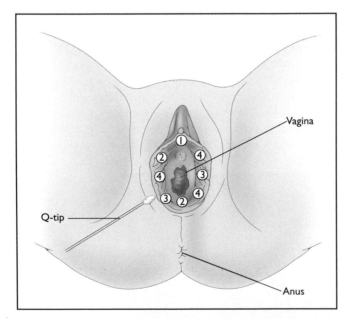

Figure 37-9. An example of the Q-tip test. All patients with chronic pelvic pain or dyspareunia should be screened with this test, which involves lightly touching these eight points of the vestibule. Patients are asked to evaluate the pain felt at each point on a scale of 0 to 4, with 0 indicating no pain and 4 indicating exquisitely painful.

The most commonly mentioned irritant responsible for vulvar vestibulitis is calcium oxalate crystals. The theory that sharp oxalate crystals are the cause of severe burning on contact with the vestibule cannot be scientifically verified despite numerous patient testimonials. However, calcium citrate and a low oxalate diet appear to give some patients relief.

There is no doubt that patients with vestibulitis experience psychological stress and dysfunction as a result of their severe dyspareunia. One study found depression in 89% of patients and suicidal ideation in 57% [10]. These psychologic symptoms are more likely secondary than primary in the etiology of vestibulitis.

The gold standard for diagnosing vestibulitis is a positive Q-tip test. All patients presenting with CPP must be screened by lightly touching the vestibule with a Q-tip. A prescribed mapping technique is used. The patient should be instructed to grade each area (Figure 37-9). A scale 0 to 4 may be used to quantify the degree of pain experienced at each location; this permits assessment of treatment response.

Treatment of vestibulitis is empiric. Some patients with vestibulitis undergo spontaneous remission. No controlled studies have compared the various treatment modalities. One systematic approach of treatment, including oral, topical, injectable, and surgical therapy is shown in Figure 37-10. Amitriptyline is the most effective oral medication. Topical agents can be added one at a time for 1 month each. Acyclovir and 5-fluorouracil have been used with limited success. The Q-tip test is used to monitor objective improvement. If topicals are not curative, injectables can be tried. Triamcinolone and interferon-α have met with limited success.

Surgical treatments include laser vaporization and vestibulectomy. The use of CO_2 laser has been discussed, but this treatment has had poor results and may cause pudendal neuralgia. Its use for vestibulitis should be condemned. The surgical removal of the vestibule is approximately 70% effective. However, this surgery is disfiguring and can result in formation of a neuroma, which is a difficult complication to overcome. Most patients respond before surgery is necessary.

DYSESTHETIC VULVODYNIA

A constant burning throughout the distribution of the pudendal nerve is characteristic of dysesthetic vulvodynia or pudendal neuralgia. The keys to diagnosing this condition are the burning quality of the pain and the involvement of the entire vulva along with the perineum and anus. These patients are more likely to be postmenopausal. They may have experienced some trauma to the pudendal nerve. CO_2 laser vaporization of the vulva, long motorcycle trips, vaginal delivery, diabetic neuropathy, and painful surgical procedures have all been reported as initiating events by patients.

Treatment with oral neuropathic medications offers most patients some relief (Figure 37-11). Shooting pain appears to respond best to carbamazepine. Burning pain often responds best to amitriptyline or gabapentin.

NEUROMA FORMATION OF THE VULVA

A neuroma may be formed any time a nerve is interrupted distal to its cell body. The terminus of this cut nerve can be exquisitely sensitive and generate spontaneous action potentials, which are perceived as pain. The patient may report a deep pain of gradual onset that becomes more intense with time. Surgical procedures or traumatic straddle injuries may be responsible. The diagnosis is made by palpation of a singularly tender area in scar tissue. Often, patients can put their finger right on the neuroma. Blocking with local anesthetics temporarily relieves the pain and confirms the diagnosis.

Currently, there is no reliable treatment. Cryotherapy, chemical ablation, surgical resection, and radiofrequency ablation have been tried with mixed results.

Adnexal Cysts

Patients and physicians usually assume that lateral pelvic pain arises from the ovary or fallopian tube. Ruptured cysts, ectopic pregnancy, adnexal torsion, or inflammatory pathology commonly cause acute pain. The production of CPP by adnexal cysts is more complex and less common. Adnexal cysts may be derived from any parametrial structure. Ovary, fallopian tube, mesospheric remnant, and encapsulating adhesions can produce this pathology.

Chronic ovarian cysts usually do not produce pain. Slow distention of the ovarian capsule can be completely asymptomatic. Ovarian cancer is a good example of this phenomenon. Mechanical pressure on adjacent organs and development of adhesions in response to ovarian cysts are more likely to be responsible for CPP.

An ovarian remnant is a fragment of ovarian tissue left behind during surgical adnexectomy. Most of these patients experience cyst formation. An intense inflammatory reaction may occur causing pain. The pain is unilateral. The patient often has a history of difficult previous surgery from adhesions or endometriosis. Symptoms may be cyclic. Diagnosis is rarely possible by pelvic examination. Ultrasound and CT scans may be helpful. Clomiphene citrate stimulation can help localize the mass if given before a CT or ultrasound scan is performed. Surgical extirpation is the treatment of choice and can be performed laparoscopically in some cases.

Recurrent pelvic pain can be produced by entrapment of ruptured ovarian cyst fluid. This is a peritoneal inclusion cyst caused by tight adhesions surrounding the ovary. Impaired

Treatment of Vestibulitis

Oral

Amitriptyline: 10–75 mg at bedtime

Topical

Acyclovir ointment: apply to tender vestibular glands twice per day

Fluorouracil: apply to vestibule for 2 hours twice per week

Injectables

Triamcinolone: 20 mg (0.5 mL) in 0.5 mL of 0.5% plain bupivacaine injected into tender vestibular points

Interferon-α-N3: 2.5 million U injected into tender vestibular points twice per week for 4 weeks, then once per week for 4 more weeks

Biofeedback

Decreasing the resting tone of the pubococcygeus muscle with diminishing superficial electromyographic variability

Surgery

Vestibulectomy

Figure 37-10. Treatment of vestibulitis.

Medications Effective for Neuropathic Pain

Amitriptyline: 10–75 mg at bedtime

Carbamazepine: 200 mg bid (titrate with blood levels)

Doxepin: 50–150 mg at bedtime

Gabapentin: 100–400 mg tid

Lamotrigine: 25 mg qod for 2 weeks, then once per day

Nortriptyline: 25 mg tid to qid

Phenytoin: 100 mg tid (titrate with blood levels)

Trazodone: 50–150 mg at bedtime

Figure 37-11. Medications effective for neuropathic pain.

ability to absorb this fluid produces mechanical pressure and pain. Ultrasonic and pelvic examinations may reveal the change in diameter as the patient's symptoms wax and wane. Surgical extirpation is the treatment of choice.

Adnexal torsion with resultant hypoxia and pain is usually an acute surgical emergency. However, intermittent, partial adnexal torsion can produce CPP. The patient complains of lower pelvic pain localized to one side. Initially, the pain is diffuse, and it localizes only if peritoneal signs develop. It may occur daily and have no relationship to cycle. It may be associated with intercourse. Laparoscopic detorsion and fixation to prevent recurrence is the treatment of choice.

Hormonal suppression of chronic pelvic cysts is unsuccessful. The aspiration of these cysts almost always results in recurrence. Surgery offers the best hope of relief from the CPP. Laparotomy is indicated for patients when laparoscopy is contraindicated.

Pelvic Floor Relaxation

The bony pelvis serves as a structure for the attachment of pelvic fascia and ligaments. The bones have no significant support function. The pelvic organs are supported by the pelvic floor musculature and the pelvic fascia (Figure 37-12). If the muscle–fascia complex is injured, pelvic organs are pulled by gravity and pushed by intra-abdominal pressure into anatomically abnormal relationships. The stretch nociceptors of both autonomic and somatic nerves are stimulated. This condition is progressive and is a common cause of CPP in women. These support defects most commonly originate from vaginal delivery but may result from trauma. The tearing of the fascial planes of the pelvis (endopelvic fascia) is consistently found on pathologic examination [11].

As the relaxation of the pelvic support continues, symptoms become more pronounced. Low back pain caused by traction on the uterosacral ligaments becomes a common complaint.

These patients have back pain after standing for long periods. Similarly, medial thigh pain and soreness are caused by traction on the cardinal ligaments.

Organ dysfunction results from loss of normal anatomic support. Stress urinary incontinence, obstipation, and dyspareunia are common. The physical examination may reveal one or all of the following: cystocele, rectocele, enterocele, increased posterior urethrovesical angle, uterocervical prolapse, and vaginal vault prolapse (Figure 37-13).

Prevention of CPP from pelvic relaxation is difficult because some patients exhibit a genetic predisposition to this condition. Cesarean section for the macrosomic fetus and the avoidance of traumatic intrapartum maneuvers may decrease fascial plane ruptures. Women should develop proper lifting techniques to decrease the stress placed on their pelvic floor. It is important to keep tissues of postmenopausal patients strong with estrogen replacement.

Successful treatment depends on the accurate appreciation of each anatomic abnormality and the restoration of normal anatomy and function. Vaginal pessaries are sometimes satisfactory to prop up stretched pelvic support. This may offer temporary relief in some patients.

Surgical correction can be conservative in patients who wish to retain fertility. Laparoscopic uterosacral plication, uterine suspension, paravaginal repair, enterocoele repair, and urethrocystopexy can be performed. Vaginal surgical procedures, such as anterior and posterior repair and vaginal vault suspension, may also be necessary. Hysterectomy is indicated along with these reparative procedures if no further pregnancies are desired. Relief of CPP and organ dysfunction by surgery is usually good.

Urinary System Causes

The urinary tract is a common site for inflammatory pathology, stones, and other conditions that can activate visceral nerves

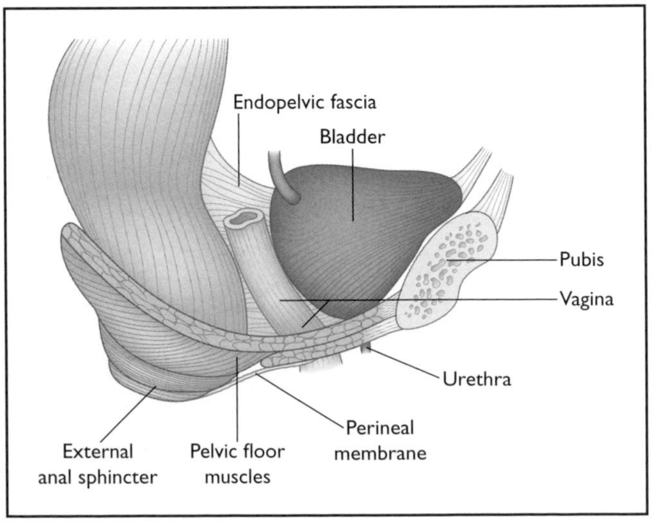

Figure 37-12. The pelvic organs are supported by the pelvic floor musculature and the endopelvic fascia.

Pelvic Relaxation

Anatomic Defect	Symptoms Produced
Cystocele	Pelvic pressure, postvoid dribbling, dyspareunia, and increased residual volume
Uterine prolapse	Pelvic pressure, dyspareunia, low back pain, medial thigh pain (symptoms exacerbated by prolonged standing or lifting)
Rectocele	Pelvic pressure, dyspareunia, and obstipation
Enterocele	Pelvic pressure
Vaginal vault prolapse	Pelvic pressure
Increased posterior urethrovesical angle	Stress urinary incontinence

Figure 37-13. Pelvic relaxation.

and cause CPP. Because visceral pain is diffuse and may be poorly localized, a history of voiding abnormalities offers the best sign of origin. The most common triggers for CPP originating from the urinary system are hypersensitivity as a result of recurrent, chronic urinary tract infections; interstitial cystitis; and urolithiasis.

RECURRENT INFECTION WITH HYPERSENSITIVITY

The urothelium is ordinarily bathed in a constant flow of sterile urine. Uropathogens, such as bacteria, fungus, and viruses, can infect this tissue and cause inflammation and pain. If the tissue injury is repetitive or chronic, the dorsal horn neurons of the spinal cord become sensitized. They can then become activated by even normal stimuli (eg, bladder filling). Visceral nerve hypersensitivity produces pelvic muscle spasm, soft tissue trigger points, and skin hyperesthesia through the convergence–projection phenomenon. These changes may persist long after the initial insult [12].

Urinary tract infections are one of the most common conditions encountered in clinical practice. In 1990, in the United States, about 5.7 million office visits were for painful urination, frequency, and urgency. Approximately 75% of all urinary tract infections occur in women. The increased susceptibility is thought to be the result of three factors: 1) the comparatively short urethra, 2) the ability of uropathogens to colonize the periurethral zone, and 3) the presence of specific receptors to the adhesive strains of bacteria on urothelial cells [13]. Patients with certain blood types (B and AB) seem more likely to have recurrent infections. Urethral obstruction and urinary stasis have also been implicated as predisposing factors. Treatment of urethral stenosis and urethral diverticulum appears to decrease the incidence of the lower urinary tract syndrome.

Lower urinary tract sensitivity produces nocturia and frequency. This may produce an inherently smaller bladder capacity, which potentiates these symptoms. Terms such as *chronic trigonitis*, *urethral syndrome*, and *chronic nonbacterial cystitis* have been applied to this condition.

Although initiated by infection, there may be no persistent infection after the cascade of events is set in motion. Neuropathic pain and myofascial pain are common. Women describe a constant burning in their urethra or bladder. Some patients complain of intermittent, shock-like pain. Pelvic floor spasm may produce postcoital aching or a sense of vaginal fullness. The diagnosis of hypersensitive lower urinary tract depends on the history of voiding dysfunction, absence of a positive culture, and absence of cystoscopic evidence of interstitial cystitis. The physical examination consists of single-digit palpation of the lower urinary tract starting at the distal urethra and proceeding proximally. The trigone and each ureteral insertion should be evaluated separately. Urodynamics, uroflowmetry, and pelvic floor electromyography can help define difficult voiding dysfunction such as vesicle–sphincter dyssynergia.

Prevention of recurrent urinary tract infections is the best way to interdict hypersensitivity of the lower urinary tract and CPP. Asymptomatic bacteriuria and cystitis should be treated promptly with appropriate antimicrobials. Relief of dysuria with phenazopyridine hydrochloride is recommended.

Frequency and nocturia can be helped by imipramine pamoate, 100 mg given at bedtime. Tolterodine, 2 mg twice a day, is usually helpful as well. When bladder capacity is reduced by chronic low-volume voiding, bladder diaries and retraining are beneficial.

Surgical therapy for chronic lower urinary tract syndrome is controversial. Repeated urethral dilations may relieve chronic nonbacterial dysuria in some patients. External urethroplasty has been used for frequency, nocturia, and slow stream [14]. Transurethral cauterization is advocated by some for chronic trigonitis. Neuroablative procedures, such as presacral neurectomy and uterovaginal ganglion excision, have been inconsistent in relieving symptoms.

Interstitial Cystitis

Some consider interstitial cystitis the end stage of lower urinary tract syndrome. Others believe that the clinical findings are distinct enough to qualify this condition as a separate disease. No infectious agents have been found associated with interstitial cystitis. In fact, cultures are consistently negative. Urinalysis may show a few red blood cells. Bladder capacities are progressively reduced. The urethra becomes extremely tender, and catheterizations are painful.

Cystoscopic examinations usually require general anesthesia because of the high degree of the patient's pain. Throughout the bladder, surface blood vessels are attenuated. After hydrodistention, multiple bleeding points are noted. Occasionally, an ulceration (Hunner's ulcer) is present.

The pathogenesis of interstitial cystitis has long been believed to be an autoimmune phenomenon. Increased mast cells in the bladder mucosa in many of these patients may be evidence of this, or mast cells may be a protective mechanism of the host. The bladder wall lacks a glycosaminoglycan layer. Urea and other noxious agents in the urine gain access to the nociceptors of the submucosa to produce pain and spasm [15].

Typically, patients with interstitial cystitis have frequency, urgency, nocturia, constant suprapubic pelvic pain, and dyspareunia. The dyspareunia may be the result of bladder tenderness, pelvic floor myalgia, or vestibulitis. Some patients have all three components. Normal sexual activity is almost impossible. Nocturia is sometimes severe, often occurring more than three times each night. Ninety percent of patients have a bladder capacity of less than 350 mL. Treatment of the CPP resulting from interstitial cystitis includes hydrodistention and diet therapy, bladder instillations, and oral therapy. Dimethylsulfoxide or sulfated polysaccharide heparin placed and held in the bladder offers some patients substantial relief. Pentosan polysulfate sodium given orally decreases symptoms in up to two-thirds of patients.

Surgical approaches to the patient who fails to respond to conservative therapy include the following: 1) cystoplasty and bladder augmentation, 2) bladder denervation procedures, and 3) cystectomy. None of these offers women assurance that the CPP will resolve.

Urolithiasis

The predominant quality of pain from urolithiasis is colic. This severe visceral pain usually leads to immediate medical intervention for analgesia and relief of obstruction. Recurrent ureteral colic can produce prolonged hyperalgesia and referred pain. Depending on the intensity and frequency of ureteral colic, musculoskeletal and dermatome-specific referred pain can present as undiagnosed CPP.

The smooth muscle of the renal pelvis and ureter are a continuous syncytium. Its intrinsic myogenic peristaltic rhythm is dominated by the renal pelvis pacemaker. The rate is altered by sympathetic efferent stimulation. There is little or no parasympathetic input. It is further modified by diuresis, obstruction, and inflammation. Colic is a function of ureteral distention, local inflammation, and ischemia. The afferent impulses are carried by renal and hypogastric autonomic nerves to the T10-L2 segments of the spinal cord [16]. There, the dorsal horn neurons receive the nociceptive signals and transmit them to the brain. These dorsal horn neuron transmission cells are shared with somatic sensory and motor peripheral nerves. Frequent stimulations of the ureteral afferent nerves by urolithiasis result in referred pain and muscle spasm through the convergence–projection phenomenon [17].

Patients with a history of recurrent lumbar pain, flank pain, and shooting pain into the genitofemoral distribution may have this type of neuropathic CPP. The prevention of this type of CPP depends on early analgesia for ureteral colic. The dietary therapy for preventing the specific type of stones formed should be instituted. Integral to urolithiasis prevention is increased water intake. Treatment consists of those medications previously discussed to be efficacious for neuropathic pain.

Bowel-related Causes

Chronic pelvic pain may be produced by a number of conditions affecting the bowel. Pathology can be divided into extrinsic and intrinsic diseases. Extrinsic conditions include intermittent bowel obstruction and endometriosis. Intrinsic conditions include dysmotility disorders and inflammatory changes (Figure 37-14).

Bowel-related Causes of Chronic Pelvic Pain

Extrinsic Disorders	Intrinsic Disorders
Endometriosis	Dysmotility
Ovarian tumors	Irritable bowel syndrome
Pelvic adhesions	Constipation dominant
	Diarrhea dominant
	Crohn's disease
	Ulcerative colitis
	Diverticulitis

Figure 37-14. Bowel-related causes of chronic pelvic pain.

Extrinsic Disorders

Intermittent, partial bowel obstruction can be a cause of CPP. The pain can be diffuse and perceived to originate low in the pelvis. Adhesive bands from previous surgery are the most common cause. Pelvic tumors can also produce this luminal compromise. Ovarian cancer may present in this fashion. Endometriosis involves the bowel in up to 37% of cases. The terminal ileum appears to be a common site of this condition, with resultant menstrual exacerbations of symptoms. Cramping, sharp pain, often accompanied by nausea and vomiting, is the most common presentation. The abdomen may be slightly distended during episodes of partial obstruction. High-pitched bowel sounds may be heard during episodes of pain. The diagnosis can be confirmed with a flat and upright abdominal radiograph. The treatment is surgical relief of the luminal compromise by adhesiolysis or partial bowel resection [18].

Intrinsic Disorders

Symptoms of intermittent bowel obstruction can originate with disorders of bowel motility (dysmotility). The most common type is irritable bowel syndrome. Although it is thought to be a disturbance of the large bowel, the small bowel function may also be abnormal. This condition affects women of all ages but is especially common in younger women experiencing school or career stresses. There are two distinct patterns: constipation dominant and diarrhea dominant. Small bowel dysmotility is most often seen in the patient complaining of diarrhea. These patients may have sharp abdominal and pelvic pain with bloating. The abdominal examination usually reveals normal bowel sounds and no point tenderness. The constipation-dominant dysmotility is manifested by infrequent, hard stool. These patients complain of intermittent, sharp lower abdominopelvic pain. There may be some discomfort to pressure over the sigmoid colon or cecum. Hard stool is often palpable on abdominal examination. Endoscopy and imaging studies are nonspecific.

Inflammatory conditions of the bowel are among the most frequently seen causes of CPP from the bowel. Early Crohn's disease and ulcerative colitis often present as pelvic pain of undetermined cause. These conditions are perplexing before the onset of bloody diarrhea. Endoscopic and radiographic studies usually yield the correct diagnosis.

In older women, CPP may be the result of diverticular disease. It is thought to occur in one third of the population older than 45 years and in two thirds of the population older than 85 years. Because the colon and sigmorectum share the same innervation as the cervix, uterus, and adnexa, it may be difficult to determine if lower abdominopelvic pain is gynecologic or enterocolic in origin. Diagnosis may be even more difficult with the presence of a pelvic mass, called a phlegmon. This can be made up of colon, diverticular abscess, bladder wall, and pelvic sidewall. The patient usually complains of cramping, lower abdominopelvic pain. Fever, nausea, and dyschezia may be present. Endoscopy and barium enemas should not be performed in patients with actively inflamed bowel for fear of perforation. CT scan is usually diagnostic. Oral antibiotics may be sufficient conservative therapy, but for recurrent bouts in younger patients, surgical resection may become necessary [19].

Musculoskeletal Causes

The pelvic musculoskeletal frame is a common source of CPP but often goes unrecognized and untreated. This can be a primary source of pain or can be a secondary response to true visceral pain. Most commonly, patients with CPP have a combination of both. Usually, the visceral pain initiates the muscular spasm, which in turn causes joint dysfunction and skeletal changes. The mechanism for this sequence of events resides in the interneuronal communications of the spinal cord (Figure 37-15). The visceral nociceptors cause reflex activation of the motoneurons, which produces muscle contraction and activation of muscle nociceptors [2]. Muscles sharing dermatome innervation with the pelvic viscera are thus susceptible to this spasm and pain reaction (Figure 37-16). These patients complain of activity-specific pelvic pain. For example, patients with piriformis muscle spasms have exacerbations when climbing stairs, and patients with pubococcygeus spasms experience dyspareunia or pain when sitting. The diagnosis of these conditions is made by careful palpation of the muscles looking for spasm and tenderness. Physical therapy is essential if progress is to be made in pain reduction. Trigger-point injections may be necessary. Only temporary improvement is realized if the site of visceral nociception is not remedied (eg, endometriosis).

Uterine Fibroids

Uterine leiomyomas are the most common tumors of the female pelvis, occurring in one in every four or five women. The size of the myoma depends on vascular supply, proximity to adjacent tumors, degenerative changes, and hormonal growth factors. These tumors may be submucous, intramural, subserosal, or pedunculated. Although most fibroids are asymptomatic, 10% to 40% may produce menorrhagia, infertility, or pain.

Chronic pelvic pain has been attributed to uterine fibroids more frequently than is justified. Special conditions, such as acute red degeneration during pregnancy and transcervical prolapse of a submucous fibroid ("aborting fibroid"), are notable exceptions. There is evidence that CPP is more likely produced by associated pathology (eg, endometriosis, adhesions) than by uterine fibroids. Impingement of leiomyomas on surrounding structures can cause a variety of symptoms. Collision dyspareunia, rectal pressure, and pelvic discomfort are likely to result from a fixed retroverted fibroid.

Diagnosis of uterine fibroids is 95% accurate by pelvic examination. Pelvic ultrasound can confirm location and size. The treatment is dependent on desire to maintain fertility and degree of symptoms produced. Medical therapy with a GnRH agonist is temporizing and usually reserved for those fibroids for which a temporary diminution of size and vascularity is desired. Abdominal myomectomy can be performed by laparotomy or laparoscopy. Transcervical resection of submucous fibroids can ameliorate the menorrhagia in some patients.

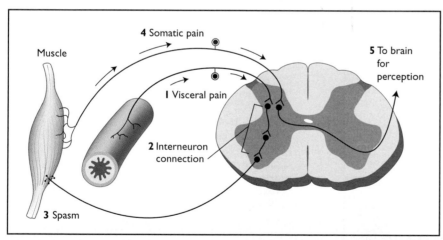

Figure 37-15. The mechanism by which visceral pain may produce pelvic floor muscle spasm. Visceral nociception (1) is transmitted to the muscle by interneuron connection (2) and produces spasm (3). Muscle nociceptors (4) transmit pain of spasm back to the spinal cord, which is perceived by the brain (5). (*Adapted from* Fields [2].)

Muscles That Share Dermatome Innervation with the Pelvic Viscera and are Subject to the Spasm-Pain Reaction

Superficial Pelvic Floor Muscles	Intermediate Pelvic Floor Muscles	Deep Pelvic Floor Muscles
Superficial transverse perineal	Levator ani	Obturator internus
Ischiocavernosus	Pubococcygeus	Coccygeus
Bulbospongiosus	Puborectalis	Piriformis
	Iliococcygeus	

Figure 37-16. Muscles that share dermatome innervation with the pelvic viscera and are subject to the spasm-pain reaction.

If fertility is no longer desired, hysterectomy may be the treatment of choice [20].

Fibromyalgia

Fibromyalgia is a common condition manifested by diffuse musculoskeletal pain and fatigue. Chronic visceral nerve nociceptive stimulation is often related to the onset of fibromyalgia and therefore may be seen in patients presenting with CPP. The cause of fibromyalgia is unknown. One hypothesis tries to explain the association of other autonomic nerve disturbances with an integrated theory [21]. Genetic predisposition may allow an inciting event (eg, endometriosis, trauma, emotional stress) to produce central nervous system hyperactivity. This causes neurogenic inflammation with increased peripheral and visceral nociception. Neuroendocrine disturbances then produce other signs, such as sleep disorders and mood swings. The sum total of these abnormal states is autonomic dysfunction. This would explain the common association of fibromyalgia and mitral valve prolapse, temporomandibular joint pain, migraine headaches, irritable bowel, interstitial cystitis, endometriosis, and other pain states.

The diagnosis of fibromyalgia is dependent on the presence of at least 11 of 16 paired tender points (Figure 37-17). If patients with CPP are not routinely checked for these tender points, the diagnosis remains obscure.

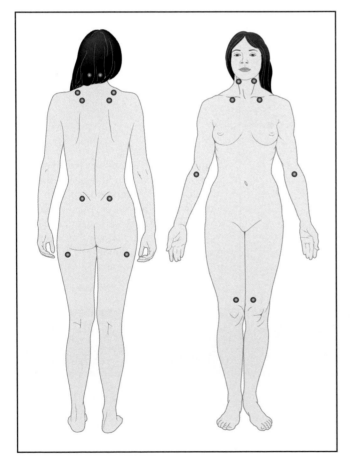

Figure 37-17. At least 11 of the 18 designated "tender points" should be diagnosed with fibromyalgia.

Treatments consist of systematic relief of all manifesting symptoms. Sleep disturbances may respond to trazodone hydrochloride, 50 to 150 mg given at bedtime. Muscle tenderness can be helped with tizanidine hydrochloride, 4 mg given at bedtime. Depression can be treated with a selective serotonin uptake inhibitor.

Physical therapy is the cornerstone of returning these patients to function that is more normal. These patients are usually physically deconditioned because exercise can be painful and they are usually too tired to do regular aerobic conditioning. Swimming-pool therapy may offer them the best opportunity to regain their stamina.

References

Papers of particular interest have been highlighted as follows:
- Of interest
- Of outstanding interest

1.•• Rogers RM: Basic pelvic neuroanatomy. In *Chronic Pelvic Pain: An Integrated Approach*, edn 1. Edited by Steege JF, Metzger DM, Levy BS. Philadelphia: WB Saunders; 1998:31–58.
This chapter represents the most current anatomic study on pelvic pain in the literature. Its illustrations offer unparalleled appreciation for the complex interaction of visceral and somatic pain perception.

2. Fields HL: Pain from deep tissues and referred pain. In *Pain*. New York: McGraw-Hill; 1987:79–97.

3. Hurst BS, Rock JA: The peritoneal environment in endometriosis. In *Modern Approaches to Endometriosis*. Edited by Thomas E, Rock J. Boston: Kluwer Academic Publishers; 1991:79–96.

4. Koninckx PR, Lesaffre E, Meuleman C, *et al.*: Suggestive evidence that pelvic endometriosis is a progressive disease, whereas deeply infiltrating endometriosis is associated with pelvic pain. *Fertil Steril* 1991, 55:759–765.

5. Kligman I, Drachenberg C, Papadimitriou J, *et al.*: Immunohistochemical demonstration of nerve fibers in pelvic adhesions. *Obstet Gynecol* 1993, 82:566–568.

6. Kresch AJ, Seifer DB, Sachs LB, *et al.*: Laparoscopy in 100 women with chronic pelvic pain. *Obstet Gynecol* 1984, 64:672–674.

7. Soper DE: Genitourinary infections and sexually transmitted diseases. In *Novak's Gynecology*, edn 12. Edited by Berek JS, Adashi EY, Hillard PA. Baltimore: Williams & Wilkins; 1996:429–445.

8. Jones KD, Lehr ST: Vulvodynia: diagnostic techniques and treatment modalities. *Nurse Pract* 1994, 4:34–46.

9. McKay M: Vulvodynia. In *Chronic Pelvic Pain: An Integrated Approach*, edn 1. Edited by Steege JF, Metzger DM, Levy BS. Philadelphia: WB Saunders; 1988:188–196.

10. Jantos M, White G: The vestibulitis syndrome: medical and psychosexual assessment of a cohort of patients. *J Reprod Med* 1997, 42:135–139.

11. Wall LL: Incontinence, prolapse, and disorders of the pelvic floor. In *Novak's Gynecology*, edn 12. Edited by Berek JS, Adashi EY, Hillard PA. Baltimore: Williams & Wilkins; 1996:619–676.

12. George NJR: Diagnostic criteria of the hypersensitive disorders. In *Sensory Disorders of the Bladder and Urethra*. Edited by George NJR, Gosling JA. New York: Springer-Verlag; 1986:17–29.

13. Kunin CM: Urinary tract infections in adults. In *Urinary Tract Infections: Detection, Prevention, and Management*, edn 5. Baltimore: Williams & Wilkins; 1997:128–164.

14. Richardson FH: External urethroplasty in women: technique and clinical evaluation. *J Urol* 1969, 101:719–723.

15. Parsons CL: Interstitial cystitis. In *Common Problems in Infections and Stones*. Edited by Drach GW. St. Louis: Mosby Year Book; 1992:23–28.

16. Bach D: The treatment of ureteric colic and promotion of spontaneous passage. In *Urolithiasis: Therapy, Prevention*. Edited by Schneider HJ. New York: Springer-Verlag; 1986:75–83.

17. Giamberardino MA, Dalal A, Valente R, *et al.*: Changes in activity of spinal cells with muscular input in rats with referred muscular hyperalgesia from ureteral calculosis. *Neurosci Lett* 1996, 203:89–92.

18. Krebs HB, Goplerud DR: Mechanical intestinal obstruction in patients with gynecologic disease: a review of 368 patients. *Am J Obstet Gynecol* 1987, 157:577–583.

19. Veidenheimer MC, Roberts PL: History, prevalence and epidemiology, natural history. In *Colonic Diverticular Disease*. Edited by Veidenheimer MC, Roberts PL. Boston: Blackwell Scientific Publications; 1991:1–14.

20. Hutchins FL: Uterine fibroids. *Obstet Gynecol Clin North Am* 1995, 22:659–665.

21. Clauw DJ: The pathogenesis of chronic pain and fatigue syndromes, with special reference to fibromyalgia. *Med Hypotheses* 1995, 44:369–378.

38 | Dysmenorrhea

Roger P. Smith

- Dysmenorrhea is cyclic menstrual pain and should be distinguished from other causes of acute and chronic pelvic pain.
- Primary dysmenorrhea is painful menses without clinically identifiable causes, whereas secondary dysmenorrhea is menstrual pain with underlying pathology.
- Primary dysmenorrhea is first treated with nonsteroidal anti-inflammatory drugs, continuous low-level topical heat, or oral contraceptives. Secondary dysmenorrhea is managed by treating the detectable underlying cause.
- Diagnostic laparoscopy is indicated when medical management fails to improve symptoms of primary dysmenorrhea or when there is a serious question regarding the diagnosis.

Dysmenorrhea is defined as cyclic pain associated with menses. It is a common gynecologic disorder affecting up to half of women in the childbearing age group. Approximately 10% to 15% of women with dysmenorrhea suffer enough to be incapacitated for 1 to 3 days a month, thereby causing significant absenteeism from work. It is also the leading cause of recurrent short-term absenteeism from school among adolescent girls. In one classic study of 19-year-old women, over 70% reported having had dysmenorrhea, with over 50% reporting loss of time from school or work [1]. Whereas dysmenorrhea is uncommon in the first 6 months of menstruation, 38% of women experience it during their first year [1].

Noncyclic pelvic pain, whether acute or chronic, has different causes than dysmenorrhea and may have different therapies. Therefore, distinguishing cyclic menstrual pain from noncyclic pain is essential in formulating a treatment plan for the patient. Furthermore, clinicians must differentiate true menstrual-related symptoms from those symptoms aggravated during the menstrual cycle.

Dysmenorrhea is divided into two categories: primary and secondary. Primary dysmenorrhea is painful menses without clinically identifiable causes, whereas secondary dysmenorrhea is menstrual pain with detectable underlying pathology.

Primary Dysmenorrhea

SYMPTOMS

Most menstruating women have experienced primary dysmenorrhea during their lifetime. It usually appears within 2 years of menarche and occurs almost exclusively in ovulatory cycles. Women seeking medical attention for primary dysmenorrhea tend to be younger, although women in their 30s and 40s may experience symptoms as well. The pain is sharp or cramping and generally occurs in the first 3 days of menstruation. The pain is usually suprapubic but may radiate to the back, inner thighs, or deep pelvis. The duration of primary dysmenorrhea is generally 48 to 72 hours, with an onset just hours before to the onset of bleeding or, more typically, just after the onset of menstrual flow. Nausea, with or without vomiting, and diarrhea also may occur. Dyspareunia, even during menstruation, is uncommon and should suggest pathology.

Pelvic examination of women with primary dysmenorrhea should be unremarkable. Therefore, the diagnosis of primary dysmenorrhea is one of exclusion; that is, there should be no other noted abnormalities on history or physical examination that might suggest the cause of the dysmenorrhea.

ETIOLOGY

During ovulatory cycles, production and release of prostaglandins by the endometrium normally occur during menstruation. Through a series of enzymatic steps, arachidonic acid from cell walls is converted to prostaglandin E2a, prostaglandin F2a, thromboxane A2, or prostacyclin. The first three prostaglandins promote strong uterine contractions and are potent vasoconstrictors whereas prostacyclin is a potent vasodilator and a smooth muscle relaxant. An alternative pathway converts arachidonic acid to leukotriene, which is also a potent vasoconstrictor and causes uterine contractions.

Women with primary dysmenorrhea have been shown to have elevated levels of prostaglandins in the endometrium and in menstrual fluid compared with women without symptoms. Prostaglandins cause uterine contractions and an increase in resting tone of the uterus. Women with primary dysmenorrhea have been shown to have resting pressures that approach 100 mm Hg and contractions that reach 400 mm Hg [2]. Subjective studies of pain and objective studies of uterine activity have established a firm connection between the two [3,4]. Excess prostaglandins may also be responsible for the smooth muscle activity noted in the gastrointestinal tract of these women. Hypermobility of the gut may be responsible for the frequent coexistence of nausea, vomiting, and diarrhea in these patients. Prostaglandins appear to act as initiators and potentiators of nociceptive pain signals, further contributing to the symptoms experienced.

MEDICAL MANAGEMENT
Prostaglandin Synthesis Inhibitors
As with most areas of medicine, the best treatment is one directed at the cause of the problem. A direct method of altering the sequence leading to discomfort comes in the form of nonsteroidal anti-inflammatory drug (NSAID) therapy. These drugs inhibit the production and/or the action of prostaglandins. Prostaglandin synthesis inhibition is an effective treatment for most patients. Nonsteroidal anti-inflammatory drugs should be taken at the first sign of pain (or the onset of menstruation for those with consistent monthly symptoms) and continued for 48 to 72 hours and taken on a regular schedule rather than on an as-needed basis. For women with a history of rapid onset of symptoms, the starting dose may be increased (although the maintenance dose can be kept the same).

There are two broad classes of NSAID compounds (carboxylic acids, enolic acids), each with subgroups (Figure 38-1). Some drugs that have the ability to inhibit prostaglandin synthesis have had little usefulness in treating dysmenorrhea. Some have weak antiprostaglandin activity, require metabolic transformation to become active, or have side effects that limit their usefulness. These drugs (such as aspirin, phenacetin, phenylbutazone, paracetamol, or indomethacin) can be used to treat dysmenorrhea but have generally been replaced by other, more effective agents.

It is the carboxylates with which most physicians are familiar. These agents have the most utility for dysmenorrhea. Within this major group, there are four families of compounds that have individual characteristics. Generally, the similarities between inhibitors within a family are such that practitioners need only be familiar with one or two agents. However, patients who have a poor or partial response to one agent may respond well to a different agent, especially if the agent chosen is from a different chemical family. Subtle differences in the site or mechanism of action are responsible for this phenomenon. Most women have significant improvement, and a 4- to 6-month course of therapy taken in a compliant manner should be tried before considering treatment a failure.

The short-term efficacy and safety of the new selective cyclooxygenase-2 inhibitors seems to be good, but several concerns remain, as evidenced by the emergence of concerns about coronary heart disease with prolonged use [5], which may not be the case with older agents [6]. (Most of these agents have been withdrawn from the market or issued with black box warnings regarding the risk of serious adverse events.) Despite a decrease in the incidence of gastrointestinal side effects with these agents, their use by patients with active gastrointestinal ulceration, infection with *Helicobacter pylori*, or inflammatory bowel disease has not been adequately studied. In the treatment of dysmenorrhea, the increased cost of these agents over the more commonly used agents, along with the lack of clinical efficacy studies, would suggest a second-line role.

If pain relief is not complete, patients should be warned not to add additional analgesics, especially other NSAIDs, because of the increased possibility of gastrointestinal and other side effects. When at least partial relief of symptoms is not achieved, a serious reappraisal of the original diagnosis of primary dysmenorrhea must be made. This reappraisal may include discussion of family, school, and other potential sources of stress. When indicated, the possibility of invasive diagnostic procedures such as laparoscopy may have to be considered to establish the diagnosis.

Whereas side effects for these medications are infrequent and generally mild, serious side effects are possible. Contraindications to NSAIDs include hypersensitivity to aspirin and gastrointestinal ulcers. Side effects include nausea, dyspepsia, and diarrhea. Generally, these side effects can be treated and the medication continued.

Continuous Low-level Topical Heat Therapy
The portability, low cost, and proven high efficacy make continuous low-level topical heat therapy an attractive option for treating women with menstrual and lower abdominal pain. This modality offers a high degree of efficacy without the systemic and other problems associated with pharmacotherapy.

The use of heat to treat dysmenorrhea has a venerated history of success but low levels of use [7]. In the past, the practicalities of rapidly cooling hot water bottles, electrical cords, and the risk of burns for heating pads have limited the utility of this option. The recent development of small wearable devices capable of supplying a continuous low level of topical heat therapy at a constant temperature over a prolonged period of time now make this modality a viable treatment option [8]. A published study by Akin *et al.* [9] demonstrated that continuous low-level topically applied heat was similar or superior to oral ibuprofen therapy for menstrual pain [9], and an even more recent report has demonstrated similar success when heat was compared to acetaminophen [10].

Oral Contraceptives
For women with primary dysmenorrhea who desire contraception, oral contraceptives are a reasonable treatment and are effective in more than 90% of cases. Multiphasic and monophasic agents have been shown to be equally effective [11], as have the new low-androgenic progestins.

The standard combination estrogen-progestin contraceptives contain potent synthetic progestins that cause the endometrium to become very thin over time. The thinned endometrium contains relatively small amounts of arachidonic acid resulting in reduced menstrual flow and less production of prostaglandins, thereby decreasing dysmenorrhea. Limited data from randomized studies confirm the benefit of these agents compared with placebo [12,13]. Unfortunately, there are no randomized trials comparing hormonal therapy and NSAIDS.

An alternative to the standard schedule for administering combination estrogen-progestin oral contraceptives is to use "long-cycle" dosing. This approach has been described as a "minipseudopregnancy" because it results in menses only a few times a year, rather than monthly. The extended cycle regimen appears to be associated with less menstrual pain than the monthly regimen, but both regimens are effective and have not been compared to each other for treatment of primary dysmenorrhea [14].

Medroxyprogesterone acetate (Depo Provera; Pfizer, New York, NY) induces light menstrual flow or amenorrhea and can be effective treatment for primary dysmenorrhea. Like oral contraceptives, this could be appropriate therapy in women who desire contraception, especially those who are not compliant with oral contraceptives.

Use of the levonorgestrel intrauterine device, which releases small amounts of a progestin directly into the endometrial cavity, has been associated with 50% reduction in the prevalence of dysmenorrhea [15]. In contrast, nonhormonal intrauterine devices, such as those containing copper, may worsen dysmenorrhea or cause secondary dysmenorrhea.

Other Conservative Treatments

Transcutaneous electrical nerve stimulation (TENS) is a nonpharmacologic modality that has been used for several types of pain conditions, including primary dysmenorrhea [16]. This modality appears to be a useful alternative in women who cannot or prefer not to take oral analgesics. The degree of pain relief obtained with TENS therapy alone is variable and sometimes less than that from drugs; however, some women may be able to lower their analgesic dose with combined therapy.

Herbal medicine, vegetarian diets, microwave diathermy treatments, and vitamins B1 and E have all been advocated for treatment of primary dysmenorrhea. Studies reporting the results of their trials found improvement over controls [17–19]. Dietary

---

Nonsteroidal Anti-inflammatory Drugs

Carboxylic acids

Acetic acids

  Aspirin

  Diflunisal (Dolobid; Merck & Co., Inc., Whitehouse Station, NJ)

Salicylic acids

  Indomethacin (Indocin; Merck & Co., Inc., Whitehouse Station, NJ)

  Tolmetin (Tolectin; Ortho-McNeil Pharmaceuticals, Inc., Raritan, NJ)

  Sulindac (Clinoril; Merck & Co., Inc., Whitehouse Station, NJ)

  Diclofenac (Voltaren; Novartis Pharmaceuticals, East Hanover, NJ)

  Zomepirac (Zomax; Ortho-McNeil Pharmaceuticals, Inc., Raritan, NJ)

Propionic acids

  Ibuprofen (Motrin; Pharmacia and Upjohn Company, Kalamazoo, MI; Rufen, BASF, Wien, Germany)*

  Naproxen (Naprosyn; Roche Pharmaceuticals, Nutley, NJ)

  Naproxen sodium (Anaprox; Roche Pharmaceuticals, Nutley, NJ)*

  Fenoprofen calcium (Nalfon; Pedinol Pharmaceuticals, Farmingdale, NY)

  Suprofen

  Ketoprofen (Orudis; Wyeth Pharmaceuticals, Philadelphia, PA)*

Fenamates

  Mefenamic acid (Ponstel; Sciele Pharma, Inc., Atlanta, GA)*

  Meclofenamate (Meclomen; Pfizer, Inc., New York, NY)

Enolic acids

Pyrazolones

  Oxyphenbutazone (Oxalid; Novartis Pharmaceuticals, East Hanover, NJ)

  Phenylbutazone (Azolid; Sanofi Aventis, Paris, France; Butazolidin; Novartis Pharmaceuticals, East Hanover, NJ)

Oxicams

  Piroxicam (Feldene; Pfizer, Inc., New York, NY)

*US Food and Drug Administration approval for primary dysmenorrhea.

Figure 38-1. Nonsteroidal anti-inflammatory drugs in the treatment of dysmenorrhea.

supplement with omega-3 fatty acids in the form of fish oil capsules has been proposed. Omega-3 fatty acids intercede in the phospholipid-to-prostaglandin cascade. By competing with the endogenous omega-6 fatty acids, less potent prostaglandins and leukotrienes are produced. A small study has demonstrated some benefit, but the role of this approach appears limited [20].

If after 4 to 6 months of compliant medical therapy, there has been no improvement, diagnostic laparoscopy may be considered to exclude pelvic pathology and secondary dysmenorrhea. If no disease is seen, other treatments may be tried. Short, judicious courses of hydrocodone or codeine may be used for 2 to 3 days per month.

Surgical Management

Dilation of the cervix has been advocated as effective treatment for primary dysmenorrhea but data is lacking and it has generally fallen out of favor. Diagnostic laparoscopy, on the other hand, has several roles in the management of dysmenorrhea. One is patient reassurance. Diagnostic laparoscopy can result in a therapeutic response in patients who may be anxious about neoplasia, infection, or other pelvic causes of their pain. The more important indication is to exclude pathology and secondary dysmenorrhea.

Laparoscopic uterosacral nerve ablation (LUNA) by cautery or CO_2 laser transects the afferent pain fibers within the uterosacral ligaments [21]. LUNA offers a secondary line of therapy for dysmenorrhea only after medical therapy options have been exhausted. Potential long-term complications have not been evaluated and may include loss of cervical support leading to uterine prolapse and creation of large denuded areas posterior to the uterus, leading to adhesion formation of the tubes and ovaries. The proximity of the ureters is also of concern to the gynecologic surgeon. Chen *et al.* [22] reported their experience with LUNA in 35 women who had poor response to medical management. There were no complications in this small series. At 3 months' follow-up, the efficacy was greater than 80%; however, at 12 months' follow-up, the efficacy had fallen to 51%.

Presacral neurectomy has also been advocated by some authors for patients with dysmenorrhea. The indications are similar to those for LUNA. Potential complications include hemorrhage (from the middle sacral vein) and ureteral injury. Chronic constipation may also be a side effect. Re-enervation is possible, and long-term effectiveness is inconsistent and may be disappointing.

Secondary Dysmenorrhea

SYMPTOMS AND DIAGNOSIS

In secondary dysmenorrhea, identifiable pathologic or iatrogenic conditions act on the uterus, tubes, ovaries, or pelvic peritoneum causing the sensation of pain. The perception of pain generally results when these processes alter pressure in or around the pelvic structures, release chemical messengers or irritants, change or restrict blood flow, or cause irritation of peritoneal surfaces. These pathologies may act in combination with normal physiologic changes to create discomfort, or they may act independently with their symptoms becoming noticeable during menstruation.

Secondary dysmenorrhea by definition has associated, clinically identifiable, intrauterine or extrauterine pathology as its cause, and the cause often colors the symptoms the patient will experience. Diffuse lower abdominal cramping, back or thigh pain, nausea, diarrhea, and headache may occur with either intrauterine or extrauterine sources of secondary dysmenorrhea. Extrauterine sources are the most likely to provide hints of their presence through additional nonmenstrual symptoms. Musculoskeletal, gastrointestinal, or urinary pathologies may cause symptoms at the time of menstruation, but their effects are rarely restricted to the time of flow.

Pelvic examination including a rectovaginal examination may reveal the nodularity and tenderness associated with endometriosis. A history of intermenstrual spotting is sometimes found in patients with endometriosis. Irregularity of the uterus in a younger woman may indicate a bicornuate uterus or blind uterine horn, whereas in an older woman, leiomyomas may be felt. Adenomyosis may result in painful menstruation and may be prevalent in the fourth or fifth decades. Pelvic examination with adenomyosis may reveal a boggy, slightly tender, but symmetric uterus.

Laboratory tests will not be cost effective without a specific indication. Some authors recommend a complete blood count, erythrocyte sedimentation rate and Venereal Disease Research Laboratory test as general screening measures. These may suggest occult organic disease. Urinalysis and culture, even when the patient has no urinary complaints, may occasionally uncover a chronic cystitis or other urologic disease.

Ultrasonography of the pelvis is usually not particularly helpful. Uterine leiomyomas are a clinical diagnosis. Furthermore, endometriosis and adenomyosis do not typically have specific ultrasonographic findings.

Laparoscopic examination under general anesthesia is indicated in women with dysmenorrhea not responding to medical therapy or when the possibility of significant pathology cannot be ruled out. Recent evidence indicates that many endometrial implants may not fit the classic description of black or blue lesions and that many conditions can simulate endometriosis. Therefore, biopsy samples should be taken of classic lesions as well as any abnormal-appearing areas of peritoneum. Pelvic adhesions and incidental ovarian cysts are rarely the source of chronic pelvic pain and are an even less likely cause of pain restricted to the time of menstruation.

MANAGEMENT

When secondary dysmenorrhea is identified, the best therapeutic approach will be directed toward the clinically identified pathology. If an intrauterine contraceptive device is the likely cause, removal is in order. If endometriosis is diagnosed, medical or surgical therapy is indicated. Only when the definitive therapy is not practical or available (eg, multiple fibroids in a patient wishing no possibility of hysterectomy or impaired fertility) are analgesics or modifications of the menstrual cycle indicated. Although these latter interventions are often adequate, they are frequently less than completely successful and are short-term at best.

Endometriosis can be treated with prostaglandin synthesis inhibitors and oral contraceptives. Other modalities may be tried (eg, gonadotropin-releasing hormone agonists, such as leprolide acetate) when fertility is to be maintained. During laparoscopy, ablation of visible endometrial implants can be performed. Presacral neurectomy, laparoscopically or through laparotomy, can provide substantial relief, but side effects are common and the procedures do not uniformly result in improvement.

Intrauterine contraceptive devices may cause dysmenorrhea. Prostaglandin synthesis inhibitors are effective in treating dysmenorrhea as well as the often accompanying menorrhagia. If symptoms persist, discontinuing the intrauterine contraceptive devices and instituting another method of birth control may be necessary.

Uterine leiomyomas also may increase prostaglandin levels. NSAIDs may only temporarily relieve dysmenorrhea, with hysterectomy being the definitive treatment. Oral contraceptives, alone or in combination with NSAIDs, may provide significant relief. If there are no contraindications, low-dose oral contraceptives are effective treatment of menorrhagia and dysmenorrhea associated with uterine leiomyomas. They may be used for short courses (3 to 4 months) or continued in the patient with no contraindications.

Adenomyosis is usually not responsive to conservative therapies. It also may be difficult to diagnose. A normal ultrasonographic and laparoscopic examination would be expected. The diagnosis is made when a woman undergoes hysterectomy for unremitting symptoms and the pathologist finds endometrial implants within the uterine musculature microscopically.

Conclusion

Primary dysmenorrhea can be distinguished from secondary dysmenorrhea by history and physical examination, although laparoscopy may occasionally be necessary. Factors such as the need for contraception, contraindications to NSAIDs, personal preferences or other factors must be considered. With the choices currently available, almost all women with dysmenorrhea should be able to expect relief from dysmenorrhea. No woman need suffer, miss work, or school. Physicians should ask specifically about painful menses and reassure their patients about the safety of treatment.

References

1. Andersch B, Milson I: An epidemiologic study of young women with dysmenorrhea. *Am J Obstet Gynecol* 1982, 144:655.

2. Smith RP, Powell JR: Intrauterine pressure changes during mefenamic acid treatment of primary spasmodic dysmenorrhea. *Am J Obstet Gynecol* 1982, 143:286–292.

3. Smith RP, Powell JR: Simultaneous objective and subjective evaluation of meclofenamate sodium in the treatment of primary dysmenorrhea. *Am J Obstet Gynecol* 1987, 157:611–616.

4. Smith RP, Heltzel J: Interrelation of analgesia and uterine activity in women with primary dysmenorrhea. A preliminary report. *J Reprod Med* 1991, 36:260–264.

5. Garcia Rodriguez LA, Varas-Lorenzo C, Maguire A, Gonzalez-Perez A: Nonsteroidal antiinflammatory drugs and the risk of myocardial infarction in the general population. *Circulation* 2004, 109:3000–3006.

6. Chan AT, Manson JE, Albert CM, et al.: Nonsteroidal antiinflammatory drugs, acetaminophen, and the risk of cardiovascular events. *Circulation* 2006, 113:1578–1587.

7. O'Dowd MJ, Philipp EE: *The History of Obstetrics and Gynaecology.* New York: The Parthenon Publishing Group; 1994:346.

8. Smith RP: The next hot topic: heat therapy. *Female Patient* 2003, 28:30–39.

9. Akin MD, Weingand KW, Hengehold DA, et al.: Use of continuous low-level topical heat in the treatment of dysmenorrhea. *Obstet Gynecol* 2001, 97:343–349.

10. Akin MD, Price-Rodriguez G Jr, Erasala G, et al.: Continuous low-level topical heat wrap therapy compared to acetaminophen for primary dysmenorrhea. *J Reprod Med* 2004, 49:739–745.

11. Milsom I, Sundell G, Andersch B, et al.: The influence of different combined oral contraceptives on the prevalence and severity of dysmenorrhea. *Contraception* 1990, 42:497–506.

12. Proctor ML, Roberts H, Farquhar CM: Combined oral contraceptive pill (OCP) as treatment for primary dysmenorrhoea (Cochrane Review). *Cochrane Database Syst Rev* 2001, 4:CD002120.

13. Hendrix SL, Alexander NJ: Primary dysmenorrhea treatment with a desogestrel-containing low-dose oral contraceptive. *Contraception* 2002, 66:393–399.

14. Edelman AB, Gallo MF, Jensen JT, et al.: Continuous or extended cycle vs. cyclic use of combined oral contraceptives for contraception. *Cochrane Database Syst Rev* 2005, CD004695.

15. Baldaszti E, Wimmer-Puchinger B, Loschke K: Acceptability of the long-term contraceptive levonorgestrel-releasing intrauterine system (Mirena): a 3-year follow-up study. *Contraception* 2003, 67:87–91.

16. Proctor ML, Smith CA, Farquhar CM, Stones RW: Transcutaneous electrical nerve stimulation and acupuncture for primary dysmenorrhoea (Cochrane Review). *Cochrane Database Syst Rev* 2002, CD002123.

17. Barnard ND, Scialli AR, Hurlock D, Bertron P: Diet and sex-hormone binding globulin, dysmenorrhea, and premenstrual symptoms. *Obstet Gynecol* 2000, 95:245–250.

18. Ziaei S, Faghihzadeh S, Sohrabvand F, et al.: A randomised placebo-controlled trial to determine the effect of vitamin E in treatment of primary dysmenorrhoea. *BJOG* 2001, 108:1181–1183.

19. Ziaei S, Zakeri M, Kazemnejad A: A randomised controlled trial of vitamin E in the treatment of primary dysmenorrhoea. *BJOG* 2005, 112:466–469.

20. Harel Z, Biro FM, Kottenhahn RK, et al.: Supplementation with omega-3 polyunsaturated fatty acids in the management of dysmenorrhea in adolescents. *Am J Obstet Gynecol* 1996, 174:1335–1338.

21. Gurgan T, Urman B, Aksu T, et al.: Laparoscopic CO2 laser uterine nerve ablation for treatment of drug resistant primary dysmenorrhea. *Fertil Steril* 1992, 58:422–424.

22. Chen FP, Chang SD, Chu KK, et al.: Comparison of laparoscopic presacral neurectomy and laparoscopic uterine nerve ablation for primary dysmenorrhea. *J Reprod Med* 1996, 41:463–466.

39 Premenstrual Syndrome

Frank W. Ling and C. James Chuong

- Premenstrual syndrome is defined as a cyclic psychologic and somatic change that occurs for 10 to 14 days during the luteal phase of the ovulatory cycle.
- As many as 70% to 90% of women of reproductive age have a certain degree of premenstrual changes, but only 20% to 41% of them report clinically significant symptoms, and only 3.2% report severe symptoms.
- PMS is considered to result from an aberration of normal cycle changes in the activity of neurohormones during the luteal phase.
- Prospective recording of symptoms is much more predictive of premenstrual changes than are retrospective reports, which tend to overdiagnose PMS.
- As PMS can be superimposed on other medical or mental disorders, it is important to identify these disorders on the basis of history, physical and psychologic evaluations, and laboratory tests.
- Effective therapeutic strategies may include a general approach such as education, lifestyle changes, medical therapy in a primary care setting, and more specific neurohormonal modification in a tertiary referral setting.

Definition, Incidence, and Epidemiology

More than 60 years have passed since various psychologic and physical symptoms that occur premenstrually were first described, yet there is little or no consensus on the pathophysiology, diagnostic criteria, optimal evaluation techniques, or effective treatment of premenstrual syndrome (PMS). PMS is defined as cyclic psychologic and somatic changes that occur for 10 to 14 days during the luteal phase of the ovulatory cycle. All the changes disappear dramatically within 2 days after the onset of menstrual flow, or after the onset of the following cycle in patients who have undergone hysterectomy, and the patients are symptom free for at least 2 weeks afterward. Psychologic changes include irritability, tension, anxiety, mood swings, emotional lability, restlessness, decreased concentration, depression, aggression, lethargy, poor coordination, craving for sweet or salty food, crying easily, and increased or decreased sexual desire. Somatic changes include generalized swelling; breast tenderness; abdominal bloating; swelling of face, hands, or feet; weight gain; change in bowel habits; headache; dizziness; hot flushes; and acne. There is a great deal of individual variability in symptomatology among women within a menstrual cycle and within menstrual cycles in the same woman.

Since 1985 PMS has been classified as "late luteal phase dysphoric disorder" in the Appendix of the *Diagnostic and Statistical Manual of Mental Disorders III* and *IV*. Those who proposed PMS as a psychiatric disorder emphasized that the principal symptoms of PMS are "psychologic and behavioral rather than physical, and the differential diagnosis is with the other mental disorder rather than with physical disorders." As a result, the current psychiatric terminology is *premenstrual dysphoric disorder* (PMDD).

The term *PMS* should be reserved for the description of adverse premenstrual changes that are of sufficient duration and severity to cause distressing impairment of the sufferer's psychic and physical well-being. As many as 70% to 90% of women of reproductive age have a certain degree of premenstrual changes, but only 20% to 41% report clinically significant symptoms, and only 3.2% report severe symptoms [1,2•]. Therefore, it is important to distinguish between PMS and the mild premenstrual changes. The PMS symptoms appear to become more pronounced during the fourth decade.

Pathophysiology

Numerous hypotheses regarding pathophysiology have been proposed in the past 60 years. Although many investigators believe that PMS, like all physical disease, arises from disordered physiology, others attempt to explain premenstrual symptoms on a psychogenic basis, and the exact pathophysiology remains elusive. Several hypotheses have been proposed and are presented for historical perspective.

PROGESTERONE DEFICIENCY AND WITHDRAWAL

It has been asserted that an unopposed estrogenic effect due to deficient progesterone production is linked to PMS based on luteal phase steroid levels, endometrial biopsies, and vaginal smears of PMS patients. However, it is possible that progesterone withdrawal rather than progesterone deficiency causes PMS because symptoms are known to be maximal as progesterone levels decrease during the late luteal phase. The rate of fall of progesterone levels has been implicated as an etiologic factor. Current thinking is that progesterone levels are normal in patients with PMS and PMDD.

FLUID RETENTION AND REDISTRIBUTION

Detailed studies have failed to reveal good evidence for the hypothesis of fluid retention in PMS, and investigations of weight change and of sodium and water balance have yielded controversial results. The phenomenon of fluid redistribution was also thought to be due to the increased capillary filtration coefficient during the luteal phase in women with PMS. Tollan *et al.* [3] measured colloid osmotic and hydrostatic interstitial pressures on the thorax and on the leg. Based on these findings, redistribution of fluid rather than water retention was suggested as a mechanism for the bloating symptoms in PMS patients. Further studies are necessary to assess the exact redistributional changes of various body fluids in these patients. Contemporary thought is that any changes are more result than cause.

OPIATE WITHDRAWAL

Central nervous system hormones have been linked to PMS by symptom similarity and by association with other emotional syndromes. These hormones include neurotransmitters and peptides with opiate receptor activity. Several pieces of information build a foundation to support the hypothesis that PMS results from luteal phase changes in one of the opiate levels, β-endorphin (β-EP). Endorphin and estrogen and progesterone levels have been shown to co-vary. Progesterone is also associated with an increase in endogenous opiate peptide activity.

Experiments with naloxone, an opiate receptor antagonist, provide more evidence in support of the endogenous opiate hypothesis. Naloxone, which achieved opiate withdrawal, was found to produce symptoms similar to those of PMS when it was administered in high doses to normal volunteers.

The plasma β-EP levels have been shown to peak at midcycle with no obvious difference between the follicular phase and the luteal phase [4] in normal ovulatory women. Patients with PMS were noted to have lower levels of plasma endorphin during the luteal phase of the menstrual cycle compared with their own levels during the follicular phase and compared with control subjects during the luteal phase [5]. In another study [6•], peripheral β-EP levels throughout the periovulatory phase were noted to be lower in PMS patients than in the controls. Based on these data, it was proposed that the premenstrual decrease of β-EP peripherally might reflect a decrease in the central levels of β-EP and be responsible for the PMS symptom complex. The data also suggested that such aberration of β-EP activity might start near the time of ovulation. Currently available techniques do not afford access to the central site of synthesis and secretion of β-EP. It has been known that failure to exhibit a naloxone-induced luteinizing hormone (LH) increase suggests a deficiency in β-EP activity. Chuong and Hsi [7] administered five naloxone infusions during the follicular, periovulatory, and luteal phases of the cycle in PMS patients but did not find significant difference in LH response between the patients and the controls. This β-EP activities theory lacks any further substantiation.

SEROTONIN DEFICIENCY

The strongest evidence is that serotonin plays a role in PMS [8••]. A significant reduction in the platelet uptake of serotonin has been reported among PMS patients during the premenstrual phase. In addition, the whole blood serotonin levels of PMS subjects were found to be significantly lower during the last 10 days of the menstrual cycle. However, serotonin levels in the blood do not indicate brain levels because serotonin is found in a variety of foods, and diet alone can alter blood levels. Despite the difficulty in the determination of brain serotonin levels, studies on the effect of nutrient intake on PMS provide evidence in support of the serotonin deficiency hypothesis. PMS patients were noted to increase calorie and carbohydrate intake significantly during the late luteal phase. Consumption of a carbohydrate-rich, protein-poor evening test meal premenstrually improved many of the mood symptoms [9]. The data suggested that the positive moods that followed intake of the carbohydrates were due to increases in the synthesis of brain serotonin. Carbohydrate consumption without protein has been shown to increase the uptake of tryptophan, the amino acid precursor of serotonin, in the brain. The consumption of protein-rich foods would inhibit brain uptake of tryptophan and prevent serotonin synthesis and release. Due to multiple investigations demonstrating the efficacy of selective serotonin reuptake inhibitors in the treatment of PMS and PMDD, serotonin is currently seen as the most likely cause.

VITAMIN AND MINERAL DEFICIENCY

Mood and behavior have been known to be influenced by biogenic amines in the central nervous system. Several vitamins and minerals are cofactors in the synthesis of the precursors of these amines. Despite the wide use of nutritional supplements in the treatment of PMS, neither an excess nor deficiency of vitamins, minerals, and other dietary factors has been well documented in patients compared with control subjects. Serum vitamin and mineral levels may assist in assessing vitamin and mineral deficiencies in patients with PMS and serve as a guideline before and during nutritional supplement therapy. Several studies [10,11] were conducted to determine whether changes in peripheral vitamin and mineral levels were associated with PMS symptoms.

No significant changes in vitamins A, B$_6$, or E or magnesium were found between the controls and the patients in either the luteal or the follicular phase. These findings cannot explain the beneficial effect of vitamin A and magnesium reported previously. Chuong and Dawson [10] suggested that the response to various vitamins and magnesium in these studies was a result of a pharmacologic response rather than correction of a deficiency state. The zinc levels were significantly lower, and the copper levels were markedly higher in the patients than those in the controls during the luteal phase. Because copper competes with zinc for intestinal absorption and serum protein–binding sites, the availability of zinc in patients premenstrually was reduced further by the elevated copper. Patients with PMS were also found to have lower serum calcium levels in the peripheral blood than controls. Whether these peripheral concentrations reflect central changes requires further study.

OTHER THEORIES
Other theories include hyperprolactinemia, abnormal prostaglandin metabolism, adrenal-cortisol dysregulation, hypoglycemia, and thyroid dysfunction. To date, however, none of these theories has been substantiated.

Diagnosis

CLINICAL EVALUATION
The proposed protocol for the diagnosis and treatment of PMS is shown in Figure 39-1. The most important approach at the first visit is to listen to the history. The physician should assess the patient's psychiatric history and explore her relationship with her family members and coworkers. External stress associated with these relationships can make the symptoms worse. Premenstrual changes may be confused with other gynecologic or psychiatric problems. The evaluation should include not only a detailed history but the formulation of a differential diagnosis of each complaint and a thorough physical and psychological examination, with laboratory and radiologic examinations if indicated and referrals when appropriate [12••]. It has been shown that PMS is associated with the number of deliveries, postpartum depression, past birth control pill use, alcohol and drug use, and history of PMS in first-degree relatives [13]. If PMS is associated with interictal dysphoric disorder, such as epilepsy, a combination of antidepressant and antiepileptic medication is indicated [14]. The data in this study suggested concordance of symptomatology between interictal and PMDD may extend to treatment. It is also important to differentiate PMS from psychiatric disorders with premenstrual aggravation. As an aid to understanding the psychologic status of patients, the Minnesota Multiphasic Personality Inventory may

be administered whenever necessary. Patients with different depression severity should be considered as having different subtypes of PMS because they may have different responses to the treatment, such as depo-leuprolide [15•]. Therefore, an accurate recognition of various subtypes of PMS cannot be overemphasized.

It is critical for the diagnosis of PMS that symptoms occur specifically during the luteal phase of the cycle and that there is a symptom-free period of at least 1 week after the cessation of menstruation. Symptoms continuing after the 5th day of the menstrual cycle are not generally considered PMS. There are still no uniformly accepted objective criteria for the diagnosis of PMS, and we have to depend on the patient's subjective report. Prospective recording of symptoms for at least 1 to 2 months using a daily diary, specific mood assessment charts, or specific visual linear analog scales is much more predictive of premenstrual changes than are retrospective reports, which tend to overdiagnose PMS. Keeping careful records is also helpful in increasing the patient's awareness of her problems.

LABORATORY EVALUATION
Thyroid dysfunction, hyperandrogenism, diabetes mellitus, hypoglycemia and hyperprolactinemia can cause somatic and affective symptoms that are occasionally mistaken for PMS. Therefore, thyroid work-up and measurement of serum PM cortisol, testosterone, glucose, and prolactin levels may be performed to exclude the underlying medical problems. However, the routine use of peripheral hormonal tests for patients with premenstrual complaints is costly and not indicated at this time [16•].

Treatment

The general approach to the patient with PMS requires a multidisciplinary team.

PATIENT EDUCATION AND LIFESTYLE CHANGES
The patient should be reassured that this is a problem common to many women. It is most important that the woman be allowed to express herself and to describe her problems. The articulate patient can be encouraged to write a diary of her moods, feelings, activities, and functions during this premenstrual period. The diary can serve as another mode of ventilation as well as a description of the pattern of the patient's premenstrual tension. A simple numerical rating of 0 to 3 for three key symptoms each day can also serve this purpose. Particularly important is the physician's sensitivity. Low-fat and low-carbohydrate diets have been shown to be helpful. Eating regular, frequent, small meals and decreasing the intake of salts and caffeine are helpful. Food made from whole grains, legumes, seeds, nuts, vegetables, fruits, and vegetable oils should be encouraged. It has been shown that women who participate in sports experience less premenstrual anxiety than nonathletic women. How exercise helps PMS is not clear, but

exercise is known to increase β-EP levels, which may explain the sense of well-being reported by some patients. If β-EP withdrawal contributes to PMS, the symptoms may be corrected at least partially by exercise.

MEDICAL THERAPY

If no improvement is reported within 1 to 2 months using the approach of education, diet, and exercise, then medical therapy is administered.

Specific Symptoms

Fatigue, Headache, and General Aches and Pains

A prostaglandin synthase inhibitor, such as 250 mg of mefenamic acid, given daily during the luteal phase significantly improved several symptoms, particularly fatigue, headache, general aches and pains, and mood swings. Nonsteroidal anti-inflammatory agents, such as acetylsalicylic acid or acetaminophen with or without codeine, are also used to relieve premenstrual headaches and muscle and joint pain. Sumatriptan, a 5-hydroxytryptamine receptor agonist, has been shown to be effective and well tolerated for menstruation-associated and nonmenstrual migraine. Women treated for menstruation-associated migraine with 6 mg of sumatriptan subcutaneously had significant headache relief after 1 hour. Other associated symptoms, such as nausea and photophobia, were

also improved. The most common adverse events were injection site reactions, dizziness, tingling, nausea, vomiting, warm sensation, and chest tightness. Most of the adverse events lasted less than 1 hour. Other forms of this medication, such as nasal spray and oral pills, are also available.

Weight Gain and Fluid Retention

Studies have shown significant improvement in reduction in weight and psychologic symptoms using spironolactone, a potassium-sparing diuretic. If the patient gains weight and experiences bloating and edema premenstrually, and if weight loss occurs dramatically after the onset of menstruation, spironolactone, 25 mg four times a day during the luteal phase, is recommended.

Breast Tenderness and Swelling

The dopaminergic agonist bromocriptine, 5 mg at night daily from days 10 to 26 of the cycle, was noted to produce a significant reduction in breast tenderness and swelling but was ineffective in controlling other symptoms of PMS. Danazol, 200 mg once or twice daily, could effectively suppress breast and other generalized symptoms.

Generalized Symptoms

Naltrexone

The β-EP withdrawal or deficiency hypothesis suggests treatment of PMS with exogenous β-EP but it is not practical

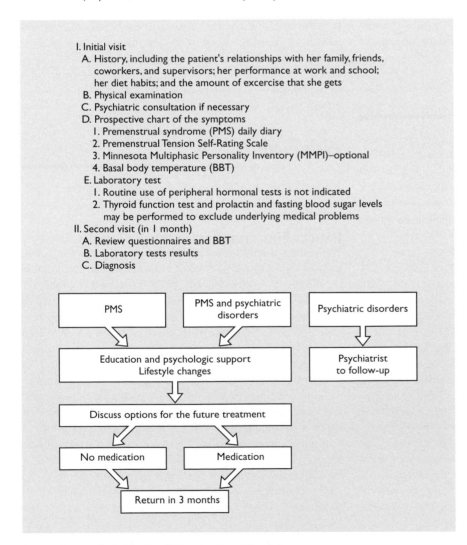

Figure 39-1. Diagnosis and treatment protocol for patients with premenstrual syndrome.

because of addiction and the route of administration (intramuscular or intravenous). An opiate antagonist, given before the periovulatory β-EP peak and withdrawal, might offer a rational treatment of PMS by keeping a constant level of β-EP. Naltrexone is an oral pure narcotic antagonist that has been used in the treatment of withdrawal symptoms for patients with heroin addiction. Unlike drugs that have mixed agonist and antagonist effects, it does not cause addiction or withdrawal.

Studies suggested that naltrexone alleviated PMS symptoms and might be developed into an effective treatment [17]. The acceptability of this medication was good, with only a low incidence of nausea, decreased appetite, dizziness, and fainting, which may be minimized by further dividing or decreasing the dosage. It is possible that naltrexone inhibited β-EP withdrawal and prevented the decrease of β-EP levels, thus reducing the severity of symptoms significantly.

D-Fenfluramine

Enhancement of serotonin synthesis and neurotransmission by administration of tryptophan or of serotonin-specific drugs has been used to treat some types of depressive illness. Administration of large doses of pyridoxine (vitamin B_6), a cofactor in serotonin synthesis, has been observed to alleviate depression, anxiety, irritability, and a number of other PMS symptoms. Wurtman et al. [9] showed that carbohydrate consumption was effective in alleviating many PMS mood changes and thus exerted a therapeutic, not a nutritional, effect. Based on these observations, a study [18] was conducted using D-fenfluramine, which acts specifically to enhance serotonin-mediated neurotransmission in PMS patients. Significant improvement of depressed mood and reduced calorie and carbohydrate intake, as compared with placebo, was noted using D-fenfluramine. These results support the hypothesis that serotonin is involved in both the affective and appetite symptoms of PMS.

Serotonin Reuptake Inhibitors

Fluoxetine is an antidepressant that is a serotonin reuptake inhibitor. It is chemically unrelated to tricyclic, tetracyclic, or other available antidepressant agents. Effects of fluoxetine in the treatment of PMS have been established [19]. Sertraline, another serotonin reuptake inhibitor, has also been used successfully in PMS [20]. Open-label pilot studies using other serotonin reuptake inhibitors, such as paroxetine [21] and fluvoxamine [22], on a daily basis also showed significant improvement of PMS symptoms. Significant improvement of symptoms by a serotonin reuptake inhibitor only during the luteal phase in patients with PMS has also been reported [23].

Vitamins and Minerals

It has been suggested that deficiencies of vitamins and minerals are related to PMS. Although deficiencies of several vitamins and minerals in PMS patients could not be demonstrated [10], a number of these supplements have appeared widely on the market during the past few years. It was reported that a combination tablet of 100 to 600 mg of vitamin B_6 and other essential micronutrients reduced the severity of many PMS symptoms. The use of daily 400 IU of vitamin E in the treatment of PMS was also reported to achieve improvement of several symptoms. Until these issues are addressed, the supplementation of vitamins and minerals can only be considered empiric therapy for PMS.

Progesterone

Progesterone vaginal suppository was not superior to placebo in several double-blind placebo-controlled studies despite higher circulating progesterone levels [24]. These data contradicted previous reports. Although many authorities question its efficacy, progesterone has remained one of the popular medications for the treatment of PMS [25].

Psychotropic Agents

Several psychotropic agents have been used in the treatment of PMS, including diazepam, alprazolam, buspirone hydrochloride, clorazepate dipotassium, clonazepam, amitriptyline hydrochloride, and tricyclic agents. Because of the required long-term therapy for PMS patients, these agents may produce undesirable side effects over time. It is recommended that these agents be given to patients with severe symptoms only as a short-term adjuvant to other therapies.

Medical Oophorectomy

In an earlier study, it was demonstrated that elimination of ovarian cyclicity through down-regulation of pituitary gonadotropin secretion with gonadotropin-releasing hormone (GnRH) agonist resulted in marked attenuation of premenstrual symptoms. The therapy was rapidly reversible, which is possible with no influence on subsequent cycles. Medical oophorectomy prevents the fluctuation and deficiency of β-EP levels as well as estrogen and progesterone by causing temporary cessation of cyclic ovarian activity. Studies using monthly depo-leuprolide [15,26] and other GnRH agonists showed similar results.

The safety and side effects of long-term medical oophorectomy remain to be determined. Studies using "add-back" synthetic sex steroid therapy to prevent bone loss in patients given GnRH agonists have been reported in patients with endometriosis [27], and similar types of studies in PMS patients are under investigation.

Surgical Oophorectomy With or Without Hysterectomy

Studies have shown that total abdominal hysterectomy and salpingo-oophorectomy with low-dose estrogen replacement is effective in relieving the symptoms in women with severe, debilitating PMS who did not respond to conventional interventions [28,29]. The surgical solution to PMS should be considered only as a last resort after careful screening of patients and after all forms of medical therapy have failed, particularly medical oophorectomy. Only those who have completed childbearing should be considered for this option. Because PMS is related to the ovarian function, bilateral oophorectomy alone by laparoscopy should be sufficient. Continuous estrogen and progestin replacement after surgery can avoid monthly withdrawal bleeding and PMS-like symptoms. Concurrent hysterectomy is also indicated if the patient has other gynecologic conditions, such as fibroid uterus, severe dysmenorrhea, or severe menorrhagia. Patients who received hysterectomy alone with intact ovaries were noted to have persistent cyclic luteal phase symptoms in the absence of menstrual flow as shown on the symptom calendar and basal body temperature chart. Endometrial ablation is not expected to improve the symptoms because ovarian function is preserved with this procedure.

Conclusion

Prospective recording of symptoms is much more predictive of premenstrual changes than are retrospective reports, which tend to overdiagnose PMS. Because the PMS population is not homogeneous and PMS can be superimposed on other medical or mental disorders, it is important to identify these disorders on the basis of history, physical and psychologic evaluations, and laboratory testing.

Premenstrual syndrome and PMDD appear to occur when there is an abnormal serotonin response to normal cyclic hormone fluctuations. Many hormones can mediate neuroendocrine dysfunction and thereby explain diverse symptoms. Effective therapeutic strategies may include a general approach, such as education, lifestyle changes, psychologic support, and general medical therapy in a primary care setting, and a more specific neurohormonal modification, such as medical and surgical oophorectomy in a tertiary referral setting.

References

Papers of particular interest have been highlighted as follows:
- *Of interest*
- •• *Of outstanding interest*

1. Johnson SR, McChesney C, Bean JA: Epidemiology of premenstrual symptoms in a nonclinical sample. *J Reprod Med* 1988, 33:340–345.

2.• Singh BB, Berman BM, Simpson RL, *et al.*: Incidence of premenstrual syndrome and remedy usage: a national probability sample study. *Altern Ther Health Med* 1998, 4:75–79.

This article reported that women were aware of symptoms related to PMS more frequently than they recognized a formalized medical syndrome.

3. Tollan A, Oian P, Fadness HO, *et al.*: Evidence for altered transcapillary fluid balance in women with the premenstrual syndrome. *Acta Obstet Gynecol Scand* 1993, 72:238–242.

4. Chuong CJ, Smith ER, Tsong Y: β-Endorphin levels in the human menstrual cycle. *Acta Obstet Gynecol Scand* 1989, 68:497–501.

5. Chuong CJ, Coulam CB, Kao PC, *et al.*: Neuropeptide levels in premenstrual syndrome. American Fertility Society-Associate Members Forum Prize Award Paper. *Fertil Steril* 1985, 44:760–765.

6.• Chuong CJ, Hsi BP, Gibbons WE: Periovulatory β-endorphin levels in premenstrual syndrome. *Obstet Gynecol* 1994, 83:755–760.

This article suggested that the aberration of β-endorphin activity in PMS patients might start around the time of ovulation.

7. Chuong CJ, Hsi BP: Effects of naloxone on luteinizing hormone secretion in premenstrual syndrome. *Fertil Steril* 1994, 61:1039–1044.

8.•• Kouri EM, Halbreich U: State and trait serotonergic abnormalities in women with dysphoric premenstrual syndromes. *Psychopharmacol Bull* 1997, 33:767–770.

This article reviewed the current data on changes in serotonergic parameters in women with dysphoric PMS.

9. Wurtman J, Brzezinski A, Wurtman RJ, *et al.*: Effect of nutrient intake on premenstrual depression. *Am J Obstet Gynecol* 1989, 161:1228–1232.

10. Chuong CJ, Dawson EB: Critical evaluation of nutritional factors in the pathophysiology and treatment of premenstrual syndrome. *Clin Obstet Gynecol* 1992, 35:679–692.

11. Chuong CJ, Dawson EB: Zinc and copper levels in premenstrual syndrome. *Fertil Steril* 1994, 62:313–320.

12.•• Keye WR, Hammond DC, Strong T: Medical and psychological characteristics of women presenting with premenstrual symptoms. *Obstet Gynecol* 1986, 68:635–640.

This article describes a general approach to PMS. Treatment should be offered by a multidisciplinary team that integrates the efforts of a gynecologist, an endocrinologist, a psychiatrist or psychologist, a social worker, and a nutritionist.

13. Chuong CJ, Burgos DM: Medical history in women with premenstrual syndrome. *J Psychosomat Obstet Gynecol* 1995, 16:21–27.

14. Blumer D, Herzog AG, Himmelhoch J, *et al.*: To what extent do premenstrual and interictal dysphoric disorder overlap? Significance for therapy. *J Affect Disord* 1998, 48:215–225.

15. Brown CS, Ling FW, Anderson RN, *et al.*: Efficacy of depot leuprolide in premenstrual syndrome: effect of symptom severity and type in a controlled trial. *Obstet Gynecol* 1994, 84:779–786.

This article showed that leuprolide reduced both behavioral and physical symptoms in the absence of severe premenstrual depression and suggested that women should be evaluated for depression before receiving a GnRH agonist.

16.• Rubinow DR, Hoban MC, Grover GN, *et al.*: Changes in plasma hormones across the menstrual cycle in patients with menstrually related mood disorder and in control subjects. *Am J Obstet Gynecol* 1988, 158:5–10.

This article demonstrated that the routine use of peripheral hormonal tests for patients with premenstrual complaints was not only costly but also not indicated.

17. Chuong CJ, Coulam CB, Bergstralh EJ, *et al.*: Clinical trial of naltrexone in premenstrual syndrome. *Obstet Gynecol* 1988, 72:332–336.

18. Brezinski A, Wurtman JJ, Wurtman RJ: D-fenfluramine in the treatment of premenstrual syndrome: a double-blind, placebo-controlled, randomized clinical trial. *Obstet Gynecol* 1990, 76:296–301.

19. Pearlstein TB, Stone AB: Long-term fluoxetine treatment of late luteal phase dysphoric disorder. *J Clin Psychiatry* 1994, 55:332–336.

20. Yonkers KA, Halbreich U, Freeman E, *et al.*: Symptomatic improvement of premenstrual dysphoric disorder with sertraline treatment: a randomized controlled trial. Sertraline Premenstrual Dysphoric Collaborative Study Group. *JAMA* 1997, 278:983–988.

21. Yonkers KA, Gullion C, Williams A, *et al.*: Paroxetine as a treatment for premenstrual dysphoric disorder. *J Clin Psychopharmacol* 1996, 16:3–8.

22. Freeman EW, Rickels K, Sondheimer SJ: Fluvoxamine for premenstrual dysphoric disorder: a pilot study. *J Clin Psychiatry* 1996, 57(Suppl):56–61.

23. Young SA, Hurt PH, Benedek DM, *et al.*: Treatment of premenstrual dysphoric disorder with sertraline during the luteal phase: a randomized, double-blind, placebo-controlled crossover trial. *J Clin Psychiatry* 1998, 59:76–80.

24. Maddocks SG, Hahn PM, Moller F, *et al.*: A double-blind placebo-controlled trial of progesterone vaginal suppositories in the treatment of premenstrual syndrome. *Am J Obstet Gynecol* 1986, 154:573–577.

25. Martorano JT, Ahlgrimm M, Colbert T: Differentiating between natural progesterone and synthetic progestins: clinical implications for premenstrual syndrome and perimenopause management. *Compr Ther* 1998, 24:336–339.

26. Freeman EW, Sondheimer SJ, Rickels K: Gonadotropin-releasing hormone agonist in the treatment of premenstrual symptoms with and without ongoing dysphoria: a controlled study. *Psychopharmacol Bull* 1997, 33:303–309.

27. Freundl G, Godtke K, Gnoth C, *et al.*: Steroidal add-back therapy in patients treated with GnRH agonists. *Gynecol Obstet Invest* 1998, 45(Suppl 1):22–30.

28. Casson P, Hahn PM, Van Vugt DA, *et al.*: Lasting response to ovariectomy in severe intractable premenstrual syndrome. *Am J Obstet Gynecol* 1990, 162:99–105.

29. Casper RF, Hearn MT: The effect of hysterectomy and bilateral oophorectomy in women with severe premenstrual syndrome. *Am J Obstet Gynecol* 1990, 162:105–109.

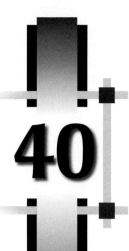

40 Amenorrhea

Christopher M. Estes

- Primary amenorrhea is defined as menarche delayed beyond 16 years of age.
- Secondary amenorrhea is defined as absent menstruation for 6 consecutive months in a patient who has had at least one menstrual cycle previously.
- The most common causes of amenorrhea in reproductive-aged women are pregnancy, anovulation, hypothalamic-pituitary disorders, and thyroid disorders.
- A history and physical examination followed by hormonal evaluation are the keys to the diagnosis of the affected step or organ responsible for amenorrhea and to guiding treatment.
- In the context of a normal physical examination, a pregnancy test, progesterone challenge test, and measurement of serum prolactin and thyroid-stimulating hormone will provide a diagnosis in the majority of patients with amenorrhea.
- Treatment should be directed toward the underlying cause of amenorrhea.
- While hormonal deficiencies and associated symptoms are treated, the patient's fertility desires should be carefully considered.

Introduction

Amenorrhea is a symptom not a diagnosis. Amenorrhea is more commonly physiologic than pathologic, occurs in the prepubertal period, during pregnancy and lactation, and after menopause. The median age of menarche in the United States is 12.8 years; 98% of women will reach menarche by age 16 [1]. Thus, the incidence of primary amenorrhea is approximately 2%. The incidence of secondary amenorrhea (cessation of menses for 6 months or more with a history of previously regular cycles) varies by age group. Women under age 20 have an annual incidence as high as 7%, whereas women over age 35 have an annual incidence as low as 3% [2].

The simplest way to approach the diagnosis of amenorrhea is to conceptualize its root cause as occurring in one of four compartments: 1) anomalies of the outflow tract, 2) disorders of the ovary, 3) disorders of the anterior pituitary and thyroid, and 4) hypothalamic and other systemic disorders. Our discussion of the topic will proceed in a logical fashion to evaluate each of these compartments in an effort to discover the root cause of the problem.

Anomalies of the Outflow Tract

As with all patient encounters, good history taking is an essential component. By doing so, a long, complicated differential diagnosis can be quickly whittled down to only the most likely pathologies. Foremost, the provider must determine if the patient's complaint is that of primary or secondary amenorrhea. If she has never had a menstrual period, and she is over age 16, then it is primary amenorrhea. If she has had even one menstrual period, then ceased menstruating for longer than 6 months, it is secondary amenorrhea. Anatomical problems are nearly always causes of primary, not secondary amenorrhea. The exception to this rule is Asherman's syndrome.

The first section of this chapter will deal primarily with the second step in any clinical encounter: the physical examination.

MÜLLERIAN ANOMALIES
Congenital Anatomic Malformations

The exact incidence of malformations of the lower genital tract that lead to primary amenorrhea is estimated to be between 0.1% and 3.8% [3•]. Generally, the patient will present with a concomitant complaint of cyclic low abdominal pain. Other associated symptoms include vaginal or vulvar pain, urinary retention, and back pain. This group of disorders results from improper formation of the müllerian system during embryogenesis. The organs of the upper genital tract (cervix, uterus, fallopian tubes, and upper one third of the vagina) are formed by the fusion of the two paramesonephric ducts, whereas the lower genital tract (vulva, hymen, and lower two thirds of the vagina) is formed from the urogenital sinus [4]. A defect at either of these levels can result in an obstruction and subsequent amenorrhea.

Imperforate hymen, transverse vaginal septum, cervical atresia, and vaginal atresia can all be diagnosed through the physical examination. The anomalous area may show marked swelling or an ecchymotic appearance, as a large quantity of blood may be concealed. If the patient has had obstructed menstrual cycles, the uterine cavity may be distended with blood. This is referred to as *hematocolpos* and may be suspected if the uterus feels enlarged and/or tender on bimanual examination. It is definitively diagnosed via pelvic imaging—sonography or MRI.

Care should be taken not to rupture an imperforate hymen or septum in the office for the sake of preventing infection and patient discomfort. No biopsy or needle aspiration is needed for the diagnosis of these conditions. Patients should be taken to the operating room for the appropriate surgical management. Preoperative work-up should also include imaging of the kidneys, ureters, and bladder, because concomitant malformations of the urinary collecting systems are present in 12% of these patients [5].

Congenital Absence of Müllerian Structures
Rokitansky-Kuster-Hauser syndrome is a rare condition whose incidence is approximately one in 4000 [5]. These individuals have normal ovaries and vulva, but no uterus or cervix and a shortened vagina. If no cervix is seen on physical examination, an ultrasound should be performed to confirm the presence or absence of the uterus. Should the uterus indeed be absent, the next step in evaluation should be a karyotype. The indication for a karyotype is to rule out the presence of a Y chromosome; because, if present, the gonads must be removed after puberty due to their increased risk of developing malignancy.

Androgen Insensitivity
Complete androgen insensitivity, or testicular feminization, occurs in an individual with a 47,XY karyotype who is phenotypically female. This is a result of a genetic defect in the androgen receptor, and it is inherited in a maternal X-linked recessive fashion [1]. As patients have no functional androgen receptors, signs of adrenarche will be absent: pubic and axillary hair will be absent or retain a downy, prepubertal character. Breast development will be that of a normal female, because circulating levels of estrogen are high, and breast development is not dependent on testosterone.

The gonads of these individuals are genetically male and may be located in an inguinal hernia. These gonads carry a significantly increased risk of malignant tumors, as high as 5% to 10% [6,7]. Depending on the location of the testis, resection may be possible laparoscopically.

Proper diagnosis and management of these patients must also proceed with appropriate psychologic counseling, as the implications for sexual identity are profound. Referral to counselors with expertise in genetic and sexual disorders is recommended.

Figure 40-1 shows the differences between müllerian agenesis and androgen insensitivity.

ACQUIRED OBSTRUCTIONS OF THE OUTFLOW TRACT
Asherman's syndrome is the accumulation of intrauterine synechiae leading to infertility, recurrent miscarriage, and secondary amenorrhea. It is generally seen in patients who have had multiple intrauterine surgeries including dilation and curettage, hysteroscopic myomectomy, and repair of intrauterine septa and has been reported in the setting of cesarean section as the only previous uterine surgery. Patients who had a postpartum curettage are at particularly increased risk, especially if they had concomitant endometritis. The incidence of Asherman's syndrome seems to be geographically dependent and has been estimated to be present in 1.5% of all patients undergoing hysterosalpingography [8].

This condition should only be suspected in cases of secondary amenorrhea in a patient with an appropriate history (prior uterine surgery) and an otherwise normal physical examination and endocrinologic work-up. The diagnosis is confirmed with hysterosalpingography or hysteroscopy. Treatment is surgical with hysteroscopic resection of the adhesions with monopolar or bipolar cautery, followed by intrauterine distention with a Foley catheter and estrogen supplementation to facilitate healing of the scarred tissue and prevent repeat adhesions.

Agglutination of the cervical canal can occur after a loop electrosurgical excision procedure or cone biopsy of the cervix. Hematometra also may be present in these patients, because the menstrual fluid will accumulate in the endome-

Differences Between Müllerian Agenesis and Androgen Insensitivity

Factor	Müllerian Agenesis	Androgen Insensitivity
Karyotype	46,XX	46,XY
Heredity	Unknown	X-linked
Sexual hair	Normal female	Sparse
Testosterone	Normal female	Normal male
Malignancy	Normal incidence	5% (gonads)

Figure 40-1. Differences between müllerian agenesis and androgen insensitivity.

trial cavity. Treatment is therapeutic dilation of the cervix. Posttreatment topical estrogen therapy is often prescribed to prevent re-agglutination.

Disorders of the Ovary

When considering amenorrhea of ovarian origin, it is useful to divide the causes into two categories: patients with abnormal karyotypes and patients with normal karyotypes. We shall consider the former group first. Figure 40-2 lists the different syndromes of gonadal dysgenesis.

ABNORMAL KARYOTYPES
Turner Syndrome
Turner syndrome is characterized by absence of one X chromosome; the karyotype is reported as (45,X) (Figure 40-3). The associated phenotype is that of short stature, webbed neck, shield chest, and increased carrying angle of the arms [1]. The ovaries of patients with Turner syndrome do not develop normally and do not produce estrogen. As such, the hypothalamic-pituitary axis has no source of negative feedback, and levels of gonadotropins will be high (we will discuss this mechanism at length in the next section). Although nonfunctional, the "streak ovaries" of a patient with a (45,X) karyotype do not present a risk for the patient. However, 40% of patients who appear to have Turner syndrome phenotypically have a mosaic karyotype [1]. These patients must be managed in a different fashion depending on the nature of the mosaicism.

Mosaicism
Mosaicism is defined as the juxtaposition in an organism of genetically different tissues [9]. The most common form of mosaicism in patients with amenorrhea is (46, XX/45, X). They have one normal, female germ line and one Turner syndrome cell line. The ovaries of these patients may produce some estrogen, and they may menstruate and even ovulate. Less common mosaics include a Y chromosome. Specialized DNA probes may be necessary to detect its presence, but it should be ruled out carefully as 30% of patients will have no clinical signs of virilization [1]. This exhaustive search for the presence of a Y chromosome has to do with the malignant potential of the gonads. If a Y chromosome is present, the gonads should be prophylactically removed after puberty to avoid the development of cancer.

Swyer Syndrome
A patient with a normal female phenotype, intact, normally developed müllerian system, and a (46,XY) karyotype has Swyer syndrome. As discussed, the gonads should be removed after puberty to avoid malignant transformation.

NORMAL KARYOTYPE
Premature Ovarian Failure
Patients with premature ovarian failure present with the same complaints as a woman entering menopause. Their complaints will include hot flashes, sleep disturbance, vaginal dryness, and absent or irregular menses—all signs of a hypoestrogenic state. The majority of the cases of premature ovarian failure are idiopathic. Some are associated with autoimmune disorders, and work-up should proceed along these lines. Ovarian biopsy or removal of the ovaries is unnecessary in these patients. Treatment is with combined hormonal replacement: estrogen and progestin. Other causes of premature ovarian failure are listed in Figure 40-4.

Iatrogenic Ovarian Failure
Chemotherapeutics and radiation therapy can cause ovarian failure. The risk of complete failure is dependent upon dose and the patient's age. Older patients who receive higher doses of radiation to the pelvis are more likely to have permanent ovarian failure [10]. This matter is of particular concern for young women who have not completed child bearing and are diagnosed with a malignancy whose treatment requires chemotherapy and/or radiation. Measures to protect the ovary (concomitant administration of a gonadotropin-releasing hormone (GnRH) agonist, leuprolide [Lupron; TAP Pharmaceuticals, Lake Forest, IL]) or pretreatment oocyte harvesting/cryopreservation should be offered to the patient.

Causes of Failure of Gonadal Development

45,X (Turner syndrome)

Mosaicism (45,X/XX, X/XX/XXX)

46,X, abnormal X (short- or long-arm deletion)

46,XX or 46,XY pure gonadal dysgenesis

Figure 40-2. Causes of failure of gonadal development.

Stigmata of Turner Syndrome

Short stature

Sexual infantilism

Somatic features (webbed neck, shield chest, cubitus valgus, short fourth metacarpal)

Associated anomalies (autoimmune thyroiditis, coarctation of aorta, renal anomalies)

Hirsutism (if mosaic karyotype with Y elements)

Figure 40-3. Stigmata of Turner syndrome.

Causes of Premature Ovarian Failure

Gonadal dysgenesis

Autoimmune disorders

Infections (mumps, bilateral tubo-ovarian abscess)

Iatrogenic (irradiation, chemotherapy, surgical)

Vascular insufficiency (bilateral ovarian torsion, posthysterectomy)

Idiopathic

Figure 40-4. Causes of premature ovarian failure.

Enzyme Deficiencies Leading to Ovarian Dysfunction

Although an individual may have a normal karyotype, this does not ensure a fully normal genome. In regards to amenorrhea, this may occur in 17-hydroxylase and 17, 20-desmolase deficiency. These enzymes are essential steps in the pathway of steroidogenesis leading the conversion of progesterone to estrogen. Deficiency of these will preclude normal sexual development entirely, and the individual will remain in a prepubertal state unless hormone therapy is initiated. As such, these deficiencies are associated with primary amenorrhea. The diagnosis is confirmed by high progesterone levels in the serum.

Ambiguous genitalia are a common associated finding among this group of patients. As such, most patients are identified in infancy. Although the external genitalia appear female, these enzyme deficiencies are more commonly seen among individuals with a 46,XY karyotype. Sexual assignment is best handled in early childhood with appropriate hormone supplementation around the time of puberty to ensure full secondary sexual development and normal bone maturation, in the hopes that the child will attain normal adult stature.

Also of note, given the abnormal hormonal milieu of these patients, circulating levels of mineralocorticoids are also present. This can lead to potassium wasting and sodium retention. Individuals will present with hypertension and altered mental status; the diagnosis is confirmed with blood and urine chemistries. Therapy with corticosteroids is needed in this group of patients in addition to replacement of sex steroids at puberty.

Disorders of the Anterior Pituitary and Thyroid

THE HYPOTHALAMIC-PITUITARY-OVARIAN AXIS

Before discussing the pathology associated with abnormal functioning in the anterior pituitary, a brief elaboration of the normal endocrine mechanisms of the region is appropriate. Given the clinical nature of this text, our attention will be focused solely on those mechanisms within the system that hold a particular relevance to a given pathology or treatment. The menstrual cycle is controlled centrally by the hypothalamus. Its basis is GnRH. GnRH is produced in the hypothalamus and travels down the pituitary stalk where it stimulates the production of luteinizing hormone (LH) and follicle-stimulating hormone (FSH). The endocrinologic mechanism of the regulation of LH and FSH secretion is a complex feedback loop, in which normal functioning is dependent on the hypothalamus, the pituitary, and the ovaries. Figure 40-5 depicts a graphic representation of this system.

Normally, GnRH is secreted in a pulsatile fashion. When it reaches the cells of the anterior pituitary, LH and FSH production increase; this is mediated by a dopamine receptor. However, if the GnRH stimulation continues in a tonic fashion, LH and FSH production will decrease over time. This paradoxical relationship, positive feedback during pulsatile stimulation, negative feedback during tonic stimulation, is the basis for all pituitary-related causes of amenorrhea. Malfunction at any one of these points can cause amenorrhea.

HYPERPROLACTINEMIA

Prolactin secreting tumors of the anterior pituitary account for approximately one third of the patients with secondary amenorrhea [1]. Galactorrhea may or may not be present. High circulating levels of prolactin cause the secretion of GnRH to cease being pulsatile and become tonic. Over time, levels of GnRH release become very low. As such, little LH and FSH are produced, and normal to low values will be noted on serum assay. FSH is the most sensitive measure and is usually sufficient to measure it alone. When a high prolactin level is first diagnosed, serum thyroid-stimulating hormone (TSH) should also be measured to rule out hypothyroidism as the primary cause of hyperprolactinemia.

Once hyperprolactinemia is established, imaging of the brain (CT or MRI) and assessment of the visual fields are indicated. Special protocols exist by which high-resolution images of the sella turcica can be obtained. Such procedures may vary by hospital; providers should discuss with a radiologist how to order such a study for matters of efficiency. Only half of the patients with hyperprolactinemia will have an abnormal imaging study of the anterior pituitary [11]. As the pituitary gland sits just above the optic chiasm, pressure from a prolactinoma can cause visual defects. The classic manifestation is bitemporal

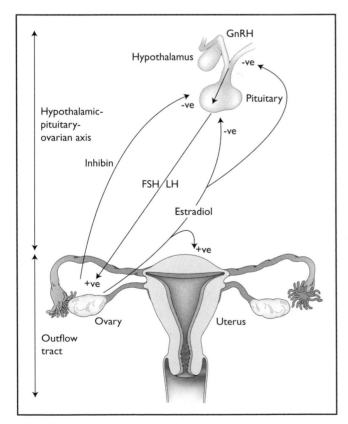

Figure 40-5. Hypothalamic-pituitary-ovarian axis. GnRH—gonadotropin-releasing hormone; FSH—follicle-stimulating hormone; LH—luteinizing hormone.

hemianopia: loss of both temporal visual fields [12]. Referral to an ophthalmologist skilled in such an evaluation is advised. Early detection and aggressive treatment of tumors that cause visual loss are essential to minimize morbidity.

Tumors greater than 10 mm in diameter are referred to as *macroadenomas*; those smaller than 10 mm are referred to as *microadenomas* [13]. First-line therapy for tumors that are not causing a mass effect or visual disturbance is medical. Dopamine agonists, cabergoline or bromocriptine, are the preferred agents. Should a mass effect, visual disturbance or tumor refractory to medication be present, transsphenoidal resection is the next option. Whereas most tumors are indolent and responsive to medical therapy [1], early intervention is essential. Patients need close follow-up; a multidisciplinary approach is appropriate.

Numerous other causes of hyperprolactinemia are also shown in Figure 40-6.

OTHER TUMORS

Other tumors, such as craniopharyngioma, have been known to cause compression of the pituitary stalk. By so doing, GnRH is unable to reach the anterior pituitary and FSH and LH are secreted in subnormal, tonic quantities. CT scan or MRI will diagnose the presence of such a lesion. One would suspect a lesion compressing the stalk of the pituitary in a patient with normal or low serum FSH, LH, and prolactin.

Sheehan's Syndrome

Infarction of the pituitary after obstetric hemorrhage has nearly become a historical entity. Thanks to blood transfusion and improved obstetrical care, hypotension and decreased circulation to the brain are rarely severe enough to cause the pituitary to die. Patients present in the early postpartum period with amenorrhea and failure to lactate.

Empty Sella Syndrome

This condition is a congenital absence of the sellar diaphragm that allows an extension of the subarachnoid space into the pituitary fossa. The pituitary is then separated from the hypothalamus and is flat in appearance. This finding is present in as many as 16% of women with abnormal findings of the sella turcica [14]. These patients will have elevated prolactin levels and may have a concurrent prolactinoma (of note, tumor infarction is one proposed mechanism of empty sella formation) [1]. Serial measurement of serum prolactin and serial radiologic evaluation to rule out the growth of a tumor is the recommended course of action. Treatment for these patients depends on the presence or absence of a prolactinoma. If absent, only hormonal regulation of menses is needed. If present, medical and/or surgical therapy for the prolactinoma is needed.

DISORDERS OF THE THYROID

Hypothyroidism is the most common thyroid state that leads to amenorrhea; though hyperthyroidism may cause it as well. TSH will be higher than normal in the former and lower than normal in the latter. The mechanism by which amenorrhea occurs in hypothyroidism has to do with the interaction between thyrotropin-releasing hormone (TRH) and the abnormal levels of TSH. As there is no thyroid hormone

being produced to negatively feedback upon the hypothalamus, TRH secretion continues in a tonic, unopposed fashion. TRH has a stimulatory effect on the anterior pituitary and thus increases prolactin. Note that the level of hyperprolactinemia is generally mild [1]. With the hormonal milieu out of balance in this fashion, ovulation and menstruation are not possible.

When a patient's TSH is abnormal, the work-up should then proceed to determine the cause of hyper- or hypothyroidism. In patients with concomitantly elevated prolactin levels, imaging of the brain remains appropriate as the stimulatory effects of TRH can lead to hyperplasia and growth of the pituitary gland. Once the thyroid disorder is corrected, this growth of the pituitary disappears, and no further treatment is necessary.

Causes of Hyperprolactinemia

Hypothalamic (through decreased hypothalamic dopamine secretion)

Trauma (stress, surgery, general anesthesia)

Hypothalamic tumors (craniopharyngioma-hamartomas)

Infectious lesions (gumma, tuberculoma, idiopathic meningoencephalitis)

Pituitary (through increased prolactin secretion)

Prolactin-secreting adenomas

Nonfunctioning adenomas

Empty sella syndrome (carotid artery aneurysm, obstruction of the aqueduct of Sylvius)

Pituitary compression

Other space-occupying lesions (gumma and tuberculoma)

Hypothyroidism (through increased thyroid-stimulating hormone, which acts as a pituitary prolactin-secreting factor)

Chest wall trauma (same neuroendocrine mechanism as prolactin release during suckling)

Chest surgery

Trauma

Burns

Herpes zoster virus infection

Breast manipulation, breast reduction, or augmentation

Renal failure (decreased clearance of prolactin)

Drugs (through depletion of dopamine or receptor blocking)

Antipsychotic medications

Anticonvulsant medications

Hormonal contraceptives

Gonadotropin-releasing hormone agonists

Antidepressants

Antihypertensives such as reserpine and methyldopa

Pregnancy (through dopamine-independent amniotic membrane prolactin release)

Figure 40-6. Causes of hyperprolactinemia.

Hypothalamic and Other Systemic Disorders

HYPOTHALAMIC AMENORRHEA

Hypothalamic amenorrhea is essentially a diagnosis of exclusion. As the normal levels of GnRH are highly variable and dependent on the time of day they are measured, checking serum levels in a patient with amenorrhea will add no useful information for her clinical care. In the presence of low circulating gonadotropins and prolactin, normal thyroid function, imaging studies, and physical examination, the hypothalamus is the only remaining culprit.

Hypothalamic amenorrhea is usually a cause of secondary, rather than primary, amenorrhea. It is most commonly a result of physical or psychological stress. Whereas the other hormonal markers are depressed (FSH, LH, prolactin), cortisol is elevated [15]. The hypothesized mechanism of amenorrhea is from corticotropin-releasing hormone direct inhibition of GnRH in the hypothalamus.

Stressors like frustration with work, a move, a divorce, or marriage are not uncommonly associated with temporary amenorrhea. Medical therapy is not necessary for these patients. However, identification of underlying psychiatric pathology, such as major depression or bipolar disorder, is essential.

Extreme, intense exercise regimens can also lead to hypothalamic amenorrhea. Young athletes and dancers are particularly prone to this problem. Physical stress combined with low body weight and low body fat mass lead to amenorrhea among these women.

Anorexia nervosa and bulimia may also lead to amenorrhea. The mortality rate associated with these diagnoses is significant (5% to 15%) [16]; they are potentially fatal illnesses that deserve close attention and specialist treatment. The mechanism of amenorrhea in these cases is similar to the corticotropin-releasing hormone–mediated pathways described earlier. Once again, other medical disorders must be ruled out before reaching this conclusion.

POLYCYSTIC OVARIAN SYNDROME

Polycystic ovarian syndrome (PCOS) is a diagnosis whose characteristics and defining criteria have gone through numerous permutations over the past three decades. Originally, the diagnosis was based on infertility complaints, later upon abnormal hormonal milieu as evidenced by FSH/LH ratios. In order to make categorization of these patients more uniform and to include the most appropriate spectrum of patients affected by PCOS, the American Society for Reproductive Medicine and the European Society for Human Reproduction and Embryology have issued the following guidelines for the diagnosis of PCOS [17]. A patient is diagnosed with PCOS if she has any two of the following three symptoms or findings: 1) clinical or laboratory evidence of oligo- or anovulation, 2) clinical or biochemical signs of hyperandrogenism, and 3) sonographic evidence of polycystic ovaries.

In the context of the current discussion, amenorrhea represents clinical evidence of anovulation. During a normal, ovulatory menstrual cycle, the feedback loops that trigger menses are, in part, mediated by events surrounding ovulation [1]. Adequate follicular development requires a decrease in circulating levels of estrogen. Most of the patients with PCOS are overweight or obese. Peripheral adipose tissue is able to convert androstenedione to estrogen, providing an extragonadal source of hormone that disrupts the ovulatory cycle [18].

Clinical signs of hyperandrogenism are sufficient to make a diagnosis of PCOS in a patient with amenorrhea. Signs of virilization include male pattern baldness, acne (especially of the chest and back), coarse facial hair, and male escutcheon. Whereas these symptoms may seem merely cosmetic, they are an indication of endocrinopathy. If no clinical signs are present, total serum testosterone and dehydroepiandrosterone sulfate can be checked. Note that the valuable test in this case is the total testosterone and dehydroepiandrosterone sulfate. Patients with PCOS will have abnormal levels of sex hormone binding globulin as well; thus the free fractions of the hormones may appear to be lower than they actually are.

The polycystic appearing ovary has a classic "string of pearls" appearance. It is defined as the presence of 10 or more follicles of 2 mm to 8 mm in diameter arranged around the periphery of one or both ovaries [11]. These small, undeveloped follicles are the consequence of sustained periods of anovulation. They are not associated with pelvic pain symptoms, are not of malignant potential, and do not require any surgical intervention. If a patient has this finding on ultrasound, special care should be taken to ensure that she understands these facts.

The role of ultrasound in the diagnosis of PCOS is a topic of debate in the literature [20]. Although the ultrasonographic appearance of a polycystic ovary remains one of the diagnostic criteria, use of ultrasound alone to establish the diagnosis of PCOS is discouraged [1]. In a patient with clinical findings consistent with PCOS who has no other pelvic symptoms, pelvic ultrasound will add little to her management. The cost and anxiety associated with additional testing outweigh the utility of this test in this scenario. However, if a provider believes a patient has an indication for a pelvic sonogram, referral to a gynecologist or radiologist who is skilled in the performance and interpretation of transvaginal sonography is recommended.

IATROGENIC AMENORRHEA

Numerous drugs are associated with amenorrhea. Foremost are contraceptives. Some patients taking 28-day, cyclic, combined oral contraceptives will have no withdrawal bleeding. The incidence depends on the formulation and duration of use [21]. If a patient presents with this complaint, pregnancy should be excluded. If she is not pregnant, she can be reassured that such an occurrence is a benign side effect. Progestin-only methods, depomedroxyprogesterone acetate, progestin-only pills, and levonorgestrel-containing intrauterine devices are also associated with amenorrhea. A patient's perception of this side effect can vary from joy to absolute disdain. Her preferences for periodic withdrawal bleeding (monthly, every 3 months, or none at all) should be considered when selecting a contraceptive method. Switching pill formulation, increasing estrogen dose, or adding 0.3 mg of conjugated equine estrogen daily in the week before the scheduled withdrawal bleed (days 14–21 of a 28-day cycle) may help regulate the withdrawal bleed.

GnRH analogs, most commonly used to treat endometriosis, are also associated with amenorrhea. The duration of the associated amenorrhea is dependent on dose, frequency of injection, and duration of use. Most women will return to normal menstrual function with 3 to 4 months of their last use of the drug. Older women may experience longer delays in returning to normal menses as their reserve levels of ovarian estrogen are significantly lower than young women.

Numerous psychotropic drugs are known to interfere with menstrual function. The action of this side effect is likely central in nature, as the hypothalamic-pituitary axis is dependent on dopamine for proper regulation. Anticonvulsant medications have also been implicated in the development of amenorrhea. Once other causes for amenorrhea have been excluded, an exhaustive drug history should be obtained to identify any potential agents that could be causing amenorrhea.

Approach to the Patient with Amenorrhea

To differentiate the cause of amenorrhea, a systematic approach based upon the compartment system outlined above will ensure a complete, cost effective, and accurate work-up. The most common cause of amenorrhea is pregnancy. As such, a pregnancy test is the first diagnostic test to consider. A urine pregnancy test is sufficient, as high-sensitivity pregnancy tests available on the market are sensitive to serum levels of beta-human chorionic gonadotropin in the range of 25 mIU. If the pregnancy test is negative, then the work-up should proceed compartment by compartment to rule out pathology.

PRIMARY AMENORRHEA

Figure 40-7 depicts the diagnostic approach to patients with primary amenorrhea. Foremost, the patient's history is important. Is this primary or secondary amenorrhea? If it is primary, anomalies of the outflow tract, genetic anomalies, and enzyme deficiencies become more suspect than in a patient with secondary amenorrhea. In the patient with primary amenorrhea and a negative pregnancy test, a thorough pelvic examination is necessary to rule out obstructions or anomalies of the outflow tract. Regardless of the findings on the physical examination, a pelvic ultrasound is nonetheless indicated to evaluate the size and shape of the ovaries and character of the uterus

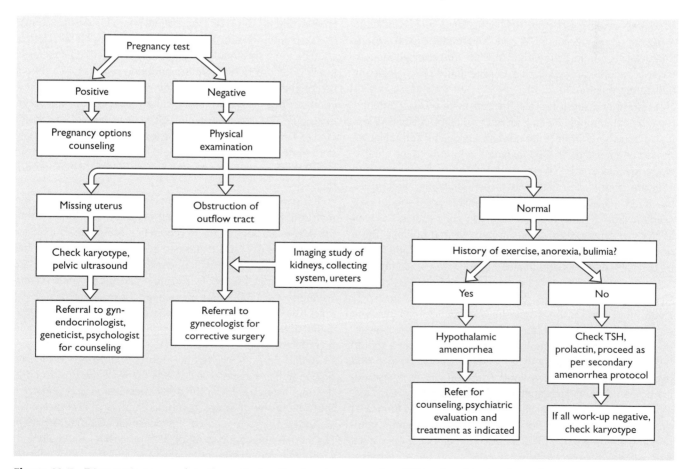

Figure 40-7. Diagnostic approach to the patient with primary amenorrhea. TSH—thyroid-stimulating hormone.

and endometrial cavity. If anomalies of the reproductive tract are noted, further work-up of the genitourinary system is indicated. Intravenous pyelography or a CT scan with contrast to evaluate the kidneys, collecting system, and bladder should be the next step in the management of the patient.

If the pelvic examination in a patient with primary amenorrhea is normal, proceed to note whether or not other secondary sex characteristics have developed. If the breasts have developed, and pubic and axillary hair are present, genetic anomalies like Turner syndrome, testicular feminization, and heritable defects in enzymes are less likely. If breast development or pubic and axillary hair are abnormal, the next step in management should be to order a karyotype. The karyotype is essential at this stage to rule out the presence of a Y chromosome (as in testicular feminization, mosaicism or female pseudohermaphroditism in the case of an enzyme deficiency). This is essential, as most of these patients will need to have a gonadectomy following puberty due to the increased risk of developing malignancy.

Moreover, psychologic counseling concerning sexual identity and future fertility is best begun at the earliest stages of diagnosis. This should involve the patient and her parents as appropriate. Delivering such a diagnosis is never easy and should be done with the assistance of a professional who is experienced in the field, as the patient and her family members will invariably have many questions once the diagnosis is explained. The provider should feel comfortable to discuss the pathology, prognosis, possibility for future fertility, and necessary treatments before delivering such serious news to a patient. Proper preparation and collaboration with experts is crucial to minimize the chances that this clinical encounter will become an awkward and potentially psychologically damaging situation.

Exercise and stress can also be causes of primary amenorrhea, but should only be considered as diagnosis of exclusion. If all of the above findings are normal, a prolactin and TSH level should be checked. An FSH level will add little to the clinical diagnosis and in this patient is not necessary. If prolactin and TSH are normal, the diagnosis of hypothalamic amenorrhea has been made. Diagnostic inquiry at this point should proceed towards carefully focused history to elicit stressors as well as signs or symptoms of anorexia nervosa and bulimia. These disorders have a higher incidence among teenagers and should be carefully ruled out and treated appropriately if identified.

SECONDARY AMENORRHEA

Figure 40-8 depicts the diagnostic approach to patients with secondary amenorrhea. If the patient's pregnancy test is negative, and the physical examination is normal, two tests should be ordered: prolactin and TSH. Hyperprolactinemia and hypothyroidism are the two most common causes of secondary amenorrhea in such a patient. If the prolactin is elevated, work-up should proceed with imaging of the sella turcica as described above to rule out a pituitary lesion or tumor compressing the stalk of the pituitary. Also remember, if the patient has complaints of headache or if a mass is noted on imaging, an ophthalmologic evaluation of the visual fields is needed. If

the TSH is abnormal, the thyroid gland should be examined, worked up, and treated appropriately.

If the patient's TSH and prolactin are normal, the next test to consider is a progestin challenge test (Figure 40-9). Essentially, this test is checking whether or not the patient is producing estrogen and if there is an occult obstruction of the outflow tract. The patient is given progestin (medroxyprogesterone) for 10 days and then told to observe for vaginal bleeding afterwards. If she has bleeding, this is evidence that her body is, indeed, producing estrogen. If she has no bleeding, that means that she is not producing estrogen or has an occult obstruction of the outflow tract. To differentiate between these two, a combined hormonal challenge test is administered. A low-dose combination oral contraceptive is administered for 7 days, and the patient again monitors vaginal bleeding afterward. If there is bleeding, this proves an intact outflow tract. If there is not bleeding, this is suspicious for an occult obstruction of the outflow tract (ie, Asherman's syndrome). At this point, the patient should have an examination under anesthesia and hysteroscopy to rule out occult lesions.

The next test to order is an FSH level. FSH may be ordered at an earlier stage if the patient describes menopause-like symptoms associated with amenorrhea. If the patient had a withdrawal bleed with progestin alone and has a normal FSH, this is indicative of anovulation. If she had a withdrawal bleed only with combined hormonal challenge, and her FSH is high, this is indicative of premature ovarian failure. Note that FSH levels may be "borderline" elevated in either of these patients. Should this be the case, the patient's fertility desires should be taken into account to guide further therapy. If she desires child bearing, she should be referred to an infertility specialist. If she does not desire fertility, hormone replacement should be commenced. This can be accomplished with low-dose oral contraceptives or other combined hormonal replacement regimens. At this stage, an autoimmune work-up should be considered. A serum assay for antinuclear antibodies is an adequate start. Further costly work-up should be reserved for patients in whom there are other associated findings suggestive of autoimmune disease.

If a patient with secondary amenorrhea has otherwise normal testing, consideration should be given to PCOS. Recall the American Society for Reproductive Medicine criteria for the diagnosis of PCOS (Figure 40-10). The patient already has one sign, amenorrhea, which is evidence of anovulation. So, if she has clinical signs of virilization (facial hair, male pattern baldness, chest hair, male escutcheon, or excessive acne), the diagnosis of PCOS is made. If these signs are absent, an ultrasound to evaluate the ovaries for polycystic appearance should be ordered.

Again, the patient's fertility desires should be considered first once the diagnosis of PCOS is made. If she desires child bearing, a referral to an infertility specialist is appropriate at this time. If she does not, combined hormonal contraceptives should be begun to regulate the menstrual cycle. If the patient has a contraindication to estrogen, a progestin-only method or levonorgestrel-containing intrauterine device may be placed. This is important as these patients are at substantially increased risk for endometrial hyperplasia, a precursor to endometrial cancer. Hormonal therapy will decrease this risk. Patients should also begin treatment with metformin. Metformin has several benefits for these individuals. Foremost, it improves their insulin sensitivity and may lessen the likelihood of developing overt diabetes. Second, it will assist weight loss. Third, it will assist menstrual cycle control.

Periodic surveillance of patients with PCOS should include measurement of fasting glucose and an oral glucose tolerance test. As these individuals are at a substantially increased risk for developing diabetes, they should be counseled to modify their diet and lifestyle to decrease any factors associated with cardiovascular risk. Though this statement could be applied to all patients, it carries special significance for this group of patients as they are predisposed to develop risk factors associated with cardiovascular disease [22].

If all other work-up is normal, the diagnosis of hypothalamic amenorrhea is made. As mentioned above, evaluation for environmental stressors, anorexia and bulimia should be pursued. If this is negative as well, the provider may consider

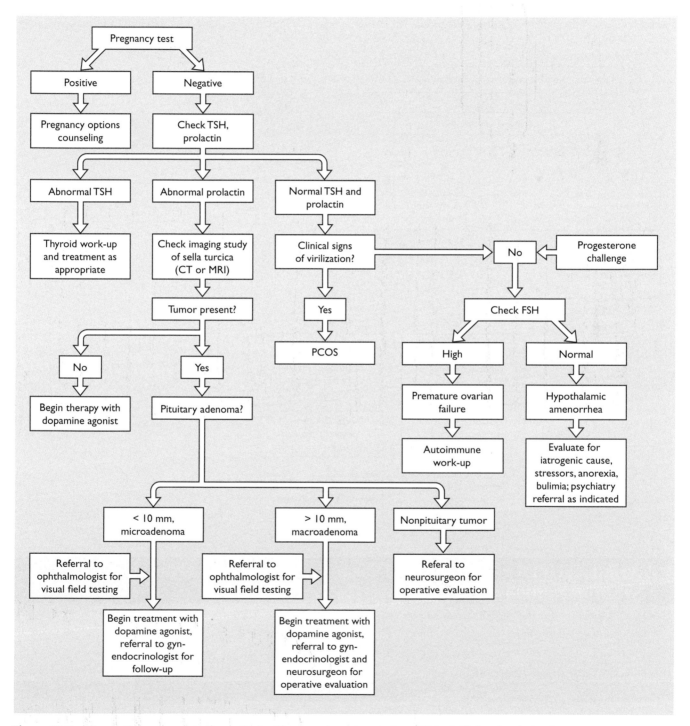

Figure 40-8. Diagnostic approach to the patient with secondary amenorrhea. FSH—follicle-stimulating hormone; PCOS—polycystic ovarian syndrome; TSH—thyroid-stimulating hormone.

ordering a karyotype. Most karyotypic anomalies would have made themselves apparent earlier in this exhaustive work-up. However, atypical presentations are not unheard of and should be at the back of the clinician's mind during evaluation.

Summary

Amenorrhea is a common presenting complaint among women of reproductive age. Most of the time, a pregnancy test, a thorough physical examination and measurement of serum TSH and prolactin are adequate to establish a diagnosis. The major-

ity of the causes of amenorrhea are benign in nature. However, tumors of the central nervous system, genetic anomalies, and conditions that predispose to the development of malignancy or coronary artery disease in the future are not unheard of. Given this, a provider should take a systematic approach to each patient who presents with this complaint in order to ferret out the root cause of amenorrhea for each patient. Never assume the simplest, benign explanation is the case.

Having a ready network for referral to specialist counselors and gynecologists skilled in endocrine anomalies and assisted reproduction is essential to the care of the patient. Such infrastructure should be in place prior to handling these complaints.

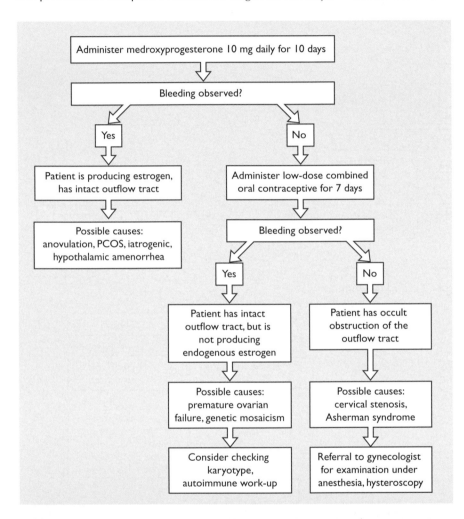

Figure 40-9. The progesterone challenge test.

ASRM/ESHRE Criteria for the Diagnosis of Polycystic Ovarian Syndrome: 2003

A patient is diagnosed with polycystic ovarian syndrome if she has two of the following:

1. Clinical or laboratory evidence of anovulation

2. Clinical or laboratory evidence of hyperandrogenism

3. Polycystic appearing ovaries on ultrasound*

*Ten or more peripheral follicles of 2 to 8 mm in diameter in one or both ovaries.

Figure 40-10. American Society for Reproductive Medicine/ European Society for Human Reproduction and Embryology (ASRM/ESHRE) criteria for the diagnosis of polycystic ovarian syndrome.

Therapies should always be directed to address the underlying pathology, while doing one's utmost to observe the patient's immediate and future desires for child bearing. Lastly, identification of serious underlying pathology must be immediately coupled with appropriate follow-up and routine health surveillance to care for the patient as a whole. Though her presenting complaint may be gynecologic, the underlying problem may be found in another system entirely.

References

Papers of particular interest have been highlighted as follows:
- Of interest
- • Of outstanding interest

1. Speroff L, Glass R, Kase N: *Clinical Gynecologic Endocrinology and Infertility*, edn 6. Philadelphia: Lippincott, Williams & Wilkins; 1999.

2. Munster K, Helm P, Schmidt L: Secondary amenorrhea: prevalence and medical contact: a cross-sectional study from a Danish county. *Br J Obstet Gynecol* 1992, 99:430–433.

3.• Nazir Z, Rizvi R, Qureshi R, *et al.*: Congenital vaginal obstructions: varied presentation and outcome. *Ped Surg Int* 2006, 22:749–753.
This article details long-term outcomes of patients with congenital anomalies of the female genital tract. It is one of the few articles that contains outcomes beyond the immediate postoperative period.

4. Sadler TW: *Medical Embryology*, edn 7. Philadelphia: Williams and Wilkins; 1995.

5. Stenchever M, Droegemueller W, Herbst A, Mishell D: *Comprehensive Gynecology*, edn 4. Philadelphia: Mosby; 2001.

6. Rutgers J, Scully R: The androgen insensitivity syndrome (testicular feminization): a clinicopathologic study of 43 cases. *Int J Gynecol Pathol* 1991, 10:126.

7. Griffin J: Androgen resistance- the clinical and molecular spectrum. *N Engl J Med* 1992, 326:611.

8. Al-Inany H: Intrauterine adhesions: an update. *Acta Obstet Gynecol Scand* 2001, 80:986–993.

9. *Steadman's Medical Dictionary*, edn 28. New York: Lippincott, Williams & Wilkins; 2006.

10. Gradishar WJ, Schilsky RL: Ovarian function following ration and chemotherapy. *Semin Oncol* 1989, 16:425.

11. Schlechte J, Sherman B, Halmi N, *et al.*: Prolactin secreting pituitary tumors. *Endocrinol Rev* 1980, 1:295.

12. Fujimoto N, Saeki N, Miyauchi O, Adachi–Usami E: Criteria for early detection of temporal hemianopia in asymptomatic pituitary tumor. *Nature* 2002, 16:731–738.

13. Molitch M, Thorner M, Wilson C: Management of prolactinomas. *J Clin Endocrinol Metab* 1997, 82:996–1000.

14. Speroff L, Levin R, Hanning R, Kase N: A practical approach for the evaluation of women with abnormal polytomography or elevated prolactin levels. *Am J Obstet Gynecol* 1979, 135:896.

15. Berga S, Daniels T, Giles D: Women with functional hypothalamic amenorrhea but not other forms of anovulation display amplified cortisol concentrations. *Fertil Steril* 1997, 67:1024.

16. Sullivan P: Mortality in anorexia nervosa. *Am J Psych* 1995, 152:1073.

17. Revised 2003 consensus on diagnostic criteria and long-term health risks related to polycystic ovary syndrome (PCOS). *Hum Reprod* 2004, 1:41–47.

18. Siiteri P, MacDonald P: Role of extraglandular estrogen in human endocrinology. In *Handbook of Physiology: Section 7, Endocrinology*. Edited by Geyer S, Astwood E, Greep R. Washington, DC: American Physiology Society; 1973.

19. Adams J, Franks S, Polson D, *et al.*: Multifollicular ovaries: clinical and endocrine features and response to pulsatile gonadotropin releasing hormone. *Lancet* 1985, 2:1375–1379.

20. Belosi C, Selvaggi L, Apa R, *et al.*: Is the PCOS diagnosis solved by the ESHRE/ASRM 2003 consensus or could it include ultrasound examination of the ovarian stroma? *Hum Reprod* 2006, 21:3108–3115.

21. *Contraceptive Technology*, edn 18. Edited by Hatcher R, Trussell J, Stewart F, *et al.* New York: Ardent Media; 2004.

22. American College of Obstetricians and Gynecologists: Polycystic ovarian syndrome. ACOG Practice Bulletin. Number 41, December 2002. *Int J Gynaecol Obstet* 2003 80:335–348.

41 Vulvar and Vaginal Dysplasia

Lisa M. Landrum, Kelly L. Molpus, and Todd D. Tillmanns

- Risk factors for vulvar and vaginal dysplasia include a prior or concomitant history of dysplasia at any site of the lower genital tract. Tobacco use, human papillomavirus infection, and chronic immunosuppression are other etiologic factors.
- Liberal use of tissue biopsy of any suspicious vulvar or vaginal lesions is the cornerstone for diagnosis.
- The goal of treatment is to prevent invasive disease and provide symptomatic relief, while preserving normal anatomy and function.
- Treatment modalities in common use include surgical excision, laser ablation, and topical application of 5-fluorouracil. Wide local excision is the treatment of choice in most cases.
- The decision regarding whether to refer depends largely on the experience and comfort level of the primary care provider. Referral should not be delayed if invasive carcinoma is suspected or confirmed.
- Counseling is focused on risk reduction, and clinical care emphasizes early diagnosis and treatment.

Incidence and Epidemiology

VULVAR DYSPLASIA

The incidence of in situ vulvar carcinoma, also called *vulvar intraepithelial neoplasia* (VIN) III, has increased 411% from 0.56 cases per 100,000 women in 1973 to 2.9 cases per 100,000 women in 2000 [1]. Peak incidence is observed in women between 40 to 49 years of age, with a gradual decline thereafter. In younger women, VIN is more likely to be multifocal and associated with human papillomavirus (HPV) subtypes 16, 18, and 31. Increased rates of HPV infection, coupled with expanded screening and detection strategies by physicians, likely contribute to the rise in incidence for a population of younger women. Despite an increase in preinvasive disease, there has been very little change in the epidemiology of vulvar cancer. The incidence has increased modestly with 1.8 cases per 100,000 women in 1973 to 2.2 cases per 100,000 women in 2000 [1]. In addition, although VIN is seen in an increasingly younger population, only 15% of vulvar carcinomas occur in women younger than 40 years [2]. Vulvar cancer remains primarily a disease of postmenopausal women between 65 and 75 years of age. HPV-related invasive vulvar carcinoma is seen in younger women who commonly have adjacent VIN. In older women, the invasive component is less likely to be HPV-related and is often found adjacent to nonneoplastic changes, such as lichen sclerosis.

VAGINAL DYSPLASIA

The incidence of vaginal intraepithelial neoplasia (VAIN) has remained at a steady state in recent years and is estimated to be 0.2 to 0.3 cases per 100,000 women in the United States [3]. Previously VAIN was most commonly noted in the sixth decade of life; however, recent studies suggest the mean age at diagnosis for VAIN, similar to VIN, is getting younger [4]. Invasive vaginal cancer is uncommon with an estimated incidence of 0.42 cases per 100,000 women. The upper third of the vagina is the region most commonly involved, but a field effect exists in the lower female genital tract, such that intraepithelial neoplasia may develop at any site lined by squamous epithelium (Figure 41-1). Accordingly, up to 80% of VAIN cases are associated with prior, concomitant, or subsequent cervical intraepithelial neoplasia (CIN) or VIN [5,6].

In epidemiologic reports, vaginal and vulvar carcinomas are typically grouped together with gestational trophoblastic disease and fallopian tube carcinoma as "other and unspecified gynecologic neoplasms" making separate analysis difficult [7••].

Pathophysiology

VULVAR DYSPLASIA

Vulvar intraepithelial neoplasia is graded as mild (VIN I), moderate (VIN II), or severe (VIN III) based on the depth of epithelial involvement. Carcinoma in situ or VIN III involves the full thickness of the epithelium, but does not invade the basement membrane. This grading system is parallel to that established for CIN and proposes that a continuum exists from preinvasive to invasive disease; however, the data that suggest a clear progression from VIN to vulvar cancer is less compelling than those for the cervix. A multifactorial etiology is probable, given that vulvar HPV infections are common, whereas intraepithelial neoplasia occurs much less frequently. HPV type 16 DNA is detected in up to 90% of cases of severe vulvar dysplasia. In addition, patients with a history of genital warts have an increased risk of VIN III and invasive carcinoma [8,9].

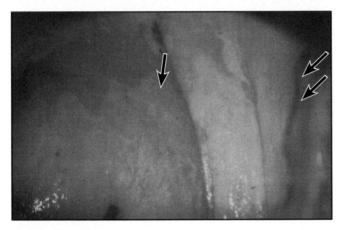

Figure 41-1. Dysplastic field defect in squamous mucosa shown by acetowhite epithelium of the cervix (*arrow*) and vagina (*double arrow*). Cervical os can be seen (*black*; *left of center*).

Based on morphologic features, grade 3 VIN lesions are classified into three types: warty (condylomatous), basaloid (usual type), and differentiated (simplex type) [10]. Grossly, the warty type is characterized by an undulating or irregular raised surface and is usually found in HPV-infected, younger women. A relatively flat, smooth surface with a thickened epithelium is seen more often in the basaloid and differentiated types, which are more common in older women. Histologically, warty lesions have large cells with nuclear pleomorphism, mitotic figures, and surface keratinocytes with koilocytes and multinucleation. Basaloid lesions are composed of atypical, immature parabasal-type cells with numerous mitoses and, less often, koilocytes. Differentiated-type lesions contain basal or parabasal cells with eosinophilic cytoplasm, enlarged nuclei, and prominent nucleoli. Superficial layers have normal maturation but may contain mild nuclear atypia. These histologic types may occur solely or in combination as a mixed pattern [10]. The relationships to malignancy are outlined herewith (Figure 41-2 and Figure 41-3) [11–13].

The natural history of VIN similar to CIN follows a pattern of persistence, potentially leading to cancer versus regression [14,15]. van Seters *et al.* [15] discovered that 9% of untreated cases of vulvar dysplasia would progress to cancer without treatment over 1 to 8 years. The recurrence rate of VIN after treatment can be as high as 46% to 70%, with positive margin status increasing the likelihood of recurrence [16]. Risk of recurrence also may be related to the multifocal nature of this disease. Long-term surveillance is required. Surveillance methods can be improved by educating patients to perform self-examination with vinegar on a monthly basis as well as recognize symptoms of persistent dysplasia or cancer.

VAGINAL DYSPLASIA

Similar to VIN, a grading system from I to III is implemented to describe preinvasive lesions of the vagina. A prior abnormal Papanicolaou smear, genital warts, and early hysterectomy

Comparison of Classic Vulvar Intraepithelial Neoplasia to Simplex

Distinctions	Classic VIN	Simplex
Age	30–40 years old	Older
Subclassification	Warty (condylomatous); basaloid (undifferentiated)	
HPV associated	Yes	No
Local recurrence	7%–32% (occult malignancy 6%–20%)	Greater potential for progression
Smoker	Yes (60%–80%)	Yes (25%)
Associated with parakeratosis	No	Yes
Condyloma, HSV, and HIV more common	Yes	No
Multifocal	Yes (20%–50%)	Can be, but less often
P53-positive cells	No	Yes

Figure 41-2. Comparison of classic vulvar intraepithelial neoplasia (VIN) to simplex. HPV—human papillomavirus; HSV—herpes simplex virus.

have been identified as risk factors for VAIN. It is unknown whether vaginal cancer has a preclinical phase that could be detected by screening, or if all invasive cancers begin with an in situ phase. At present, there is no way to predict accurately the clinical behavior of VAIN lesions. Regression of VAIN has been demonstrated in some cases, but others have progressed to invasive cancer. Combined results of two studies addressing the natural history of VAIN in 35 women showed disease regression in 24 (68%), persistent disease in nine (26%), and progression to invasive cancer in two (6%) [6,17].

Differential Diagnosis

DIFFERENTIAL DIAGNOSIS OF VULVAR LESIONS

Among the most commonly seen vulvar lesions are nonneoplastic dermatoses such as lichen sclerosis and lichen planus. The most common symptom is pruritis, which is often severe, resulting in scratching and subsequent ulceration. On examination, lichen sclerosis is characterized by thin, hypopigmented skin that is classically described as parchment-like. Lichen sclerosis is often found in a distribution encompassing the vulvar and perianal areas. The labia minora may atrophy beyond recognition, and introital stenosis may occur. Microscopic features include hyperkeratosis, flattening of the rete pegs, and cytoplasmic vacuolization of the basal layer. Lichen planus is less common and is characterized by erosive, erythematous lesions originating in the vestibule and extending up the vaginal canal. If left untreated, agglutination of the labia and vagina may result, producing significant dyspareunia. Other dermatoses include the entire spectrum of skin disorders, such as contact dermatitis, infective dermatitis including *Candida* and tinea, psoriasis, and lichen simplex chronicus [18].

Pigmented lesions account for approximately 10% of all vulvar lesions, the most common of which is lentigo. Pigmentation is derived from a concentration of melanocytes in the basal cell layer. Although rare, melanoma is the second most common primary vulvar malignancy (2%) [19]. Characteristics that should raise suspicion of melanoma include asymmetry, irregular borders, color variation, change in size or shape of nevi, bleeding, diameter greater than 6 mm, and pruritus [20•]. Excisional biopsy of a pigmented lesion needs no additional therapy if it is a nevus of junctional, compound, or intradermal type. Special attention is also paid to areas of induration, ulceration, fissures, and to elevated lesions. Paget disease of the vulva is most often an intraepithelial lesion, but investigation to exclude an underlying adenocarcinoma is necessary. Basal cell carcinoma may present as a waxy, scar-like nodule or as papules with a smooth, pearly appearance [20•].

Biopsy confirmation of diagnosis is mandatory before any extended medical treatment. When premalignant and malignant lesions have been ruled out, medical therapy to alleviate symptoms is initiated. High potency corticosteroids such as clobetasol have proven most effective in treating lichen sclerosis and may provide enhanced therapeutic benefit with reduced side effects.

DIFFERENTIAL DIAGNOSIS OF VAGINAL LESIONS

Vaginal intraepithelial neoplasia is generally asymptomatic but occasionally causes postcoital bleeding or vaginal discharge. A frequently encountered patient profile is a woman who has undergone prior hysterectomy for high-grade CIN. The clinical appearance of VAIN is varied and may include subtle or striking areas of leukoplakia, erythematous mucosa (Figure 41-4), or acetowhite lesions with increased vascularity. Punctation (colposcopic visualization of small vessels on end) is more common in VAIN than is mosaicism (colposcopic visualization of small vessels longitudinally). Suspicion for invasive disease increases as the vascular atypia worsens from punctation to mosaicism to atypical vessels. Atypical vascularity is the primary harbinger of invasive carcinoma [7••].

Atrophy of the postmenopausal vaginal epithelium is a frequent cause of VAIN-like changes on Papanicolaou smear. A trial of local or systemic estrogen therapy will often resolve abnormal cytologic findings. Follow-up Papanicolaou smear and colposcopic examination should be performed in several months versus HPV testing. Lesions suspicious for invasive carcinoma should undergo biopsy at the initial visit to avoid delay

Two Etiologic Types of Vulvar Carcinoma: Vulvar Intraepithelial Neoplasia and Basaloid/Warty and Keratinizing

Distinctions	VIN and Basaloid/Warty	Keratinizing
Age	Variable	Older women: 70–80 years old
VIN associated	Yes	No
HPV associated	Yes (75%–100%)	No (2%–23%)
Two or more sexual partners	81%	43%
Smoker	94%	29%
Associated with lichen sclerosis	No	Yes (present 25%–60%)
Condyloma, HSV, and HIV more common	Yes	No
Multifocal	Yes (15%–50%)	No

Figure 41-3. Two etiologic types of vulvar carcinoma: vulvar intraepithelial neoplasia (VIN) and basaloid/warty and keratinizing. HPV—human papillomavirus; HSV—herpes simplex virus.

in diagnosis. Endometriosis may present as a vaginal lesion, but the marked variation in clinical presentation requires biopsy for confirmation (Figure 41-5).

Possible causes of vaginal erythema, ulceration or discharge may be of infectious etiology such as *Candida*, bacterial vaginosis, *Chlamydia*, *Trichomonas*, or herpes simplex virus or foreign body reaction. Treatment for infectious etiology is with the appropriate antibiotic, antifungal, or antiviral medication.

DIAGNOSTIC STUDIES

A thorough history and physical examination are the basis of diagnostic evaluation. Liberal use of biopsies for all suspicious areas to establish histopathologic diagnosis cannot be overemphasized. Topical cleansing with povidone-iodine (Betadine) solution and local infiltration of lidocaine provide adequate preparation. Small lesions can be completely removed using techniques of wide local excision (Figure 41-6). Large, diffuse, or multifocal lesions may be sampled using variously sized punch biopsies (Figure 41-7) that provide 2- to 6-mm diameter tissue

samples. Vaginal biopsy samples are best obtained using tissue biopsy forceps (eg, Eppendorfer or Kevorkian biopsy forceps). After biopsy, hemostasis may be acquired by application of silver nitrate, Monsel's solution (ferric subsulfate), or direct pressure. DiSaia and Creasman [21] use a Keyes punch to remove a piece of Gelfoam that is placed in the biopsy defect and covered with a sterile dressing for 24 hours.

Vulvar Lesions

Vulvar examination is carried out in bright light because clinically significant lesions can usually be seen on gross examination. Visualization may be enhanced by the addition of acetic acid or toluidine blue or by shaving the vulva. Only dilute acetic acid solution should be used (3%–5%), because glacial (nondilute) acetic acid causes severe burns. Acetic acid may need to be left in place for 5 minutes or longer to enhance visualization of all lesions. This dehydrates dysplastic cells, which have relatively less cytoplasm than normal cells, and results in acetowhite epithelial changes (Figure 41-8). Toluidine blue 1% aqueous solution may be applied and allowed to dry for 2 to 3 minutes, then cleansed with 1% to 2% acetic acid solution. Areas suspicious for increased mitotic activity stain a royal blue, in contrast to normal skin, which is relatively unstained. High false-positive and false-negative rates occur in situations of excoriation and hyperkeratosis, respectively [20•].

Lesions may be present at any site on the vulvar region; the most commonly affected areas are the labia minora, perineum, and clitoral hood. The anal mucosa is involved with intraepithelial neoplasia in approximately 20% of women with VIN [22•]. Anoscopy may be necessary to evaluate extension into the anal canal. An algorithm for the evaluation of vulvar lesions is provided in Figure 41-9.

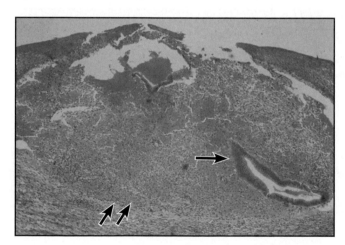

Figure 41-4. Vaginal carcinoma in situ presenting as a friable, erythematous lesion on gross examination (*arrows*).

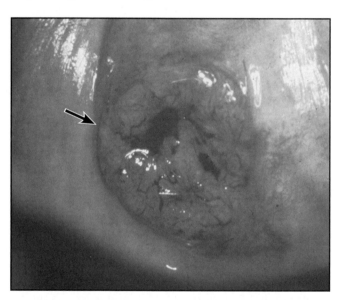

Figure 41-5. Vaginal endometriosis with ectopic endometrial glands (*arrow*) and stroma (*double arrows*).

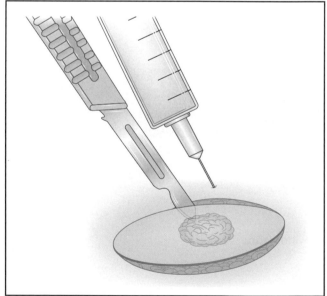

Figure 41-6. Wide local excisional biopsy technique.

Vaginal Lesions

Evaluation includes visual inspection, Papanicolaou smear of the vaginal apex, and colposcopy with directed biopsies of all suspicious areas. VAIN lesions tend to be multifocal, necessitating inspection of the entire vaginal mucosal surface. Examination and colposcopy should include rotation of the speculum because anterior and posterior lesions can be obscured by standard speculum placement. Addition of dilute acetic acid (Figure 41-10) or Lugol's solution may be used to enhance visibility. Glycogen-rich vaginal epithelium stains dark on application of Lugol's solution, whereas dysplastic epithelium resists staining.

Visibility of all mucosal surfaces is often more difficult in the posthysterectomy patient because of deep angles at the vaginal apex. Speculum manipulation, skin hooks, forceps, and dental mirrors are among the suggested assistance techniques used in an effort to visualize all tissue surfaces [21]. Multifocal sampling is imperative because of the multifocal nature of VAIN. On gross inspection, erythema, thickened epithelium, and ulcerations raise suspicion for invasive disease. On colposcopic examination, abnormal vascular patterns are highly associated with invasive carcinoma. Currently, there is no role for routine laboratory testing or radiographic imaging in the diagnostic evaluation of preinvasive vulvar and vaginal lesions. An algorithm for the evaluation of vaginal lesions is given in Figure 41-11.

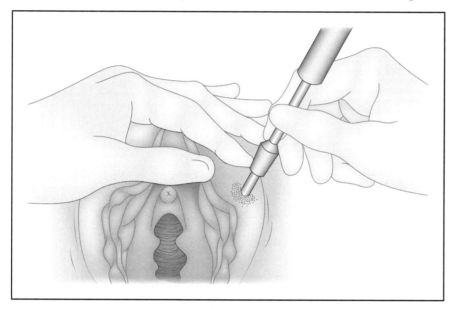

Figure 41-7. Punch biopsy technique.

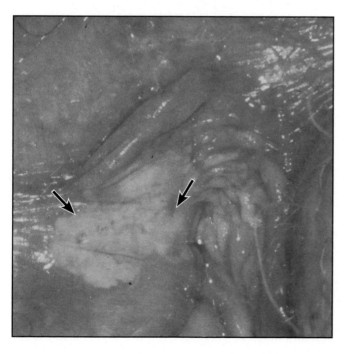

Figure 41-8. Acetowhite changes of high-grade vulvar intraepithelial neoplasia (*arrows*).

Treatment

VULVAR INTRAEPITHELIAL NEOPLASIA

The goal of treatment is to prevent invasive disease and relieve symptoms, while preserving normal anatomy and function. Surgical excision of the affected area is the mainstay of treatment because most lesions are amenable to excision. A wide local excision should include a disease-free border of at least 5 mm. The principal advantage over destructive therapy or chemotherapy is that excision provides a biopsy specimen of the entire lesion for complete histopathologic assessment. This prevents inadequate treatment of an unrecognized invasive lesion, which has been reported with a rate near 20% within a field of VIN III [23]. The vulvar skin and underlying tissue are lax and usually permit primary reapproximation, even after extensive resection.

Despite removal of up to 1 cm of normal-appearing surrounding skin and mucosa, the resected specimen margins often are involved (Figure 41-12). Recurrence rates are significantly higher with multifocal disease and with margins positive for intraepithelial neoplasia, in which the recurrence rate approximates 50% [22•]. Accordingly, some clinicians advocate liberal use of frozen-section analysis to assess margin status. An intraoperative finding of marginal extension would necessitate additional resection.

Many physicians consider laser therapy the treatment of choice, especially in the setting of multifocal disease. The

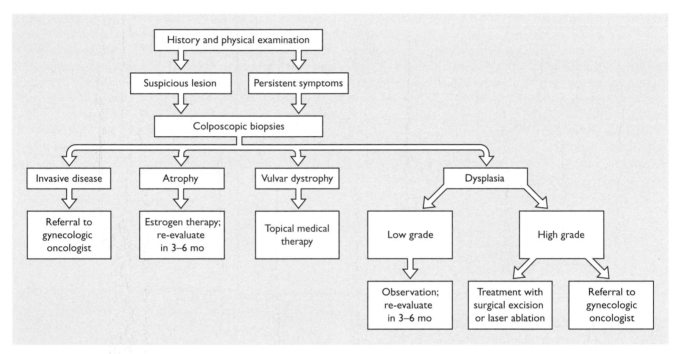

Figure 41-9. Algorithm for evaluation of vulvar lesions.

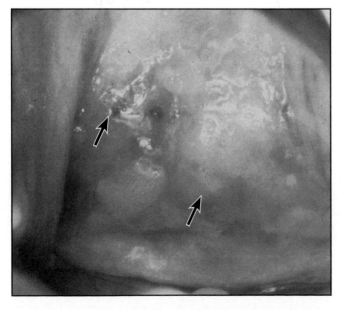

Figure 41-10. Acetowhite changes of high-grade vaginal intraepithelial neoplasia (*arrows*).

carbon dioxide laser is well suited for ablation of vulvovaginal lesions. The greatest benefit to laser vaporization is the ability to conserve the anatomy near the urethra, clitoris, and perianal areas. Benedet et al. [24] evaluated 122 women with severe VIN and found the mean thickness of vulvar epithelium to be 0.52 mm (range, 0.1–1.9 mm). Only 19 cases had skin appendageal involvement. In cases of dysplasia extending into hair follicles, the mean depth of involvement was 1.9 mm (range, 1.0–3.4 mm) (Figure 41-13). Based on their findings, 1-mm depth of destruction for nonhair-bearing epithelium is considered adequate treatment, and 2.5- to 3-mm depth is required if skin appendages are involved [24]. These depths correspond to the first three laser surgical planes defined by Reid [25]. Nonhair-bearing skin may be treated to the first or second plane, composed of surface epithelium with basement membrane, and dermal papillae, respectively. Healing is rapid, with good cosmetic results. Involvement of epithelial skin appendages requires ablation into the third plane. This affects the upper and middle reticular areas containing pilosebaceous ducts. Destruction of deeper tissues is not necessary with VIN and would result in delayed healing with increased scar formation.

Pain during initial postlaser healing is the primary complaint. Therapy is directed at symptomatic relief and adequate healing. Perineal care includes frequent sitz baths—two to three times daily—and vulvar rinsing, followed by drying the area with a hair dryer. We have found that patients have decreased burning during urination if they simultaneously irrigate the vulvar area with water. Topical corticosteroids, silvadine cream, or both, with topical and systemic analgesics, provide additional relief. Analgesia is especially important during the first 3 to 4 days after treatment, which is when discomfort is most intense.

Medical management of VIN with modalities such as 5-fluorouracil, corticosteroids, interferons, photodynamic therapy, and immune modulators is an attractive option particularly given the rising incidence in younger women; however, the results at present have been less successful compared with excision.

5-Fluorouracil is generally effective in 40% to 75% of cases with VIN [26,27]. Imiquimod cream (Aldara; Graceway Pharmaceuticals, Bristol, TN) is a cream that can be applied to the vulvar area weekly or 3 times weekly. The mechanism of action is an immune response modifier that stimulates cytokine production from local macrophages and upregulates T cells and NK cells. It is US Food and Drug Administration approved for the treatment of external genital and perianal warts/condyloma acuminata in individuals 12 years old and older. In one study, the cream was self-administered three times per week for periods of 6 to 34 weeks, with remission in 29% to 43% of patients [28].

Prevention: Prophylactic Vaccine

All forms of genital dysplasia are related to infection with HPV. Seventy-five percent to 80% of sexually active women

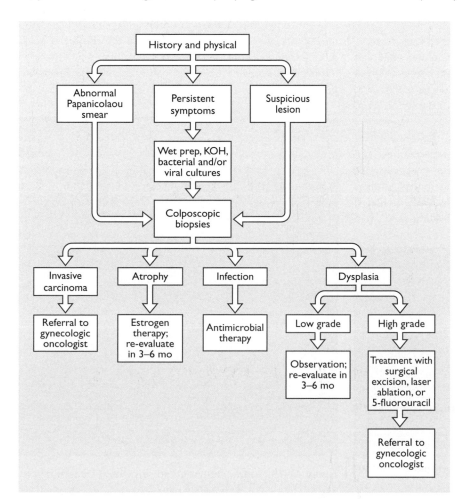

Figure 41-11. Algorithm for the evaluation of vaginal lesions.

have been exposed to HPV. Other than HIV, there is no other sexually transmitted disease that is more expensive to diagnose and treat than HPV. HPV 16 and 18 are the most common causes of high risk HPV for vaginal dysplasia. Of note, 70% of VAIN II and III and VIN III are caused by HPV 16 and 18. Approximately 50% of VAIN I and VIN I are caused by HPV 6, 11, 16, or 18. HPV 6 and 11 cause over 95% of the cases of genital warts. Gardasil (quadrivalent HPV types 6, 11, 16, 18, recombinant vaccine), is a new investigational vaccine from Merck & Co. (Whitehouse Station, NJ). The US Food and Drug Administration approved Gardasil for vulvar precancers (VIN II and III); and vaginal precancers (VAIN II and III) caused by HPV types 16 and 18. Gardasil is also approved for the prevention of genital warts caused by HPV types 6, 11, 16, and 18. Gardasil is approved for 9- to 26-year-old girls and women.

VAGINAL INTRAEPITHELIAL NEOPLASIA

Excision is also suitable for vaginal lesions. Depending on the extent of disease, a wide local excision to complete vaginectomy may be required. The denuded vaginal tissue is quite vascular, and extensive resection may result in substantial blood loss. Small areas may be closed primarily with absorbable suture. Larger areas may be allowed to heal by secondary intent. Occasionally, a split-thickness skin graft tailored to a vaginal form is used in cases of vaginectomy. Postoperative estrogen therapy and dilation may be necessary to prevent stenosis.

Vaginal lesions are commonly amenable to laser therapy. The depth of tissue destruction is tailored to the epithelial thickness, with a mean thickness of 0.46 mm (range, 0.1–1.4 mm) [29]. Therefore, laser destruction to a depth of 1 mm to 1.5 mm should provide dysplastic epithelial destruction without damage to underlying tissue [25,29].

In extensive, multifocal disease, topical 5-fluorouracil may be used. The optimal dosing and treatment regimen have not been established. Some clinicians advocate a short course of treatment, followed by a period of rest and repeat application. Regimens that have been used and reasonably tolerated include 5% 5-fluorouracil inserted into the vagina each night

for 7 to 10 days, followed by a 10- to 14-day rest period. The application cycle is repeated if necessary. Alternatively, vaginal insertion of approximately 1.5 g of 5-fluorouracil weekly for 10 consecutive weeks may result in less toxicity and better compliance [21]. Caution is necessary when using 5-fluorouracil. Intense local inflammatory and desquamative reactions can occur, resulting in prolonged discomfort, scarring, and vaginal stenosis. Additionally, 5-fluorouracil is teratogenic; therefore, its use in reproductive-aged women must be judicious. The aforementioned side-effect profile makes the use of 5-fluorouracil less appealing in comparison to surgical excision or laser ablation. Cure rates for extensive lesions treated by vaginectomy, laser therapy, and 5-fluorouracil are comparable (80%–90%) [30].

Cryotherapy has not been successfully incorporated into treatment of VAIN. In contrast to cryotherapy of the cervix, a satisfactory freezing contact is difficult because of the geometry of the vagina and the compliance of the vaginal wall. Similarly, vulvar cryotherapy has had disappointing results. As with other destructive methods, the risk of obscuring an underlying invasive process exists. Visibility of new lesions on follow-up examination may be obscured, resulting in diagnostic delay. Cavitron ultrasonic surgical aspirator, loop electrosurgical excision procedure, and topical or intralesional interferon have all been investigated to lesser degrees such that recommendation for clinical use at this time is reserved.

Potential new treatments under investigation are chemopreventive agents, such as micronutrients, retinoids, eflornithine, and anti-inflammatory drugs. The therapeutic effect is directed at reversing precancerous changes, with reversion to normal tissue [7••]. The clinical utility of these agents has not been defined.

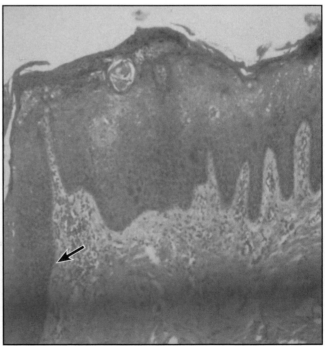

Figure 41-13. Vulvar carcinoma in situ with increased depth adjacent to hair follicle (*arrow*).

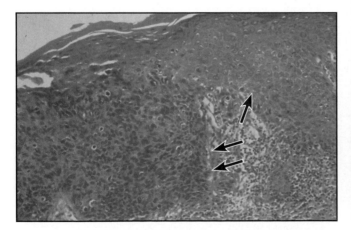

Figure 41-12. Normal vulvar epithelium (*arrow*) with transition into carcinoma in situ (*double arrows*).

Referral

The decision regarding whether to refer depends largely on the experience and comfort level of the clinician. To provide care in cases of VIN and VAIN, training in the diagnosis and management of dysplastic lesions is necessary. The primary care provider should have resources available for colposcopic examination and biopsy as well as access to pathologists familiar with vulvar and vaginal disease. Additionally, a reasonable prevalence of these disorders should exist in the patient population to maintain a high level of clinical acumen. Referral to a gynecologic oncologist should not be delayed if invasive carcinoma is suspected or confirmed. Excision of an invasive lesion need not be performed before referral.

Prevention

Primary care providers have a good opportunity to detect VIN, VAIN, and carcinoma early in their progressive courses. It is yet unresolved whether vulvar and vaginal cancer have a premalignant phase that could be detected with routine screening. Because of the low incidence of vulvovaginal intraepithelial neoplasias and carcinomas, screening for these disorders in the general population is probably not warranted. Preferably, a high-risk population should be defined and considered for screening. Increased risk factors include tobacco use, immunosuppression, HPV infection, and past or current history of preinvasive vulvar, vaginal, cervical, or perianal disease.

Counseling is focused on risk reduction and prevention of recurrence. The two major modifiable risk factors are tobacco use and sexually transmitted diseases. Furthermore patients with vulvar dysplasia may have an increased risk for sexual dysfunction after resection of the dysplasia [31]. Discussion with patients before surgery may decrease postoperative misconceptions regarding appearance and future function for the patient and her partner. Use of barrier contraceptives (condom, diaphragm, or both) may reduce the chance of sexually transmitted diseases, but it is improbable that diaphragm use provides any protection against vulvovaginal exposure. The clinician should provide prompt treatment of women and their partners, with education regarding vulvar self-examination. Compliance with follow-up examinations is encouraged in an effort to diagnose and treat in a timely fashion.

The ultimate goal in prevention of vulvar and vaginal dysplasia is to prevent potential development of invasive carcinoma (Figure 41-14). Although vulvar and vaginal cancers are uncommon, the morbidity associated with disease and treatment is substantial. Diagnostic delay adversely affects prognosis by permitting disease progression.

References

Papers of particular interest have been highlighted as follows:
- Of interest
- Of outstanding interest

1. Judson PL, Habermann EB, Baxter NN, et al.: Trends in the incidence of invasive and in situ vulvar carcinoma. Obstet Gynecol 2006, 107:1018–1022.

2. Rutledge FN, Mitchell MF, Munsell MF, et al.: Prognostic indicators for invasive carcinoma of the vulva. Gynecol Oncol 1991, 42:239–244.

3. Henson D, Tarone R: An epidemiologic study of cancer of the cervix, vagina, and vulva based on the Third National Cancer Survey in the United States. Am J Obstet Gynecol 1977, 129:525–532.

4. Dodge JA, Eltabbakh GH, Mount SL, et al.: Clinical features and risk of recurrence among patients with vaginal intraepithelial neoplasia. Gynecol Oncol 2001, 83:363–369.

5. Benedet JL, Sanders BH: Carcinoma in situ of the vagina. Am J Obstet Gynecol 1984, 148:695–700.

6. Petrilli ES, Townsend DE, Morrow CP, et al.: Vaginal intraepithelial neoplasia: biologic aspects and treatment with topical 5-fluorouracil and the carbon dioxide laser. Am J Obstet Gynecol 1980, 138:321–328.

7.•• Wharton JT, Tortolero-Luna G, Linares AC, et al.: Vaginal intraepithelial neoplasia and vaginal cancer. Obstet Gynecol Clin North Am 1996, 23:325–345.
A comprehensive review of vaginal dysplasia and carcinoma.

8. Newcomb PA, Weiss NS, Daling JR: Incidence of vulvar carcinoma in relation to menstrual, reproductive, and medical factors. J Natl Cancer Inst 1984, 73:391–396.

9. Brinton LA, Nasca PC, Mallin K, et al.: Case-control study of in situ and invasive carcinoma of the vagina. Gynecol Oncol 1990, 38:49–54.

10. Kurman RJ, Norris HJ, Wilkinson EJ: Atlas of Tumor Pathology: Tumors of the Cervix, Vagina, and Vulva: 3rd series, vol 4. Washington, DC: Armed Forces Institute of Pathology; 1992:183.

11. Trimble CL, Hildesheim A, Brinton LA: Heterogenous etiology of squamous carcinoma of the vulva. Obstet Gyn 1996, 87:59–64.

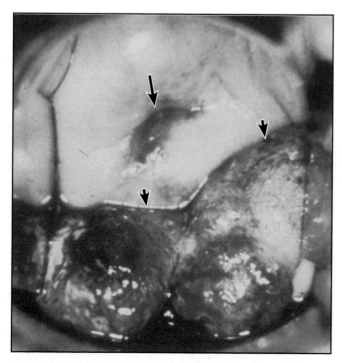

Figure 41-14. Invasive vaginal carcinoma (*arrowheads*) distorting the cervix. Cervical os (*arrow*).

12. Gillison ML, Shah KV: Role mucosal human papilloma-virus in nongenital cancers. *J Natl Cancer Inst Monogr* 2003, 31:57–65.

13. Brinton LA, Nasca PC, Mallin K: Case-control study of cancer of the vulva. *Obstet Gynecol* 1990, 75:859–866.

14. Jones RW, McLean MR: Carcinoma in situ of the vulva: a review of 31 treated and five untreated cases. *Obstet Gynecol* 1986, 68:499–503.

15. van Seters M, van Beurden M, de Craen AJ: Is the assumed natural history of vulvar intraepithelial neoplasia III based on enough evidence? A systematic review of 3322 published patients. *Gynecol Oncol* 2005, 97:645–651.

16. Hart, WR: Vulvar intraepithelial neoplasia: historical aspects and current status. *Int J Gynecol Pathol* 2001 1:16–30.

17. Aho M, Vesterinen E, Meyer B, *et al.*: Natural history of vaginal intraepithelial neoplasia. *Cancer* 1991, 68:195–197.

18. Foster DC: Vulvar disease. *Obstet Gynecol* 2002, 100:145–163.

19. Wechter ME, Reynolds RK, Haefner HK, *et al.* :Vulvar melanoma: Review of diagnosis, staging and therapy. *J Low Genit Tract* 2004, 8:58–69.

20.• Edwards CL, Tortolero-Luna G, Linares AC, *et al.*: Vulvar intraepithelial neoplasia and vulvar cancer. *Obstet Gynecol Clin North Am* 1996, 23:295–324.

A comprehensive review of vulvar dysplasia and carcinoma.

21. DiSaia PJ, Creasman WT: In *Clinical Gynecologic Oncology*, edn 5. St. Louis: CV Mosby; 1997:45.

22.• Kaufman RH: Intraepithelial neoplasia of the vulva. *Gynecol Oncol* 1995, 56:8–21.

A thorough review of preinvasive vulvar disease.

23. Modesitt SC, Waters AB, Walton L, *et al.*: VIN III: Occult cancer and the impact of margin status on recurrence. *Obstet Gynecol* 1998, 92:962–966.

24. Benedet JL, Wilson PS, Matisic JP: Epidermal thickness and skin appendage involvement in VIN. *J Reprod Med* 1993, 38:108–112.

25. Reid R: Superficial laser vulvectomy. *Am J Obstet Gynecol* 1985, 152:504–509.

26. Sillman FH, Sedlis A, Boyce JG: A review of lower genital intraepithelial neoplasia and the use of topical 5-fluorouracil. *Obstet Gynecol Surv* 1985, 40:190–220.

27. Krupp PJ: 5-fluorouracil topical treatment of in situ vulvar cancer. *Obstet Gynecol* 1978, 51:702–706.

28. Di Renzo GC, Mignosa MM, Gerli S, *et al.:* Reply. *Am J Obstet Gynecol* 2006, 194:594.

29. Benedet JL, Wilson PS, Matisic JP: Epidermal thickness measurements in VAIN. *J Reprod Med* 1992, 37:809–812.

30. Mitchell MF: Preinvasive disease of the female lower genital tract. In *Operative Gynecology.* Edited by Gershenson DM, DeCherney AH, Curry SL. Philadelphia: WB Saunders; 1993:231.

31. Likes WM, Stegbauer C, Hathaway D, *et al.*: Use of the female sexual function index in women with vulvar intraepithelial neoplasia. *J Sex Marital Ther* 2006, 32:255–266.

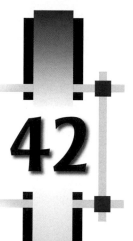

42 Cervical Dysplasia

Todd D. Tillmanns

- Regular Papanicolaou smears are the key to preventing cervical cancer. Since the introduction of the Papanicolaou smear in North America, cervical cancer has decreased from the number one cause of female cancer deaths to number eight.
- Regular Papanicolaou smears should begin at the onset of sexual activity, or no later than 18 years of age, and continue into senescence; they should be accompanied by risk evaluation and education.
- Papanicolaou smears and colonoscopy are essential components of a full evaluation for cervical disease.
- In women who do not have a Papanicolaou smear for greater than 3 years, the incidence of invasive cervical cancer rises.
- A significant population of women remain unscreened. An estimated 11 million women in the United States have not had a Papanicolaou smear within the past year; 1 million women older than 18 years of age have never had a Papanicolaou smear.

Cervical dysplasia is the precursor lesion to cervical cancer. Cervical cancer was responsible for more female cancer deaths and morbidity than any other malignant etiology before the 20th century. Currently, cervical cancer remains a significant source for cancer morbidity and mortality, though primarily in developing nations. The substantial reduction in cervical cancer in developing nations has been one of the greatest public health achievements in the last century. There were almost 10,000 cases of invasive cervical cancer diagnosed in the United States, and almost 4000 women died of cervical cancer in 2006. On a global scale, cervical cancer claims an estimated 288,000 lives, and 510,000 women will be diagnosed over the same time period [1]. Cervical cancer is second only to breast cancer in incidence, and 80% of all cases are in developing countries [1].

The prevalence of cervical cancer in the United States from January 1, 2003 Surveillance, Epidemiology and End Results Program (SEER) data is 253,781 for all ages, and women less than 49 years of age were 67,739; 50 to 69 years of age 103,498; and greater than 70 years of age were 82,544 [2]. Essentially all cases of cervical cancer are preventable as they are related to infection with the human papillomavirus (HPV). HPV typically causes a preinvasive lesion, described as cervical intraepithelial neoplasia (CIN). There are approximately

500,000 of these CIN II and III precursor lesions diagnosed every year in the United States [3]. As a result of early diagnosis, preventative methodology, and treatment of these precursor lesions, the morbidity and mortality of cervical cancer have declined substantially in the later part of the 20th century. The cost to society of HPV regarding loss of work and sexual dysfunction and anxiety is substantial and is second only to HIV regarding sexually transmitted infections.

Nomenclature

Abnormalities revealed on close examination of the cervix can be ascertained by review of cytology and/or histology. Cytology is generally obtained by examination of the traditional Papanicolaou smear or evaluation of liquid based cytology obtained most often through the use of ThinPrep (Cytyc Corporation, Marlborough, MA). The Bethesda classification (Figure 42-1) defines the methods of reporting cytology [4].

Histologic definitions include mild, moderate, and severe dysplasia. These have been broken down for reporting purposes into CIN. CIN I refers to dysplasia confined to the lower or basal third of the epithelium. CIN II describes lesions confined to the basal two-thirds of the epithelium. CIN III is confined to the full thickness of the epithelium. CIN III was referred to as severe dysplasia or CIS, carcinoma in situ (Figures 42-2 and 42-3).

Incidence and Epidemiology

Cervical cancer is almost entirely the result of infection with the human papillomavirus (HPV). HPV infection in itself will not result in malignancy. The second process in the carcinogenic episodes must be incorporation of HPV DNA into the host DNA. Concomitantly, the host immune system must be overwhelmed, incapacitated, or unable to recognize the HPV infection. This results in a long-term process that eventually results in the process of carcinogenesis occurring within the glandular or epithelial cells of the cervix.

Worldwide, more than 500,000 cervical cancers are diagnosed yearly. In the United States, more than 10,000 new cervical carcinomas are diagnosed every year. Numerous studies have now confirmed that HPV is the cause of this cervical cancer in over 98% of the cases. Cervical cancer is the third most common cause of cancer death in women worldwide. There are approximately 200,000 deaths due to cervical cancer [5]. Eighty percent of global cervical cancer deaths are in developing countries, which reveals a stark contrast to developed countries in that developing countries lack effective screening programs. Because of the efforts of George Papanicolaou

and numerous investigators since the initial identification of cervical changes related to suspect development of cervical carcinoma, we are now able to largely prevent cervical cancer in appropriately screened populations.

Infection with one of the 13 cancer-associated HPV types measured by hybrid capture II (16, 18, 31, 33, 35, 39, 45, 51, 52, 56, 58, 59, and 68) is clearly recognized as necessary for the development of cervical cancer [6–8]. These HPV types can be identified with the use of liquid-based screening obtained at the time of a Papanicolaou smear. Of the 3.5 million women who have an abnormal Papanicolaou smear in the United States each year, the most common abnormality is atypical squamous cells. This abnormality accounts for approximately 2 million cases. Any of the squamous intraepithelial lesions result in 1.25 million of the abnormalities, of which almost one fourth are of the high grade variety. In all, approximately 7% of all Papanicolaou smears are considered to be abnormal [9].

Risk Factors for Development of Cervical Dysplasia

Increased sexual activity or sexual activity with high-risk partners has been demonstrated to increase transmission of high-risk HPV types. It has been estimated that 60% to 80% of women that are sexually active will have been exposed to HPV

The Bethesda System for Reporting Cervical Cytologic Diagnoses

Specimen adequacy
Satisfactory for evaluation
Presence or absence of endocervical or transformation zone components or other quality indicators such as partially obscuring blood or inflammation
Unsatisfactory for evaluation (specify reason)
Specimen rejected or not processed (specify reason)
Specimen processed and examined, but unsatisfactory for evaluation of epithelial abnormalities (specify reason)
General categorization (optional)
Negative for intraepithelial lesion or malignancy
Epithelial cell abnormality
Other
Interpretation/result
Negative for intraepithelial lesion or malignancy
Organism
Trichomonas vaginalis
Fungal organisms morphologically consistent with *Candida* species
Shift in flora suggestive of bacterial vaginosis
Bacteria morphologically consistent with *Actinomyces* species
Cellular changes consistent with herpes simplex virus
Other non-neoplastic findings (optional to report)
Reactive cellular changes associated with:
  Inflammation (includes typical repair)
  Radiation
  Intrauterine contraceptive device
  Glandular cells status posthysterectomy

Interpretation/result
Atrophy
Epithelial cell abnormalities
Squamous cell
Atypical squamous cell
Atypical squamous cell of undetermined significance
Atypical squamous cell cannot exclude high-grade squamous intraepithelial lesion
Low-grade squamous intraepithelial lesion
  Encompassing: human papillomavirus, mild dysplasia, and cervical intraepithelial neoplasia I
High-grade squamous intraepithelial lesion (HSIL)
  Encompassing: moderate and severe dysplasia, carcinoma in situ, cervical intraepithelial lesion II and III
Squamous cell carcinoma
Glandular cell
Atypical glandular cells
  Specify endocervical, endometrial, or glandular cells not otherwise specified
Atypical glandular cells, favor neoplastic
  Specify endocervical or not otherwise specified
Endocervical adenocarcinoma in situ
Adenocarcinoma
Other (list not comprehensive)
Endometrial cells in a woman 40 years of age or older
Automated review and ancillary testing (include if appropriate)
Educational notes and suggestions (optional)

Figure 42-1. The Bethesda System for reporting cervical cytologic disease. (*Adapted from* Solomon *et al.* [27].)

by the age of 50 [10]. Sexual risk factors include sexual activity at an early age, intercourse with a partner that has previously had a partner with cervical cancer or high-isk cervical dysplasia, and multiple sexual partners. Approximately 25% of young women develop low-grade squamous intraepithelial lesion (LSIL) after an HPV infection [11]. Women with the cytologic diagnosis of atypical squamous cells of undetermined significance or LSIL that were found to be HPV16 (+) had a 2 year cumulative absolute risk for a greater than CIN III of 32.5% and 39.1% respectively [12]. Other risk factors include cigarette smoking, multiparity, and immunodeficiency (HIV, lupus, and diabetes). Low socioeconomic status and low educational level have also been implicated for developing cervical dysplasia and concomitantly cervical cancer. Racial ethnicities including African-Americans, Hispanics, and Native Americans all have an increased risk for cervical dysplasia and cancer. Despite these risk factors, more than 90% of HPV infections resolve in 2 years. Resolution rates are currently determined most definitively by hybrid capture assays and polymerase chain reaction. Despite sensitive assays, it remains unclear whether the HPV infections are cleared or are undetectable only to become active at a later date.

Human Papillomavirus Subtypes and Classifications

There are low-risk types including HPV-6, -11, -40, -42, -43, -44, -54, -61, -70, -72, and -81. There are likely high-risk types of HPV-26, -53, and -66, and then there are the high-risk types of HPV-16, -18, -31, -33, -35, -39, -45, -51, -52, -56, -58, -59, -68, -73, and -82 [13].

DIAGNOSTIC MODALITIES

Infection with HPV is asymptomatic in males and females. In fact, the most common symptoms that would alert a patient that they previously were infected are the abnormal vaginal bleeding that often occurs with intercourse in patients that have an advanced cervical cancer. Once HPV infection has occurred, on average it takes years to develop into frank malignancy. Therefore, the detection of HPV and early dysplastic changes to the cervix are of paramount importance to prevent cervical cancer.

Cervical cytology screens for cervical dysplasia using conventional Papanicolaou smear or liquid-based methods (ThinPrep or SurePath [TriPath Imaging, Burlington, NC]) [14]. Guidelines are currently in the process of reevaluation to supplant routine Papanicolaou smear follow-up as previously recommended to HPV testing in specific situations. These recommendations will be published when the new American Society for Colposcopy and Cervical Pathology (ASCCP) guidelines are adopted. Currently, we recommend ASCCP guidelines and the modifications made to the algorithm in Figure 42-4.

Colposcopy allows visualization and magnification of the cervix, vagina, vulva, and perianal areas from two times to 25 times. The use of 3% to 5% acetic acid assists in visualizing dysplasia. The acetic acid typically denatures the protein

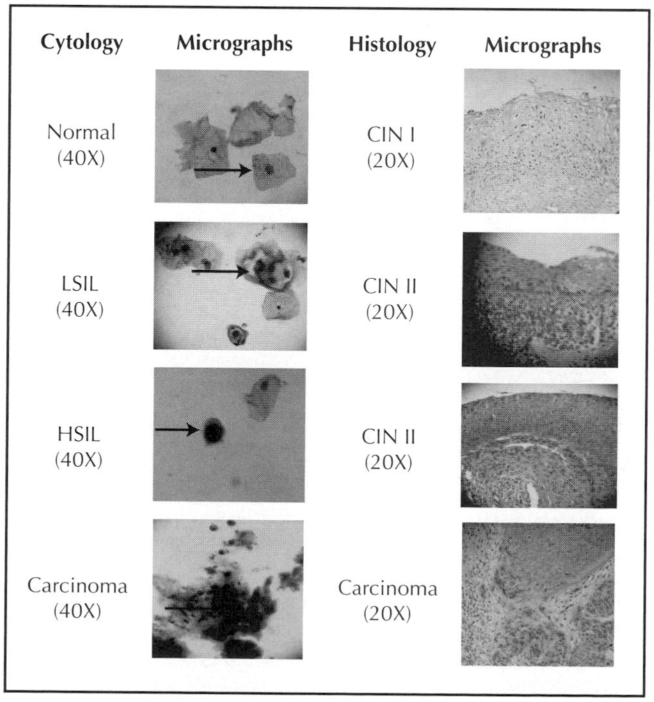

Figure 42-2. Cytologic and histologic cervical variants. CIN—cervical intraepithelial neoplasia; HSIL—high-grade squamous intraepithelial lesion; LSIL—low-grade squamous intraepithelial lesion. (*Courtesy of* David Spencer, MD.)

Staging of Cervical Intraepithelial Neoplasia and Cervical Carcinoma

Stage	Definition
CIN I	Cytologic changes limited to lower one third of epithelium
CIN II	Cytologic changes limited to lower two thirds of epithelium
CIN III	Cytologic changes seen in upper one third of epithelium
CA stage 0	Carcinoma in situ; intraepithelial neoplasia (CIN I, II, and III)
CA stage I	Carcinoma strictly confined to the cervix (disregard extension to the corpus)
CA stage II	Involvement of the upper two thirds of the vagina, or infiltration of the parametria, but not to the sidewall
CA stage III	Involvement of the lower one third of the vagina, or extension to the pelvic sidewall; all cases of hydronephrosis
CA stage IV	Extension outside the reproductive tract

Figure 42-3. Staging of cervical intraepithelial neoplasia (CIN) and cervical carcinoma (CA).

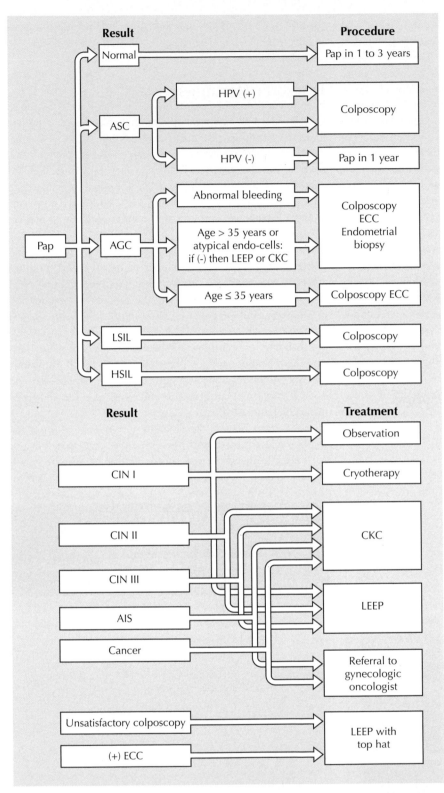

Figure 42-4. Current guidelines for management of abnormal Papanicolaou (Pap) smears with treatment options based on recommendations from American Society for Colposcopy and Cervical Pathology with modifications. AGC—atypical glandular cells; AIS—endocervical adenocarcinoma in situ; ASC—atypical squamous cells; CIN—cervical intraepithelial neoplasia; CKC—cold-knife conization; ECC— endocervical curettage; HPV—human papillomavirus; HSIL—high-grade squamous intraepithelial lesion; LEEP—loop electrosurgical excisional procedure; LSIL—low-grade squamous intraepithelial lesion.

within cells causing cells with increased protein (dysplastic cells) to turn white. More severely dysplastic cells will often change color first within 10 seconds on the cervix, and the color change usually lasts for 90 seconds or less. Other notable colposcopic findings that may indicate dysplasia include mosaicism, punctuations, hairpin loops, and coarse or thickened patterns. Reids colposcopic index defines dysplastic areas by interpretation of lesion margin, color of acetowhitening, blood vessels, and iodine staining and may be quite helpful for less experienced colposcopists [15]. More recently, an optical density system (MediSpectra, Inc., Lexington, MA) was able to improve the detection of CIN II and III by 25% among women with atypical squamous cells of undetermined significance and low-grade squamous intraepithelial lesion cytology referred for colposcopy [16]. This optical density system is easy to use and allows for a colored visual printout of areas more concerning for dysplasia. Risks for progression, persistence, and regression of cervical dysplasia have been published with two notable studies found in Figures 42-5 and 42-6.

TREATMENT

Treatment options for cervical dysplasia (confirmed by cervical biopsy) include ablation techniques such as cryotherapy, electrocautery, laser ablation, or chemotherapeutic desquamative modalities. Excissional modalities are primarily by the Loop electrosurgical excisional procedure (LEEP), cold knife conization, or rarely, laser conization. Laser conization will not be discussed as it has become obsolete and is no more therapeutically effective than other techniques at a much greater cost.

LEEP was originally used to treat patients eligible for ablative procedures. The LEEP procedure was modified and referred to as a LEEP-Cone. The LEEP-Cone is completed by initially performing the traditional LEEP followed by a second pass or top-hat. The top-hat removes more cervical tissue in the endocervical canal, mimicking a cold-knife cone biopsy. This LEEP-Cone has been shown to be equivalent to a cold-knife conization if performed properly [17]. The LEEP-Cone is now often used to supplant the cold-knife cone using the same traditional indications, including two-step discrepancies (two-grade difference between cytology and colposcopic biopsy), positive endocervical curettage (positive ECC), and unsatisfactory colposcopy [18].

The 2001 Consensus Guidelines for the Management of Women with Cervical Intraepithelial Neoplasia supports the use of the LEEP for treatment of CIN I, CIN II, or CIN III [19]. The guidelines confirm that other ablative modalities are acceptable and have similar efficacy to treat all grades of CIN if the colposcopy is adequate, the ECC is negative, and there is no discrepancy between cytology and histology [20]. Other excisional modalities to treat CIN in this context are also equal, including laser conization and cold-knife conization. Indications that we favor for cold-knife conization

include adenocarcinoma in situ and suspicion for malignancy of the cervix. Generally if there is any suspicion for persistent severe dysplasia or malignancy, consultation with a gynecologic oncologist should be considered, especially before a hysterectomy is chosen for definitive management.

The modality chosen for cervical excision must take into account physician training, expertise, patient resources, availability, and patient preference. Overtreatment can be a significant issue in young, fertile women that wish to avoid the potential risks of excisional procedures [21]. Traditional indications for excisional procedures are now being questioned with increasing adoption of more conservative strategies. We expect the soon-to-be-published updated ASCCP guidelines to recommend conservative approaches for previously indicated excisional or ablative recommendations. Follow-up after excisional procedures should occur at 3 to 6 month intervals generally with cytology or HPV testing. Strong consideration for ECC should be entertained if the squamocolumnar junction is not visualized. If margins are positive after an excisional procedure, then options are to re-excise the remaining cervical tissue or follow-up with observation. Reports of negative cytology with positive margins have been as high as 70% to 99% [21–23].

Prevention

A new era in prevention of cervical dysplasia is at hand. The prophylactic vaccines currently available and those under development will allow for the prevention of both communicative and acquisition of the type-specific HPV through sexual and nonsexual contact. These vaccines are largely being developed by Merck and GlaxoSmithKline. Currently available vaccines include Gardasil (Merck & Co., Whitehouse Station, NJ) (HPV-16, -18, -6, and -11) and Cervarix (GlaxoSmithKline, Philadelphia, PA) (HPV-16 and -18). These two vaccines utilize virus-like particles (VLPs) , which are self-assembled viral particles of the main structural HPV-L1 protein, in the absence of any viral genetic material. Thus, whereas these capsid particles structurally resemble HPV virions, they are noninfectious. Recently Gardasil prevented nearly 100% of high-grade cervical dysplasia associated with HPV types 16 and 18 in a phase III study. These vaccines seem to stimulate the immune system of the subject to produce immunoglobulin G antibodies thought to be responsible for prevention of the type-specific HPVs in the genital tract and also in the vulvar area. Guidelines for the utilization of the Gardasil vaccine are summarized in Figure 42-7. Other less successful, but potentially more broadly HPV-type efficacious methods, are utilization of vaginal and penile condoms [24]. At this time the vaccines are only indicated for prophylaxis; however, further research and development of newer vaccines may demonstrate a therapeutic potential.

Rates of Progression and Regression of Cervical Dysplasia Over 2 Years [25]

Dysplasia	Regress to Normal, %	Unchanged, %	Progress to > CIN II, %	Progress to > CIN III, %
CIN I	44	45	11	2
CIN II	33	51	N/A	16

Figure 42-5. Rates of progression and regression of cervical dysplasia over 2 years [25]. CIN—cervical intraepithelial neoplasia; N/A—not applicable.

Rates of Progression and Regression of Cervical Dysplasia Over 2 Years [26]

Dysplasia	Regress to Normal, %	Persistence, %	Progress to CIN III, %	Progress to Cancer, %
CIN I	60	30	10	1
CIN II	40	40	20	5
CIN III	33	55	N/A	> 12

Figure 42-6. Rates of progression and regression of cervical dysplasia over 2 years [26]. CIN—cervical intraepithelial neoplasia; N/A—not applicable.

Summary of American Cancer Society Recommendations for Human Papillomavirus Vaccine Use to Prevent Cervical Cancer and Its Precursors

Routine HPV vaccination is recommended for girls aged 11 to 12 years

Girls as young as age 9 may receive HPV vaccination

HPV vaccination also is recommended for girls aged 13 to 18 years to catch up missed vaccine or complete the vaccination series

There are currently insufficient data* to recommend for or against universal vaccination of women aged 19 to 26 years in the general population. A decision about whether a woman aged 19 to 26 years should receive the vaccine should be based on an informed discussion between the woman and her health care provider regarding her risk of previous HPV exposure and potential benefit from vaccination. Ideally, the vaccine should be administered before potential exposure to genital HPV through sexual intercourse because the potential benefit is likely to diminish with increasing number of lifetime sexual partners

HPV vaccination is not currently recommended for women over the age of 26 or for men

Screening for cervical intraepithelial neoplasia and cancer should continue in vaccinated and unvaccinated women according to American Cancer Society early detection guidelines

*Insufficient evidence of benefit in women aged 19 to 26 years refers to 1) clinical trials data in women with an average of two, and no more than 4, lifetime sexual partners, indicating a limited reduction in the overall incidence of cervical intraepithelial neoplasia II/III; 2) the absence of efficacy data for the prevention of HPV-16/-18–related cervical intraepithelial neoplasia II/III in women who had more than four lifetime sexual partners; and 3) the lack of cost effectiveness analyses for vaccination in this age group.

Figure 42-7. Summary of American Cancer Society recommendations for human papillomavirus (HPV) vaccine use to prevent cervical cancer and its precursors.

References

1. Pagliusi S: World Health Organization: human papillomavirus infection and cervical cancer. Available at: http://www.who.int/vaccines/en/hpvrd.shtml. Accessed 1–25–07.

2. Hayat MJ, Howlader N, Reichman ME, Edwards BK: Cancer statistics, trends, and multiple primary cancer analyses from the Surveillance, Epidemiology, and End Results (SEER) Program. *Oncologist* 2007, 12:20–37.

3. Clifford GM, Smith JS, Aguado T, Franceschi S: Comparison of HPV type distribution in high grade cervical lesions and cervical cancer: a metaanalysis. *Br J Cancer* 2003, 89:101–105.

4. The 1988 Bethesda System for reporting cervical/vaginal cytological diagnoses. National Cancer Institute Workshop. *JAMA* 1989, 262:931.

5. Parkin DM, Pisani P, Furlay J: Global cancer statistics. *CA Cancer J Clin* 1999, 49:73.

6. Bosch FX, Manos M, Munoz N, et al.: Prevalence of HPV DNA and cervical cancer: a worldwide perspective. *J Natl Cancer Inst* 1995, 87:796–802.

7. Walboomers J, Jacob M, Mananos M, et al.: Human papilloma Virus is a necessary cause of invasive cervical cancer worldwide. *J Pathol* 1999, 198:12.

8. Munoz N: Human papilloma and cancer: the epidemiological evidence. *J Clin Virol* 2000, 19:1–5.

9. Jones BA, Davey DD: Quality management in gynecologic cytology using interlaboratory comparison. *Arch Pathol Lab Med* 2000, 124:672.

10. ACOG Practice Bulletin: Clinical management guidelines for obstetrician-gynecologists: number 61, April 2005. Human papillomavirus. *Obstet Gynecol* 2005, 105:905.

11. Moscicki AB, Hills N, Shiboski S, et al.: Risks for incident human papillomavirus infection and low–grade squamous intraepithelial lesion development in young females. *JAMA* 2001, 285:2995–3002.

12. Castle PE, Solomon D, Shiffman M, Wheeler CM: Human papillomavirus type 16 infections and 2-year absolute risk of cervical precancer in women with equivocal or mild cytologic abnormalities. *JNCI* 2005, 97:1066–1071.

13. Munoz N, Bosch FX, de San Jose S, et al.: Epidemiologic classification of human papillomavirus types associated with cervical cancer. *N Engl J Med* 2003, 348:518–527.

14 ACOG Practice Bulletin: Clinical management guidelines for obstetrician-gynecologists: number 45, August 2003. Cervical cytology screening (replaces committee opinion 152, March 1995). *Obstet Gynecol* 2003, 102:417.

15. Ferris DG, Greenberg MD: Reid's colposcopic index. *J Fam Pract* 1994, 39:160–169.

16. Huh WK: Presentation at the Fourth International Conference on Cervical Cancer. MD Anderson Cancer Center, Houston, TX; May 19–22, 2005.

17. Gold M, Dunton CJ, Murray J, et al.: Electrocautery Excisional Procedure: therapeutic effectiveness a an ablation and conization equivalent. *Gynecol Oncol* 1996, 61:241–244.

18. Duggan BD, Felix JC, Muderspach LI, et al.: Cold–knife conization versus conization by the loop electrosurgical excision procedure: a randomized, prospective study. *Am J Obstet Gynecol* 1999, 180:276–282.

19. Saslow D, Runowicz CD, Soloman D, et al.: American Cancer Society Guideline for the Early Detection of Cervical Neoplasia and Cancer. *CA Cancer J Clin* 2002, 52:342–362.

20. Mitchell MF, Tortolero–Luna G, Cook E, et al.: A randomized clinical trial of cryotherapy, laser vaporization, loop electrosurgical excision for treatment of squamous intraepithelial lesions of the cervix. *Obstet Gynecol* 1998, 92:737–744.

21. Tillmanns TD, Falkner CA, Engle DB, et al.: Preoperative predictors of positive margins after loop electrosurgical excisional procedure-cone. *Gynecol Oncol* 2006, 100:379–384.

22. Reich O, Pickel H, Lahousen M, et al.: Cervical intraepithelial neoplasia III: long term outcome after cold knife conization with clear margins. *Obstet Gynecol* 2001, 97:428–430.

23. Reich O, Lahousen M, Pickel H, et al.: Cervical Intraepithelial Neoplasia III: long term outcome after cold knife conization with involved margins. *Obstet Gynecol* 2002, 99:193–196.

24. Baldwin SB, Wallace DR, Papenfuss MR, et al.: Condom use and other factors affecting penile human papillomavirus detection in men attending a sexually transmitted disease clinic. *Sex Transm Dis* 2004, 31:601–607.

25. Holowaty P, Miller AB, Rohan T, To T: Natural history of dysplasia of the uterine cervix. *JNCI* 1999, 91:252–258.

26. Ostor AG: Natural history of cervical intraepithelial neoplasia: a critical review. *Int J Gynecol Pathol* 1993, 12:186–192.

27. Solomon D, Davey D, Kurman R, et al.: The 2001 Bethesda System: terminology for reporting results of cervical cytology. *JAMA* 2002, 287:216.

43 Common Office Procedures

Roger P. Smith

- To perform safe and effective office procedures, the clinician must know the basis of the procedure, its indications, contraindications, expected outcome, and possible complications. This is also true for the routine Papanicolaou smear and for laser surgery.
- The Papanicolaou smear may be inaccurate or misleading if not performed correctly.
- Colposcopy complements the Papanicolaou smear and allows the identification of changes suggestive of underlying abnormality.
- The use of cold to produce tissue damage can provide a convenient office modality for the destruction of cervical, vaginal, or vulvar lesions, but if used incorrectly, inadvertent damage or ineffective treatment may result.
- Despite the ease with which the loop electrosurgical excision and the large loop excision of the transformation zone procedures may be performed, they remain surgical procedures with all the attendant risks and caveats.

Many gynecologic procedures are appropriate in the primary care setting; some have always been part of this care, others are new technologies or procedures traditionally reserved for the specialist. The keys to the performance of any procedure are an understanding of its technical details, as well as awareness of potential pitfalls to be avoided. The first is readily available from a number of sources; the latter is often only gained through experience. In this chapter, we attempt to provide both.

Papanicolaou Smear

Although the Papanicolaou smear is a fundamental procedure generally learned early in the physician's medical training, it must be performed correctly to have any value as a screening test for cervical cancer. Liquid-based cytology techniques have replaced the older glass-slide methods of collecting and analyzing cervical cytology. The choice of methods is driven by a number of factors, including cost, but both continue to be acceptable. The method of obtaining the cytologic sample differs for the two.

EQUIPMENT
For the traditional Papanicolaou smear, one or more clean glass microscope slides, an Ayre spatula (plastic or wood), an endocervical sampling brush or a cotton-tipped applicator (the first

is preferred, but an applicator is acceptable), and a spray or liquid fixative agent are required. A pencil is used to label the slide. If a liquid-based cytologic method is to be used, a container of transport liquid supplied by the cytology laboratory and a collection brush will be used.

TECHNIQUE
The speculum should be selected based on the anticipated anatomy and the planned procedures to be accomplished. Most commonly used is the Graves speculum. Whichever type and size of speculum is selected, it should be inspected for integrity and functionality and warmed before use. Warming may be accomplished with a warmer, a heating pad, or the use of warm water. (Before using a heating pad to warm the speculum, check local fire and electrical codes. In many areas, the use of heating pads, especially inside storage drawers, is against fire regulations.) Water provides a modicum of lubrication and avoids the problem of water-soluble lubricants interfering with cultures and the Papanicolaou smear. If water is used to warm the speculum, excess should be gently shaken off and the temperature checked against the physician's hand or wrist, or the patient's thigh, before insertion.

Once the cervix is located, the blades of the speculum should be held open by adjusting one or both screws or ratchets. The entire cervix should be visible, with the os centrally located.

When a traditional method of cytology is to be used, endocervical and ectocervical samples are obtained separately. Although there remains some debate about the sequence, most authors recommend obtaining the ectocervic sample first (using the Ayre spatula; Figure 43-1). To obtain this sample, the protrusion of the spatula is placed into the cervical os and the entire spatula is rotated through 360° while gentle pressure is maintained. The patient may experience some sensation when this is performed, but it should not be uncomfortable. The spatula is immediately smeared on the previously labeled microscope slide. If more than one slide is to be used, the first slide should be immediately fixed using a fixative spray or immersion in a fixative liquid.

An endocervical sample is obtained next using a specially made brush or a cotton-tipped applicator. The chosen instrument is inserted into the cervical os and gently rotated. The material obtained is immediately placed on the microscope slide and fixed. The endocervical and ectocervical cells are sensitive to air-drying, which may result in a smear that cannot be interpreted. The endocervical cells are slightly more sensitive, making rapid fixation imperative.

Some mild bleeding may result from taking the endocervical sample; this suggests the possibility of cervicitis, although bleeding can occur in many healthy patients as well.

When liquid-based cytology is used, a broad brush (or "broom") is used to obtain the ectocervical and endocervical samples at the same time. This is placed at the cervix with the protrusion of the brush (center) gently inserted into the cervical os. This is rotated through 360° while gentle pressure is maintained. The brush is withdrawn, and the head is detached and placed within the transport liquid recommended (or supplied) by the cytology laboratory.

Colposcopy

Colposcopy and exfoliative cytology complement each other, improving the diagnostic accuracy of each. The colposcope permits the identification of normal landmarks, finds changes suggestive of underlying abnormality, and aids in the selection of sites for biopsy that will yield the greatest information.

EQUIPMENT

A colposcope is a stereoscopic operating microscope with magnifications of four to 40 times. Other tools needed are an endocervic speculum, biopsy forceps (eg, Tischler or Kevorkian), endocervic curette, large-tipped cotton swabs, and cotton balls or small gauze sponges. (Any instrument that will enter the endocervical canal or will be used for biopsy should be sterilized before use.) Containers of acetic acid (3%–5%, white vinegar), Monsel's solution (ferric subsulfate), and Lugol's (5%) solution (supersaturated iodine) also should be available.

TECHNIQUE

Colposcopy requires a wider field of exposure than routine screening or cytologic examinations. Therefore, the physician should use the largest warmed, but unlubricated, speculum that the patient can comfortably accommodate. With the cervix satisfactorily in view, the cervix and the vaginal fornices should be inspected for lesions.

The colposcope should be positioned to provide an unobstructed view of the cervix. With the focus of the colposcope at the middle of its range, the position of the entire instrument should be adjusted so that the cervix is in focus, permitting further fine adjustments to be made using only the instrument's focusing mechanism.

Acetic acid (3%–5%) should be liberally applied to the cervix. (A sensation of cold or stinging may be experienced, and the patient should be warned of this before the application.) The changes brought on by the application of acetic acid are only temporary, requiring periodic reapplication at roughly 5-minute intervals. Lesions exposed by the application of the acetic acid should be noted for further evaluation.

The transformation zone should be identified and inspected in its entirety. Any areas of white change, vascular abnormality, or mosaicism should be inspected under greater magnification. Any acetowhite area and areas of thickening, abnormal vascular pattern, or mosaicism should be sampled using any one of several different types of biopsy forceps available. When multiple abnormalities are present, biopsies of the most severe areas take precedence. Whenever possible, the biopsy should include the edge or border of the lesion. Biopsies should be placed in a buffered formalin solution for transport to the pathology laboratory.

Endocervical canal curettage must be included in the colposcopic examination to exclude the possibility of endocervical lesions above the limits of visibility. To perform endocervical canal curettage, the curette is passed into the endocervical canal to the level of the inner os. If resistance does not provide an indication of the location of the inner os, the curette should not be advanced more that approximately 2 cm from the external os. The entire endocervical canal should be sampled in all directions. Tissue obtained should be placed in a buffered formalin solution, as with any other histologic specimen.

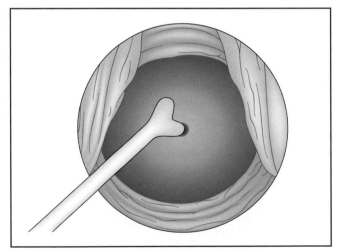

Figure 43-1. The Ayre spatula is designed to provide good contact between the cervix and the spatula edge, increasing the likelihood of obtaining cells from the transformation zone.

If bleeding from a biopsy site persists or is heavy, Monsel's solution may be applied. Monsel's solution should only be applied after all specimens have been obtained. Because Monsel's solution can delay healing, it should be used sparingly.

For a colposcopy to be considered adequate, the entire transformation zone must be visualized. The full extent of any lesion present must also be visible for the study to be considered adequate. If the colposcopy is inadequate, diagnostic conization is required.

Cryosurgery

The use of cold to produce tissue damage can provide a convenient office modality for the destruction of cervical, vaginal, or vulvar lesions. The equipment necessary to perform cryosurgery is simple to operate and relatively inexpensive to purchase and maintain.

EQUIPMENT
Cryosurgical units come in many types, although the most common are based on the release of pressurized gas (nitrous oxide). In addition to the cryosurgical unit, the procedure requires an assortment of cryosurgical tips and some water-soluble lubricant.

TECHNIQUE
The cervix should be brought into view using a standard speculum. If any cultures or cytologic smears are to be obtained, they should be taken at this point. A cryoprobe tip should be selected so that the freezing effect will extend approximately 5 mm beyond the extent of the lesion (Figure 43-2). Whenever possible, the probe should be flat or slightly conical to minimize the risk of extensive endocervic freezing. The selected tip should be attached to the cryocautery handle following the manufacturer's directions.

A water-soluble gel or lubricant is applied to the tip of the cryoprobe. The tip of the probe should be placed against the cervix, covering the lesion, taking care that the probe is not in contact with the vaginal side walls. The cryosurgical unit should be activated, and after approximately 5 seconds, the tip will adhere to the cervix. Once the tip has adhered to the cervix, the tip is bought outward and away from the vaginal sidewalls to avoid damage to the vaginal wall.

Freezing should continue for 3 minutes, resulting in an iceball that extends 5 mm beyond the cervical lesion. The freezing mechanism is then deactivated to permit a 5-minute thaw. After thawing for 5 minutes, the lesion is refrozen as above for an additional 3 minutes.

The patient should be informed that postoperative vaginal discharge can be expected for several weeks, and a follow-up sequence of Papanicolaou smears should be discussed with the patient. The first Papanicolaou smear should be delayed at least 3 months to allow for complete healing.

When cryosurgery is applied to other lesions, the lesions should be moistened with water or a water-soluble gel. A fine tip should be chosen and placed in contact with the moistened lesion. Once the tip has become adherent to the lesion,

traction should be supplied to lift the tip (and lesion) away from the surrounding skin. The same freeze-thaw-freeze sequence used for cervical lesions should be used.

Conization

For selected patients, the loop electrosurgical excision procedure and the large loop excision of the transformation zone conization procedures may provide diagnosis or therapy in a more convenient, less expensive, and less threatening environment than the traditional conization. Despite the ease with which they may be performed, they remain surgical procedures with all the attendant risks and caveats.

EQUIPMENT
The loop electrosurgical excision procedure requires an electrosurgical generator with the following features: output capability of at least 50 watts in coagulation and cutting modes, a variety of waveform outputs (pure cut, blended current, and coagulation current), patient grounding pad monitor, and isolated circuitry. Additional equipment required includes a variety of electrodes, a smoke evacuator with odor and viral filter, Monsel's paste (ferric subsulfate solution allowed to evaporate to the consistency of paste), a Kevorkian or similar endocervic curette, histology fixative (10% formalin) in containers, a syringe with 25- or 27-gauge 1.5-inch needle for anesthetic injection, 1% or 2% lidocaine with or without 1:100,000 epinephrine, a 12-inch needle holder, 2-0 suture material (or similar), and a vaginal pack (optional).

TECHNIQUE
Once informed consent has been obtained, position the patient, undressed from the waist down, on the examination table as for a speculum examination. Attach the return

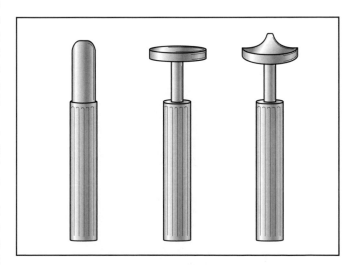

Figure 43-2. The cryosurgery tip chosen should be of a size and shape that complete coverage of the lesion is assured. The tip should provide good contact to the surface of the cervix, but not extend far into the endocervical canal. (*Adapted from* Smith and Ling [1 • •].)

electrode ("grounding pad") to patient's thigh with the long edge directed toward the hip. This is then connected to the electrosurgical generator.

The cervix should be visualized using a nonconductive speculum with smoke evacuator attachment. If any cultures or cytologic smears are to be obtained, they should be taken at this point. Acetic acid or Lugol's solution should be applied to the cervix to delineate the area of abnormality.

The local anesthetic should be injected submucosally into the cervix at the 3-, 6-, 9-, and 12-o'clock positions. These injections should be approximately 3 to 5 mm deep. As the anesthetic takes effect, the appropriate loop should be selected based on the size of the lesion to be treated. Lesions confined to the portio are most often treated with a round loop, 2 cm in width and 0.8 cm deep. For a nulliparous, small cervix, a loop 1.5 cm in width and 0.7 cm in depth is used. For lesions extending into the endocervix, a square loop electrode 1 by 1 cm can be used.

The power setting for the electrosurgical generator depends on the manufacturer of the generator as well as the diameter of the loop. The 2 cm × 0.8 cm loop requires 35 to 45 watts of power, whereas the 1 cm × 1 cm loop requires 20 to 30 watts of power. A blended current should be used.

The physician holds the loop several millimeters lateral to the edge of the lesion and simulates passing the loop over the lesion to ensure that there are no obstacles. The electrosurgical generator is then activated in the "cut" mode. The loop is pressed perpendicular into the tissue to a depth of 5 to 8 mm and then is dragged laterally across and through the endocervix. The loop should be pulled to a point several millimeters past the lesions or beyond the transformation zone, whichever is further (Figure 43-3). The resultant specimen should be dome shaped with the endocervic canal visible in the middle (Figure 43-4). The loop should not be pressed greater than 4 or 5 mm deep at the lateral borders of the cervix because of the arterial blood supply to the cervix entering at the 3- and 9-o'clock positions.

If the lesion is too large to be removed in a single pass, the central portion of the lesion is removed first using a 2-cm wide loop as described above. Additional passes are then made using the same loop to remove remaining lesion and the transformation zone (Figure 43-5).

If a blended current is used, bleeding from the base of the excision site is generally minimal. If necessary, fulguration of bleeders using the ball electrode at the "coagulation" setting may be performed; Monsel's solution may also be applied if needed.

The patient should be instructed to avoid intercourse, the use of tampons, and douching for 2 to 3 weeks. She should also be instructed to contact the physician if bleeding equals or exceeds a normal period, if bleeding lasts more than 2 weeks from the time of the procedure, if the vaginal discharge becomes foul smelling, or if she develops a fever.

Endometrial Biopsy

The availability of simple endometrial sampling systems makes this quick, easy, inexpensive, and safer than the traditional dilation and curettage.

EQUIPMENT

A number of devices (Accurette, Explora, Gynocheck, and Pipelle; CooperSurgical, Trumbull, CT; Z-Sampler; BEI Medical Systems International, Gembloux, Belgium; and others) have been shown to provide adequate tissue for diagnosis in 90% to 100% of cases. In addition to the sampling device itself, this procedure requires skin preparation materials (generally an iodine-based antibacterial solution such as betadine) and buffered formalin or other histologic fixative. A tenaculum and probe are often desirable as well.

TECHNIQUE

After the cervix has been visualized, it is disinfected with a topical antiseptic. If the patient is parous, endometrial sam-

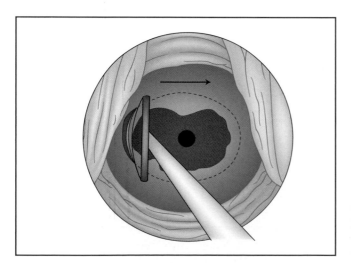

Figure 43-3. For small superficial ectocervical lesions, the loop electrode may be used in a single pass to remove the lesion. (*Adapted from* Smith and Ling [1••].)

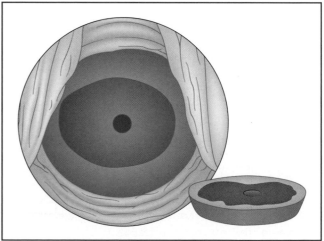

Figure 43-4. When correctly performed, the specimen removed has a dome-shaped contour and completely contains the lesion identified by colposcopy. (*Adapted from* Smith and Ling [1••].)

pling may be accomplished without stabilizing or dilating the cervix. The sampling device is gently introduced into the uterine cavity and the depth noted. For suction devices such as the Pipelle or Z-Sampler, the piston is withdrawn (producing a vacuum), and the curette is gradually withdrawn using a spiral or twisting motion. If an adequate tissue sample is obtained, it should be placed in fixative, completing the procedure. If additional tissue is needed, the piston may be advanced to a point just short of expelling the already obtained sample, the device again advanced into the uterine cavity, and the procedure repeated. An open curette, such as the Novak (Medicon, Tuttlingen, Germany), or a rigid suction cannula should be

gently inserted to the apex of the uterine cavity and then withdrawn in a straight line, using light pressure against the uterine wall. Tissue obtained may be removed from the opening of the curette using the point of a broken (but still sterile) wooden cotton-tipped applicator.

Diaphragm Fitting

The diaphragm remains an important reversible contraceptive method for the well-motivated patient. Its effectiveness in preventing pregnancy and reducing upper genital tract infection

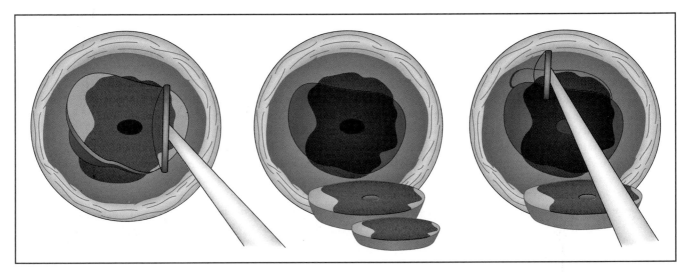

Figure 43-5. Large lesions may require two or more passes to ensure complete removal. The size and shape of each pass may be adjusted based on the lesion present. (*Adapted from* Smith and Ling [1●●].)

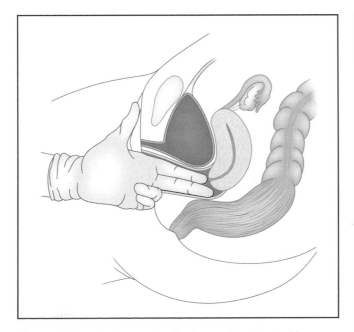

Figure 43-6. The size of the diaphragm is estimated by measuring the distance from the pubic symphysis to the posterior fornix (behind the cervix). (*Adapted from* Smith and Ling [1●●].)

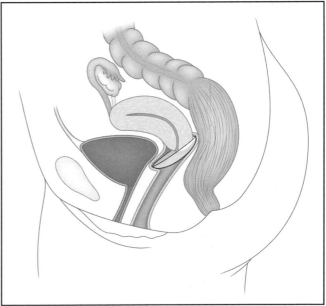

Figure 43-7. The correctly fitting diaphragm should sit comfortably behind the symphysis and in the posterior vaginal fornix, with the cervix covered and in contact with the spermicidal cream or jelly that has been applied to the dome. (*Adapted from* Smith and Ling [1●●].)

is predicated on the proper selection of size and type and on careful instructions to the patient to ensure correct positioning of the device when in use.

EQUIPMENT

Fitting a diaphragm requires a selection of fitting rings in sizes from 65 to 90 mm in diameter.

TECHNIQUE

Diaphragm fitting begins with a bimanual vaginal examination. The examining fingers of the vaginal hand are advanced until they touch the posterior fornix, just posterior to the cervix (Figure 43-6). The distance from under the symphysis to the posterior fornix is measured. A fitting ring with this diameter is selected and the size confirmed by measuring the ring against the fingers.

The selected ring is next lubricated and folded by compressing the sides between the fingers of one hand. The folded ring is gently inserted into the vagina and guided to the posterior fornix by the tips of the fingers. Once the ring has been placed in the posterior fornix, behind the cervix, the opposite side should be placed behind the symphysis anteriorly (Figure 43-7). The ring should fit snugly but allow a finger to pass easily between it and the vaginal wall in all directions. A correctly fitted diaphragm should be unnoticed or noticed only with concentration or effort. The patient should be asked to perform Valsalva's maneuver, cough, or move around to check for comfort and to ensure against displacement with normal activities. After the size has been determined, the fitting ring should be removed by sliding a finger between the ring and the symphysis anteriorly, displacing the ring downward, and withdrawing the ring with the hooked finger.

Diaphragm springs come in several different types. The type of spring used in the construction of the diaphragm determines its behavior when compressed by the fingers or the lateral vaginal walls. The type of spring chosen for the individual patient is often a matter of preference, although some broad guidelines are helpful (Figure 43-8). Parous patients, those with early pelvic relaxation, and those with a broad pubic arch do best with the arching type spring. Those with a narrow, poorly defined arch do better with a flat spring. Most patients can successfully use any of the three types and may try different styles as desired.

Pessary Fitting

As our population ages, the prevalence of pelvic relaxation will increase. As an alternative to surgery, pessaries may effectively provide mechanical support for the pelvic organs. These useful

Characteristics of Three Diaphragm Types

Spring Type	Shape When Compressed	Introducer	Advantages
Arching	Arch	Not needed	Firm rim; good when pelvic support is poor
Coil	Flat (will curve to fit the body)	Optional	Soft; best with good support and with the cervix on midplane or anterior position
Flat	Flat	Optional	Soft; remains in flat plane; best for women with narrow pubic angle or shallow retropubic space

Figure 43-8. Characteristics of the three diaphragm types. (*Adapted from* Smith and Ling [1••].)

Indications for Common Pessaries

Malposition
 Lever-type (Hodge)
Prolapse
 Uterine: Gellhorn, ring, doughnut, cube
 Vaginal: Doughnut, cube, ball (Gehrung)
 Cystocele or rectocele: Gehrung
Incompetent cervix
 Lever, ring
Incontinence
 Doughnut, lever, ring incontinence
Preoperative
 Based on defect
Drug delivery
 17 β-estradiol, medroxyprogesterone

Figure 43-9. Indications for common pessaries. (*Adapted from* Smith and Ling [1••].)

devices work well only when they have been carefully chosen and fitted to the individual patient.

EQUIPMENT

Fitting a pessary requires examples of appropriate pessaries in a variety of sizes (generally, the "average size" and at least one size larger and smaller).

TECHNIQUE

Before fitting a pessary, a careful determination of the anatomic defects present must be made. The presence or absence of normal pelvic support helps to determine the type of pessary best suited for the individual patient. The type chosen for a given patient is determined by the anatomic defect and the symptoms that the patient is experiencing. The indications for various types of commonly used pessaries are shown in Figure 43-9. The most commonly used forms of pessary for pelvic relaxation are the ring (or doughnut), the ball, and the cube.

Pessaries are fitted and placed in the vagina in much the same way as the contraceptive diaphragm. The depth of the vagina and the integrity of the supporting structures of the vagina are gauged as a part of the pelvic examination, and the size of pessary to be fitted is based on these findings. The selected pessary is lubricated with a water-soluble lubricant, folded or compressed, and inserted into the vagina. The pessary is adjusted so that it is in the proper position based on the type. Ring and lever pessaries should sit behind the cervix (when present) and rest in the retropubic notch; the Gellhorn pessary should be contained entirely within the vagina, with the plate resting above the levator plane; the Gehrung pessary must bridge the cervix with the limbs resting on the levator muscles on each side; and the ball or cube pessary should occupy and occlude the upper vagina. All pessaries must permit the easy passage of an examining finger between the pessary and the vaginal wall in all areas.

Patients should be instructed on proper insertion and removal techniques. Ring pessaries should be removed by hooking a finger into the pessary's opening, gently compressing the device, and then withdrawing the pessary with gentle traction; Gellhorn and Gehrung pessaries are removed by a reversal of their insertion procedures; cube pessaries must also be compressed, but the suction created between the faces of the cube and the vaginal wall must be broken by gently separating the device from the vaginal side wall. (The locator string often attached to these pessaries should not be used for traction.) Inflatable pessaries should be deflated before removal.

Patients fitted with a pessary require careful initial monitoring. Examination 5 to 7 days after initial fitting is required to confirm proper placement, hygiene, and the absence of pressure-related problems (vaginal trauma or necrosis). Earlier evaluation (in 24 to 48 hours) may be advisable for patients who are debilitated or require additional assistance.

References

Papers of particular interest have been highlighted as follows:
• Of interest
•• Of outstanding interest

1.•• Smith RP, Ling FW: *Procedures in Women's Health Care.* Baltimore: Williams & Wilkins; 1997.
A large number of procedures that may be performed as a part of women's health care are reviewed with equipment lists and tips on coding.

Recommended Reading

Ang MS, Kaufman RH, Adam E, *et al.*: Colposcopically directed biopsy and loop excision of the transformation zone: comparison of histologic findings. *J Reprod Med* 1995, 40:167–170.

• Chambers JT, Chambers SK: Endometrial sampling: when? where? why? with what? *Clin Obstet Gynecol* 1992, 35:28–39.
An easy reading overview.

• Curry SL, Pfenniger JL, Sarma S: Colposcopy: when? why? how? *Patient Care* 1994, 15:167.
Another excellent overview.

Deger RB, Menzin AW, Mikuta JJ: The vaginal pessary: past and present. *Postgrad Obstet Gynecol* 1993, 13:1.

•• Dunton CJ, Sedlacek TV: *Comprehensive Review of Colposcopy.* Washington, DC: American College of Obstetricians and Gynecologists and American Society for Colposcopy and Cervical Pathology; 1996.
One of many excellent texts that cover the field of colposcopy.

Ferris DG: Lethal tissue temperature during cervical cryotherapy with a small flat cryoprobe. *J Fam Pract* 1994, 38:153–156.

•• Greenhill JP: The nonsurgical management of vaginal relaxation. *Clin Obstet Gynecol* 1972, 15:1083.
One of the classic texts dealing with pessaries and their use.

Johnson BA: The colposcopic examination [review]. *Am Fam Physician* 1996, 53:2473–2482; 2487–2488.

Lipscomb GH, Lopatine SM, Stovall TG, *et al.*: A randomized comparison of the Pipelle, Accurate, and Explora endometrial sampling devices. *Am J Obstet Gynecol* 1994, 170:591–594.

Mathevet P, Dargent D, Roy M, *et al.*: A randomized prospective study comparing three techniques of conization: cold knife, laser, and LEEP. *Gynecol Oncol* 1994, 54:175–179.

Nolan TE, Smith RP, Smith MT, *et al.*: A prospective evaluation of an endometrial suction curette. *J Gynecol Surg* 1992, 8:231–234.

• Reid PC, Brown VA, Fothergill DJ: Outpatient investigation of postmenopausal bleeding. *Br J Obstet Gynaecol* 1993, 100:498.
A good general review.

Shier RM: The colposcopy unit: instrumentation, colposcopic technique, recording of findings, and terminology [review]. *Obstet Gynecol Clin North Am* 1993, 20:47–67.

Sulak PJ, Kuehl TJ, Shull BL: Vaginal pessaries and their use in pelvic relaxation. *J Reprod Med* 1993, 38:919–923.

Townsend DE: Colposcopy, cryosurgery, carbon dioxide laser, and loop electrosurgical excision procedure (LEEP). In *Office Gynecology*, edn 4. Edited by Glass RH. Baltimore: Williams & Wilkins; 1992:133–161.

Zeitlin MP, Lebherz TB: Pessaries in the geriatric patient. *J Am Geriatr Soc* 1992, 40:635–639.

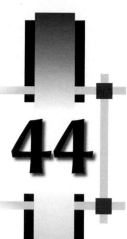

Sexual Dysfunction in Women

Candace Brown

- The female sexual response is circuitous and includes emotional intimacy, sexual stimuli, and relationship satisfaction.
- The etiology of female sexual disorders may be related to medical conditions, medications, psychologic factors, or a combination of these components.
- Assessment of female sexual disorders always includes a sexual history and may require a physical examination in selected disorders.
- Female sexual dysfunction includes sexual desire disorders, sexual arousal disorders, orgasmic disorders, and sexual pain disorders.
- Management of female sexual disorders includes general treatment guidelines for all women, hormone therapy for selected postmenopausal women, and referral to a psychologist or sex therapist for more difficult cases.

Normal Female Sexual Response

Most clinicians are aware of the traditional human sexual response cycle of Masters and Johnson [1] and Kaplan [2]. This cycle depicts a linear sequence of discrete events, including desire, arousal, plateau of constant high arousal, peak intensity arousal and release of orgasm, possible repeated orgasms, and then resolution. An alternative sexual response model has been suggested by Basson [3]. This model incorporates the importance of emotional intimacy, sexual stimuli, and relationship satisfaction. It acknowledges that compared with male sexual functioning, female sexual functioning proceeds in a more complex and circuitous manner and is affected by psychosocial issues. Women may enter the cycle at multiple points and their goal is not necessarily orgasm, but personal satisfaction, which may include physical or emotional satisfaction or both.

Etiology

MEDICAL CONDITIONS

Numerous medical conditions are associated with sexual dysfunction (Figure 44-1) [4]. Women with spinal cord injuries may experience anorgasmia and reduced genital vasocongestion and lubrication depending on the degree and type of injury.

Insufficient blood flow resulting from arterial diseases, such as hypertension, may cause vaginal wall and clitoral smooth muscle fibrosis, resulting in vaginal dryness and dyspareunia. Blunt trauma and surgical disruption also may lead to a decreased vaginal and clitoral blood flow.

Gynecologic malignances, radiation, and chemotherapy may produce physiologic changes, which lead to dyspareunia and reduced sexual arousal. Psychologic effects, related to an impaired self-image, particularly after a mastectomy or from chemotherapy-induced hair loss, may significantly impair sexual desire.

Hormonal changes associated with menopause and aging often cause important physical and psychologic effects on sexual function. Vaginal atrophy often results in vaginal dryness and pain during intercourse, whereas stress and urge incontinence may affect a women's level of comfort during sexual activity for fear of leakage. Other hormonal imbalances that may affect sexual functioning include diabetes mellitus, hyperprolactinemia, hypothyroid and hyperthyroid states [4].

MEDICATIONS

The most common medications associated with female sexual dysfunction are the selective serotonin reuptake inhibitors (SSRIs) (Figure 44-2). Delay or absence of orgasm with reduced sexual desire occurs in up to 70% of women taking SSRIs [5••,6•]. Those antidepressants least likely to interfere with sexual response include non-SSRI antidepressants such as nefazodone, mirtazepine, bupropion, venlafaxine, duloxetine, and buspirone [5●●,6●]. Other centrally acting medications including antipsychotics, barbiturates, benzodiazepines, opiates, and antihistamines also may affect sexual function [5●●,6●].

Antihypertensives that penetrate the blood-brain barrier, such as beta blockers and centrally acting antihypertensives, as well as diuretics may reduce sexual desire [5●●,6●]. However, calcium channel blockers, angiotensin-converting enzyme inhibitors, and angiotensin II receptor blockers (ARBs) are generally not considered to have sexual side effects [5●●,6●] Other cardiovascular agents such as antilipemics may also induce sexual problems [5●●,6●].

A subgroup of women using oral contraceptives or estrogen therapy report low sexual desire, which may be caused by reduced free testosterone production and an increased level of sex hormone-binding globulin [5●●,6●]. Progestins may induce sexual dysfunction by their mood-altering effects [6●]. Some selective estrogen receptor modulators such as raloxifene and tamoxifen may have estrogen antagonistic activity in the vagina, resulting in vaginal dryness and dyspareunia [5●●,6●].

PSYCHOLOGIC FACTORS

Low libido often occurs in women with major depression. Women who report mood changes, sleep disturbance, fatigue, decreased concentration, low self-esteem, reduced interest in activities, decreased energy and motivation, and appetite or weight changes may improve in sexual function if their depression is effectively treated (Figure 44-3).

Women who are under tremendous stress often feel they do not have time for sexual activity and may view it as just "another responsibility." Those who work full-time, take care of children, and carry the majority of domestic activities may hold resentment toward their partner. In addition, assuming the role of "mother" and "wife" may reduce a woman's feeling of being sexual, in both her eyes and in those of her partner.

Although alcohol and other recreational substances may temporarily produce a "disinhibiting" effect on women who are anxious about sexual activity, chronic substance abuse impairs sexual function. Women who have a history of sexual abuse during childhood or in adult relationships may develop an aversion toward sexual activity.

One of the most common contributors to sexual dysfunction in women is relationship difficulties, stemming from poor communication skills, infidelity, control issues, partner substance abuse, and parental conflicts. Lack of privacy because of the presence of children or relatives living with a couple also may affect a woman's comfort level in engaging in sexual activity. In addition, any partner dysfunction such as erectile dysfunction or premature ejaculation can reduce a woman's motivation to be sexual.

Women who were raised in a very restrictive religious background or culture, where sexual activity was considered wrong before marriage, may find it difficult to automatically transition into feeling sexual once she becomes married. Finally,

Medical Causes of Female Sexual Dysfunction

Neurologic problems
  Spinal cord injuries
Cardiovascular disease
  Hypertension
  Hypercholesterolemia
  Peripheral vascular disease
Cancer
  Ovarian cancer
  Endometrial cancer
  Breast cancer
Urogenital disorders
  Stress and urinary incontinence
  Uterine prolapse
Hormonal loss or abnormalities
  Natural and surgical menopause
  Diabetes mellitus
  Hyperprolactinemia
  Hypothyroid and hyperthyroid states

Figure 44-1. Medical causes of female sexual dysfunction. (*Adapted from* Bachmann and Avci [4].)

Medication-induced Sexual Dysfunction

Psychoactive medications
  Antipsychotics
  Barbiturates
  Benzodiazepines
  Selective serotonin reuptake inhibitors
  Tricyclic antidepressants
Opiates
Anticholinergics
Antihistamines
Antihypertensives
  Beta-blockers
  Centrally acting (clonidine, methyldopa)
  Diuretics
Antilipid medications
Hormones
  Oral contraceptives
  Gonadotropin-releasing hormone agonists
  Medroxyprogesterone
  Selective estrogen receptor modulators

Figure 44-2. Medication-induced sexual dysfunction. (*Adapted from* American College of Obstetrician Gynecologists [5●●] and Phillips [6●].)

many women may not have received any education about sex, including basic knowledge of female and male anatomy and a woman's sexual response.

Assessment

SEXUAL HISTORY

A comprehensive sexual history is the first step in establishing the diagnosis of a female sexual disorder. Sexual inquiry should aim at exploring the areas of the patient's concerns, moving from general to more specific areas.

Figure 44-4 identifies the components of a thorough sexual history. Questions that should be asked during the history of the present illness include chief sexual complaints (in the patient's own words), eliciting information on the onset, duration, precipitating factors, and other sexual complaints. It should be determined whether the symptoms are situational (occur in only one setting) or are generalized (present in all settings) and whether they are lifelong (have always been present) or acquired (there was a time in which there was normal sexual functioning). The clinician should determine the patient's and the partner's explanation for the symptoms because their thoughts may add significant insight into the cause of the problems. It is important to know why the patient is seeking treatment now, the amount of distress, and the woman's motivation for seeking treatment, as these factors may affect patient compliance with therapy. Information should be elicited on type of previous treatment and its success.

Patients should be asked to describe a typical sexual encounter. This allows the patient to "tell their story" and to feel heard. The typical encounter should evaluate all phases of sexual response, including desire, arousal, orgasm, and pain. The frequency and types of sexual activity should be determined and which partner initiates the activities. It is important to keep in mind that women often do not "initiate" sexual activity but their desire is more related to their "receptivity" to their partner. The significance of contextual factors, such as time of day, location, fatigue, privacy, atmosphere, and foreplay should be elicited. Both the patient and their partner's response to the symptoms should be determined because they may involve misinterpretation and lead to communication difficulties.

PHYSICAL EXAMINATION

Physical examination is crucial for diagnosing some sexual disorders such as dyspareunia. A very careful genital examination should be performed, especially of the introitus, because in most cases of dyspareunia, the pain is introital. Careful detailed inspection for vulvar atrophy or dystrophy or posterior fourchette scars (often facilitated by allowing the woman to see the examination using a mirror) and testing for allodynia around the hymenal edge with a cotton swab are needed. Resting vaginal tone and voluntary muscle contraction can be assessed approximately by the examining finger(s), and/or with the use of perineometry. Tenderness, often focal from pressing on the deep levator ani ring, can be checked along with pain and discomfort by palpating the uterus and adnexa. Fixed retroversion can be determined, along with any nodularity suggestive of endometriosis. Bladder and urethral sensitivity can be assessed by palpating the anterior vaginal wall.

Differential Diagnoses

The definitions of female sexual dysfunction have been defined by the International Consensus Development Conference on Female Sexual Dysfunction (Figure 44-5) [7••]. The

---

Psychologic Causes of Female Sexual Dysfunction

Interpersonal
  Depression/anxiety
  Stress
  Alcohol/substance abuse
  Prior sexual or physical abuse
Relationship
  Relationship quality and conflict
  Lack of privacy
  Partner performance and technique
Sociocultural
  Conflict with religious, personal, or family values
  Societal taboos
  Inadequate sexual education

Figure 44-3. Psychologic causes of female sexual dysfunction. (*Adapted from* Bachmann and Avci [4].)

Sexual History

History of present illness
Typical encounter
Current medications
Past medications
Medical history
Social history
Psychiatric history
Family history
Developmental and sexual history
Relationship history
Stressors
Psychiatric examination
Mental status
Physical examination
Diagnosis

Figure 44-4. Sexual history.

consensus conference panel built on the existing framework of the World Health Organization International Classification of Disease-10 [8] and the Diagnostic and Statistical Manual of Mental Disorders IV of the American Psychiatric Association [9]. The former Diagnostic and Statistical Manual of Mental Disorders IV classifications were expanded to include psychogenic and organic cause of desire, arousal, orgasm, and sexual pain disorders. An essential element of this new diagnostic system is the personal distress criterion, meaning that a condition is considered a disorder only if it creates distress for the woman experiencing the condition.

SEXUAL DESIRE DISORDERS

Approximately 30% of women experience hypoactive sexual desire disorder [10•]. Hypoactive sexual desire disorder, also known as sexual desire/interest disorder, is defined as "the persistent or recurrent deficiency (or absence) of sexual fantasies/thoughts, and/or desire for or receptivity to sexual activity, which causes personal distress" [7••].

SEXUAL AROUSAL DISORDER

Sexual arousal disorder is defined as "the persistent or recurrent inability to attain or maintain sufficient sexual excitement, which in turn causes personal distress" [7••]. Women with the problem report a lack of subjective excitement and/or lack of genital (lubrication/swelling). Up to 20% of women experience lubrication problems with sexual exchange [10•].

Classification of Sexual Dysfunction Disorders According to the International Consensus Development Conference on Female Sexual Dysfunction

Sexual desire disorders (sexual desire/interest disorder)

  Hypoactive sexual desire disorder

  Sexual aversion disorder

Sexual arousal disorder

  Combined sexual arousal disorder

  Subjective sexual arousal disorder

  Genital arousal disorder

Orgasmic disorder

Sexual pain disorders

  Dyspareunia

  Vaginismus

Other sexual pain disorders

  Generalized vulvodynia

  Vestibulodynia

Figure 44-5. Classification of sexual dysfunction disorders according to the International Consensus Development Conference on Female Sexual Dysfunction. (*Adapted from* Basson *et al.* [7••].)

ORGASMIC DISORDER

Orgasmic disorder is defined as "the persistent or recurrent difficulty, delay in, or absence of attaining orgasm following sufficient sexual stimulation and arousal, which causes personal distress" [7••]. Primary orgasmic disorder refers to a woman's inability to achieve an orgasm under any circumstances. A secondary orgasmic disorder most often refers to an inability to reach climax during intercourse, but otherwise can be achieved with masturbation or during sexual foreplay. Inability to have orgasm via intercourse is common, occurring in approximately one third of women and is only problematic if it distresses the woman. Studies of the general population and sex therapy clinic populations indicate the prevalence of female orgasmic disorder ranges from 24% to 37% [10•].

SEXUAL PAIN DISORDERS

Dyspareunia is defined as "the recurrent or persistent genital pain associated with sexual intercourse" [7••]. When looking at both pre- and postmenopausal populations, 14.4% of all women report pain during sexual activity [10•]. This percentage appears to increase with the onset of menopause, where up to 34% of postmenopausal women report pain during coital exchange.

Vaginismus is defined as "the recurrent or persistent involuntary spasm of the musculature of the outer third of the vagina that interferes with vaginal penetration and causes personal distress" [7••]. Generalized vaginismus is characterized by involuntary vaginal spasms, which occur in all situations. Situational vaginismus refers to a dysfunction that is apparent only in a specific situation such as vaginismus triggered by intercourse but not with tampon insertion.

OTHER SEXUAL PAIN DISORDERS

Noncoital sexual pain disorder is the new category of sexual pain disorders, which was added to the classification system after the 1998 International Consensus Development Conference [7••]. Essential dysesthetic vulvodynia (also known as generalized vulvodynia) is associated with a constant diffuse pain affecting the labia majora, labia minora, and/or vestibule. Vulvar vestibulitis (also known as vestibulodynia), however, is characterized by focal pain aggravated by touch and pressure. Vaginal penetration is often painful or impossible for most women with this condition. Women with vulvodynia may see several clinicians and undergo a range of treatments before receiving the correct diagnosis.

Management

GENERAL TREATMENT GUIDELINES

Women should be provided information and education about normal anatomy, sexual function, and normal changes of aging, pregnancy, and menopause. To enhance stimulation and eliminate routine, the clinician should encourage communication during sexual activity; recommend use of vibrators; discuss varying positions, times of day or places; and suggest making a "date" for sexual activity. Distraction techniques should also be discussed, including encouraging erotic or nonerotic fantasy; recommending pelvic muscle contracting and relaxation (similar to Kegel exercise) with intercourse; recommending use of background music, and videos or television. The clinician should encourage noncoital behaviors and recommend sensual massage, sensate-focus exercises (sensual massage with no involvement of sexual areas), where one partner provides the massage and the receiving partner provides feedback as to what feels good (aimed to promote comfort and communication between partners), and oral or noncoital stimulation, with or without orgasm. To minimize dyspareunia, the clinician should recommend sexual positions including female superior or side-lying for control of penetration depth and speed and use of lubricants, topical lidocaine, and warm baths before intercourse.

HORMONE THERAPY

Estrogen and androgen therapy may play a key role in the peri- and postmenopausal woman. Estrogen therapy is helpful in relieving dyspareunia and may be helpful in treating arousal disorders by decreasing coital pain and improving clitoral sensitivity [6•].

Although testosterone replacement has not yet been approved by the US Food and Drug Administration for low libido, it has been shown to improve sexual function in some postmenopausal women [6•]. In addition to decreased sexual desire, symptoms of androgen insufficiency include fatigue and decreased well-being [11••].

No guidelines for testosterone replacement therapy exist for women with desire disorders, and there is no consensus on "normal" or "therapeutic" levels. Many clinicians are concerned about the lack of safety data on testosterone in breast cancer and on hepatic side effects; however, hepatocellular damage or carcinoma is rare at prescribed dosages, and the development of breast cancer has not been reported clinically. Side effects of testosterone, which occur in 5% to 35% of patients, include lower levels of high-density lipoprotein, acne, hirsutism, clitoromegaly, and voice deepening [6•]. Alteration of lipoprotein levels is rarely significant if estrogen and testosterone are coadministered, and most other side effects are reversible with discontinuation of testosterone or a dosage adjustment [6•]. Before starting testosterone therapy, clinicians should establish a baseline of acne, hirsutism, and other androgenic signs and counsel the women on potential androgenic changes. In general, patients with current or previous breast cancer, uncontrolled hyperlipidemia, liver disease, acne, or hirsutism should not receive testosterone therapy. Treatment guidelines are provided in Figure 44-6. It should be reiterated that testosterone is not formally approved by the US Food and Drug Administration for the treatment of desire disorders in women.

COMPOUNDED BIOIDENTICAL HORMONES

Compounded drugs are agents that are prepared, mixed, assembled, packaged, or labeled as a drug by a pharmacist [12]. Unlike drugs that are approved by the US Food and Drug Administration to be manufactured and sold in standardized dosages, compounded medications often are custom made for a patient according to a clinician's specifications.

Bioidentical hormones are plant-derived hormones that are biochemically similar or identical to those produced by the ovary or body and most commonly include dehydroepiandrosterone, testosterone, pregnenolone, progesterone, estrone, estradiol, and estriol [12]. They are available in oral, sublingual, percutaneous, or as implants, injectables, and suppositories. Currently there is no scientific evidence to support claims of increased efficacy or safety for bioidentical hormones. Purchases of compounded hormones are not typically reimbursed by insurance companies.

Referral

Typical reasons for referring a patient include: 1) if she has a complex history, including physical and psychologic symptoms; 2) if she has not responded to traditional therapy (eg,

Androgen Therapy for Treatment of Female Androgen Insufficiency*

Screening

  Baseline testosterone levels[†] (free and total), estradiol levels[‡], DHEA-S[§], baseline lipid profile, baseline liver enzyme levels, mammography, Papanicolaou smear

Initiate therapy[¶]

  Combination product (Estratest or Estratest H.S., Solvay Pharmaceuticals, Brussels, Belgium)

  Testim 1% (5 g/5 mL per tube); apply 0.5 mL every other day to every day

  DHEA 25 mg 1 capsule by mouth daily

  Compounded testosterone vanishing cream**

Reevaluation at 3 months

  Repeat androgen levels, DHEA-S, estradiol, lipid profile, liver enzyme levels

  Monitor symptom side effects

Continued therapy

  Taper to lowest effective dose

  Monitor lipid levels and liver enzyme levels once or twice yearly

  Routine Papanicolaou smear and mammogram schedules

*These are recommendations; no evidence-based protocols are available on androgen therapy for the treatment of women with desire disorders.
†Many authors recommend that total levels remain in "normal" range for premenopausal women.
‡Metabolic pathway of testosterone metabolism ends with estradiol.
§Dehydroepiandrosterone sulfate.
¶None of these medications are labeled by the US Food and Drug Administration for treatment of desire disorders.
**Use in conjunction with compounding pharmacist.

Figure 44-6. Androgen therapy for treatment of female androgen insufficiency. DHEA-S—dehydroepiandrosterone sulfate. (*Adapted from* Phillips [6•].)

antidepressants); 3) if it appears there are major relationship issues (eg, infidelity); 4) a history of sexual abuse or domestic violence; 5) multiple medical conditions are present with coexisting medications; 6) if the clinician does not have adequate knowledge in treating sexual disorders; and 7) if the clinician does not have adequate time or desire to treat sexual disorders. The best way to determine the location of a qualified certified sex therapist is to go to the web site of the American Association of Sex Educators, Counselors, and Therapists (AASECT) (www.AASECT.org).

References

Papers of particular interest have been highlighted as follows:
• Of interest
•• Of outstanding interest

1.   Masters WH, Johnson VE: *Human Sexual Response*. Boston: Little & Brown; 1987.

2.   Kaplan H, Passalacqua D: *Illustrated Manual of Sex Therapy*, edn 2. New York: Routledge; 1988.

3.   Basson R: A model of women's sexual arousal. *J Sex Marital Ther* 2002, 28:1–10.

4.   Bachmann GA, Avci D: Evaluation and management of female sexual dysfunction. *Endocrinologist* 2004, 14:337.

5.•• American College of Obstetrician Gynecologists: Sexuality and sexual disorders. In *Clinical Updates in Women's Health*. Washington DC: American College of Obstetricians and Gynecologists: 2003.
Comprehensive overview of the diagnosis and treatment of female sexual disorders.

6.•   Phillips NA: Female sexual dysfunction: Evaluation and treatment. *Amer Fam Physician* 2000, 62:127.
Provides clinical guidelines for the use of testosterone in women.

7.•• Basson B, Berman JR, Burnett AL, *et al.*: Report of the International Consensus Development Conference on female sexual dysfunction: definitions and classifications. *J Urol* 2000, 163:888.
Most current classification of female sexual disorders.

8.   World Health Organization: *International Statistical Classification of Diseases and Related Health Problems (ICD-10)*, edn 10. Geneva: World Health Organization; 1994.

9.   American Psychiatric Association: *DSM-V: Diagnostic and Statistical Manual of Mental Disorders*, edn 4. Washington, DC: American Psychiatric Press; 1994.

10.• Laumann EO, Paik A, Rosen RC: Sexual dysfunction in the United States: prevalence and predictors. *JAMA* 1999, 281:537.
Largest community-based sample on the prevalence of female sexual dysfunction.

11.•• Bachmann G, Bancroft J, Braunstein G, *et al.*: Female androgen insufficiency: the Princeton consensus statement on definition, classification, and assessment. *Fertil Steril* 2002, 77:660.
Provides algorithm for the treatment of female androgen deficiency.

12.   American College of Obstetrician Gynecologists: Compounded bioidentical hormones. In *Committee Opinion*. Washington, DC: American College of Obstetrician Gynecologists; 2005.

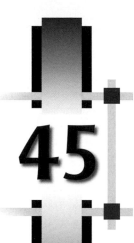

45 | Dyspareunia

Frank W. Ling and John A. Lamont

- Dyspareunia is the most common sexual symptom affecting women who seek gynecologic care.
- Community surveys report that 8% of women have dyspareunia and 17% more admit to vaginal dryness.
- Etiologic factors include intrapsychic, organic, and interpersonal problems.
- Pathophysiology of dyspareunia includes lack of arousal, vaginismus, and pathology of the pelvic tissues.
- The PLISSIT model of treating sexual problems (permission, limited information, specific suggestions, intensive therapy) encourages primary care practitioners to deal effectively with the majority of sexual problems in the office setting.

Comfortable coitus in a heterosexual relationship may foster a sense of personal competence and affirm the partners' intimacy. Dyspareunia, or painful intercourse, results in disappointment, loss of self-esteem, a sense of sexual incompetence, and a loss intimacy in the relationship. Dyspareunia is the most common sexual symptom affecting women who seek gynecologic care [1]. The term *dyspareunia* is derived from ancient Greek and means "bad or difficult mating." During the 20th century, dyspareunia has been used to describe orgasmic dysfunction, lack of simultaneous orgasm, or coital pain with an organic cause [2,3]. In this chapter, *dyspareunia* is used to refer to female coital pain, including recurrent or persistent discomfort associated with coitus. Dyspareunia can be primary, secondary, situational, or complete. Primary dyspareunia refers to pain that is experienced with each and every attempt at coitus. Secondary dyspareunia occurs when a woman has experienced comfortable coitus for a period of time, followed by the occurrence of pain with coitus. Situational dyspareunia describes a woman who consistently experiences discomfort with coitus in a specific situation or with a specific partner but does not experience it in other situations or with other partners. Complete dyspareunia refers to discomfort (primary or secondary) that is experienced in all coital situations.

The term *vaginismus* needs clarification here because of the role it plays in the cause of dyspareunia. Vaginismus is an involuntary spasm of the pelvic floor muscles and the perineal muscles, involving the outer third of the vagina, resulting in painful intercourse or prohibiting intromission. This spasm is a reflex contraction, induced by "imagined, anticipated, or real attempts at inserting something into the vagina." In severe cases, the pelvic floor spasm can be accompanied by contraction of the adductors of the thighs, the rectus abdominus muscle, and the gluteus muscles [4]. Similarly, vaginismus can be primary or secondary. It also can be situational or complete. Secondary vaginismus is often a component of secondary dyspareunia. The original pain may have been initiated by an organic cause (episiotomy or infection), which has been treated effectively without resolution of the pain during intromission. Careful examination is necessary to determine that the initial cause of discomfort is resolved but that its presence had induced a reflex involuntary contraction of the pelvic floor that has become the source of the ongoing dyspareunia (Figure 45-1).

Incidence and Epidemiology

In a community survey, 33% of women said they had experienced sexual dysfunction [5]. Eight percent of the total surveyed acknowledged the presence of dyspareunia, and a further 17% acknowledged vaginal dryness. Several gynecologic studies suggested a prevalence of sexual dysfunction in women that ranges from 10.6% to 46% [2,6–8]. The prevalence in other clinics ranged from 4% to 33.5% [5,9–11]. The actual figures are hard to obtain because most women who have painful intercourse do not present this as their chief complaint [6]. Women who have pain with coitus as a major complaint often present with other symptoms or for routine care, with the hope that the health professional will take the initiative in exploring sexual issues [2,5–7].

Comfortable coitus occurs with the right blend of emotional and physiologic responses. This requires an atmosphere of privacy and safety; physiologic sexual response, including vaginal lubrication and vaginal expansion; and relaxation of the pelvic floor muscles [1]. Etiologic factors that interfere with these physiologic and emotional responses include intrapsychic, interpersonal, and organic factors [12]. Intrapersonal issues are the main contributing factors in 43% of patients presenting with dyspareunia (Figure 45-2). Individual assessment requires careful questioning about sexual socialization, gender role socialization, and history of sexual trauma. Elements of fear, anxiety, and dysphoria are often identified. Women who participate in coitus only for reproductive purposes or who are unable to accept responsibility for their own sexual pleasure often experience dyspareunia.

Interpersonal conflict is the primary contributing factor in 27% of cases of dyspareunia. These relationships are characterized by unresolved anger and poor communication, with special difficulty in talking about sex and about feelings [13]. "Struggle for control" is identified as a relationship issue that can adversely affect the physical relationship and result in a decrease in sexual desire and loss of sexual response for many women. The expectation of sexual accommodation by the woman and of sexual entitlement for the man is a common attitude produced by sexual role socialization in monogamous heterosexual relationships. Men who commit to a monogamous heterosexual relationship may feel entitled to sexual access on demand, and women may feel obliged to accommodate coitus to ensure the man's monogamous commitment. This contributes to a differential of power and loss of intimacy in the couple's relationship as well as inhibition of sexual desire in many women. Sexual performance pressure can be present when intercourse is the primary or sole method of sexual contact and when coital orgasm is necessary as a measure of intimacy for one or both partners.

Assessment of the relationship is best carried out with both partners present to determine the quality of communication, the ability to negotiate, and the degree of mutual support between the partners. Sexual factors can be assessed in the same situation, including interest, range of behavior, satisfaction, and a congruency of reproductive goals.

Organic problems present in 30% of new cases of dyspareunia. The etiologic factors in these cases include previous obstetric or gynecologic trauma to the vagina, menopausal or radiation atrophy; inflammation of the urinary tract, rectum, or vagina; or limited mobility of pelvic tissues resulting from a gynecologic pathology (Figure 45-3).

Pathophysiology

The pathophysiology of dyspareunia can be considered in three categories. The first results from lack of normal physiologic sexual response, the second is a result of vaginismus, and the third results from pathology of the vulva, vagina, or pelvis that produces discomfort from touching, stretching, or motion.

Sexual signals result in a marked vasocongestive change in the pelvis, producing vaginal lubrication, an expansion of the inner two thirds of the vagina, and the formation of an "orgasmic platform" involving the outer third of the vagina. These changes are thought to be related to a preparation of the vulva, vagina, and pelvic organs to accommodate intromission and ensure that coitus is comfortable. These changes do not occur if the woman is distracted or is feeling any negative emotion that causes aversion. If coitus is attempted in this circumstance, the vagina is dry and contracted, resulting in discomfort.

Vaginismus is the involuntary contraction of the pelvic floor, or levator ani muscle, with attempts at intromission. This response can be primary in the case in which a woman has been unable to insert anything in her vagina, including tampon, speculum, finger, or penis [4]. In a less severe situation, a tampon, finger, or penis may have been inserted successfully into the vagina but never without pain (primary dyspareunia). Secondary vaginismus occurs when the woman has experienced

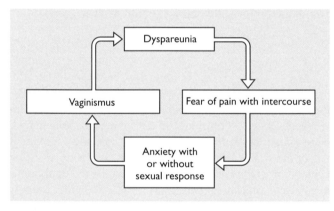

Figure 45-1. Dyspareunia and vaginismus cycle.

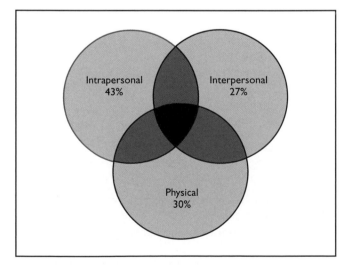

Figure 45-2. Factors associated with female dyspareunia.

comfortable intromission, but at some point in her life physical or psychologic trauma has resulted in the establishment of the involuntary muscle response, which produces painful intromission (secondary dyspareunia).

The third source of discomfort is an organic problem affecting the vulva, vagina, or pelvis. The vulva can be the source of exquisite discomfort caused by infection, inflammation, or atrophy or by a vulvar dystrophy, such as lichen sclerosus, lichen planus, or lichen simplex chronicus. Vulvar vestibulitis and vulvodynia are other common complaints. Vulvar and vaginal scarring from episiotomies or vaginal repair can result in fibromas or neuromas in the scar, producing point tenderness when the introital or vaginal scar is stretched.

Pelvic structures contribute to the discomfort directly or indirectly. The uterus can produce discomfort on deep thrusting through retroversion or large fibroids. Fixation of the adnexa with adhesions from a tubo-ovarian abscess or posthysterectomy scarring can also produce pain with deep thrusting. Extrauterine sources of discomfort include endometriosis (scarring), adhesions from previous inflammation, interstitial cystitis, trigonitis of the bladder, chronic constipation, inflammatory bowel disease, and vascular pain from pelvic congestion and pelvic varicose veins.

Differential Diagnosis

Establishing a differential diagnosis is best accomplished by remembering the impact of sexual response on pelvic structures and by keeping a three-dimensional image of the pelvis in mind while the history is taken. In a sexual medicine practice, the most common causes of pain with intercourse are vulvodynia (plus vulvar vestibulitis) and secondary vaginismus. The patient seen with vulvodynia most often has a history of discomfort all or most of the time, which is made worse by attempts at insertion of anything into the vagina, resulting in a secondary vaginismus. Patients presenting with pain occurring only at attempts at intromission and having secondary vaginismus on examination often have underlying pelvic abnormalities, such as a tender retroverted uterus, a rectum and sigmoid full of hard stool, or pelvic varicose veins that are aggravated by sexual arousal. The third common source of discomfort with intercourse is lack of response based on lack of desire, history of sexual trauma, or aversion to sexual activity.

The three most uncommon causes of painful intercourse are extrauterine pelvic scarring following gynecologic surgery or pelvic inflammatory disease, scarring of the vulva or vagina after episiotomy or vaginal repair, and vulvovaginitis. Each of these can be the primary cause of discomfort in a specific patient; however, in a clinical setting, they are relatively infrequent compared with those causes listed in the previous paragraph.

Diagnostic Studies

HISTORY
A careful patient history is the most important diagnostic tool in assessing a complaint of dyspareunia. The primary care phy-

sician should include routine questions about sexual function and satisfaction in any patient's systems review, so that patients will view the primary care setting as a safe environment for discussion of sexual health issues or concerns about sexual dysfunction. Each health professional must develop his or her own approach to sexual history taking, making sure to project an air of comfort that permits the patient to relax and feel confident in continuing the discussion. The presenting complaint must be carefully explored to understand the onset and course of the symptom. What impact has the problem had on the woman's sexual response (desire, arousal, orgasm), and what impact has it had on her relationship? Has the discomfort been present on each occasion in which intromission has been attempted, and does it affect the use of tampons or speculum examination as well as coitus? Is there any similar discomfort experienced at times other than during intromission? Past gynecologic history, history of pelvic surgeries, and careful systems review add

Summary of Primary and Secondary Problems Associated with Dyspareunia

Primary Physical Problem	Number		Secondary Problems, n
Trauma			
Episiotomy	10		
Vaginal tears	8	19	2
Vaginal septum	1		
Atrophy			
Postmenopausal			3
Surgical castration	14		
Radiation	2	19	
Neovagina	1		
Vulvar dystrophies	2		
Inflammation			
Vulvitis			
Vaginitis	8		
Urethritis and caruncle	1	10	2
Pessary	1		
Obstruction or fixation			
Constipation	5		1
Retroversion and congestion	9		6
Endometriosis	3	20	3
Prolapse	1		
Adhesions	1		5*
Intact hymen	1		

Tender adnexa—no diagnosis.

Figure 45-3. Summary of primary and secondary problems associated with dyspareunia.

useful information to understanding the potential sources of discomfort during intercourse. Review of past and present mood disorders provides essential information to help complete the overview of sexual function. Many antidepressant medications interfere with physiologic sexual response by decreasing desire, delaying arousal, and inhibiting orgasm. Sexual energy is excess energy. Depression eliminates sexual interest or desire by destroying physical and emotional energy.

PHYSICAL EXAMINATION

Careful physical examination with particular focus on the gynecologic examination helps to isolate specific causes of dyspareunia [14•]. This involves visual inspection of the vulva with the addition of a colposcopic assessment when indicated. Palpation of the vestibule, hymen, and pelvic floor is necessary to elicit the vaginismus response. A one-finger examination with gentle pressure on the edge of the levator muscle reproduces the pain of vaginismus. A cotton-swab assessment of the vestibule elicits a positive response for vestibulitis. A one-finger examination of the vaginal barrel permits assessment of scars from a vaginal repair or episiotomy. Speculum examination permits visualization of the upper two thirds of the vagina and the cervix. Bimanual examination permits a full assessment of the pelvic structures, looking for obstruction or fixation within the pelvis that can cause pain. Rectovaginal examination permits complete assessment of abnormalities in the cul-de-sac.

Laboratory investigation is indicated when the history and physical examination suggest the need for assessment of pituitary or gonadal hormone levels, or when the presenting complaint may suggest some underlying disease (multiple sclerosis or diabetes).

Imaging of the abdomen or pelvis is useful in excluding pelvic pathology that may be the source of discomfort. A transvaginal ultrasound performed with the patient in the sitting position may identify the presence of pelvic varicosities lateral to the cervix. The identification of pelvic varicosities may be followed by a venogram and embolization of the varicosities.

Indications for an Educational Pelvic Examination

Patients undergoing first pelvic examination

Patients with gynecologic abnormalities

Patients who are highly anxious about a pelvic examination

Pediatric patients

Patients with dyspareunia and vaginismus

Patients requiring assessment of sexual dysfunction (a conjoint examination may involve an educational genital examination of the male, as well)

Patients who need to be taught self-insertion and removal of vaginal pessaries or diaphragms

Patients with a history of sexual trauma

Figure 45-4. Indications for an educational pelvic examination.

Laparoscopy can be used to add useful information to the assessment. It is a simple and safe procedure that permits clear visualization of the pelvic structures. Laparoscopy is useful in cases in which pelvic fixation or adhesions are suggested on physical examination and the cause needs visualization or treatment. Care needs to be exercised in the interpretation of abnormal findings, which may not explain the pain, and in determining how to interpret a negative result in the further management of the patient.

Treatment

Treatment must be directed at the underlying pathophysiology. Sexual function and sexual relationships are a complex interaction of personal, relationship, and medical issues that may require multiple therapeutic approaches simultaneously [13]. When a medical problem has been present for a long time without resolution, it can often lead to intrapsychic and interpersonal issues that will not disappear by treating the underlying medical problem. Primary care practitioners should be familiar with the PLISSIT model (permission, limited information, specific suggestions, and intensive therapy) for treating sexual problems, which is helpful in addressing their anxiety and fear about getting involved in helping resolve intrapsychic and interpersonal issues [15••].

The most important aspect of therapy for dyspareunia involves the quality of the doctor–patient relationship. A physician with knowledge and personal comfort with sexual issues will provide an environment that encourages disclosure by the patient. Patients identify sexual problems as problems of physical function, and physicians are their first choice for treatment [11].

PATIENT EDUCATION

All patients require sexual information, which may be factual information to correct myths and misinformation, an outline of physiologic sexual response to reassure the patient of normal bodily function, or an educational pelvic examination, which is particularly helpful in assessing and treating vaginismus (Figure 45-4) [15••].

THE PLISSIT MODEL

The PLISSIT model is a theoretic model intended to reassure primary care professionals who may have some reservations about their skills in providing individual or couples therapy for intrapsychic problems, relationship conflict, or sexual problems. The model is reassuring because it acknowledges that most cases presenting as sexual dysfunction can be handled with the proper knowledge, attitude, and listening skills in the primary care setting. The elements of permission, limited Information, and specific suggestion can be appropriately delivered by any primary care professional.

INDIVIDUAL PSYCHOTHERAPY

Although many sexual issues are best addressed using couples therapy, a number of issues having a direct impact on sexual comfort and function can be addressed in individual psychotherapy. Women suffering from sexual aversion or disinterest as a result of domestic violence or adult or childhood sexual abuse may best respond during an individual assessment. In long-term relationships, the partner may resist change and stifle the personal growth that is necessary in the patient to overcome the residual effects of her abuse. Primary anorgasmia readily responds to individual therapy using self-pleasuring techniques. This newly acquired skill can then easily be taught to the partner in several brief conjoint visits. Primary vaginismus may represent complex intrapsychic conflicts, such as autonomy, differentiation, and boundary issues, which are best addressed at least initially in individual therapy [16••,17••].

CONJOINT RELATIONSHIP AND SEX THERAPY

Many sexual problems are the result of long-standing relationship conflict. Restoring enjoyable sexual function requires that both partners participate in change to correct a power imbalance, to develop constructive communication patterns, or to restore intimacy, sensuality, and enriching sexual interaction. If the goals of the two partners are different (eg, one wants to focus on sex and the other on communication), relationship and sexual issues can be confronted simultaneously.

MEDICAL AND SURGICAL PROBLEMS

Any medical or surgical problems identified during the assessment should be treated appropriately. Vulvovaginal infections require appropriate assessment and treatment of positive cultures. Vulvar dermatoses need to be treated with the appropriate topical agent, such as hormone cream or high-potency steroid cream. If underlying pathology, such as endometriosis, is identified, appropriate medical therapy should be instituted. Chronic bowel dysfunction may require expert assessment. Chronic constipation is managed with a high-fiber diet and the use of stool softeners until adequate bowel function is restored. If painful scars are identified, injection with steroids or a long-acting local anaesthetic may reverse the problem or may help to identify the potential benefits of a scar revision if symptoms are relieved temporarily with these injections. Depression and treatment of depression may require reassessment and change in medication if sexual desire and response are adversely affected by the depression or its treatment.

TREATMENT OF VAGINISMUS

This section is added because of the benefits of office management of this problem. Primary vaginismus often requires individual psychotherapy to address some of the major issues outlined earlier in this chapter. Secondary vaginismus is often treated with simple exercises described in the office after the diagnosis has been confirmed by vaginal examination. The patient is instructed to perform Kegel exercises as a first step to overcoming the involuntary muscle spasm. After she can contract these muscles with ease, she is instructed to reverse the exercise, initiating a 1-second pelvic floor contraction followed by 5 seconds of relaxation. Biofeedback is also used; the patient places her finger in the vagina so that she can feel the contraction and relaxation of the pelvic floor. This allows the use of the finger to massage the muscle, facilitate relaxation, and reinforce the relaxation part of the cycle. After

comfortable insertion of one finger, the woman moves on to two fingers. After three fingers can be introduced comfortably, the patient is instructed to perform these exercises in the female-superior position. When relaxation can be accomplished in this position, the patient is instructed to slide the vagina over the lubricated penis to accomplish full intromission. After this exercise has been completed on several occasions, coitus can be attempted in a variety of different positions.

Referral

Most sexual complaints in the primary care setting can be addressed adequately within that setting by a comfortable and knowledgeable primary care physician. A small minority of cases may be too complex, too time consuming, or outside the area of interest or level of skills of the primary care physician. These few cases require referral to an appropriate secondary or tertiary care practitioner. The problem may require referral for in-depth individual or couple psychotherapy. Specific couple sexual problems may require in-depth relationship or sexual therapy. The final situation in which referral is indicated relates to the usefulness of a colleague for a second opinion. This exercise may benefit the primary care practitioner and the clients by reassuring both that the issues are clearly identified and the course of treatment is appropriate.

Prevention

Primary care practice provides a golden opportunity for preventive sexual health care by incorporating sexual health issues into everyday practice. This can be accomplished by including routine questions in every general assessment, every initial assessment, and every systems review. Exposing patients to these routine questions and issues helps them to develop an association between their sexuality and their health care. This "advertising" invites the patient to address sexual issues with the primary care health practitioner. This approach is welcomed by patients and is an effective way to encourage them to express their concerns, which may otherwise go unnoticed. Primary care physicians are also in a key position to encourage education between parents and their children or to act as a surrogate educator on behalf of the parents to help inform children about their sexuality. The physician can create a comfort zone in which young people can address issues of sexual abuse, sexual function, masturbation, and sexually transmitted diseases and learn to be responsible for their sexual health.

References

Papers of particular interest have been highlighted as follows:
• Of interest
•• Of outstanding interest

1. Lamont JA: Female dyspareunia: when making love hurts. *Contemp Obstet Gynecol* 1994, 3:41–42.

2. Jeffcoate TNA: *Principles of Gynecology*, edn 3. London: Butterworth; 1967.

3. Harlow RA, McCluskey CJ: Introital dyspareunia. *Clin Med* 1972, 79:25.

4. Lamont JA: Vaginismus. Am J Obstet Gynecol 1978, 131:632.

5. Osborn M, Hawton K, Gath D: Sexual dysfunction among middle aged women in the community. *Br Med J* 1988, 296:959–962.

6. Bachmann GA, Leiblum SR, Grill J: Brief sexual inquiry in gynecologic practice. *Obstet Gynecol* 1989, 73:425–427.

7. Frenken J, Van Tol P: Sexual problems in gynecological practice. *J Psychosom Obstet Gynecol* 1987, 6:143–155.

8. Jamieson DJ, Steege JF: The prevalence of dysmenorrhea, dyspareunia, pelvic pain, and irritable bowel syndrome in primary care practices. *Obstet Gynecol* 1996, 87:55–58.

9. Glatt AE, Zinner SH, McCormack WM: The prevalence of dyspareunia. *Obstet Gynecol* 1990, 75:433–436.

10. Dickinson RL: *Human Sexual Anatomy*. Baltimore: Williams & Wilkins; 1949.

11. Shein M, Zyzanski SJ, Levine S, *et al.*: The frequency of sexual problems among family practice patients. *Fam Pract Res J* 1988, 7:122–134.

12. Lamont J: Female dyspareunia. *Am J Obstet Gynecol* 1980, 136:282–285.

13. Rust J, Golombok S, Collier J: Marital problems and sexual dysfunction: how are they related? *Br J Psychol* 1988, 152:629–631.

14.• Steege JF, Ling FW: Dyspareunia: s special type of chronic pelvic pain. *Obstet Gynecol Clin North Am* 1993, 20:779–793.

An in-depth review of the subject using brief and easy-to-read sections of the chapter.

15.•• Lamont JA: Office sexual counseling and the educational pelvic examination. *Gynecol Obstet* 1996, 6:1–11.

A review of current issues and strategies for providing sexual health care in the office setting.

16.•• Silverstein JL: Origins of psychogenic vaginismus. *Psychother Psychosom* 1989, 52:197–204.

Presents a theory that vaginismus is protection against violation.

17.•• Shaw J: Treatment of primary vaginismus: a new perspective. *J Sex Marital Ther* 1994, 20:46–55.

Primary vaginismus is viewed as a somatic boundary needed in the struggle for differentiation.

46 Sexual Assault and Abuse

Emily Jackson, Joquetta D. Paige, Dalia Brahmi, Adjoa B. Duker, and Marji Gold

- Approximately one in six women and girls in America experience sexual assault; most of these incidents occur before the victim is 20 years old and are perpetrated by someone known to the victim.
- A history of sexual assault is associated with long-term physical and mental health complications, including chronic pain syndromes, depression and anxiety, substance abuse, and other self-destructive behaviors.
- Only 25% to 35% of sexual assaults are reported to criminal justice authorities or medical professionals; therefore, in the health care setting, most are discovered only through routine, direct questioning.
- The medical examination of a rape victim should focus on the evaluation and treatment of injuries and the prevention or identification and treatment of pregnancy and sexually transmitted infections.
- The forensic examination is best performed by a trained sexual assault examiner and should follow state protocols for the collection, storage, and maintenance of forensic specimens.

Violence in the lives of girls and women has a profound effect on short- and long-term health. It may present obviously or be hidden behind nonspecific complaints acutely or long after the abuse has occurred. Whether recent or remote, most cases of sexual abuse and assault are not disclosed to the health care provider but are discovered only when directly and specifically addressed by the clinician. For this reason, the primary health care provider is in an optimal position to identify and address violence in the lives of adolescent and adult women and to offer preventive strategies that can reduce the complicated and costly sequelae.

This chapter first addresses the identification and management of adult or adolescent patients who have a past history of sexual assault. Then, the acute management of a sexual assault victim is reviewed with an emphasis on the clinician's responsibilities in the areas of medical care and evidence collection. Finally, recommendations for follow-up are made, and prevention strategies are discussed.

Definitions

The terms *rape* and *sexual assault* are legal terms with definitions that vary from state to state. All definitions, however, include the following three basic components: 1) sexual penetration, 2) lack of consent, and 3) the use of force, threat of force, or intimidation. In all states, the definition of sexual penetration implies penetration of the vulva (not necessarily the vagina), mouth, or anus. In most states, lack of consent also includes the inability to provide consent because of physical or mental limitations, including impairment caused by alcohol or other substance use.

The use of force is obvious when physical force or a weapon is used, but it is also implied when a victim is coerced or intimidated into having sexual intercourse by a person in a position of authority over the victim. The term *statutory rape*, or criminal sexual conduct with a minor, refers to sexual activity with a child or adolescent who is under the age of consent as defined by state laws.

The age of consent varies considerably among states as does the legal requirement to report such cases. All states, however, have mandatory reporting laws for cases of childhood sexual abuse. Because of the variation in definitions and reporting mandates, it is critical that clinicians who care for children and adolescents are familiar with their state's reporting requirements; these are generally available through state medical associations or local rape crisis centers. A complete discussion of statutory rape and child sexual abuse is beyond the scope of this chapter.

For legal and medical purposes, different types of sexual assault have been defined. Figure 46-1 lists the various types of sexual assault, their definitions, and relevant issues for each type of assault. There is significant overlap between the various types of assault described, but these classifications hold particular importance in addressing the psychologic impact and emotional recovery from rape.

Epidemiology

The problem of violence against women has been recognized as a serious public health epidemic in the United States [1]. It is estimated that more than 300,000 women and 93,000 men are sexually victimized every year, and more than 18 million women and 3 million men in the United States have experienced at least one sexual assault during their lifetime [2•]. Population-based studies indicate that about 1 in 6 women and girls experience sexual assault [2•]. Rape occurs to men and women, but almost 86% of victims are female, and the majority of perpetrators are men.

The incidence of rape increased rapidly in the United States through the 1980s and early 1990s, peaking at 42.8 reported sexual assaults per 100,000 people in 1992. Recent trends indicate a steady decline with sexual assaults being reported at a rate of 31.7 per 100,000 people in 2005 [3]. However, these estimates likely underrepresent true numbers as rape remains woefully underreported, with only 25% to 35% of rapes ever reported to law enforcement or medical professionals [3,4]. There are many reasons a rape victim may not report the crime, including embarrassment, feelings of guilt, fear of retribution, lack of faith in the legal system, and lack of knowledge of victims' legal rights. For adolescent girls in particular, additional barriers include concerns about confidentiality, lack of funding, and limited access to health care, leading to incomplete or significantly delayed reporting when compared with older women [5•]. In date rape or acquaintance rape cases, the victim may not identify the event as rape because it does not fit the stereotypic definition of rape. Furthermore, some victims

Types of Sexual Assault

Type of Assault	Definition	Significance
Stranger rape	The victim is suddenly overtaken by an unknown assailant and sexually assaulted	Accounts for approximately 15% to 20% of all sexual assaults; victims face recovery issues related to regaining a sense of safety
Acquaintance rape	Sexual assault that is perpetrated by a person whom the victim does not know well, but with whom the victim had a nonviolent interaction and established some trust before the intent to rape became apparent	Commonly follows judgment errors or risk-taking behaviors, such as accepting a ride or a social encounter in an isolated setting; among adolescent girls, commonly involves a male acquaintance that is 5 or more years older; victims often encounter difficulties with trust and relationship issues
Date rape	Sexual assault that is perpetrated by a person with whom the victim voluntarily accompanied on a date; can be a type of acquaintance or partner rape	Can be similar to acquaintance rape or partner rape; frequently not reported because may think she contributed in some way; victims often develop problems with self-esteem, and trust and relationship issues; often occurs during alcohol or other substance use
Marital or partner rape	Sexual assault perpetrated by a partner or spouse	Often occurs in combination with physical abuse; occurs in most domestic violence relationships; legal definitions make it difficult to prove in a court of law
Statutory rape	Sexual intercourse with a minor (with or without consent) who is under the age of majority as defined by the state in which the incident occurs	Statutory rape charges may be made by the minor's parent or guardian or by the state; by law, the victim is too young to give consent, thus her consent is irrelevant
Aggravated sexual assault	Sexual assault that occurs with excessive force to cause physical injury, or when the victim is elderly, physically handicapped, or mentally handicapped	Can be a component of any category of sexual or physical assault
Incest	Sexual assault perpetrated by a family member	Most commonly occurs in the setting of childhood sexual abuse

Figure 46-1. Types of sexual assault.

may avoid telling authority figures about an assault because the surrounding circumstances of the assault may incriminate the victim.

Sequelae

The sexual assault victim is at risk for acute and long-term complications that affect physical and mental health. Acutely, rape victims are at risk for physical injury, sexually transmitted infections (STIs), and pregnancy. Among rape victims who seek medical attention within 72 hours of their assault, physical (nongenital) injuries occur in 25% to 45%, and grossly visible genital trauma occurs in 15% to 30% [6,7•]. When a colposcope is used for a magnified view, up to 87% of acute sexual assault victims have evidence of genital trauma [8].

The rate of STI transmission related to a rape is difficult to determine because of the possibility of pre-existing infections, the incubation period of some STIs, the interim sexual behaviors of victims between the assault and follow-up testing, and poor follow-up among victims [9]. Findings from a population-based study indicate that about 5% of sexual assault victims become pregnant as a result of their assault [10]. Most of these pregnancies occur among women who do not receive immediate attention after the assault, and many occur in settings of recurrent assault, such as occurs in child sexual abuse or domestic violence.

Extensive research has elucidated the mental health consequences of sexual assault. During a sexual assault, victims generally experience total loss of control, intense anxiety and fear, and serious threats of injury or death. After a sexual assault, post-traumatic stress disorder (PTSD) is common. The diagnosis of PTSD requires an antecedent event in which there is actual or threatened injury or death, intense fear, helplessness or horror, followed by symptoms of re-experiencing, avoidance, or hyperarousal persisting for at least

6 months [11]. Most rape survivors experience these types of symptoms immediately following their assault; 30% to 65% go on to meet the diagnostic criteria for PTSD [12]. A subcategory of PTSD has also been described as rape trauma syndrome, which describes a predictable course of emotional recovery that occurs after the assault [13]. This information, outlined in Figure 46-2, can help victims understand that their emotional reactions and certain behaviors are a normal part of the recovery process. The recovery process is largely influenced by several other factors, including the victim's self-esteem and support system, episodes of past assault, and the relationship with the assailant.

More common and difficult to treat are the long-term complications related to sexual assault. Compared with women who have not experienced sexual assault, women with such a history exhibit higher rates of chronic pain syndromes; lowered self-perception of health; increased-self destructive behaviors; increased symptoms across most body systems; and long-term increases in their use of medical services [14]. Similar comparisons between nonvictimized and victimized women reveal more frequent diagnosis and treatment of the diseases listed in Figure 46-3 [15]. The treatment of these long-term complications is difficult, and the most effective management is early identification of the experience of sexual assault and prevention of these complex sequelae through counseling, education, and preventive health care.

Care of the Woman with a History of Sexual Assault or Abuse

ROUTINE SCREENING
Population-based research has established that most sexual assault victims never report the crime to police or a health care provider. Routine screening in the primary care setting, where continuity of care has established a trusting relationship

Rape Trauma Syndrome: Emotional Recovery After Sexual Assault		
Phase	**Time Frame**	**Process**
Acute disorganization	Immediate to 6 months	Emotional reactions: fear, flashbacks, embarrassment, anger, loss of freedom, lack of trust
		Physical reactions: wound healing, soreness, vaginal or throat irritation, disturbances in sleep, appetite, and sexuality, flashbacks, nightmares, heightened startle reflex
Denial	1 to 3 months	Avoids discussions and thoughts about incident; is resistant to counseling
Reorganization	6 to 12 months	Often exhibits need to "get away"; flashbacks and nightmares recur; experiences defensive reactions to the circumstances of the rape, such as fear of indoors or outdoors, fear of the dark, fear of being alone, and sexual fears
Integration and recovery	Variable	Experiences resolution with appropriate placement of blame on the perpetrator; regains sense of safety and ability to trust; exhibits righteous anger and advocacy

Figure 46-2. Rape trauma syndrome: emotional recovery after sexual assault.

between patient and provider, can help to identify many cases. Most patients approve of physician inquiries about sexual abuse and believe that physicians can help them with problems related to abuse [16].The key to detecting sexual assault as early as possible after it occurs is routine, direct questioning in a sensitive manner [17]. Conversely, failure to question patients about violence can communicate lack of permission to discuss such issues in the medical setting. Additionally, for those who do not have a history of sexual assault, routine inquiry can establish that such an event is an important element in the medical history and should be reported to a health care professional. If there is a future sexual assault, the victim may then be more inclined to report the incident and receive early assessment and treatment.

For adolescent patients, the American Medical Association, in its *Guidelines for Adolescent Preventive Services*, recommends annual health visits that include routine screening for any history of sexual abuse as well as other types of abuse and assault [18]. These recommendations also include guidelines that address primary and secondary prevention of sexual assault and abuse, all provided within the framework of anticipatory guidance. For adult patients, many professional organizations have made similar recommendations for routine screening of past or ongoing sexual or physical violence [19, 20].

More than 70% of women and girls who have had an experience that would legally qualify as "rape" do not use that term to describe that event [21], thus screening questions are more effective when they avoid the use of terms such as *rape,*

Disorders That Are More Common In Women With A History of Sexual Assault

Chronic pelvic pain

Vaginitis

Sexual dysfunction

Premenstrual syndrome

Vaginismus

Chronic headaches

Chronic back pain

Temporomandibular joint pain, bruxism

Irritable bowel syndrome

Other gastrointestinal pain

Depression and anxiety

Phobias

Sleep disturbances

Substance abuse

Eating disorders

HIV risk factors

Suicide

Figure 46-3. Disorders that are more common in women with a history of sexual assault.

molestation, or *violence.* Instead, questions using behavioral descriptions will help patients to disclose life experiences that they may not have understood as assault (*see* Figure 46-4) [17]. It is important to establish a method for routine screening that allows the patient sufficient privacy to answer honestly. She should be screened in a private area, away from anyone who has accompanied her. In a busy office setting, a questionnaire may be more time efficient, although patients may be less likely to report assault via this method. Questionnaires and interviews can be effective in eliciting a violence history if proper measures are taken to ensure privacy and trust.

Addressing Disclosure

After a woman is identified as having a history of sexual assault, the most helpful response is to acknowledge the experience and validate it as being traumatic for her. Because many have never discussed their assault experience, the simple act of disclosing can be therapeutic. Information to be ascertained at this time includes circumstances of the assault, including sexual acts, physical violence and ejaculation, and relationship of alleged perpetrator to the patient [22]. Relevant medical history includes injuries from the assault, last menstrual period, previous sexual history and STIs, and possibility of pregnancy. At this time, women should be evaluated for physical and mental health symptoms, and providers can assess and facilitate patients' use of personal and community supports. Among women beyond their late 20s, sexual assault occurs most often within the setting of domestic violence or intimate partner violence [2•]. Eliciting a history of sexual violence should prompt further inquiry regarding physical violence and vice versa. If recent or ongoing domestic violence or abuse is identified, the clinician should make a safety assessment and help establish an exit plan. The screening, identification, and management of domestic violence are beyond the scope of this chapter, but a thorough review is available elsewhere [23•,24].

A physical examination should be performed, with a specific focus on any physical trauma that may have occurred and the detection of STIs and pregnancy. Screening for STIs should include appropriate testing for gonorrheal, chlamydial, and trichomonal infection, bacterial vaginosis, vaginal yeast infection, hepatitis B, syphilis, and HIV infection, if desired. Testing for HIV and syphilis may need to be repeated depending upon the time from assault and baseline results. Testing for herpes simplex virus or human papillomavirus should be performed if indicated by the finding of genital lesions. If the assault was remote, prophylactic antimicrobial therapy for STIs is not necessary, and it is appropriate to wait for test results. If there is reason to believe that there will be difficulty contacting the patient subsequently, prophylaxis may be appropriate.

The patient with a recent or past history of sexual assault will probably have underlying fears or concerns that she does not communicate. Rape victims commonly worry about STIs, HIV, pregnancy, and changes in their body that could have been caused by the assault. Counseling should address all of these areas to provide as much reassurance and education as possible. In many cases, early identification and assessment may also help demystify nonspecific somatic complaints by providing the patient with reassuring information about her anatomy and physiology, particularly her reproductive system.

REFERRALS

Finally, the patient should be offered referrals for counseling and community support resources. The short- and long-term complications of sexual assault should be reviewed with the patient, and she should be reminded of the importance of counseling and support to achieve a healthy recovery. Clinicians should develop links with colleagues and community resources that can provide trauma-specific counseling and therapy for women with a history of sexual assault or abuse. State or local rape crisis agencies can provide these services directly or can provide information on available resources.

Many physicians, especially in the current managed care environment, may argue that such screening and disclosure requires inordinate amounts of time, but with an established protocol and referral system, very little time is required. In addition, if a history of sexual assault is identified and appropriately addressed, one can provide the most appropriate treatment, save patients from further negative consequences of delayed disclosure, and potentially save large amounts of time that would have otherwise been required for repetitive visits for vague or superficial complaints [25].

Acute Care of the Sexual Assault Victim

REPORTING

In most states, a sexual assault must be reported to law enforcement before the evidentiary examination can be performed. For reporting victims, many state crime victim compensation programs offer additional victim support services and also pay the uncovered costs of related medical care. Although some states allow anonymous reporting, most victims who choose not to report the crime also do not receive acute medical attention.

In the period immediately after a sexual assault, it is important to encourage the victim to report the crime to law enforcement. State laws regarding reporting requirements vary, and health care professionals are responsible for knowing their state's reporting mandates. Timely reporting ensures the greatest likelihood of retrieving useful evidence and also improves the criminal justice system's ability to apprehend and convict sex offenders. Most protocols recommend collecting evidence within 72 hours of a sexual assault.

HISTORY AND PHYSICAL EXAMINATION

In caring for the woman who is reporting a rape, the clinician is asked to serve multiple roles: as a medical provider, as a source of support, and as a collector of forensic evidence. To ensure that evidence is collected and maintained properly, most states have established clear step-by-step guidelines or kits for the forensic examination and evidence collection. Furthermore, many areas of the country offer specific training through Sexual Assault Nurse Examiner (SANE) or Sexual Assault Response Team (SART) programs throughout the country. These training programs produce nurses and other health care professionals with expertise in acute crisis intervention, medical care, forensic evidence collection, evidence preservation, collaboration with law enforcement, and expert testimony in the courtroom. When available, professionals with this training can be helpful to any medical center that is called on to treat sexual assault victims in the acute setting.

It should be the goal of the examining clinician to minimize the emotional and physical trauma to the victim and to maximize the probability of collecting and preserving physical evidence for potential use in the legal system [26]. The sexual assault examiner also plays an important role in the victim's emotional recovery. The immediate experiences and reactions that follow the assault have a powerful impact on the victim's

Screening for Sexual Assault

Screening for sexual assault

"Has anyone ever tried to touch you in a sexual way when you did not want them to?"

"Has anyone ever forced you to have sex?"

"Has anyone ever had sex with you when you were unable to say 'no' to them?"

"Did anyone ever try to have sex with you when you did not want them to?"

"Does your partner or boyfriend sometimes make you feel scared?"

"Some of my patients have talked to me about experiences like _____, have you ever been through anything like that?"

Supporting patients after disclosure

"That must have been a very difficult experience."

"These things are hard to talk about, and I am glad that you told me about this."

"Has there been anyone who has helped you during this time? Would you like to have that person here while we discuss this?"

"This was not your fault."

Figure 46-4. Screening for sexual assault.

level of emotional distress. By following the suggestions listed in Figure 46-5, the clinician can help the victim regain a sense of control and reduce immediate postassault distress. It is critical that the sexual assault examiner remains sensitive and nonjudgmental. Whether the victim appears calm, frightened, or hostile, it is important for the clinician to provide reassurance, clearly communicate what should be expected, and allow the victim control over the history and physical examination.

The initial assessment should include a brief history and evaluation for serious injuries. When the patient is stable from a medical standpoint, the clinician should obtain a history, which should be limited to pertinent issues that may influence treatment or affect evidence collection. Important components of the history include allergies, current medications, chronic illnesses, last menstrual period, contraceptive use, time since last voluntary sexual intercourse, relevant past gynecologic surgery, and relevant psychiatric history that could influence her emotional recovery. In order to protect the patient during future legal action, historical components that do not need to be documented include virginity, sexual history, gravidity, parity, abortions, and any major psychiatric illness or history of substance abuse. These issues may be of great importance to the patient, however, and should be addressed by the primary care physician or mental health professional outside of the acute setting. A detailed history of specific assault events is not necessary and should be left to the law enforcement team [26].

For the sexual assault examiner, important components of the forensic history include elements such as the use of physical force (to look for evidence of bites, strangulation, or ligatures), the types of penetration that occurred (oral, vaginal, rectal), if and where ejaculation occurred, and if any kissing or licking occurred (to obtain saliva specimens). Additionally, the victim should be asked about her activities since the assault that may have affected the presence of evidence

(eg, changing clothes, eating, drinking, urinating, bathing). State protocols vary in the amount of assault history and medical history that is requested.

In the absence of serious injuries, the medical and forensic examinations should take place simultaneously. The required steps of evidence collection, physical examination, and medical testing should follow a logical sequence that prevents multiple genital examinations or repetitive exposure of the victim. The components of the medical and forensic portions of the sexual assault examination vary by state and the examiner must be aware of local protocols but include the following components [27]: obtaining written consent; a history of the forms of violence used and where and whether penetration occurred; medical history including allergies, last menstrual period, and pregnancy status; physical examination for trauma; examining orifices for trauma and seminal fluid; collecting any foreign matter; combing pubic hair for foreign hair and matter; blood type and DNA screen; fingernail scrapings; collection of torn or stained clothing; and collecting saliva for secretor status.

The areas of variation in these protocols include the amount of documentation, the collection of additional blood specimens for drug and alcohol analysis, and if head and pubic hairs are plucked. Pulling of pubic hairs is considered very traumatic by many victims of sexual assault and can be collected at a later date if needed.

Ideally, the examination is done by a trained sexual assault forensic examiner using an evidence collection kit. This has been shown to increase collaboration with law enforcement, decrease examination time in the emergency department, and improved the quality of the evidence collected [28•,29].

Documentation of injuries is particularly important, with an emphasis on findings that support the use of force. Using a magnifying lens or colposcope can greatly enhance visualization of genital trauma and increase the rates of detection [8]. Some centers have the availability to take colposcopic photographs for

Helping a Victim Become a Survivor: Advice for the Clinician

To help the victim gain a sense of control:

Obtain informed consent

Minimize the number of times the victim must tell what happened

Allow the victim to make choices whenever possible

Always ask permission before touching the victim or performing any physical examination

Give the victim permission to pause or stop the examination at any point

Respect the victim's confidentiality

Do not discuss the victim's case with anyone else without the victim's explicit permission

To diffuse self-blame, communicate the following ideas:

"I'm sorry this happened to you"

"It was not your fault"

"You did what you needed to do to survive"

"I'm glad you are alive"

Figure 46-5. Helping a victim become a survivor: advice for the clinician.

documentation purposes, but if that is not available, a simple diagram can be used to indicate any lacerations, erythema, or other abnormalities. In fact, unless the examiner is experienced taking magnified photographs, a diagram may be preferable because in court, a simple illustration can be much more convincing to a jury than a poorly taken photograph.

After the examination, it is important to provide reassurance about physical findings. Even if there is minor trauma, the victim can be reassured that the physical injuries will heal rapidly and should not interfere with future reproductive function. The decision to obtain swabs from the cervix and all penetrated orifices for detection of pre-existing or acquired STIs at the time of the assault should be made on an individual basis. Although all 50 states have laws that strictly limit the use of survivors' previous sexual and STI history as a means to undermine their credibility, in rare instances STI results may later be accessed by the legal system. For this reason, the survivor and clinician may opt to defer testing until the follow-up examination [30]. Vaginal swabs should be obtained for microscopy to detect vaginitis but not necessarily to look for motile sperm. Semen evidence should be carefully collected and preserved, but microscopic examination for motile sperm is not as accurate as the highly sensitive testing used in forensic analysis. It has actually been recommended that the examiner abandon the practice of looking for sperm because conflicting testimony from the sexual assault examiner and the forensic scientist regarding the presence, absence, number, or motility of spermatozoa can undermine the strength of the prosecution [26].

Finally, blood samples are obtained for both forensic and medical purposes. Most forensic laboratories request blood samples for DNA or blood group antigen testing. Additional specimens are used for baseline testing for syphilis and hepatitis B. Baseline testing for HIV should also be offered after appropriate counseling. Other laboratory testing, such as serum pregnancy testing, is ordered as clinically indicated.

HANDLING THE EVIDENCE

After the examination, evidence must be properly labeled and stored. Most criminal justice jurisdictions provide evidence collection kits that have detailed instructions and contain materials for the proper collection and storage of forensic specimens. These kits also optimize the maintenance of the chain of custody, which ensures that the evidence has not been contaminated or tainted. In the absence of an evidence kit, the examiner should take care to package each specimen in a dry envelope that is clearly labeled with the site, the type of evidence (eg, suspected semen stain), the victim's name or number, the collector's name, and the date and time that it was collected. To prevent decay and loss of potential evidence, wet specimens, such as clothing, saliva specimens, or genital swabs should be completely air-dried before packaging. Finally, all evidence should be properly sealed, and documentation of the chain of custody should be maintained on the packaging. When complete, the evidence kit should be handed directly to the investigating law enforcement official.

POST-EXAMINATION TREATMENT AND COUNSELING

After the physical assessment, prophylaxis or treatment should be offered as clinically indicated or desired by the victim. Antimicrobial agents are prescribed according to current recommendations of the Centers for Disease Control and Prevention to prevent or treat STIs [30,31]. Figure 46-6 lists appropriate prophylactic treatments. If the victim is at risk for pregnancy, and her pregnancy test is negative, she should also be offered emergency contraception to prevent rape-related pregnancy. Figure 46-7 details several possible emergency contraception regimens [32].

Finally, a list of all the tests performed, treatments received, prescriptions provided, and follow-up instructions should be supplied to the victim in written form. Standard patient education forms can be easily made to provide a checklist of items that can be individualized for each patient. The educational material should also provide a telephone number to call for questions and for test results. A space for documentation of follow-up appointments should be included. Most rape victims do not remember the treatments they received or recommendations that were made to them, and having this information in written form can alleviate post-examination anxiety. Furthermore, because follow-up rates are low for rape victims, this may be the only time to provide the victim with prevention-focused information, such as what to expect emotionally during the recovery process (see Figure 46-2) and the availability of community resources.

Follow-Up Care

For women who undergo either an acute evidentiary examination or a delayed medical examination related to a sexual assault, follow-up is important to provide test results, assess mental health functioning, reiterate health-related recommendations, and provide additional preventive education. For the victim seen in the acute care setting, recommendations for the timing of follow-up visits vary, but in general, repeat testing for STIs is recommended 6 weeks after the assault. Testing at that time should include tests for gonorrhea, chlamydial infection, trichomonal infection, syphilis, HIV infection, and hepatitis B infection. HIV testing should be repeated at 3 to 6 months and again at 1 year. If the patient received the first hepatitis B vaccine at the initial examination, the importance of follow-up to complete the vaccination series should be stressed.

For all victims, the expected stages of recovery listed in Figure 46-2 can be reviewed, and the importance of counseling should be re-emphasized. If the victim is accompanied by a family member or significant other, it is a good time to provide preventive education for those who accompany her as well. The suggestions listed in Figure 46-5 should help those close to the victim assist in her recovery. Additionally, those in the victim's support network, particularly parents or partners, may also need counseling to address their own emotional reactions to their loved one's assault. They should be encouraged to seek counseling or support separately from the victim.

Prevention

The formidable task of sexual assault prevention involves collaboration between educators, health care professionals, the criminal justice system, parents, and communities in general. Primary health care providers are in a key position to implement prevention strategies aimed at decreasing sexual violence against women and children and decreasing the complicated sequelae that often result when victims remain unidentified and untreated. However, no single specialty can be charged with this task, and the optimal approach is a continuum of prevention efforts that are provided from childhood through maturity, with several points reiterated at all developmental levels.

Educational efforts and anticipatory guidance are important in the primary prevention of rape. Beginning in childhood, healthy respect for the body and for privacy should be the focus. Clinicians can model this respect by always asking permission before initiating any physical contact with children. This also includes discussing child sexual abuse with parents and encouraging age-appropriate parent-child communication regarding sexual abuse. Issues that should be addressed with parents include surveillance of children's media viewing and leisure activities, warning signs of risk-taking behaviors, and continued parent-child communication, particularly in the area of sexuality. It is important to educate boys as well as girls regarding healthy attitudes about sexuality, respect for the body, avoidance of violence, and appropriate knowledge regarding sexual abuse and assault.

Prevention efforts are especially important when adolescents begin to consider dating relationships. Many adolescents lack the skills necessary to recognize and avoid potentially violent dating situations, and some even believe that violence in a dating relationship is justifiable in certain situations. Given a sociocultural context in which male dominance, female victimization, and power imbalances in relationships are highly visible, dispelling common myths about rape is important in the education of both boys and girls [33]. The most vulnerable population is adolescent girls, as half of all females who experience sexual assault are between 12 and 24 years of age [34]. Assaults usually happen in familiar surroundings; those involving older adolescents most commonly occur in social circumstances, such as a date, whereas extended family members are the most common assailants in assaults of younger adolescents [33].

It is important to stress that sexual assault affects girls and women of all socioeconomic classes and is pervasive in most cultures. Parents of adolescents and adolescents themselves should be educated about the typical setting for acquaintance or date rape. Parents should be encouraged to have discussions with their adolescent children regarding warning signs in dating relationships, the importance of limit-setting for sexual activity, the role of drug and alcohol use in sexual assault, and rape-resistance strategies. Figure 46-8 offers some suggestions for parent-teen discussions or discussions between health care professionals and adolescent patients. During routine health visits or through other types of health education, adolescents can be presented with hypothetical accounts of difficult dating scenarios and helped with developing a plan or solution. This type of skills development and rehearsal can help teens recognize and avoid potentially violent situations in the future.

Prevention education and counseling are particularly relevant for the adolescent or adult who has already experienced a sexual assault because a history of previous victimization is a

---

Medical Prophylaxis for Sexual Assault

Sexually transmitted diseases

Gonorrhea (and incubating syphilis)

Ceftriaxone sodium 125 mg IM

Cefixime 400 mg PO

If allergic to cephalosporins, may substitute a single dose of the following:

Spectinomycin 2 g IM*

Chlamydia

Azithromycin 1 g PO single dose or

Doxycycline 100 mg PO BID for 7 days

Trichomoniasis

Metronidazole 2 g PO single dose or

Tinidazole 2 g PO single dose

Hepatitis B

Begin hepatitis B vaccination series if not previously done

HIV

Postexposure prophylaxis within 72 hours, although no definitive evidence of benefit exists

Injuries

Tetanus booster 0.5 mL IM if > 10 years of age

*Expensive. Not currently available in the United States; check http://www.cdc.gov for updates.

Figure 46-6. Medical prophylaxis for sexual assault. IM—intramuscularly; PEP—post-exposure prophylaxis; PO—by mouth.

Emergency Contraception

Plan B (levonorgestrel 0.75 mg [Duramed Pharmaceuticals, Pomona, NY])

Two tablets PO STAT

May be used up to 120 hours after unprotected intercourse

Combined oral contraceptives

If Plan B is not available, combined oral contraceptives containing levonorgestrel may be substituted

Go to http://ec.princeton.edu for more information.

Figure 46-7. Emergency contraception. PO—by mouth.

significant independent risk factor for experiencing another in the future [35]. Unfortunately, all adolescent girls can be considered at increased risk for sexual assault because the highest incidence of attempted or completed sexual assault occurs during this time, with lifetime prevalence rates approaching 42% [36]. Those from vulnerable populations, such as women with developmental delays, history of child abuse, family home environmental problems, or substance use are at even higher risk [37].

After a sexual assault has occurred, secondary prevention efforts can reduce the incidence of some of the long-term sequelae. Victims should be advised of the psychologic and behavioral changes that are common, such as increases in substance use, risky sexual behaviors, eating disturbances, relationship problems, and psychologic reactions, such as anxiety, panic attacks, and depression [37]. Counselors who have experience treating patients with PTSD and sexual assault victims can use simple and brief behavioral modification techniques to teach the patient how to deal with these problems and prevent them from becoming established and severe. It is not necessary for the primary care provider to offer in-depth counseling, but referrals should be made to local resources that can further assess and address the sexual victimization history (see Figure 46-9).

Prevention and early detection are now vital components in the provision of comprehensive primary health care. By applying these methods to the issue of sexual assault, significant positive effects on the overall health status of women are likely. Primary care physicians and other health care providers are in a unique position to provide medical services and to reduce the emotional and physical trauma related to sexual assault. This can be accomplished by establishing a professional, safe, and supportive environment for women and girls and by promoting prevention strategies that target the prevention of rape or the prevention of the complex complications that are associated with sexual assault.

Sexual Assault Prevention Strategies

For young women in dating relationships

Don't date someone who is much older than you are

Set limits before going out on a date, and tell your date what those limits are

Plan to meet your date in a public place, and arrange your own transportation home

Try group or couple dating if you don't feel comfortable going out with someone

Communicate clearly when you do not want to be hugged, touched, or kissed

Do not let alcohol or drugs cloud your thinking

If a date has been drinking or using drugs, do not let him drive you home

Always have a back-up plan for getting home if needed

If a date shows disrespect to you or other women, do not go out with him

For all women

Be alert to what is happening to you at all times

Avoid alcohol and drugs when you are with people you do not know well

Do not let someone you don't know drive you anywhere

Trust your instincts

Figure 46-8. Sexual assault prevention strategies.

Sexual Assault Resources

Support services readily available in the emergency department

Sexual assault nurse examiners in select hospitals nationwide

Follow-up appointment with primary care provider 1 to 2 weeks after assault has occurred

Encourage presence of immediate family, partner, friends, or loved ones

Referral to community rape crisis centers

Religious clergyperson, if requested

Referral to local department of public health as needed

Local police department rape victims contact person

State Attorney General office contact

Additional resources

Rape Abuse & Incest National Network (R.A.I.N.N.); www.rainn.org provides extensive services for victims of sexual assault and since 1994 operates the National Sexual Assault Hotline (1-800-656-HOPE); live volunteers provide 24-hour services to survivors including immediate confidential rape crisis counseling, support, and locations for over 600 local rape crisis centers throughout the country

National Sexual Violence Resource Center; www.nsvrc.org (1-877-739-3895)

National Center for Victims of Crimes, includes Teen Victim Project; www.ncvc.org (1-800-FYI-CALL and 1-800-394-2255)

Office for Victims of Crime: US Department of Justice; www.ojp.usdoj.gov/ovc

Center for the Prevention of Sexual and Domestic Violence (Faith Trust Institute); www.faithtrustinstitute.org

Physician training resources

Sexual Assault Forensic Examiner Training; www.safeta.org (1-877-819-SART); national training standards for licensed health professionals including physicians, registered nurses, nurse practitioners, and physician assistants performing sexual assault physical examinations

Sexual Assault Training & Investigations (SATI); www.mysati.com

Figure 46-9. Sexual assault resources.

References

Papers of particular interest have been highlighted as follows:
• Of interest
•• Of outstanding interest

1. U.S. Department of Health and Human Services. *Healthy People 2010: With Understanding and Improving Health and Objectives for Improving Health*, vol 2, edn 2. Washington, DC: US Government Printing Office; 2000.

2.• *Extent, Nature and Consequences of Rape Victimization: Findings From the National Violence Against Women Survey: A Research Brief from the National Institutes of Justice and the Centers for Disease Control and Prevention.* Washington, DC: US Government Printing Office; 2006.
Comprehensive report of most recent national survey of the United States population on sexual assault.

3. Federal Bureau of Investigation: *Crime in the United States: Uniform Crime Reports for the United States, 2005.* Washington, DC: Federal Bureau of Investigation; 2006.

4. Rennison CM: *Rape and Sexual Assault: Reporting to Police and Medical Attention, 1992–2000.* Washington, DC: US Department of Justice; 2002.

5.• Lessing J: Primary care provider interventions for the delayed disclosure of adolescent sexual assault. *J Pediatr Health Care* 2005, 19:17–24.
Useful review of delayed disclosure of sexual assault and how to approach this issue in the primary care setting.

6. Mein JK, Palmer CM, Shand MC, *et al.*: Management of acute adult sexual assault. *Med J Austr* 2003, 178:226–230.

7.• Martin SL, Young SK, Billings DL, Bross CC: Health care-based interventions for women who have experienced sexual violence: a review of the literature. *Trauma Violence Abuse* 2007, 8:3–18.
This meta-analysis provides a comprehensive review of clinical sexual assault programs and services in the emergency and outpatient settings located in the United States and globally. It uniquely includes a review of articles documenting these perspectives from patients and clinicians.

8. Mancino P, Parlavecchio E, Melluso J, *et al.*: Introducing colposcopy and vulvovaginoscopy as routine examinations for victims of sexual assault. *Clin Expl Obstet Gynecol* 2003, 30:40–42.

9. Reynolds MW, Peipert JF, Collins B: Epidemiologic issues of sexually transmitted diseases in sexual assault victims. *Obstet Gynecol Surv* 2000, 55:51–57.

10. Holmes MM, Resnick HS, Kilpatrick DG, Best CL: Rape-related pregnancy: estimates and descriptive characteristics from a national sample of women. *Am J Obstet Gynecol* 1996, 175:320–325.

11. American Psychiatric Association: *Diagnostic and Statistical Manual of Mental Disorders*, edn 4. Arlington, VA: American Psychiatric Association; 1994.

12. Conoscenti LM, McNally RJ: Health complaints in acknowledged and unacknowledged rape victims. *J Anxiety Disord* 2006, 20:372–379.

13. Burgess AW, Holmstrom LL: Rape trauma syndrome. *Am J Psychiatry* 1974, 131:981–986.

14. Stein M, Lang A, Laffaye C, *et al.*: Relationship of sexual assault history to somatic symptoms and health anxiety in women. *Gen Hosp Psychiatry* 2004, 6:178–183.

15. Koss MP, Heslet L: Somatic consequences of violence against women. *Arch Fam Med* 1992, 1:53–59.

16. Friedman LS, Samet JH, Roberts MS, *et al.*: Inquiry about victimization experiences. A survey of patient preferences and physician practices. *Arch Intern Med.* 1992, 152:1186–1190.

17. Diaz A, Edwards S, Neal WP, *et al.*: Obtaining a history of sexual victimization from adolescent females seeking routine health care. *Mt Sinai J Med* 2004, 71:170–173.

18. American Medical Association: *Guidelines for Adolescent Preventive Services (GAPS), Recommendations and Rationale.* Baltimore: Williams & Wilkins; 1994.

19. Family violence: an AAFP white paper. The AAFP Commission on Special issues and Clinical Interests. *Am Fam Physician* 1994, 50:1636–1640, 1644–1646.

20. Council on Scientific Affairs, American Medical Association: Violence against women: relevance for medical practitioners. *JAMA* 1992, 267:3184–3189.

21. Fisher BS, Daigle LE, Cullen FT, Turner MG: Acknowledging sexual victimization as rape: Results from a national-level study. *Justice Quarterly* 2003, 20:535–574.

22. New York State Department of Health and Department of Social Services: Appendix K. In *Child and Adolescent Sexual Offence: Medical Protocol.* New York, NY: New York State Department of Health; 1997.

23.• Brown R: *Roadmaps for Clinical Practice: Case Studies in Disease Prevention and Health Promotion—Intimate Partner Violence.* Chicago, IL: American Medical Association; 2002.
Review of literature on domestic violence as well as diagnosis, intervention, and treatment.

24. American College of Obstetricians and Gynecologists: *Domestic Violence.* ACOG Technical Bulletin 209. Washington, DC: American College of Obstetricians and Gynecologists; 1995.

25. Katon W, Sullivan M, Walker E: Medical symptoms without identified pathology: relationship to psychiatric disorders, childhood and adult trauma, and personality traits. *Ann Intern Med* 2001, 134:917–925.

26. State of New York Department of Health: *Protocol for the Acute Care of the Adult Patient Reporting Sexual Assault.* New York City: State Department of Health; 2004.

27. Ledray L: Evidence Collection and Care of the Sexual Assault Survivor: the SANE-SART Response. Violence Against Women Online Resources; 2001.

28.• Campbell R, Patterson D, Lichty LF: The effectiveness of sexual assault nurse examiner (SANE) programs: a review of psychological, medical, legal, and community outcomes. *Trauma Violence Abuse* 2005, 6:313–329.
This article reviews the benefits of sexual assault nurse examiner (SANE) programs in accurately collecting forensic evidence in the emergency setting. It further describes the effectiveness of such programs in improving prosecution while providing effective medical and psychologic care.

29. Girardin B: The sexual assault nurse examiner: a win-win solution. *Top Emerg Med* 2005, 27:124–131.

30. Centers for Disease Control and Prevention: Sexually transmitted disease guidelines 2006. *MMWR* 2006, 55:No. RR-11.

31. Centers for Disease Control and Prevention: Update to CDC's sexually transmitted diseases treatment guidelines, 2006: fluoroquinolones no longer recommended for treatment of gonococcal infections. *MMWR* 2007, 56:332–336.

32. Stewart F, Trussell J, Van Look PFA: Emergency contraception. In *Contraceptive Technology*, edn 18. Edited by Hatcher RA, Trussell J, Stewart F, *et al.* New York, NY: Ardent Media; 2004.

33. Kaplan DW, Feinstein RA, Fisher MM, *et al*.: Care of the adolescent sexual assault victim. *Pediatrics* 2001, 107:1476–1479.

34. Bachman R, Saltzman LE: *Violence Against Women: Estimates From the Redesigned Survey*. Washington, DC: US Department of Justice, Office of Justice Programs; 1995.

35. Smith PH, White JW, Holland LJ: A longitudinal perspective on dating violence among adolescent and college-age women. *Am J Public Health* 2003, 93:1104–1109.

36. Rickert VI, Wiemann CM, Vaughan RD, White JW: Rates and risk factors for sexual violence among an ethnically diverse sample of adolescents. *Arch Pediatric Adol Med* 2004, 158:1132–1139.

37. Danielson CK, Holmes MM: Adolescent sexual assault: an update of the literature. *Curr Opin Obstet Gynecol* 2004, 16:383–388.

47 Common Pediatric Problems

Abbey B. Berenson

- The examination of children's genitals requires a patient, gentle approach by the clinician. Open communication with caregiver and child is essential.
- Vaginal discharge is the most common gynecologic problem seen in children.
- Vaginitis may result from specific or nonspecific causes.
- Nonspecific vaginitis usually is a result of chemical irritation.
- Specific vaginitis may be spread from an infection of the pharynx, skin, ear, intestine, or urinary tract.
- No specific cause of vaginal discharge can be determined in approximately 70% of cases. In these cases, treatment should include instruction in proper hygiene, loose clothing, Sitz baths, and avoidance of irritants.
- A foul-smelling bloody discharge suggests a foreign body in the vagina, the most common of which is toilet paper.
- Most vulvar disorders in children can be diagnosed by visual inspection. Biopsy usually requires general anesthesia in young patients.

The most common problems encountered by the pediatric gynecologist are vaginal discharge and bleeding, and vulvar disorders, including candidal infection, vulvar warts (human papillomavirus [HPV]), labial agglutination, molluscum contagiosum, urethral prolapse, lichen sclerosus, and contact dermatitis. Young patients also may present with menstrual irregularities or congenital anomalies or as a result of sexual abuse; these diagnoses are addressed elsewhere in this text.

A standard approach to evaluation includes questions concerning previous home remedies as well as prescribed medications. In addition to determining prior medical or surgical problems, the clinician should address prior skin infections, family history of diabetes, allergies, eczema, and contact sensitivities. Next, possible exposure to chemical irritants, including soaps, powders, and shampoos, is explored. Questions about social context are appropriate, especially with regard to identifying the primary caregiver, home or day care arrangements, and other adults or older children who may have regular contact with the patient [1•]. After questions about social setting, the clinician may ask the caregiver if there is any possibility of sexual abuse. This evaluation should be handled expeditiously to avoid child management problems. A questionnaire may be completed by the care-

giver in the waiting room, or the clinic staff may ask the questions in the examining room.

Regarding the examination of children's genitals, the physician must achieve a balance that includes a consideration of the information needed and the comfort level of the child. Even nonabused children who undergo an examination of the genitalia may experience fear or embarrassment. In preverbal or early verbal children, the caregiver may give assurances to the child. With fully verbal children, the physician should speak directly to the child: first, the child should be informed that her caregiver has requested and approved the examination. Then, she should be told by the physician that she will not be hurt. Lastly, the procedure is explained step by step. As the examination proceeds, the explanation is reiterated to decrease anxiety [2].

Permitting the child to view the examination with a mirror may give her a sense of control and help her relax. Talking to the child, singing songs, or providing other pleasant distractions have been demonstrated to decrease anxiety. Sedation may be necessary in cases of abuse or severe trauma. Forcible restraint is never indicated [2,3].

The examination should be approached in a gentle, patient manner. A child younger than 4 years of age is placed in the supine position with hips fully abducted and feet together in the "frog-leg" position. The child may also sit on the caregiver's lap and straddle her thighs. If sexual abuse is suspected, the knee-chest position exposes the inferior portion of the hymen, where most injuries occur. This position is also helpful when a foreign body is suspected because much of the vagina is exposed. A pelvic examination table with stirrups may be used when examining children older than 4 years.

Vaginal Discharge and Bleeding

Vaginal discharge is the most common gynecologic problem seen in children. Children are susceptible to developing a vaginal discharge because they lack labial fat pads and pubic hair [4]. Additional reasons that children may present with this problem include lack of estrogen during the prepubertal years, inadequate or overzealous hygiene, scratching, or masturbation.

Nonspecific vaginitis may be caused by chemical irritants, such as shampoo, creams, perfumes, or soap; tight-fitting or nylon clothing; diapers; poor hygiene; or allergens. In general, irritation from any source is the root cause of nonspecific vaginitis. The symptoms—pruritus, irritation, burning, soreness, and variable discharge—are indistinguishable from those of specific or infectious vaginitis. Management includes identifying and eliminating the cause [5].

Specific vaginitis may be spread from an infection of the pharynx, skin, ear, intestine, or urinary tract (eg, streptococcal, pneumococcal, nongonorrheal neisserial, meningococcal, or *Shigella* species infection). Pinworms can infect the vagina as well as the rectum and cause a discharge. The presence of gonorrhea or chlamydial infection suggests sexual abuse. Trichomoniasis usually indicates sexual abuse as well but may be transmitted by wet towels and washcloths [6••].

Discharge can vary in quantity, color, and effect: from slight to copious; white or yellow to bloody; no effect to secondary vulvitis. Gynecologic evaluation should include examination of the vulva and vagina in the supine and knee-chest positions. Cultures for aerobic organisms may be obtained from the vaginal wall with a moistened swab.

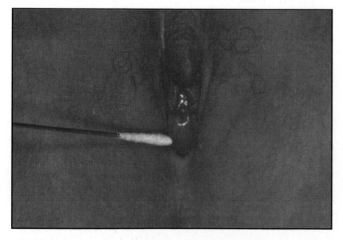

Figure 47-1. Urethral swab, moistened to reduce pain or trauma, should be used to obtain cultures.

Because of the sensitivity of the thin, red epithelium, a small, moistened cotton-tipped swab, such as a urethral swab, should be used (Figure 47-1.) Cultures are preferable to DNA probes in children because of the risk of false-positive results with the latter [3].

A foul-smelling bloody discharge suggests a foreign body in the vagina, the most common of which is toilet paper. A KUB (kidneys, ureter, bladder) film is rarely helpful because the object is usually not radio-opaque. If a foreign body is suspected but not visible on inspection of the genitalia, a vaginoscopy is indicated.

No specific cause of vaginal discharge can be determined in approximately 70% of cases [6••]. In these cases, treatment should include instruction in proper hygiene, loose clothing, Sitz baths, and avoidance of irritants. If a specific pathogen is identified from the cultured swab, antibiotics should be administered. For guideline to the treatment of specific vaginitis, see Figure 47-2 [6••].

In addition to a foreign body, bloody discharge or frank vaginal bleeding may be caused by urethral prolapse, polyps, neoplasms, precocious puberty, sexual abuse, or trauma. Treatment varies with cause.

Urethral prolapse involves a complete circular eversion of urethral mucosa through the external meatus, resulting from poor attachments between smooth muscle layers of the urethra in association with episodic increase in intra-abdominal pressure. This condition is rarely associated with other urinary tract anomalies (Figure 47-3).

Children most commonly present with vaginal bleeding. Dysuria, urinary retention, or urinary frequency may also be present. Several studies have suggested that this disorder is most common in black girls younger than 10 years [7]. On visual inspection of the genitalia, a cherry-red doughnut of tissue or a fungating mass 2 to 3 cm in diameter is apparent. Although the lesion extends from the urethra, it may appear to extend from the vagina when large [8••,9]. When in doubt of its cause, place a small Foley catheter through the lesion. Passage of urine is consistent with the diagnosis of urethral prolapse.

Conservative management is indicated: topical estrogen cream with or without antibiotics is the treatment of choice. Sitz baths may also be used. Recurrence necessitates surgical management.

Sarcoma botryoides account for 73% of cases of vaginal bleeding caused by a neoplasm in prepubertal children. A characteristic grapelike structure may be seen protruding from the vagina and is usually visible before age 5 years. Neoplasms require biopsy for diagnosis [3].

Precocious puberty, or sexual development before 8 years of age, is categorized by etiology as isosexual precocity, with the child presenting with normal pubertal development, or heterosexual precocity, with evidence of virilization with or without development. Isosexual precocity may be considered if there is evidence of breast budding or pubic hair. Its cause is related to early activation of the hypothalamus and pituitary gland. Organic disorders that may bear an effect are cerebral disorders, including brain tumor; neurofibromatosis; tuberous sclerosis; suprasellar cyst; carcinoid granuloma; hydrocephalus; and postinfectious, posttraumatic, or post-irradiation conditions. Congenital adrenal hyperplasia and primary hypothyroidism should also be considered. Pseudo-precocious puberty may indicate ovarian tumors, adrenal disorders, use of estrogen-containing creams, or ingestion of medications, such as birth control pills [6••].

Heterosexual precocious puberty occurs as a result of excess androgen production from adrenal glands or ovaries producing acne, hirsutism, or virilization. Breast development alone, uterine bleeding alone, or development of pubic hair alone may be apparent, but no other signs of estrogenization are present.

Treatment of early onset puberty begins with reassurance of parents and referral to a pediatric endocrinologist or pediatric gynecologist for consultation [6••].

Straddle-type injuries account for 75% of genital injuries in children and may produce hematomas or tearing. Apply pressure with ice packs if a vulvar hematoma results from trauma. Expanding hematomas may require vessel ligation under general anesthesia. Exploratory laparotomy may be required to determine the extent of injury to the retroperitoneal area (Figure 47-4) [6••].

Vulvar Disorders

The most common vulvar disorders observed in female children are vulvitis caused by candidal infection, vulvar warts (HPV), labial agglutination, molluscum contagiosum, lichen sclerosus, and contact dermatitis.

VULVITIS

Candida species, a common cause of diaper rash, prefers an estrogenic environment. Thus, vulvitis during the prepubertal years usually is not a result of candidal infection unless there are other risk factors, such as use of antibiotics or diabetes mellitus. Initially, it may present as mild erythema and edema with pruritus. Severe cases result in intense, red, macerated, weeping, eczematous dermatitis with satel-

Treatment of Vulvovaginal Infections in the Prepubertal Child

Etiology	Treatment
Streptococcus pyogenes	Penicillin V 250 mg tid po for 10 d
Haemophilus influenzae	Amoxicillin 20–40 mg/kg/d po for 7 d
	For resistant strains: amoxicillin-clavulanate, cefixime, cefuroxime axetil, trimethoprim-sulfamethoxazole, erythromycin-sulfamethoxazole
Staphylococcus aureus	Cephalexin 25–50 mg/kg/d po for 7–10 d
	Dicloxacillin 25 mg/kg/d po for 7–10 d
	Amoxicillin-clavulanate 20–40 mg/kg/d (of amoxicillin) po for 7–10 d
	Cefuroxime axetil oral suspension 30 mg/kg/d po divided bid (maximum 1 g) for 10 d (tablets: 250 mg bid)
Streptococcus pneumoniae	Penicillin*, erythromycin, trimethoprim-sulfamethoxazole, clarithromycin
Shigella species	Trimethoprim 8 mg/sulfamethoxazole 40 mg per kg/d po for 5 d
	For resistant organisms: cefixime, ceftriaxone
Chlamydia trachomatis	Erythromycin 50 mg/kg/d po for 10–14 d; or azithromycin 20 mg/kg (maximum 1 g), single dose
	Children 8 years of age or older: doxycycline 100 mg bid po for 7 d
Neisseria gonorrhoeae	Ceftriaxone 125 mg IM† (alternative: spectinomycin 40 mg/kg [maximum 2 g] IM) once, plus treatment for *Chlamydia* species infection as above
	Children 45 kg or heavier and 8 years of age or older can be treated with adult regimens
Candida species	Topical nystatin, miconazole, clotrimazole, or terconazole cream; possibly fluconazole po in immunosuppressed children
Trichomonas species	Metronidazole 15 mg/kg/d given tid (maximum 250 mg tid) for 7–10 d, or 40 mg/kg (maximum 2 g), single dose
Pinworms *(Enterobius vermicularis)*	Mebendazole 1 chewable 100-mg tablet, repeated at 2 wk

*With increased resistance, high-dose penicillin or alternative therapy may be added.
†Given the effectiveness of oral therapies in adults, it is likely that the same regimens can be used in children.

Figure 47-2. Treatment of vulvovaginal infections in the prepubertal child. bid—twice daily; IM—intramuscularly; po—orally; tid—three times daily. (*Adapted from* Emans *et al.* [6••].)

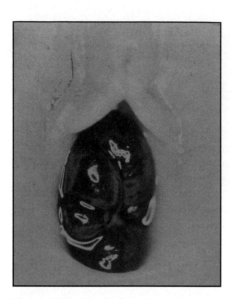

Figure 47-3. Urethral prolapse in a 4-year-old white girl.

Differential Diagnosis of Vaginal Bleeding in the Prepubertal Girl

Trauma

  Accidental

  Sexual abuse

Vulvovaginitis

  Irritation, pinworms

  Nonspecific vulvovaginitis

  Streptococcus pyogenes, Shigella species infection

Endocrine abnormalities

  Newborn bleeding due to maternal estrogen withdrawal

  Isosexual precocious puberty

  Pseudoprecocious puberty

  Precocious menarche

  Exogenous hormone preparations

  Hypothyroidism

Dermatoses

  Lichen sclerosis

Condyloma acuminata (human papillomavirus)

Foreign body

Urethral prolapse

Blood dyscrasia

Hemangioma

Tumor

  Benign

  Malignant

Figure 47-4. Differential diagnosis of vaginal bleeding in the prepubertal girl. (*Adapted from* Emans *et al.* [6••].)

lite pustules. A chronic state results in thickened red-brown skin, patches of excoriation, or rarely, persistent granuloma (Figure 47-5).

Diagnosis is usually made by visual inspection but may be confirmed by KOH smear or culture. Treatment is with nystatin cream given two to four times daily for 2 weeks. Severe refractory cases may be treated topically with 3% amphotericin B cream, two to four times daily for 2 weeks, or systemically with intravenous amphotericin B, 0.5 to 1 mg/kg/d. The differential diagnosis of vulvitis includes candidal dermatitis, impetigo, seborrhea, psoriasis, and acrodermatitis enteropathica [10•].

Vulvar Warts

Vulvar warts may be transmitted by vaginal delivery or close sexual or nonsexual contact with an HPV-infected person or object. More than 80 distinct types of HPV have been identified, and HPV types 6 and 11 are the most common to cause benign low-risk genital lesions [11–13]. Moderate risk of malignant transformation is carried in types 33, 35, 39, 40, 42 to 45, 51 to 56, and 58. A high risk of oncogenic potential is ascribed to types 16 and 18 [12,13]. Of children with genital warts, 25% also have cutaneous warts caused by HPV type 2 (Figure 47-6).

Diagnosis is usually apparent on visual inspection. Application of 3% to 5% acetic acid may reveal mucosal lesions as white plaques (acetowhite change). If sexual abuse is suspected, biopsy of the lesion is recommended to confirm the diagnosis. DNA typing can be used to determine the strain present but is not considered the standard of care, nor is it readily available to most clinicians.

Asymptomatic vulvar warts in young children may be treated by benign neglect because spontaneous resolution or a significant decrease in the size of lesions may occur over several months. Warts in sexually active adolescents or symptomatic lesions in young children require active treatment. Chemical destruction methods include application of 25% podophyllin in tincture of benzoin or trichloroacetic acid.

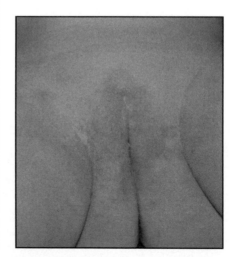

Figure 47-5. Vulvitis as a result of *Candida* species infection. (*Courtesy of* Stanley Inkelis, MD, Harbor/ UCLA Medical Center, UCLA School of Medicine.)

Cryosurgery may also help. The procedure is most useful for any lesion that may be covered completely with refrigerant, most commonly liquid nitrogen applied with a cotton-tipped swab. Warts are frozen until a circle of ice is visible around their outer edges; they are subsequently allowed to thaw, then refrozen [14]. Response rates are high for the procedure (83% reported in a comparison study of current treatments), but it may produce pain and some scarring [12].

These methods may not be tolerated by young children in the office setting. CO_2 laser or KTP excision results in minimal scarring but requires general anesthesia [3]. Regardless of the method used, warts recur in approximately 50% of cases.

LABIAL AGGLUTINATION

Labial agglutination, or the adherence of the adjacent edges of the labia minora, is common in prepubertal girls because of the thinness of the epithelium in the absence of estrogen. The labia may adhere anywhere along the vestibule, but adhesions are most common posteriorly.

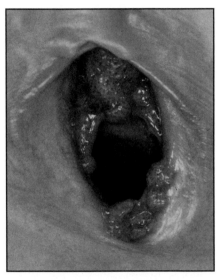

Figure 47-6. Vulvar warts (human papillomavirus) in an 8-year-old white girl.

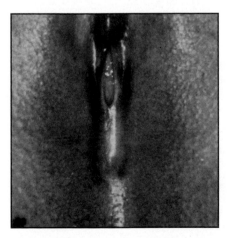

Figure 47-7. Partial labial agglutination in an 8-year-old African-American girl.

Extensive agglutination with the labia adhered from the fourchette to the urethra has been demonstrated to occur in 5% of prepubertal girls and in up to 10% of girls 12 months of age or younger [15]. Symptoms of labial agglutination include urinary dribbling or retention, urinary tract infection, and urethritis (Figure 47-7).

Children who have mild to moderate agglutination without symptoms do not require treatment because up to 80% of cases resolve spontaneously over time. When symptoms are present or extensive agglutination is noted, medical therapy should be the first line of treatment. Estrogen cream is applied to the affected area twice daily for 2 weeks. A Calgiswab may be used to lyse thin residual adhesions in the office after anesthetizing the area with 5% Xylocaine (AstraZeneca, Wilmington, DE) ointment. Traumatic separation should not be attempted, however, because it is painful and usually results in recurrence. After lysis of adhesions, vitamins A and D ointment may be applied nightly to the vulva to decrease risk of recurrence. Surgical treatment is indicated only if medical interventions are unsuccessful.

MOLLUSCUM CONTAGIOSUM

Molluscum contagiosum, a viral infection of the pox group, can result from autoinoculation or contact with others. Most prevalent in school-aged children, its spread is enhanced by conditions of poverty, overcrowding, and poor hygiene. The virus prefers a tropical climate, where it occurs in about 10% of children. Children most commonly present with pruritus, although lesions may be asymptomatic.

Inspection of the external genitalia reveals discrete, skin-colored, dome-shaped, smooth papules with a central cheesy plug (Figure 47-8).

Diagnosis usually is made by visual inspection. A warmed KOH smear under 10% magnification reveals ballooned keratinocytes. On occasion, a biopsy may be necessary.

The object of treatment is to remove the central core. Curettage of lesions is effective but requires general anesthesia in children. Cryosurgery is considered the treatment of choice because of its efficacy, painlessness, and good cosmetic result. Each lesion is frozen for 6 to 10 seconds, and this procedure is repeated every 3

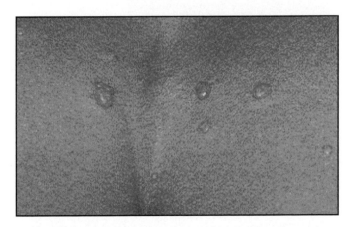

Figure 47-8. Molluscum contagiosum. (*Courtesy of* David Kerns, MD, Santa Clara Valley Medical Center, San Jose, CA.)

weeks as needed. Chemical destruction methods include retinoic acid, phenol, salicylic acid, lactic acid, and cantharidin.

LICHEN SCLEROSUS

Lichen sclerosus (formerly *lichen sclerosus et atrophicus*) is a benign chronic condition of the vulvar perianal or perineal skin, which affects prepubertal children and perimenopausal women [16]. Ten to 15% of all cases occur in children.

The condition produces a sclerotic, atrophic plaque with crinkly ivory-colored skin encircling the vagina and anus in an hourglass or figure-of-eight pattern [17,18]. Lesions usually begin as small, off-white, flat papules that later merge into larger plaques [10•]. The finely wrinkled affected skin is clearly demarcated from the normal skin by its pale, paper-like appearance. The thinned skin becomes fissured, and minimal pressure may result in bruising and bleeding.

Thus, most children present with bleeding. Perineal itching, soreness, dysuria, and painful defecation are also common presenting symptoms. In 20% of cases, a secondary infection of the vagina occurs and precedes appearance of vulvar lesions. The condition typically does not involve the vagina or urethra. When chronic, it may result in atrophy of the labia majora or clitoris, constriction of vaginal introitus or urethral meatus, anal stenosis, or anal fissures. The condition has been mistaken for trauma, especially sexual abuse (Figure 47-9) [19].

The cause of lichen sclerosus is unknown but may be related to autoimmune disorder or familial association [16].

Diagnosis is often apparent on visual inspection. The differential diagnosis includes vitiligo, morphea, perianal dermatitis, and postinflammatory hypopigmentation as well as advanced scleroderma, morphea, lupus erythematosus, advanced lichen planus, and radiation fibrosis [16,19]. When necessary, biopsy may be performed to confirm the diagnosis, but it requires general anesthesia in young children.

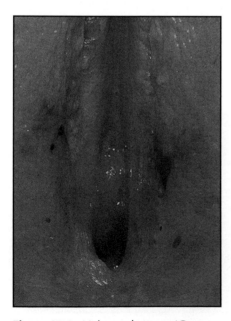

Figure 47-9. Lichen sclerosus. (*Courtesy of* David Kerns, MD, Santa Clara Valley Medical Center, San Jose, CA.)

Treatment of the symptoms may be accomplished with topical application of 1% to 2.5% hydrocortisone ointment for 1 to 3 months.

Recent studies of children with lichen sclerosus indicate high response rates produced by application of potent topical corticosteroids, and thus it has been suggested that this regimen should be used in children as well as adults. Dosage should be limited to avoid local and systemic side effects. For example, clobetasol propionate 5% may be used but should be limited to less than 30 g in 6 months [18].

Testosterone cream is usually not recommended for use in children because of possible systemic effects. Topical estrogens have no proven efficacy [16]. Hydroxyzine hydrochloride (Atarax; Pfizer, Inc., New York, NY) may be applied nightly to relieve itching. Secondary infections are common and should be treated with oral antibiotics. Caregivers should be instructed in good hygiene practices for the young patient and to avoid irritants, such as harsh soaps or nylon underwear. Two thirds of affected girls experience spontaneous clearing of lesions at or near menarche.

CONTACT DERMATITIS

Contact dermatitis is caused by irritation and usually occurs in children during the diaper period. Irritation results from too little or too much cleansing of the anogenital area with products such as treated wipes or cleaning agents. The condition is characterized by erythema, intense itching, and loss of skin markings. Scaling, crusting, or blistering with noticeable edema may be present.

Treatment should attempt first to identify and discontinue the irritant. Application of topical steroids gives relief until the skin barrier function has been restored [10•,20••].

Summary

Gynecologic problems in a child may cause anxiety for the parent, the caregiver, and the patient. Proceeding in a calm systematic manner with open communication permits the clinician to inspect the genital area and the discharge or disorder; to culture and diagnose; and to determine causes of the presenting condition. Bleeding in the prepubertal child is always a matter of concern. After a thorough evaluation, caregivers may be reassured, and the young patient may be referred for consultation if needed.

References

Papers of particular interest have been highlighted as follows:
• *Of interest*
•• *Of outstanding interest*

1.• Farrington PF: Pediatric vulvovaginitis. *Clin Obstet Gynecol* 1997, 40:135–140.
A crisply written article with special attention to the evaluation of young children.

2. Hairston L: Physical examination of the prepubertal girl. *Obstet Gynecol* 1997, 40:127–134.

3. Berenson AB: Pediatric gynecology. In *Precis: An Update in Obstetrics & Gynecology/Reproduction Endocrinology.* 1998:36–40.

4. Altcheck A: Pediatric vulvovaginitis. *J Reprod Med* 1984, 29:359–375.

5. Sobel JD: Vaginitis. *N Engl J Med* 1997, 3:1896–1903.

6.•• Emans SJH, Laufer MR, Goldstein DP: *Pediatric and Adolescent Gynecology,* edn 4. Philadelphia: Lippincott-Raven; 1998.

A comprehensive reference, including charts, photographs, and lists of resources.

7. Rimza ME: Common problems in pediatric gynecology. *Urol Clin North Am* 1994, 22:161–176.

8.•• Baldwin DD, Landa HM: Common problems in pediatric gynecology. *Urol Clin North Am* 1994, 22:161–176.

A well-written review with substantial references.

9. Rudin JE, Geldt VG, Alecssev EB: Prolapse of urethral mucosa in white female children: experience with 58 cases. *J Pediatr Surg* 1997, 32:423–425.

10.• Dodds ML: Vulvar disorders of the infant and young child. *Clin Obstet Gynecol* 1997, 40:141–152.

A well-written article supported by excellent photographs.

11. Tyring S: Perspectives on human papillomavirus infection. *Am J Med* 1997, 102:1–2.

12. Mayeaux EJ Jr, Harper MB, Barksdale W, *et al.*: Noncervical human papillomavirus genital infections. *Am Fam Physician* 1995, 52:1137–1146, 1149–1150.

13. Beutner KR, Tyring S: Human papillomavirus and human disease. *Am J Med* 1997, 102:9–15.

14. Bourke JF, Berth-Jones J, Hutchinson PE: Cryotherapy of common viral warts at intervals of 1, 2, and 3 weeks. *Br J Dermatol* 1995, 132:433–436.

15. Berenson AB, Heger AH, Hayes JM, *et al.*: Appearance of the hymen in prepubertal girls. *Pediatrics* 1992, 89:387–391.

16. ACOG educational bulletin: vulvar nonneoplastic epithelial disorders. *Int J Gynaecol Obstet* 1998, 60:181–188.

17. Fischer G, Rogers M: Treatment of childhood vulvar lichen sclerosus with potent topical corticosteroid. *Pediatr Dermatol* 1997, 14:235–238.

18. Ridley CM: Vulvar disease in the pediatric population. *Semin Dermatol* 1996, 15:29–35.

19. Loening-Baucke V: Lichen sclerosus et atrophicus in children. *Am J Dis Child* 1991, 145:1058–1061.

20.•• Siegfried EC, Frasier LD: Anogenital skin diseases of childhood. *Pediatr Ann* 1997, 26:321–331.

Excellent color photographs.

Index

Fertility.
See also Infertility
endometrial cancer and, 231–232
injectable/implantable contraceptives and, 119
intrauterine devices and, 127
Fetal demise, 36
Fibroadenoma
breast, 2, 16, 18
Fibrocystic breast disease, 2, 15–16, 18
Fibromyalgia
in chronic pelvic pain, 332, 332f
Fine needle aspiration
of breast masses, 17
Fluid retention
in premenstrual syndrome, 342, 344
Follicle-stimulating hormone
in diminished ovarian reserve, 164
Forensic examination
after sexual assault and abuse, 403–405
Frozen embryos
in infertility treatment, 199–200
Fungal infections
vulvar, 147

G

Galactography, 11
Galactorrhea
differential diagnosis of, 10f–12f, 10–11
incidence and epidemiology of, 7
pathophysiology of, 7–9, 8f–9f
prevention of, 13
treatment of, 11–12
Gardasil, 57, 368, 374, 376, 376f
Genetics
of breast cancer, 15, 16f
of endometrial cancer, 225–226
infertility treatment and, 200
Genital herpes, 59–63, 60f–63f
Genital warts, 53–57, 54f–56f
pediatric, 414–415, 415f
Germ cell tumors, 242, 242f
Gestational trophoblastic disease, 249–253, 250f–252f
Gonadal failure
in delayed puberty, 153–154, 154f
Gonadotropins
in infertility treatment, 196f, 196–197
Gonorrhea, 39–43
clinical features of, 41
diagnosis of, 41–42
epidemiology of, 39–40, 40f
pathophysiology of, 40
pelvic inflammatory disease from, 68, 73
treatment and prevention of, 42–43

H

Heat therapy
in dysmenorrhea, 336
Hereditary endometrial cancer, 221
Herpes simplex virus infection, 59–63
classification and epidemiology of, 59–60
clinical presentation and diagnosis of, 60f–61f, 60–61

in pregnancy, 63, 63f
treatment and prevention of, 61–63, 62f
vertical transmission of, 63
virology of, 59–60
vulvar, 148
Hirsutism, 171–174, 172f–173f
HIV infection
barrier contraceptives and, 102–103, 107
gonorrhea and, 40
intrauterine device use in, 127–128
pelvic inflammatory disease in, 70
Hormonal therapy
breast cancer risk and, 16
for breast pain, 4
endometrial cancer risk and, 220
menopausal, 300f–303f, 300–303
Hot flashes
menopausal, 296, 298
Human chorionic gonadotropin
in ectopic pregnancy, 21, 22f–23f, 23–24, 26
in infertility treatment, 196f, 196–197
Human papillomavirus infection, 53–57, 54f–55f
cervical dysplasia in, 373f, 373–376, 375f–376f
vaccine against, 56f, 57, 367–369, 374, 376, 376f
Hydatidiform moles, 250f–251f, 250–251
Hyperinsulinemia
hirsutism in, 173
Hyperplasia
endometrial, 187, 224, 224f
Hyperprolactinemia, 9, 10f, 11, 11f, 352–353, 353f
Hypertension
oral contraceptives and, 81–82
Hypothalamic amenorrhea, 354
Hypothalamic-pituitary-ovarian axis, 352, 352f
Hypothyroidism
galactorrhea in, 11, 11f
Hysterectomy
for abnormal bleeding, 189
for endometrial cancer, 226–229
in fallopian tube cancer, 246
in ovarian cancer, 239
for uterine leiomyoma, 318
Hysterosalpingogram
in infertility evaluation, 164–165
Hysteroscopy
in abnormal uterine bleeding, 183–184, 184f, 188–189
in infertility evaluation, 165
in tubal sterilization, 98

I

Idoxifene, 303
Imipramine
in stress urinary incontinence, 259
Imiquimod
in vulvar cancer, 211
Implantable contraceptives, 115–119, 116f–117f
In vitro fertilization, 199f, 199–202, 201f–202f
Incontinence
stress urinary, 255–250, 256f–258f

Infants
chlamydial infection in, 50
herpes simplex virus infection in, 63
human papillomavirus infection in, 53–54
Infections.
See also Sexually transmitted diseases; specific infections
intrauterine devices and, 130f, 130–131
urinary tract, 263–269, 264f, 266f–267f
vaginal, 137–139
vulvar, 147
Infertility
cervical factors in, 199
from chlamydial infection, 47
evaluation of, 159–168, 160f–163f, 165f–167f
anatomic, 164–165
environmental factors in, 160
history in, 159–160, 161f
male factors in, 160f, 165f–167f, 166–168, 198
ovarian reserve in, 164
ovulation in, 161–163, 162f–163f
pathophysiology of female, 160–161
polycystic ovary syndrome in, 163f, 163–164
normal fertility *versus,* 159, 160f
overview of, 159, 160f, 195
from pelvic inflammatory disease, 70
treatment of, 195–202, 202f
assisted technologies in, 199f, 199–200, 202f
ovulation induction agents in, 196f, 196–197
risks of, 200–201, 201f
unexplained, 197–198, 198f
tubal factors in, 197
uterine factors in, 198
Injectable contraceptives, 115–119
advantages of, 116–117, 117f
disadvantages of, 117–119
drug interactions with and contraindications to, 119
efficacy of, 116
pharmacology and dosing of, 115–116, 116f
Insulin
polycystic ovary syndrome and, 195
Intrauterine devices, 123–133
cost of, 132f, 133
ectopic pregnancy and, 126, 126f
efficacy of and satisfaction with, 125–127, 131
history of, 123–124, 124f
indications for referral with, 131f
mechanism of action of, 125
noncontraceptive benefits of, 126–127, 187–188
patient selection for, 127f–128f, 127–129
pelvic inflammatory disease and, 68, 72, 73f–74f
for postcoital contraception, 126
problems with, 129–133, 130f–131f, 339
removal of, 131–133
types of, 125, 125f
Irving sterilization technique, 92–93, 93f